THIS BOOK BELONGS TO:

NAME: ______________________________

PGR: ______________

PHONE: ______________

EMAIL: ____________________________

INTERNAL MEDICINE: INTERN SURVIVAL GUIDE ISBN: 978-0-9890657-3-3

NOTICE

Medicine is an ever-changing, rapidly advancing field. Standard safety precautions must be followed, and allowances must be made for new discoveries, drugs, and changes to standards of care. Though every effort has been made to ensure that the information in this book is accurate and up to date, readers are advised to verify for themselves, relying on their experience and knowledge of their patient to determine if the recommendations made are actually the best for their individual patient. Reviews have been performed to confirm the accuracy of the information presented in this book and often describe generally accepted practices, or "pearls". The author is not responsible for errors or omissions or for any consequences from application of the information in this book and make no warranty, expressed or implied, with respect to the currency, completeness, or accuracy of the contents of the publication. Furthermore, readers are encouraged to confirm the information contained herein with other sources. Neither the author nor the Department of Medicine assume any liability for any injury and/or damage to persons or property arising from use of this handbook. Some drugs and medical devices presented in this publication have Food and Drug Administration (FDA) clearance for limited use in restricted research settings. It is the responsibility of health care providers to ascertain the FDA status of each drug or device planned for use in their clinical practice. When prescribing medication, health care professionals are advised to consult the product information sheet (the manufacturer's package insert) accompanying each drug to verify, among other things, conditions of use, warnings, and side effects, and identify any changes in dosage schedule or contraindications, particularly if the medication to be administered is new, infrequently used, or has a narrow therapeutic range. Unless otherwise stated, all medications are for the non-pregnant, non-breast feeding adult who has reasonable liver and renal function. The publisher has made every effort to trace copyright holders for borrowed material. If there is any information that may have inadvertently been overlooked, the publisher will be pleased to make the necessary arrangements as soon as possible.

Previous editions copyrighted 2019, 2018, 2017, 2016, 2015, 2014, 2013

For details on ordering additional copies, contact the publisher through Amazon.

Printed in the United States of America

Third Edition

Library of Congress Control Number: 2018915303

Internal Medicine:

Intern Survival Guide

3rd Edition

Jacob Mathew, Jr. DO FACOI

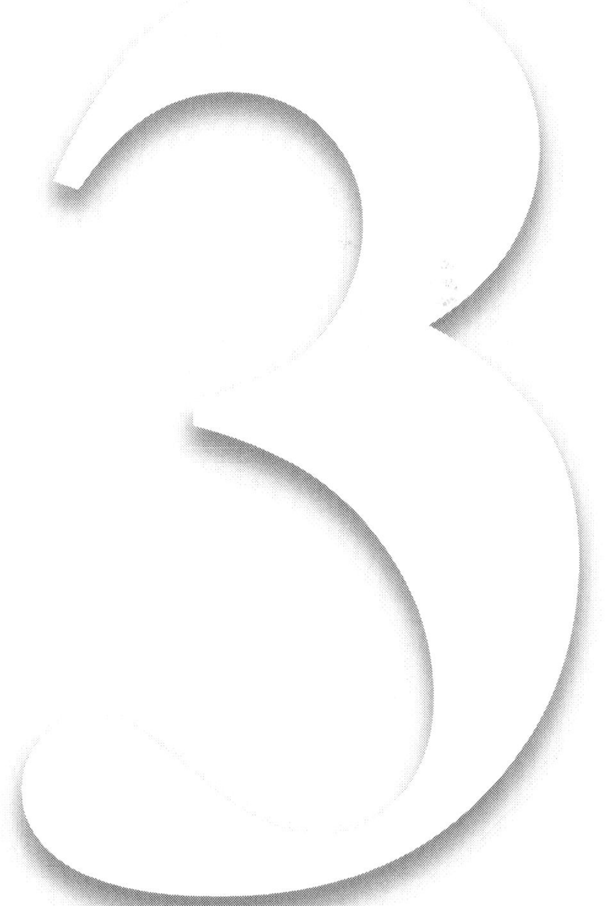

PREFACE

I started this book as a way to organize the notes I took as a third year medical student during rotation. I then added the numerous pearls I learned as an intern and the common conditions I was paged on, so it would be easier for me to not "recreate the wheel" and continue to look up the same information over and over. As I conglomerated these notes, I realized that I could transform this now 100-200 page document into to a resource that could help others that I knew had to also be in my unenviable position: to lonely night float intern who is expected to have the answer to everything! I bring to you the conglomeration of over 8 years of work, Internal Medicine: Intern Survival Guide. No matter your background, I hope you find it helpful and it allows you to provide the best care possible for the most important person in the world: **your patient**.

Jacob Mathew Jr. DO FACOI

CONTENTS

Wards

Dermatology

Gastroenterology

Quick ACLS

Infectious Disease

Cardiology

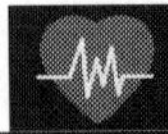

Endocrinology

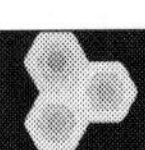

Geriatrics

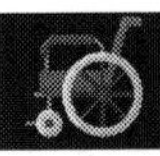

Hematology/Oncology

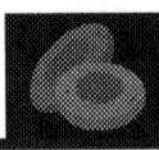

Ophthalmology

Radiology

Musculoskeletal

Neurology

Pulmonology/Critical Care

Nephrology

Otolaryngology

Rheumatology

Psychiatry

Perioperative Care

Toxicology

Women's Health

Urology

Nutrition/Diet

Fluids

Pain Management

WHAT / WHO	DEPARTMENT	PHONE NUMBER

WARDS

ADMITTING PATIENTS

- Check if patient has contact precautions
- **Call appropriate bed manager**
  - Page bed manager if general medical floor
  - Page supercharge if progressive care unit or ICU
  - Have the following information ready for them:
    - Name
    - Age
    - Last 4 SSN
    - Dx
    - Code Status
    - Location now
    - Transfer to location (and justification)
      - 6C2 for O2 requirement and telemetry
    - Accepting Team
      - Color
      - Attending
    - Contact precautions?
    - Patient ambulatory? A&Ox3?
    - ADLs?
    - O2 requirement?
    - Fall risk?
    - Disposition
- **How to Present Patient to Bed Manager / Supercharge**
  - Patients Name and Age
  - Last 4 of SSN
  - Diagnosis
  - Code Status

- Location now
- Transferring to and why
- Your name and pager #
- Ward Team and Attending
- Patient ambulating, A&O status
- ADLs or with assistance
- Contact precautions?
  - Check homepage link "Look up admissions requiring isolation"
- Disposition

NIGHT FLOAT COMMON SCENARIOS

- **Altered mental status** – see page 387
- **Fever**
  - *Fever is defined as T>100.4F for at least one hour or any temperature above 101F*
  - At night time, it is safest to assume a fever is infectious in etiology and consider broad spectrum treatment if necessary; day team coverage can always narrow down if necessary.
    - If giving antibiotics, confirm allergies, then you should always perform a FFWU (see page 94) to include cultures (blood, sputum, urine)
    - If patient is already on antibiotics, consider broadening
  - Rule out non-infectious causes like medications, NMS, or SS (see page 562)
  - For high fevers being treated (or known source), consider treating with Tylenol. If infectious in etiology however, consider avoiding Tylenol (masking).
  - For FUO, see page 94
- **Hyperglycemia** - see page 231
- **Hypoglycemia** - see page 247
- **Chest pain** - see page 150
- **Shortness of breath**
  - Get a full set of vitals to determine if the patient is subjectively SOB or if they have a low oxygen saturation.
  - The big 3 tests of dyspnea
    - ECG
    - ABG
    - Portable CXR
  - If the patient has a low oxygen saturation, administer O2:
    - Nasal cannula→venti mask→non-rebreather→NIPPV→intubation
      (if the patient requires NRB/NIPPV/Intubation then MICU should be notified)
    - Remember in general, CPAP should be used for **hypoxia** and BiPAP for **hypercapnia** or **mixed hypoxia/hypercapnia**.
    - See page 481 for supplemental oxygen options and page 471 for BiPAP vs CPAP
  - Pulmonary causes of SOB:
    - Obstructive (COPD, asthma, foreign body), pneumothorax, pneumonia, aspiration, ILD, pleural effusions, DAH, PE
    - Cardiovascular causes of SOB: ACS, cardiac arrhythmia (e.g. Afib, VT), pulmonary HTN, cardiac tamponade, acute decompensated HF
    - Non-pulmonary and non-cardiac causes of SOB: anemia, metabolic acidosis, carboxy/sulph/met-Hgb, diaphragmatic paralysis (e.g. in ALS), abdominal HTN
  - Additional tests to consider: CBC, RFP, D-dimer, CT PE, troponin and BNP
- **Hypertension** - see page 188
- **Pain management** - see page 639

DIFFERENTIAL DIAGNOSIS

Vascular
Infective/Inflammatory
Traumatic
Autoimmune
Metabolic
Iatrogenic/Idiopathic
Neoplastic
Anogenital
Degenerative/Developmental
Endocrine/Environmental
Functional

LONG-TERM CARE

Type	Description	Coverage	Cost / Day	Coverage
Post-Acute[1]				
Inpatient Rehabilitation	Facilities specifically licensed to provide active rehabilitation. Patients must receive at least 3 h a day of PT and/or OT and must show progress to be kept on Medicare	Medicare	1000-2000	Physician
Skilled Nursing (SNF)	Many nursing homes certified to provide post hospital care under Medicare. Skilled needs include complex medication schedules, wound care, or rehabilitation	Medicare Medicaid	150-300	Primary care clinician (physician, nurse practitioner, both), medical director
Long-term care Hospital	Facility certified by Medicare to handle complex care (eg, ventilator care and weaning) of patients discharged from hospitals	Medicare	1500-3000	Hospitalist
Home health care	Medicare-certified care supervised by registered nurses. Other core staff: physical, occupational, and speech therapists, and social workers	Medicare Medicaid	100-300	Primary care clinician
Outpatient Rehabilitation	May be certified to conduct active rehabilitation	Medicare Medicaid	100-200	Primary care clinician
Hospice/	Intended for those at	Medicare	200-300	Primary

palliative care	terminal phase of life with expected prognosis <6 mo. Hospice care is a specific benefit under Medicare; as such, it is predicated on primarily nonhospital care. Palliative care provides active support like hospice care but without the expectation of avoiding other medical care.	(hospice; palliative care options vary)		care clinician or palliative care specialist
Long-Term Care				
Home care/ personal care	Services to support frail person who needs assistance in meeting various ADL or IADL care	Medicaid (state plan and waivers)	75-150	PCP
Nursing home	Certified to provide long-term care; some offer specialized units for persons with dementia	Medicaid	75-300	Primary care clinician (physician, nurse practitioner, both), medical director
Assisted living	Institutional care with self-contained units including living quarters, a private bathroom, and some modest cooking and food storage facilities; heterogeneous and minimally regulated. Serve less disabled clientele than nursing homes. Some offer specialized units for persons with dementia	Medicaid in some states (waivers)	60-300	PCP
Day care or adult day health center	Care provided in centralized facilities for various periods of the day. Some also have medical or nursing services (ie, adult day health care vs social adult day care).	Medicaid (in some states)	60-120	PCP
Adult foster care	Small group living settings with care by nonprofessionals; more homelike than larger institutions	Medicaid in some states (waivers)	50-100	PCP
Independent living	Room and board and some housekeeping; may have social activities and amenities	None	50-100	PCP

FAMILY MEETINGS

- **SPIKES**[2]
  - **S**et up the situation
    Arrange for privacy; include all appropriate members, introduce everyone minimize interruptions
  - **P**erception/Assess Family's
    Use open-ended questions to assess family's perception of medical situation
  - **I**nvitation
    Ask family how much they would like to know
  - **K**nowledge
    Speak simple; stop and check for understanding, warn them that bad news is coming
  - **E**mpathetic statements
  - **S**trategy and summary
    Summarize and create a follow-through plan; end-of-life discussion

ACCIDENTAL NEEDLE STICK

- **General**
  - Confirm that all identified personnel go to the ER for proper initial treatment per protocol
    - HIV positive
      - Combivir or Truvada plus Kaletra or Boosted Lexiva
    - HIV unknown
      - Combivir or Truvada
  - Obtain source patient information from nurse
  - Can call National Clinicians' Post-Exposure Prophylaxis Hotline, PEPline: 1-888-448-4911
- **Examination**: clean wound with alcohol-based agent (viricidal to HBV, HCV, and HIV)
- **Labs**
  - Lab order exists for needle stick, otherwise:
    - HIV AB/RB with gold tube
    - HepB surface Ag
    - HepB Core IGM
    - Hep C surface Ab
    - Syphilis RPR
    - ALT
- **Follow up**
  - Notify nurse involved of above results so treatment can be d/c or continued as necessary

DECLARING PATIENT DECEASED

- You will be informed by nurse that patient has passed away and needs to be declared.
- Be prepared to encounter the family at bedside; explain that you need to examine the patient and that they may stay and that the body can stay in the room as long as the family needs
- **Diagnosis is based on 4 areas:** [3]
  - Meeting prerequisites
  - Performing the clinical examination
  - Using ancillary testing if necessary

  - Consideration for organ donation
- **Knowledge of the proximate cause**
  - Intoxication
  - Metabolic abnormalities
  - ↓Temp
- **Bedside Examination:**
  - Clinical Criteria Required:
    - Clinical and/or imaging evidence of CNS destruction
    - Absence of drug intoxication (ie. EtOH)
    - Absence of severe electrolyte abnormalities
    - Core temperature >32C
    - They cannot be declared dead until 4-5 half-lives of the suspected substance have passed. Note that substances we give patients such as paralytics, benzos, sedatives, etc. also fall under this category.
  - Exam:
    - Brainstem function (check for reflexes: pupillary, oculocephalic, oculovestibular)
    - Absent motor reflexes
    - Absent cough on tracheal suction
    - Observe for spontaneous breathing or movements
    - Auscultate for heart tones
    - Assess for response to pain by pinching finger nail or skin while auscultating (sternal rub can be done as well)
- **All above are present**
  - Apnea Test
    - Preoxygenate then disconnect from ventilator
    - Absence of response for 10 minutes with PaCO2>60 (or >20 change from baseline) and arterial PH <7.2 confirms
  - Repeat clinical exam second time to confirm no changes
- **Not all criteria present but brain death still suspected...**
  - Ancillary Testing
    - An isoelectric EEG for 30 minutes with the machine set at high gain.
    - SSEP and BAEP (absence of evoked potentials)
    - MRA/CTA (absence of intracranial blood flow)
    - Carotid angiography to document lack of flow (**gold standard**)
    - Transcranial doppler
- **Note time, offer condolences, and ask family if they would like an autopsy.**
  - Inform them of benefits of autopsy (will help in the education of house staff and may identify incidental inherited diseases and thus benefit surviving family). The autopsy will not interfere with an open casket funeral; there is the option of limited autopsy, and costs are covered by the hospital.
  - Also ask if the patient was an organ donor, if so, ask nurse to call donor hotline and obtain organ donor # (required for electronic registration)
  - Contact the chaplain if family wishes
- **Call or page attending physician!**
- **Paperwork**
  - EMR
    - Death Note
    - Discharge Summary
  - Checklist (front only)
  - Death summary (paper form)
    - Time and date of death
    - Hospital dx
    - Total # of HD's
    - Describe exam

        - Mention that the family, chaplain and attending were informed
- **Death requiring autopsy/medical examiner (family request; death <24 hrs of admission)**
    - Contact the local medical examiner
        - Leave a message if after business hours
    - Have the following information ready:
        - Time on arrival to hospital (Check T-System à Event Log)
        - Time of death
        - PMHx
        - Hospital course
        - Home address
        - DPOA/Wife/Husband name and contact #
        - Ask if they will examine patient in hospital, or if okay to take patient to morgue
- **Input case into online local health system (if applicable)**

DISCHARGING PATIENTS

1. The following items are necessary to discharge a patient:
    - Discharge Summary: R1 completes e-Discharge form, arranges follow-up, and completes prescriptions; R2/3 dictates/types a complete discharge summary with the following elements:
        - Date of admission
        - Date of discharge
        - R1, R2/3, attending on discharge
        - **Admitting diagnoses (i.e. what the patient had prior to coming to the hospital)**
        - **Discharge diagnoses (i.e. what the patient was diagnosed with during this hospital stay only) → first should always be the admitting diagnosis**
        - Procedures
        - Consults
        - Brief history of present illness
        - Hospital course
        - Physical exam (same length as a SOAP note)
        - Discharge medications:
            - New
            - Changed (any prehospital medications with dose/frequency changes)
            - Unchanged (any prehospital medications to be continued without changes)
            - Stopped (any prehospital medications that should be stopped)
        - Pending studies/labs
        - Outpatient workup needed (i.e. anemia workup, repeat CT chest, etc.)
        - Disposition (i.e. where the patient is going)
        - Diet
        - Code status
        - Activity
        - Home health/PT/wound care (if applicable)
    - Follow-up
        - *Note that all discharge summaries should be completed and signed within 24 hours of the patient's discharge. This is to ensure proper physician communication during this important transition of care.*
2. **Patient Discharge Instructions** (printed from e-Discharge system)
3. **Prescriptions** (either printed from e-Discharge system and signed, or hand written)
    - Narcotics require security Rx, either from the resident or attending
    - All Medi-CAL prescriptions need to be on security paper (ask Chiefs for this paper)
4. **D/C home, D/C IV order**
5. **Notify patient's PMD of discharge or schedule a post-discharge appointment with them in IMS clinic with a member of your team**

6. If the patient needs a primary care doctor, try to see them yourself, set them up with a member of your team, or verbally communicate with whomever they are intended to establish care.

CODE STATUS

- **Discussion**[4,5]
    - Beginning
        - Establish an appropriate setting for the discussion
            - I'd like to talk with you about possible health care decisions in the future.
            - I'd like to review your advance care planning. Would you like your daughter to be here with you?
            - I'd like to discuss something I discuss with all patients admitted to the hospital
        - Ask the patient and family what they understand
            - What do you understand about your current health situation?
            - Tell me about how you see your health.
            - What do you understand from what the doctors have told you?
        - Find out what they expect will happen.
        - Discuss a DNR order, including context
            - If you should die despite all of our efforts, do you want us to use "heroic measures" to bring you back?
            - How do you want things to be when you die?
            - If you were to die unexpectedly, would you want us to try to bring you back?
        - Respond to emotions.
        - Establish and implement the plan.
- **Options**
    - Full Code
        - **Do** everything (CPR, Intubation if necessary)
    - DNR-Comfort Care Arrest
        - Do everything until pt goes into Cardiac or Respiratory Arrest.
        - Pt receives treatment **INCLUDING resuscitative efforts** if necessary until they experience C/R Arrest. Once an arrest is confirmed, all resuscitative and treatment efforts are withdrawn, and Comfort Care alone is initiated. May continue respiratory assistance (O2) and IV medications, etc that have been a part of the patient's ongoing treatment for underlying disease.
    - DNR-Comfort Care
        - Pt receives any care that eases pain and suffering in the final days of life, but **NO RESUSCITATIVE EFFORTS** to save or sustain life.
        - **Do:** Suction airway, administer O2, Position for comfort, splint or immobilize, control bleeding, provide pain medication, provide emotional support, given antibiotics, Contact other appropriate health care providers.
            - **Do Not:** administer chest compressions, insert artificial airway, administer resuscitative drugs, defibrillate or cardiovert, provide respiratory assistance (other than those listed under DO category), initiate resuscitative IV or Initiate cardiac monitoring

DERMATOLOGY

STEROIDS

Corticosteroid potency chart (in order of popularity)		
Generic	Brand	Uses
High Potency (Class I, II)		
Fluocinonide 0.05% cream, ointment	Lidex	
Clobetasol 0.05% cream, ointment, solution	Temovate	
Clobetasol 0.05% foam	Olux	
Medium Potency (Classes III, IV, V)		
Triamcinolone 0.1% cream, ointment	Aristocort	
Hydrocortisone valerate 0.2% cream, ointment	Westcort	
Triamcinolone 0.025% cream; 0.015% spray	Aristocort	
Desonide 0.05% ointment	DesOwen	
Desonide 0.05% lotion	DesOwen	
Low Potency (Classes VI, VII)		
Hydrocortisone 1% cream	Westcort	Sensitive skin; eyelids; face; scrotum; intertriginous areas
Desonide 0.05% cream	DesOwen	
Fluocinolone 0.01% solution	Synalar	
Betamethasone 0.05% lotion	Betaloan	

Adapted from Steroids. Portland (OR): National Psoriasis Foundation; 1998.

Treatment Formulations	
Formulation	Description / Indication
Cream	Water based; low occlusion risk; No greasy feel; best for hairy intertriginous areas and wet lesions
Ointment	Preferred for dry or scaly lesions; areas with thicker skin such as palms and soles, ↑skin hydration; avoid in intertriginous areas; considered to be the most potent

Lotion	Oil-in-water emulsion; good for scalp lesions

ACNE

- **Definition**[6]
  - Common skin disease characterized as a chronic inflammatory dermatosis composed of open and closed comedones (blackheads and whiteheads) and inflammatory lesions.
- **Overview**
  - Acne vulgaris is the most common of all skin disorders.
  - It is a chronic inflammatory process that affects the pilosebaceous unit
  - D/t recessive sebum production secondary to androgen stimulation
- **Physiology**
  - The primary lesion of acne vulgaris is the microcomedone
  - The closed comedo (whitehead) is the first visible acne lesion
  - The open comedo (blackhead) is a 0.1- to 3.0-mm noninflammatory lesion that looks like a black dot
- **Etiology**
  - The prevalent bacterium implicated in the inflammatory phase of acne is *Propionibacterium acnes (P acnes)*
- **Types and Progression**
  - Comedones (blackheads or whiteheads) → papules/pustules +/- inflammation → nodules/cysts (refer to Derm)
- **Classification**
  - Mild
  - Moderate
  - Severe
- **DDx**
  - Rosacea (generally older than are acne patient)
  - Perioral dermatitis (most commonly in young adult women, clinically it is characterized by a combination of eczematous and acneiform features)
  - Hydradenitis suppurative, bacterial folliculitis, drug-induced acne, miliaria

Acne Treatment Options

Class	Options	Indication
Topical Retinoids	tretinoin (0.025-0.1% in cream, gel, or microsphere gel vehicles) *(Pregnancy Category C)* adapalene (0.1%, 0.3% cream, or 0.1% lotion) *(Pregnancy Category C)* tazarotene (0.05%, 0.1% cream, gel or foam) *(Pregnancy Category X)*	Help address the development and maintenance of acne; monotherapy for primarily comedones acne
Topical Antibiotics	Clindamycin 1% solution or gel Erythromycin 2% cream, gel, lotion, pledget	Effective overall tx for mild/moderate **and should always be combined with benzoyl peroxide**

	Dapsone 5-7.5% applied BID for 6-12 months	Dapsone has no ↑ risk in G6PD deficiency pts. Best for pts with inflammatory acne.
Oral Antibiotics	Doxycycline 20mg BID or 40mg/d Minocycline ER 1mg/kg Azithromycin TMP-SMx	Effective for moderate/severe acne; good for those patients unresponsive to topical ABx Macrolides should be limited to pregnancy or young kids (<8) due to risk for bacterial resistance
Wash	Benzoyl Peroxide 5%	Decrease risk for bacterial resistance developing
Hormonal Agents	Spironolactone, OCP (w/ estrogen), Flutamide	Effective as alternative tx options

- **Treatment (gels preferred over other vehicles)**
  - Mild-moderate:
    - Benzoyl peroxide 5% or combinations with erythromycin or clindamycin are effective acne treatments and are recommended as monotherapy for mild acne, or in conjunction with a topical retinoid, or systemic antibiotic therapy for moderate to severe acne.
      - Benzoyl peroxide is effective in the prevention of bacterial resistance and is recommended for patients on topical or systemic antibiotic therapy
      - Always combine topical Abx with benzoyl peroxide
      - Tretinoin cream (Retin-a 0.01% gel, 0.025% gel/cream, 0.1% cream qHS) + clindamycin lotion (1% applied nightly or twice daily) + OTC BPO (5% twice daily)
      - Combination benzoyl peroxide topical clindamycin (BenzaClin) +/- Topical Retinoid
    - **Adapalene (Differin 0.1% cream, 0.3% gel qHS)** + clindamycin/BPO combination
    - if not responsive after 3 months...
      - Add doxycycline (50-100 mg orally once or twice daily)
  - Moderate-severe:
    - Doxycycline + tretinoin cream + OTC BPO wash
    - Doxycycline + adapalene/BPO combination
    - If not responsive after 3 months...
      - refer to dermatology for Accutane
    - Topical dapsone 5% BID a good option for **inflammatory acne in patients who cannot tolerate benzoyl peroxide+Abx combination**. Be aware of patients with G6PD deficiency however trials did not suggest ↑ risk.
    - **Post inflammatory dyspigmentation** is best treated with azelaic acid
  - Hormonal

    Suspect in females with irregular periods with cyclic acne
    - topical retinoin + combined OCP (must contain estrogen; options include Yaz, Yasmine. Avoid Sronyx)
      - OCP: ethinyl estradiol/ norgestimate, ethinyl estradiol/norethindrone acetate/ferrous fumarate, ethinyl estradiol/drospirenone, and ethinyl estradiol/drospirenone/levomefolate
    - if not responsive after 3 months...
      - add Aldactone

- if not responsive after 3 months...
  - reassess

Acne Treatment by Severity

Severity	Almost Clear	Mild	Moderate	Severe
First Line Treatment	Benzoyl Peroxide -or- Topical Retinoid	Benzoyl Peroxide plus Topical Retinoid (start 1-2x/week then ↑ to daily as tolerated)	Topical Combination tx > BP+TABx > BP + TR > TR+BP+TABx -or- Oral Abx (Doxy) +TR+BP	Oral Abx (Doxy)+BP+TR -or- Isotretinoin (if risk of scarring high)
Second Line Treatments (if failure after 3 months)	Benzoyl Peroxide plus Topical Retinoid	Add TR or BP (if not on already) -or- PO Abx (doxycycline) + BP + TR	Consider alternative combination therapy -or- PO Isotretinoin -or- Add combined OCP or PO Spironolactone (females)	Consider PO isotretinoin
Maintenance Therapy				
> Tretinoin or adapalene or BP daily > OCP in women with acne options: must contain levonorgestrel such as Mirena (second line would be norgestimate such as Ortho-Tri cyclin)				

ABx = antibiotic
TABx = topical antibiotic
BP = benzoyl peroxide
OCP = oral contraceptive
TR = topical retinoid

- **Treatment**[7,8]
  - Mild Acne
    - Use topical antibiotics (clindamycin and erythromycin) and benzoyl peroxide gels (2%, 5%, or 10%).
      - Best combined with benzoyl peroxide-erythromycin gels.
    - Topical retinoids (retinoic acid, adapalene, tazarotene) require detailed instructions regarding gradual increases in concentration from 0.01% to 0.025% to 0.05% cream/gel or liquid.
      - Mild irritation may occur at the start of treatment (1-2 weeks)
      - Use pea-sized dose to apply thin layer to affected areas
      - Apply every other day for first 2-4 weeks (apply to face for 60 min then wash off), then apply a gentle , non-comedogenic moisturizer
  - Moderate Acne
    - Add PO ABx to the above regimen. Limit duration to 3-4 months and always combine with topical retinoid!
      - Doxycycline, 50-100 mg twice daily, tapered to 50 mg/d as acne lessens.
      - Minocycline is most effective, 50-100 mg/d (beware risk for DRESS)
      - Use of oral isotretinoin in moderate acne **to prevent scarring** has become much more common and is effective.
        - Topical dapsone 5% recommended for inflammatory acne
  - Severe Acne
    - Indicated for: cystic or conglobate acne or for any other acne refractory to treatment.
    - Precautions:
      - Concurrent tetracycline and isotretinoin may cause pseudotumor cerebri
      - Determine blood lipids, transaminases (ALT, AST) before therapy.
    - Isotretinoin, 0.5-1 mg/kg given in divided doses with food.
      - Most patients clear within 20 weeks with 1 mg/kg.
      - Recent studies suggest that 0.5 mg/kg is equally effective.
    - **Photodynamic Therapy (PDT)**
      - MOA: With exposure to the visible spectrum of light and in the presence of oxygen, the activated photosensitizer then generates reactive oxygen species and may induce selective phototoxicity of the targeted sebaceous units.
      - Emerging treatment option for all stages of acne (inflammatory and non-inflammatory), still considered off-label
      - An additional therapy option the standard acne regimen for patients with mild acne who are not responding to topical retinoids and benzyl peroxide, or in patients with moderate acne who cannot tolerate or do not respond to oral antibacterial or hormonal therapies
      - S/E: transient hyperpigmentation, erythema, swelling
  - Post Inflammatory Dyspigmentation
    - Add azelaic acid

Pharmacologic Treatment of Acne

Name	Indication	Dosage	S/E
Topical Retinoid			
Adapalene	Mild/moderate	• Cream, lotion (0.1%) • Gel (0.3%) • Adapalene/benzoyl peroxide (Epiduo) gel (0.1%/2.5%)	• Local erythema • peeling • dryness • pruritus • stinging
Tazarotene	Mild/moderate	Cream, gel (0.05%, 0.1%)	
Tretinoin (Retin-A)	Mild/moderate	• Cream (0.025%, 0.1%) • Gel (0.01%, 0.025%, 0.05%) • Microsphere gel (0.04%, 0.1%)	
Combination (Adapalene/Benzoyl Peroxide) Epiduo	Moderate	• Adapalene 0.3% Benzoyl Peroxide 0.025%	
Topical Antibiotics			
Clindamycin	Mild/moderate	• Foam, gel, lotion, solution (1.0%) • Clindamycin/benzoyl peroxide (BenzaClin) gel (1%/5%, 1.2%/2.5%) • Clindamycin/tretinoin gel (Veltin, Ziana; 1.2%/0.025%)	Local erythema, peeling, dryness, pruritus, burning, oiliness
Erythromycin	Mild/moderate (can be considered in pregnancy)	• Gel, solution, ointment (2%) • Erythromycin/benzoyl peroxide (Benzamycin) gel (3%/5%)	
Other Topicals			
Benzoyl Peroxide	Mild/moderate	• Bar, cream, gel, lotion, pad, wash (2.5% to 10%)	
Dapsone	Mild/moderate	• Gel (Aczone, 5%)	
Oral Antibiotics *Advised not to use for longer than 3 months*			
Doxycycline	Moderate	50-100mg/d or BID	Photosensitivity, Esophagitis

Minocycline	Moderate	50-100mg/d or BID	Photophobia, hepatotoxicity
Erythromycin	Moderate	250-500mg BID or QID	GI sx
Isotretinoin			
Isotretinoin	Severe	0.5 to 1.0 mg per kg per day for about 20 weeks, or a cumulative dose of 120 mg per kg Patients with moderate acne may respond to lower dosages (0.3 mg per kg per day) and experience fewer adverse effects.	

COMMON SKIN CONDITIONS

- **Acne** *(see above)*
- **Seborrheic Dermatitis**[9]
  - Characterized by redness and scaling and occurring in regions where the sebaceous glands are most active, such as the face and scalp
  - Management
    - First-line:
      - Clobetasol 0.05% TID/QID
      - Desonide 0.05% cream on face 2-3x/week
      - Ketoconazole topical 2% shampoo; lather can be used on face and chest during shower.
      - Ketoconazole topical 2% to face 2/3x/week
    - Alternative
      - 1% or 2.5% hydrocortisone cream
      - In more resistant cases → clobetasol propionate, 2% ketoconazole cream, 1% pimecrolimus cream, and 0.03% or 0.1% tacrolimus ointment
      - Pimecrolimus, 1% cream, is very beneficial
- **Atopic Dermatitis**
  - Overview
    - Dry skin and pruritus; consequent rubbing leads to increased inflammation and lichenification and to further itching and scratching: *itch-scratch cycle.*
    - Eczema is the itch that rashes
    - Predilection for the flexures, front and sides of the neck, eyelids, forehead, face, wrists, and dorsa of the feet and hands
  - Labs
    - Cultures to include bacterial (staph), viral (HSV), IgE, ↑eos, HSV antigen
  - Management
    - Dilute bleach baths (may ↓ severity after 6 weeks)
    - Topical steroids:
      - Corticosteroids
      - Pimecrolimus
      - Tacrolimus
    - Baseline therapy of dryness with emollients
    - Oral and topical antibiotics to eliminate *S. aureus*
    - Hydroxyzine 10-100mg QID to suppress pruritus
    - UVA-UVB phototherapy
- **Stasis Dermatitis**
  - Often due to chronic venous insufficiency
  - Symptoms
    - Pain (aching, cramping, heaviness, ↓ w/walking)
    - Edema
    - Venous dilation
    - Erythema & serosanguinous seepage
    - Brawny discoloration
    - Ulcerations most often seen at the medial malleoli
  - Treatment
    - Sequential compression therapy
    - Elevation (20-30m TID to QID)
    - Impact of intermittent pneumatic devices is unclear
    - ASA improves ulcer healing process
- **Perioral Dermatitis**

- Age of Onset: 16-45 years; can occur in children and the old.
- Females predominantly
- 1- to 2-mm erythematous papulopustules on an erythematous background irregularly grouped, symmetric.
- Perioral distribution with rim of sparing around the vermilion border of lips
- Management:
  - *Topical*:
    - Metronidazole, 0.75% gel two times daily or 1% once daily; erythromycin, 2% gel applied twice daily.
    - Avoid topical glucocorticoids
  - *Systemic*
    - Minocycline or doxycycline, 100 mg daily until clear, then 50 mg daily for another 2 months or Tetracycline, 500 mg twice daily until clear, then 500 mg daily for 1 month, then 250 mg daily for an additional month.

SKIN BIOPSY

Biopsies for different conditions

Indication[10]	Clinical presentation	Possible diagnosis	Biopsy technique
Diagnosis	Rashes or blisters involving dermis	Drug reaction, cutaneous lymphoma, deep tissue infection, erythema multiforme, Kaposi sarcoma, lupus erythematosus, pemphigoid, pemphigus, vasculitis	Partial/perilesional punch
	Processes Involving the subcutis	Erythema nodosum, panniculitis	Elliptical excision; saucerization
Diagnosis and treatment	Atypical moles and pigmented lesions	Dysplastic nevi, malignant melanoma	Elliptical excision; saucerization, punch for 1- to 4-mm lesions with 1- to 3-mm margins

- **Procedure**
  - Shave
    1. Obtain consent.
    2. Clean skin.
    3. Anesthetize skin.
    4. Superficial shave:
       - For macular or raised nonsuspicious lesions, hold blade parallel to the skin and shallowly remove a thin disk or the lesion itself, if raised
    5. Saucerization:
       - For pigmented lesions, measure a 1- to 3-mm margin before shaving

- Anesthetize, creating a wheal to make the lesion easier to shave and squeeze skin between the thumb and forefinger of the nondominant hand to further elevate the lesion.
- Hold blade at a 45-degree angle to the skin, bend or bow the blade depending on the width of lesion, and remove a disk of tissue well into the subcutaneous fat
- If a nidus of pigment remains after saucerization, a punch or elliptical biopsy must be performed, and the sample sent in the same specimen container.
- Use a hemostatic agent or electrocautery and wipe clean.

6. Dress with petrolatum and instruct the patient to keep the area moist and covered for at least one week to minimize scarring.
7. Cauterization with **Drysol**

GASTROENTEROLOGY

ABDOMINAL PAIN BY LOCATION

Differential Diagnosis of Abdominal Pain		
Right Upper Quadrant[11]	Epigastric	Left Upper Quadrant
Cholecystitis	Peptic ulcer disease	Splenic infarct
Cholangitis	Gastritis	Splenic rupture
Pancreatitis	GERD	Splenic abscess
Pneumonia/empyema	Pancreatitis	Gastritis
Pleurisy/pleurodynia	Myocardial infarction	Gastric ulcer
Subdiaphragmatic abscess	Pericarditis	Pancreatitis
Hepatitis	Ruptured aortic aneurysm	Subdiaphragmatic abscess
Budd-Chiari syndrome		

	Esophagitis	
Right Lower Quadrant	**Periumbilical**	**Left Lower Quadrant**
Appendicitis Salpingitis Inguinal hernia Ectopic pregnancy Nephrolithiasis Inflammatory bowel disease Mesenteric lymphadenitis Typhlitis	Early appendicitis Gastroenteritis Bowel obstruction Ruptured aortic aneurysm	Diverticulitis Salpingitis Inguinal hernia Ectopic pregnancy Nephrolithiasis Irritable bowel syndrome Inflammatory bowel disease
Diffuse Nonlocalized Pain		
Gastroenteritis Mesenteric ischemia (↑lipase, amylase) Bowel obstruction Irritable bowel syndrome Peritonitis Diabetes Malaria Familial Mediterranean fever Metabolic diseases Psychiatric disease		

ASCITES

- **Pathophysiology**[12]
  - Cirrhosis and portal hypertension leads to nitrous oxide (NO) development which causes splanchnic vasodilation. The dilation leads to:
    1) Arterial underfilling causing the heart to respond by ↑CO and ↑plasma volume. To do this, it:
      - Stimulates renin-angiotensin-aldosterone system→renal na and water retention is then caused. This retention is a part of what causes ascites.

    2) Increase in the splanchnic pressure (hepatic sinusoids and vessels) which ↑ lymph accumulation. That accumulation of lymph is what causes ascites to develop.
  - 3 most common causes in US are (1) cirrhosis (2) malignancy and (3) heart failure
- **Clinical signs and symptoms**
  - Medium/large volume ascites can be detected on physical exam generally by a distended abdomen, shifting dullness or a fluid wave
- **Staging**
  - **1**: ascites is only detectable with US
  - **2**: ascites is moderate with some abdominal distention; treat with diuretics and 2g sodium restriction
  - **3**: massive ascites with marked abdominal distention; treat as above with diuresis, Na restriction, therapeutic paracentesis, and consider TIPS
- **Workup**
  - New onset: needs diagnostic paracentesis to determine cause (even if admitted for other reason)
  - If you suspect ascites but none is apparent on physical exam, get an abdominal ultrasound to detect fluid and mark ascites for paracentesis

- Looking for infected ascites is part of the workup in a patient with cirrhosis and fever/leukocytosis/altered mental status.
- Send ascitic fluid for:
  - Cell count and differential
  - Albumin (also send serum albumin)
  - Total protein (<1g/dl increases risk of SBP)
    - Optional:
      - Culture in blood culture bottles
      - Glucose
      - LDH
      - Amylase
      - Gram stain
      - Cytology
      - AFB

- **Etiologies**
  - Classification by serum ascites albumin gradient (SAAG= serum albumin – ascites albumin)
    >95% accuracy

Differential Diagnosis based on SAAG value	
SAAG	
High gradient ≥ 1.1 g/dl	Low gradient < 1.1 g/dl
• Etiology: Portal HTN	• Nephrotic syndrome
• Cirrhosis (often low ascitic total protein level <2.5)	• Peritoneal carcinomatosis (high ascitic total protein)
• Alcoholic hepatitis	• Pancreatic ascites
• CHF (elevated ascitic total protein ≥2.5)	• Tuberculous peritonitis
• Fulminant hepatic failure	• Biliary ascites
• Budd-Chiari syndrome	• Collagen vascular disease serositis
• Massive hepatic metastases	• Infection
• Veno-occlusive disease	• Malignancy
• Portal vein thrombosis	
• Myxedema	
• Fatty liver of pregnancy	

Figure. Flow chart in the evaluation of ascites

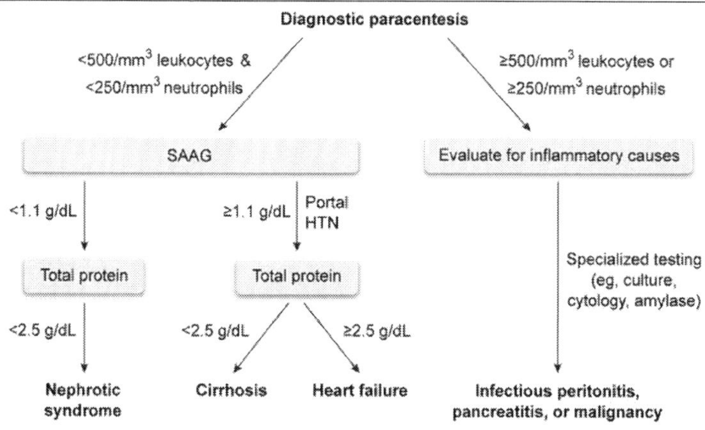

Child-Turcotte-Pugh scoring			
	1 point	2 point	3 point
Ascites	Absent	Nontense	Tense
Encephalopathy	Absent	Grades 1-2	Grades 3-4
Bilirubin (mg/dl)	<2.0	2-3	>3.0
Albumin (mg/dl)	>3.5	2.8-3.5	<2.8
Pt (sec over normal)	1-3	4-6	>6
Classification			
Score	Class	3-yr survival	
5-6	A	>90	
7-9	B	50-60	
10-15	C	30	

MELD Score[13]

MELD = 3.78xln[serum bilirubin (mg/dL)] + 11.2xln[INR] + 9.6[Ln serum creatinine (mg/dL)] + 6.43

- MELD 10: 90 percent waiting list survival versus 83 percent 1-year post-liver transplant survival (p<0.05)
- MELD 15: 81 versus 80 percent, respectively (p = 0.70)
- MELD 20: 63 versus 78 percent, respectively (p<0.05)
- MELD 25: 42 versus 74 percent, respectively (p<0.05)
- MELD 30: 21 versus 71 percent, respectively (p<0.05)

- When using the original meld score formula (which includes liver disease etiology), patients with a meld score of less than eight generally do well after tips, while those with a score greater than 18 have a poorer outcome.
- Using the meld score as modified by unos, the best outcomes occur among patients with a meld score less than 14.

- As a general rule, TIPS should be avoided if possible, in patients with a meld score greater than 24, unless the procedure is being used as salvage therapy to control active variceal bleeding

- **Treatment**
  - See staging above
  - Salt restriction
  - Fluid restriction (free water <1L/d)
  - Therapeutic Paracentesis
    - Indicated in Stage 2 ascites and above
    - Large volume paracentesis (LVP) can be done to remove 5L at one time. The most common complication is paracentesis-induced circulatory dysfunction (PICD). If >5L is removed, IV plasma expander indicated yet controversial. Consider albumin IV 8g/L of ascitic fluid removed. It should be given **during** LVP.
  - Diuretic Sensitive
    - Consider therapeutic paracentesis if tense ascites noted (will req 5L removal)
      - Large volume paracentesis (≥5L) should be combined with albumin 6-8g per L removed
    - SAAG > 1.1
      - **If Na < 120 mEq/L**
        - Fluid restriction
        - Hypertonic Saline
        - Vasopressin Receptor Antagonists
      - **If Na >120 mEq/L**
        - Lasix (40mg, BID in AM and at 3pm; max 160mg), spironolactone 100mg (max 400mg), salt restriction (<2g/day)
          - Increase diuretics q1w with maintenance of the 40:100 ratio to maintain normokalemia. If ↓K, then avoid Lasix and give spironolactone alone.
        - Max spironolactone: 400mg; max furosemide: 160mg
        - **If hypotension develops, administer Midodrine and consider TIPS or liver transplantation**
      - Cease alcohol if applicable
    - SAAG < 1.1
      - **Not due to cardiac or intrinsic liver pathology**
      - Do not respond to salt restriction and diuretics
    - Start referral for liver transplant
    - Avoid NSAIDs
  - Diuretic Resistant/Refractory Ascites
    - Unresponsive to sodium restriction and high dose diuretics (>400mg spironolactone; furosemide 160mg) or ascites that reoccurs after paracentesis
    - Options
      - Serial therapeutic paracentesis
      - Liver transplant
      - **TIPS**[14]
        - Indications
          - Acute bleeding refractory to endoscopic therapy
        - Workout prior to referral for a TIPS includes:
          - CBC, T&C, Coombs, BMP, LFT, Coag panel
          - Doppler US liver to ensure portal and hepatic veins are patent
          - TTE to evaluate pulmonary pressures and R heart fxn

- Contraindications include CHF, severe TR, severe PHTN, active hepatic encephalopathy

CIRRHOSIS

- **Types**
  - Compensated
  - Decompensated → patient should be placed for liver transplant; often have ascites, esophageal varices,
    - Loss of function → ↑INR, ↓PLT, jaundice, ↓albumin
    - Should have screening EGD for varices
      - **Variceal Prophylaxis**
        - Cirrhosis without varices = no BB; EGD q2-3y or q1y if decompensated
        - Small nonbleeding varices = no BB; EGD q1-2y if compensated and yearly if decompensated
        - Medium/Large varices = EVL or BB; q1y EGD
        - Small varices with red whale sign or decompensated cirrhosis = BB with yearly EGD
- **Etiologies**
  - Alcoholism
  - Hepatitis C
  - AIH
  - NASH
  - Inherited: Hemochromatosis, Wilson, Alpha-1
  - Hepatitis B
- **Physical Exam**
  - Palmar erythema
  - Spider angioma
  - Fluid wave
  - HJR
  - Clubbing
  - Muscle wasting
  - Hepatosplenomegaly
- **Labs/Work-up**
  - EtOH
  - H/H (anemia likely 2/2 to splenomegaly, hemolysis, IDA)
  - Hemoccult
  - LFTs
  - Albumin
  - AFP
  - RUQ US with portal flow
  - Sodium
  - HCV Ab, HBs Ag, anti-HBs, HBeAg, HCV genotype
  - Antinuclear or Antismooth muscle Ab (r/o AIH)
  - NH3
- **Severity**
  - Child-Pugh scoring
  - MELD
- **Complications**
  - PHTN → Ascites, variceal hemorrhage, and portal vein thrombosis (high suspicion if fever, abdominal pain, lower extremity edema) → tx with anti coag
  - Infection → might not mount fever or leukocytosis

- ↑INR → does not respond to Vitamin K
- SBP
- Hepatorenal syndrome
- Variceal hemorrhage
  - Screening[15]
    - All patients diagnosed with cirrhosis should have screening EGD.
    - If initial endoscopy shows no varices, then re-evaluation can be done in 2-3 years
  - Grading
    - Small (<5mm) → Repeat endoscopy q1-2y
    - Large (>5mm) → Repeat endoscopy in 1 year
    - Presence of 'red whale' or 'spots' is considered high risk for bleeding events. Other high risk features include alcohol abuse, decompensated liver failure. These patients should also have repeat endoscopy on a **yearly** basis
  - Prophylaxis
    - Nonselective BB (propranolol, nadolol)
    - Endoscopic variceal ligation
- Hepatic encephalopathy
  - Precipitating Causes
    - Drugs (sedatives)
    - ↓Volume (diarrhea, vomiting, diuretics)
    - ↑Nitrogen (GIB, constipation, ↑protein)
    - ↓K, MetAlk
    - ↓O2 ↓gluc
    - Infxn (PNA, UTI, SBP)
    - Shunting (surgical)

- **Management**
  - Ascites (see separate section on page 31)
    - ↓sodium diet (<2g)
    - 1.5L fluid restriction (if hyponatremic)
    - Lasix 40mg and spironolactone 100mg
    - Lack of response to above → TIPS or therapeutic paracentesis
  - SBP[16]
    - 2/2 bacterial translocation (E.coli, s. viridans, s. aureus) however consider perf organ if 2+ organisms
    - Diagnosed when ascitic PMN count is ≥ 250 with symptoms of fever, abdominal pain, general malaise, loss of appetite, nausea, and/or vomiting.
    - Treat with cefotaxime 2g IV daily + albumin @ 1.5 g/kg on admission and 1 g/kg on day 3
      - Alternative to cefotaxime is Augmentin 1.2g QID x5 days
  - Variceal bleed
    - Always treat for SBP as prophylaxis in these patients for 4-7 days:
      - ceftriaxone 1g/preferred
      - IV ciprofloxacin 750mg/week
      - PO norfloxacin 400mg BID x 7d
    - *Acute Bleed*
      - Initial Management
        - Fluid resuscitation (0.9NS) ideally through large bore (18G) x2
          - Aggressive hydration can actually be detrimental as it may increase portal pressures
        - CBC, T&C with consideration of blood transfusion to keep HGB≥7
        - INR to ensure correction of concurrent coagulopathy (ie. FFP)

  - PLT to ensure treatment of thrombocytopenia
  - PPI (IV vs. PO)
  - IV Octreotide 50mcg IV bolus f/b 50-mcg/hr infusion
  - IV ABx (Ceftriaxone 1g q24h x7d) (alternatives: ciprofloxacin, norfloxacin)
- <u>Upper Endoscopy</u> (within 12 hours of admission)
  - Controlled with above interventions? Stop
  - Uncontrolled with above interventions? Balloon tamponade → TIPS (see page 34)
    - Balloon tamponade can be utilized in patients who do not respond to endoscopic therapy (should not be maintained for more than 24 hours) but rather as an adjunct to TIPS vs. repeat endoscopy
- <u>TIPS</u>
    - Marked survival benefit noted in those with Child-Pugh class C disease, known cirrhosis, and high risk for treatment failure. In a study by Hernández-Gea V et al. Hepatology 2018 Jul 16, among 671 patients, those receiving a pre-emptive TIPS had higher survival at 6 weeks (92% vs. 77%) and at 1 year (78% vs. 62%) compared with those receiving standard treatment. This was associated with lower rates of recurrent bleeding and better control of ascites without increased encephalopathy rates.

Figure. Management flow chart for suspected variceal hemorrhage

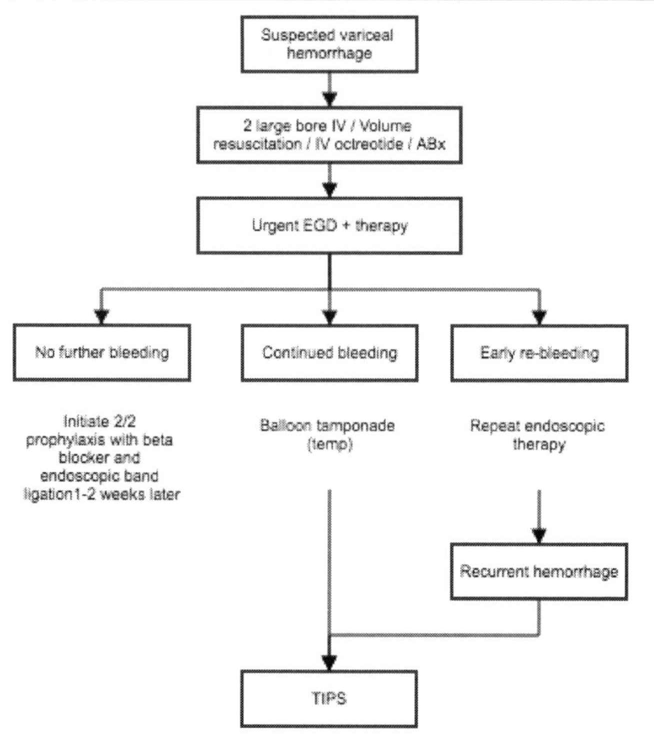

- <u>Vaccinations</u>: Hepatitis A, B, and pneumonia
- <u>Screening</u>: EGD for varices once, r/o HCC with US q6m
- <u>HRS</u>
  - Due to reflex renal vasoconstriction
  - Diagnosis is based on exclusion of other potential causes of renal failure. Major criteria include ↓GFR, absence of shock physiology, volume depletion, and nephrotoxic drugs. UA should show no proteinuria or obstructive uropathy. Minor criteria include a urine volume <500cc/d and urine sodium <10 mmol/L.
  - Types 1 and 2
    - Type 1
      - Treatment includes:
        - Stopping diuretics
        - Volume challenge with IV albumin @ 1g/kg or 1-1.5L of normal isotonic saline
        - Consider initiating midodrine, octreotide
    - Type 2
      - Usually due to refractory ascites, see separate management of refractory ascites
- <u>Hepatic Encephalopathy</u>
  - Rifaximin first line; consider lactulose titrated to 2-3 soft BM/day

IRRITABLE BOWEL SYNDROME

- **Types**[17,18,19]
  - IBS-C, IBS-D, IBS-M, IBS-U
- **Diagnosis**
  - *ROME III guidelines:*
    - Recurrent abdominal pain for at least 3d/month in the last 3 months that started at least 6 months ago associated with 2+ of the following:
      1) Improvement with defecation
      2) Onset associated with change in frequency of stool
      3) Onset associated with change in form of stool
      4) Not associated with a structural cause
- **Treatment**
  - Consider, overall a diet low in FODMAP (fermentable oligosaccharides, disaccharides, monosaccharides, and polyols) can decrease IBS symptoms
  - <u>IBS-M</u>
    - Mixture of Lactobacillus and Bifidobacterium sp appx 20-40 billion CFU/d for 4-6 weeks
    - Soluble fiber of 15g/d
    - Dicyclomine (40mg/QID x2w), Hyoscyamine (10mg QID x 4w), Peppermint Oil (200-500mg x 4w)
    - TCA (Amitriptyline 10-75mg/d x12w)
    - Rifaximin
  - <u>IBS-D</u>
    - Loperamide
    - Alosetron
    - Eluxadoline 75mg/100mg BID
  - <u>IBS-C</u>
    - Polyethylene glycol
    - Linaclotide
    - Lubiprostone

CONSTIPATION

- **Types**: Functional (see below) and Secondary (medication or 2/2 condition)
- **Definition**[20]
  - Must include two or more of the following:
    - Straining during at least 25 percent of defecations
    - Lumpy or hard stools in at least 25 percent of defecations
    - Sensation of incomplete evacuation for at least 25 percent of defecations
    - Sensation of anorectal obstruction/blockage for at least 25 percent of defecations
    - Manual maneuvers to facilitate at least 25 percent of defecations (e.g., digital evacuation, support of the pelvic floor)
    - Fewer than three defecations per week
- Avoid PO agents if pt is impacted or obstructed (KUB & DRE can assess this)
- Rule out secondary causes:
  - Hypothyroidism
  - Neurologic disorders (ie. PD, MS, spinal cord injury, amyloidosis, DM, ↑Ca, low fiber intake)
- PE involves confirming good sphincter tone exists, and relaxation possible when prompted

- **Indications for Endoscopy**
  - Age older than 50 years with no previous colorectal cancer screening
  - Before surgery for constipation
  - Change in stool caliber
  - Heme-positive stools Iron deficiency anemia
  - Obstructive symptoms
  - Recent onset of constipation
  - Rectal bleeding
  - Rectal prolapse
  - Weight loss
- <u>Mainstay Treatment</u>

  (1) Senna Docusate (2) MiraLax/Lactulose (3) Laxatives
  - ↑exercise, ↑dietary fiber (25-30g), adequate H2O, bulk laxatives (psyllium, methylcellulose)
  - MOM 30 ml PO Q 12 hours prn constipation
    - Caution in pts with renal dysfunction
  - MgOH
  - Magnesium Citrate 8 oz (240 ml) bottle PO
    - Caution in pts with renal dysfunction d/t risk of ↑Mg
  - Senna 1-2 tabs hs + docusate 100-240 mg PO bid
- <u>If no BM by day 3</u>
  - Give Fleet enema or Bisacodyl suppository PR
    - Fleet's caution in pts with renal dysfunction or CHF
  - Avoid all the above in dialysis patient's d/t hyper MG and PO4
  - Mineral Oil enema
  - Psyllium indicated for **chronic** constipation
  - Lactulose 30 ml PO
  - Bisacodyl 10 mg PO/PR
    - Not for chronic use d/t risk of ↓K and ↑Na
  - Dulcolax suppository PR x1
    - Causes contraction of intestine by stimulating mesenteric plexus
  - Glycerine Suppository PR x1
  - Colace 100mg PO daily

COLON CANCER

- **Screening**
  - Normal population with no history of familial colon cancer should start at age 45 with a colonoscopy, repeated every 10 years through age of 75 if life expectancy is 10 years or more
  - Screening is discouraged for those >85
  - If family history of colon cancer (diagnosis before age 60) or 2+ family members who have biopsy showing high grade dysplasia should receive screening start at 40 (10 years before normal population) or 10 years from diagnosis (whichever is earlier)
    - Repeat colonoscopies will occur at 5 year intervals
  - Repeat in 3 years if:
    - 3 or more adenomas of any size are found
    - 2 or more adenomas >1cm in size are found
    - Any adenoma that is villous or high grade in dysplasia
    - Can return to 5 year intervals if repeat shows no abnormalities

Screening Options for CRC[21]		
Method	Advantages	Disadvantages
Colonoscopy	• Ability to detect and remove polyps • Visualizes the entire colon	• Requires comprehensive bowel preparation • Takes 20 to 30 minutes plus recovery time • Patient may not drive or return to work if sedation is given
CT Colonoscopy	• 10-15 min • Noninvasive • No sedation • Can drive and work same day	• Same bowel prep reqd • Radiation • May miss small polyps + test → colonoscopy
FIT	• At home • Safe • No diet affects	• Reqd yearly • + test → colonoscopy
Flex Sigmoid	• Safer than colo • 10 minutes • May still drive and go to work same day	• Req bowel prep • Only distal 1/3 of colon seen • +test → colonoscopy
FOBT	• At home • Easy • Convenient	• Yearly • Diet changes • +test → colonoscopy
FIT-DNA	• At home • Safe • Convenient • No dietary changes	• Expensive • +test → colonoscopy

Follow-up Guidelines	
Number/Size/Histopathology	Surveillance Colonoscopy
Hyperplastic polyps	10 yrs
1-2 small (<1cm) tubular adenomas with no high grade dysplasia	5 yrs
3+ adenomas High grade dysplasia Villous features Any adenoma of 1cm or larger	3 yrs

DIARRHEA

- **Acute**[22,23]
  - Defined: <2 weeks
  - Etiology
    - Appearance of the stool: blood (inflammatory or invasive ulceration), mucus (IBS), or oil (malabsorption).
    - Infectious (viral, bacterial, parasitic)
    - Food exposure (onset 12h to 10d after eating)
    - Medications antibiotics, alcohol, illicit drugs, laxatives, magnesium-containing antacids, digoxin, quinidine,
      colchicine.

- Ischemia (RF: HTN, DM, chronic afib, HLD)
- Proctitis and rectal discharge suggest gonorrhea, syphilis, lymphogranuloma venereum, and herpes simplex
- History of gastrectomy, vagotomy, intestinal resection (short gut syndrome).

Bacterial Causes of Diarrhea

Etiology	Incubation Period	Signs/Sx	Duration	Associated Foods	Labs	Clinical Features & Treatment
Salmonella	1-3d	Diarrhea, fever, abdominal pain, vomiting (if associated with HA, constipation, malaise, chills, myalgias consider Typhoid)	4-7d	Contaminated eggs, poultry, unpasteurized milk or juice, cheese, contaminated raw fruits and veggies	+/- fecal WBCs	Supportive care. ABx are not indicated unless Typhoid during which use TMP-SMX or gentamycin
Shigella	1-2d	Abdominal cramps, fever, diarrhea. Stool may have blood+mucous	4-7d	Food or water contaminated with fecal material; often person to person	Stool cx +fecal WBCs	Supportive care; TMP-SMX if organism is susceptible; Fluoroquinolone x3d
B cereus (preformed)	1-8h	↑↑↑vomiting + diarrhea no fever	1d	Reheated fried rice causes vomiting or diarrhea.	Food and stool can be tested for toxin. - fecal WBCs	Acute onset, severe nausea and vomiting lasting 24 hours. Supportive care.
S.aureus	1-8h	Sudden onset of severe nausea and vomiting. Abdominal cramps. Diarrhea and fever may be present	1-2d	Unrefrigerated or improperly refrigerated meats, potato, and egg salads, cream pastries	Normally a clinical diagnosis; stool, vomitus, and food can be tested for toxin - fecal WBCs	Abrupt onset, intense nausea and vomiting for up to 24 hours, recovery in 24-48 hours. Supportive care.

Etiology	Incubation Period	Signs/Sx	Duration	Associated Foods	Labs	Treatment
Vibrio parahaemolyticus	2-48h	Watery diarrhea, abdominal cramps, nausea, vomiting	2-5d	Undercooked or raw seafood, such as fish, shellfish	Stool cx, vibrio requires special media - fecal WBCs	Supportive care. ABx recommended if severe (ie. Tetracycline 500mg QID x3d)
Yersinia enterocolitica	1-2d	Appendicitis-like symptoms (diarrhea, vomiting, fever, and abdominal pain) occur primarily in older children/young adults. May have scarlatiniform rash	1-3w	Undercooked pork, unpasteurized milk, contaminated water	Stool, vomitus or blood cx +/- fecal WBCs	Supportive care, usually self-limiting
Listeria monocytogenes	9-48h for GI sx; 2-6w for invasive disease	Fever, muscle aches, and nausea or diarrhea.	Variable	Fresh soft cheeses, unpasteurized milk, inadequately pasteurized milk, ready-to-eat deli meats	Blood or cerebrospinal fluid cx; stool cx usually not helpful	Supportive care
ETEC	1-3d	Watery diarrhea, abdominal cramps, some vomiting	3-7d	Water or food contaminated with human feces	Stool cx; ETEC requires special lab techniques. - fecal WBCs	Supportive care; Abx rarely indicated
EHEC (including E.coli O157:H7)	1-8d	Severe diarrhea, often bloody, abdominal pain and vomiting	5-10d	Undercooked beef, unpasteurized milk and juice	Stool cx; O157:H7 requires special media and reporting to	Supportive care, monitor renal fxn, H/H, and PLT closely; if ABx necessary then TMP-SMX 160-800mg BID x3d

					local agencies. +fecal WBCs	
Clostridium perfringens	8-16h	Watery diarrhea, nausea, abdominal cramps, fever rare	1-2d	Meats, poultry, gravy, or dried precooked foods	Stools can be tested for enterotoxin	Supportive care
C. jejuni	2-5d	Diarrhea, cramps, fever, and vomiting, diarrhea may be bloody	2-10d	Raw and undercooked poultry, unpast. Milk, contaminated water	Routine stool cx; campy req. special agar +fecal WBCs	Supportive care; early in dz course can use FLQ
Norwalk	1-2d	Nausea, vomiting, watery large-volume diarrhea, rare fever	24-60h	Poorly cooked shellfish; ready-to-eat foods touched by infected workers	Clinical dx; negative bacterial cx; negative fecal leukocytes. - fecal WBCs	Supportive care Bismuth sulfate
Rotavirus	1-3d	Vomiting, watery diarrhea, low-grade fever. Temporary lactose intolerance	4-8d	Fecally contaminated foods	ID of virus in stool immunoassay. - fecal WBCs	Supportive care
Cryptosporidium	7 days	Cramping, abdominal pain, watery diarrhea, fever and vomiting may be present	Days to weeks	Contaminated water, veggies	Must be specifically requested	Supportive care

Etiology	Incubation Period	Signs/Sx	Duration	Associated Foods	Labs	Treatment
E. histolytica	2-3d to 1-4w	Bloody diarrhea, frequent bowel movements	Months	Fecal-oral	Examination of stool for cysts and parasites	Metronidazole
Giardia	1-4w	Acute or chronic diarrhea, flatus, bloating	Weeks	Drinking water from other sources	Examination of stool for O&P. +/- fecal WBCs	Metronidazole

Etiologies To Consider with Acute Diarrhea	
Clinical Presentation	Potential Causes to Consider
Vomiting primarily (little diarrhea)	Viral gastroenteritis Rotavirus Norwalk Preformed toxin (staph, B. cereus, clostridium perfringens) Enterotoxin (vibrio, ETEC, klebsiella, Aeromonas)
Noninflammatory diarrhea (acute watery diarrhea without fever/dysentery)	Can be caused by all pathogens (bacterial, viral, parasitic) but most commonly performed toxin causers (bacillus, staph aureus, clostridium) and enterotoxin causers (vibrio, ETEC, klebsiella)
Inflammatory diarrhea (invasive GI, gross blood in stool)	Shigella, Salmonella, Campylobacter, EHEC, Vibrio, Yersinia, C. diff, entamoeba
Chronic diarrhea (≥14d)	Evaluate for parasites Consider Cyclosporacyetanesis Crypto E. histolytica Giardia
Systemic sx	Listeria Brucella Toxoplasma Vibrio HepA
Fever predominant	Shigella Salmonella Entamoeba Campylobacter Yersinia
Abdominal pains predominant	C. diff EHEC Rotavirus, Norovirus Salmonella, Campylobacter

- Symptoms
  - Nocturnal diarrhea suggests infectious or inflammatory cause
  - Admit patients with:
    - Severe diarrhea with dehydration
    - Bloody diarrhea
    - Fever
    - Duration > 2 days
    - With abdominal pain in elderly (r/o mesenteric ischemia)
- **Red Flags That Require Prompt Evaluation**
  - Inflammatory diarrhea: fever (> 38.5°C), WBC ≥ 15,000/mcL, bloody diarrhea, or severe abdominal pain
  - Passage of six or more unformed stools in 24 hours

- Profuse watery diarrhea and dehydration
- Frail older patients
- Immunocompromised patients (AIDS, post transplantation)
- Exposure to antibiotics
- Hospital-acquired diarrhea (onset following at least 3 days of hospitalization)
- Systemic illness

- Labs
  - Stools for markers of inflammation (leukocytes, guaiac)
    - Stool cultures positive in < 3%; therefore, initial symptomatic treatment is given for mild symptoms
  - Bacterial cultures
  - Ovocytes and Parasites (O&P) (in patients who have traveled recently)
  - C. difficile toxin (in patients with recent institutionalization and/or antibiotic or chemotherapy exposure)
  - Campylobacter, microsporidia, Isospora, and cryptosporidia. Also consider Giardia antigen.
- Management
  - Treat electrolyte abnormalities with IV or PO rehydration (sports drinks)
  - Avoid antimotility agents if suspecting infectious cause (febrile dysentery)
  - Stop newly started medications
  - Antibiotics are not recommended in nontyphoid Salmonella, Campylobacter, Aeromonas, Yersinia, or Shiga-toxin producing E coli infection except in severe disease. When indicated, consider treatment below:
    - *Empiric Regiments*
      - Fluoroquinolones (eg, ciprofloxacin 500 mg BID, ofloxacin 400 mg, or levofloxacin 500 mg once daily) for 1–3 days
      - Trimethoprim-sulfamethoxazole, 160/800 mg twice daily orally
      - Doxycycline, 100 mg twice daily orally
      - Metronidazole 250mg QID x7d for giardiasis
      - For Traveler's Diarrhea: Azithromycin, 1000 mg single dose or 500 mg daily for 3 days

- **Chronic**[24]
  - Definition – loose stools for more than 4 weeks
  - History
    - Onset – congenital, acute, gradual onset
    - Continuous or intermittent pattern
    - Duration
    - Recent travel, other sick family members, ingestion of contaminated water
    - Stool characteristics – watery, bloody, fatty
      - Small frequent bowel movements with tenesmus and bleeding suggest proctitis
      - Larger volume stools that are less frequent suggest a small bowel source
      - Steatorrhea suggest fat malabsorption or fat maldigestion
    - Concurrent incontinence?
    - Abdominal pain? More suggestive of IBS, IBD,

Differential diagnosis of chronic diarrhea based on osmolar gap		
Classification	Causes	Clinical Symptoms
Stool Osmolarity → stool analysis by calculating (Measured Stool Osmolarity-2([Na]+[K])) ▫ Calculate gap by comparing actual to calculated above ▫ Gap>75→osmotic • Upon fasting if symptoms improve, then likely ingestion of lactose or gluten → can do hydrogen breath test to r/o lactose intolerance ▫ Gap<75→secretory • Stool O&P, colonoscopy to r/o microscopic colitis, urine metanephrine, TSH, ACTH		
Osmotic	Lactase deficiency Medications: antacids, lactulose, sorbitol, olestra Gluten or FODMAP diet intolerance Factitious: magnesium-containing antacids or laxatives (Mg, PO4, SO4)	• Abdominal distention • Flatulence
Secretory	Hormonal: Zollinger-Ellison syndrome (gastrinoma), carcinoid, VIPoma, medullary thyroid carcinoma, adrenal insufficiency Laxative abuse: cascara, senna Medications Bowel resection SIBO Pancreatic insufficiency (w/ steatorrhea) Microscopic colitis (no steatorrhea)	• High-volume (> 1 L) watery diarrhea leading to dehydration • Electrolyte imbalance
Inflammatory conditions	Inflammatory bowel disease Cancer with obstruction and pseudo diarrhea Radiation colitis GI malignancies Collagenous colitis	• Abdominal pain • Fever • ↓Weight • Hematochezia • Pus • ↑stool wt (>200g)
Malabsorption	Small bowel: celiac disease, Whipple disease, tropical sprue, eosinophilic gastroenteritis, small bowel resection, Crohn disease Pancreatic insufficiency: chronic pancreatitis, cystic fibrosis, pancreatic cancer Bacterial overgrowth	• ↓ weight • Osmotic diarrhea • Steatorrhea • Nutritional deficiencies
Motility	IBS Post-surgical DM, thyroid Caffeine/EtOH	
Steatorrhea	Pancreatic exocrine insufficiency s/p Bariatric surgery Liver dz Celiac sprue Whipple's disease	

- <u>Differential</u>
  - *Osmotic*
    - Stool volume ↓ with fasting

        - ↑ stool osmolar gap (see below)
        - Often due to medications, lactose intolerance, or factitious intake
    - *Secretory*
        - Large volume stools despite fasting
        - Normal stool osmolar gap (see below)
        - Can be from myriad of causes to include hormone induced, malabsorption, and from medications
    - *Inflammatory*
        - Patients will often have a fever, hematochezia, and abdominal pain
        - Common causes include UC, Crohn's, microscopic colitis, radiation colitis
    - *Malabsorption*
        - Look for weight loss, abnormal metabolic panel, ↑ fecal fat (>10g in 24h)
        - Common causes include pancreatic insufficiency, SIBO, scleroderma, celiac, Crohn's
    - *Motility*
        - Often associated with recent abdominal surgery, IBS, DM, or ↑thyroid
- Exam
    - Rash (c/w IgA deficiency)
    - Thyroid mass (hypothyroidism)
    - Ascites (cirrhosis)
    - Fistulas (IBD)
- Labs
    - **Testing is indicated in the presence of alarm features**
    - CBC, CMP, LFTs, Ca, PO4, albumin, TSH
    - **Infectious** → CBC with leukocytosis (eosinophilia→neoplasm, eosinophilic colitis, parasitic infection, allergies, collagen disorder)
    - INR, ESR, and C-RP should be obtained in most patients
    - Fecal calprotectin to exclude Crohn's, fecal lactoferrin can be used as a surrogate for fecal leukocytes
    - *Clostridium difficile* toxin
    - **Malabsorption**
        - Obtain serum folate, B12, iron, vitamin A and D, prothrombin time.
        - Consider hydrogen breath testing or dietary removal of lactose/carbohydrates if suspecting lactose insufficiency.
        - Consider fecal elastase or chymotrypsin for fat malabsorption (ie. pancreatic d/o)
    - 24-hour stool collection for weight and quantitative fecal fat
        - Stool weight < 200–300 g/24 h excludes diarrhea and suggests a functional disorder such as irritable bowel
        - Stool weight > 200 g/24 hours confirms diarrhea
        - Stool weight > 1000–1500 g/24 hours suggests secretory diarrhea, including neuroendocrine tumors
        - Fecal fat > 10 g/24 hours indicates a malabsorption syndrome
    - R/O **Celiac**→ ↑alk phos; vitamin A, B_{12}, D, K deficiencies; iron level (deficiency expected), serum albumin (often low), anti-transglutaminase ab (IgA)
    - R/O **microscopic colitis** → ↑ESR, +ANA
    - Screening → folate, Fe, 25-hydroxyvitamin D
- Imaging
    - Imaging is mostly indicated in patients with steatorrhea (r/o pancreatic dz) and secretory or inflammatory diarrhea
        - Evaluate for strictures, fistulae, and diverticula.
        - Degree of inflammation if IBD suspected

    - CT enterography – consider as initial evaluation method for suspicion of Crohn's
  - Procedures
    - Consider colonoscopy to r/o CRC in patients with altered bowel habits +/- BRBPR
    - Small bowel disorders can be evaluated with MR enterography or video capsule endoscopy.
    - Breath tests for carbohydrate malabsorption and SIBO
  - Treatment
    - Bulk Forming: Psyllium 1-2 tsp bid-tid
    - Imodium 4 mg PO Q 4 hours x 16 hours (Max=16 mg in 24 hours)
      - Don't give with blood in stool or fever
    - Lomotil 2.5-5 mg PO tid-QID (Max=20mg in 24 hours)
      - Avoid in Hepatic failure or cirrhosis

CLOSTRIDIUM DIFFICILE

- **Overview**[25,26]
  - G+ obligate anaerobic bacillus that can exist in both vegetative and spore forms
- **Diagnosis**
  - Lab options: toxigenic culture, NAAT, glutamate dehydrogenase, cell culture cytotoxicity, toxin A+B, EIA
  - Nucleic acid amplification tests (NAAT) for *C. difficile* toxin genes such as PCR are superior to toxins A+B EIA testing as a standard diagnostic test for CDI; do not solely perform NAAT for diagnosis.
  - Insufficient data to support testing for fecal lactoferrin or any other biologic markers
  - When in doubt, perform EIA (and if you can, combine/confirm with NAAT)
- **Risk Factors**
  - PPI
  - Older age likely due to change in gut microbiota
  - Severity of underlying illness
  - Long-term care facility
  - Recent abdominal surgery
  - Recent ABx use
- **Treatment**
  - See table on prior page
  - Testing for cure should not be done.
  - If a patient has strong a pre-test suspicion for CDI, empiric therapy for CDI should be considered regardless of the laboratory testing result, as the negative predictive values for CDI are insufficiently high to exclude disease in these patients.
  - Contact precautions should be continued for 48 hours after last occurrence of diarrhea
  - In patients in whom oral antibiotics cannot reach a segment of the colon, such as with Hartman's pouch, ileostomy, or colon diversion, vancomycin therapy delivered via enema should be added to treatments above until the patient improves.
  - Probiotics[27]
    - No sufficient evidence to support concurrent treatment with probiotics
- **Patients Requiring Antibiotics**[28]
  - In patients who have a history of CDAD or cannot safely stop the antibiotics that precipitated their condition, IDSA recommends concurrent treatment for CDAD.
    - **Already on Abx and present with CDAD**
      - Extend CDAD treatment by providing a "tail" coverage with an agent effective against CDAD for 7-10 days following the completion of the inciting antibiotic.
    - **Prior history of CDAD and require Abx for another condition**

- Concurrent prophylactic doses of oral vancomycin have been found to be effective in preventing recurrence. The IDSA/SHEA recommend using low

Treatment regimen based on severity/occurrences		
Severity	Clinical Manifestations	Treatment
Carrier	no discernible clinical symptoms or signs	No treatment Is indicated
Initial Episode/Non-severe *WBC≤15k* *-and-* *SCr<1.5 mg/dL*	• Mild diarrhea < 12 stools/day • Afebrile • Mild to Moderate discomfort or tenderness • Nausea With rare or absent vomiting • With or without hospitalization • Not in ICU • Dehydration • WBC < 15k • SCr<1.5 mg/dL	• Discontinuation of predisposing antibiotics • Hydration • Monitor clinical status • Isolation • Oral vancomycin 125 mg QID x10d -or- Fidaxomicin 200mg BID x 10d • *Alternative: Metronidazole 500mg TID x10d* *No ↑in morbidity or mortality seen with Metronidazole in mild/moderate C. diff* • *consider extending to 14d of therapy if improvement in symptoms or worsening*
Initial Episode / Severe *WBC≥15k* *-or-* *SCr >1.5 mg/dL*	• Severe or bloody diarrhea >12 stools/day • Pseudomembranous colitis • N/V • Ileus • Temp > 38.9 C • Age > 60 YO • In ICU • Renal failure Criteria: • WBC ≥ 15k or SCr>1.5	No Distention • Oral Vancomycin 125mg QID x10d or Fidaxomicin 200mg BID x10d *consider extending to 14d of therapy if improvement in symptoms or worsening*
Initial Episode / Fulminant	• Hypotension / Shock • Toxic megacolon • Peritonitis	• Surgical consultation • Vancomycin 500 mg QID PO or by nasogastric tube. • If ileus, consider adding rectal instillation of Vancomycin

↓BP/shock *Ileus* *Megacolon*	• Ileus	• IV metronidazole 500 mg q8h should be administered together with oral or rectal vancomycin, particularly if ileus is present
First Recurrence / Fulminant	As above	• Vancomycin 125 mg QID for 10 days if metronidazole was used for the initial episode OR • Use a prolonged tapered and pulsed VAN regimen if a standard regimen was used for the initial episode (eg, 125 mg 4 times per day for 10–14 days, 2 times per day for a week, once per day for a week, and then every 2 or 3 days for 2-8 weeks) OR • Fidaxomicin 200 mg BID for 10 days if Vancomycin was used for the initial episode
Subsequent Recurrence / Fulminant	As above	• Vancomycin in a tapered and pulsed regimen OR • Vancomycin 125 mg QID PO for 10 days followed by rifaximin 400 mg TID for 20 days OR • Fidaxomicin 200 mg BID for 10 days OR • Fecal microbiota transplantation

doses of vancomycin or fidaxomicin (e.g., 125 mg or 200 mg, respectively, once daily) while systemic antibiotics are administered.

- **Recurrent CDI**
  - RCDI is a therapeutic challenge because there is no uniformly effective therapy.
  - After treatment of an initial episode of *C. difficile*, the chance of RCDI within 8 weeks is 10–20%,
  - Recurrence can be due to the same strain or to a different strain.
  - <u>First Reoccurrence</u>
    The first recurrence of CDI can be treated with the same regimen that was used for the initial episode. If severe, however vancomycin should be used
    - 14d of Oral Vancomycin 125mg QID OR Metronidazole 500mg TID
    - Probiotics (lactobacillus and Saccharomyces bouldardii)
  - <u>Second Recurrence</u>
    The second recurrence should be treated with a pulsed vancomycin regimen
    - Tapered dose regiment of oral vancomycin
    - 125mg QID x 7 days THEN
    - 125mg BID x 7 days THEN
    - 125mg DAILY x 7 days THEN
    - 125mg QOD x 7 days THEN
    - 125mg qTHIRDday x 14 days WITH probiotics for 30 days beginning on first day
  - <u>Third/Subsequent Recurrences</u>
    - Tapered dose oral vancomycin with probiotics
    - Followed by:
      - 14d course of rifaximin (400-800mg daily)
      - Consider IVIG (200-500 mg/kg/day)
      - Consider fecal transport through colonoscopy (first degree relative, collect 1L, instill 200-400cc total during operation)
      - Consider chronic low dose vancomycin (not metronidazole d/t s/e) in elderly
    - Consider fecal transplantation (capsule vs. colonoscopy)
- **Prevention**
  - Common probiotics include Lactobacillus, Bifidobacterium, and Saccharomyces bouldardii.
  - Growing evidence supports the benefits of probiotics in preventing CDI in patients requiring hospitalization, who are at the highest risk of CDI infection.
  - Probiotics are most effective when given within 2 days of antibiotic initiation compared with later administration.

DIVERTICULITIS

- **Classification**[29]
  - <u>Hinchy's Criteria (mortality)</u>
    - Stage 1 (<5%) – small confined, pericolic or mesenteric abscess
    - Stage 2 (<5%)– larger abscesses often combined to pelvis
    - Stage 3 (13%)– perforated diverticulitis due to diverticular rupture → peritonitis
    - Stage 4 (43%)– free rupture leading to fecal contamination
- **Diagnosis**
  - Computed tomography (CT) is recommended as the initial radiologic examination.
  - High sensitivity (approximately 93 to 97%)
  - Specificity approaching 100%
  - Look for diverticula, inflammation of pericolic fat, bowel-wall thickness > 4mm, abscess formation
- **When to Hospitalize**
  - Outpatient therapy reasonable with 7-10 days of PO Ciprofloxacin + Metronidazole
  - Admit it:
    - No PO intake

        - Pain requiring narcotics
        - Sx failure to improve after outpatient tx
- **Treatment**
    - NPO
    - NG tube if obstruction or ileus present
    - Repeat CT if sx do not improve in 72 hrs
    - Perform colonoscopy 2-6 weeks post recovery to rule out atypical colorectal carcinoma in patients with no documented colonoscopy in past 3 years.
- **Surgical consult if:**
    - Stage 4 / Peritonitis
    - Treatment does not respond to medical management in 72 hrs
    - Perforation
    - Abscess
    - Fistula
    - Repeated attacks (2+)
    - Sepsis
    - Approach
        - First operation - the diseased colonic segment is drained, and a diverting ostomy (usually a transverse colostomy) is created proximally.
        - Allows for fecal diversion and drainage of infection.
        - During the second operation, the diseased colon is resected, and a primary anastomosis of the colonic segments is performed.
        - The ostomy is reversed during the third and final operation to reestablish bowel continuity. The three-stage procedure is rarely performed and should be considered only in critical situations in which resection cannot be performed safely
        - Percutaneous Drainage
        - Bowel rest and broad-spectrum ABx if abscess <4cm and Hinchey Stage 1
        - CT-guided percutaneous drainage if >4cm (Stage II)

Treatment Regimen for Diverticulitis (5-7days)	
Medication	Dosage
Oral	
Metronidazole and a quinolone	Metronidazole – 500 mg every 6 to 8 hr Quinolone (e.g., ciprofloxacin – 500-750 mg every 12 hr)
Metronidazole and trimethoprim-sulfamethoxazole	Metronidazole – 500 mg every 6 to 8 hr Trimethoprim-sulfamethoxazole – 160 trimethoprim and 800 mg sulfamethoxazole every 12 hrs
Amoxicillin-clavulanate	Amoxicillin-clavulanate – 875 mg every 12 hr
IV	
Metronidazole and a quinolone	Metronidazole – 500 mg every 6 to 8 hr Quinolone (e.g., ciprofloxacin 400 mg every 12 hr)
Metronidazole and a third-generation cephalosporin	Metronidazole – 500 mg every 6 to 8 hr Third-generation cephalosporin (e.g., ceftriaxone – 1-2 g every 24 hr)
Beta-lactam with a beta-lactamase inhibitor	Beta-lactam with a beta-lactamase

	inhibitor (e.g., ampicillin-sulbactam – 3 g every 6 hr)

- **Complications**
  - Abscess
  - Fistula
  - Obstruction
  - Peritonitis
  - Stricture
- **Follow-up**
  - Colonoscopy 6 weeks after acute process to r/o cancer and IBD

GI BLEED

- **Classification**[30]
  - Upper (above ligament of Treitz)
  - Lower (below ligament)
- **History**
  - Prior bleeds, diverticular disease, prior GI or aortic surgery, trauma, coagulopathy, medications (ASA, NSAIDs, anticoagulants, steroids, antiplatelet medications), liver disease, alcohol abuse, renal insufficiency, poor cardiac output, hypertension, hypotension, recreational drugs (cocaine, amphetamines), rectal foreign objects (sexual activity or used to disimpact), history of STDs
- **Etiology**
  - Upper GI Bleeds (UGIB):
    - Peptic ulcer disease (H. pylori or NSAIDs)
    - Portal hypertensive gastropathy
    - Varices
    - Mallory-Weiss tear
    - Erosive esophagitis (especially alcoholics)
    - Vascular malformations
    - Dieulafoy's lesion (an abnormally large submucosal artery located in the proximal stomach)
    - Neoplasm
    - *Note that gastritis is not a cause of bleeding (possibly occult blood loss but not acute bleeding)*
  - Lower GI Bleeds (LGIB):
    - Diverticular disease
    - Hemorrhoids
    - Solitary rectal ulcer syndrome
    - Ischemic colitis
    - Infectious colitis
    - Inflammatory bowel disease (IBD)
    - Angiodysplasia
    - Neoplastic disease
    - Post polypectomy bleeding
    - NSAID ulcerations
    - CMV ulcerations (immunosuppressed)
    - Portal hypertensive colopathy and rectal varices (cirrhosis)
- **Clinical Signs and Symptoms**
  - Suggestive of UGIB: nausea, vomiting, hematemesis, melena, epigastric pain, liver disease, EtOH abuse, NSAID use, peptic ulcer disease, syncope

- Suggestive of LGIB: hematochezia (BRBPR), diarrhea, diverticulosis, colon cancer
    - Risk factors for adverse outcomes (recurrent bleeding, need for intervention, or death) in patients presenting with presumed acute lower gastrointestinal bleeding include hypotension, tachycardia, ongoing hematochezia, an age of more than 60 years, a creatinine level of more than 1.7 mg per deciliter, and unstable or clinically significant coexisting conditions.

- **Physical Exam**
    - Vital Signs:
        - Tachycardia (at10 % volume loss)
        - Orthostatics (at 20% volume loss)
        - Hypotension (at 30% volume loss)
    - Pallor, stigmata of liver disease, localized abdominal tenderness
    - Rectal:
    - Stool may appear bright red, maroon, black and tarry, or brown
        - Look for evidence of hemorrhoids or fissures
        - No guaiac necessary if concern of acute bleed. Guaiac should be used for colon cancer screening and workup of iron deficient anemia of unclear etiology not for acute hemoglobin drops.
            - 1 cc of blood loss will result in a positive guaiac; 50 cc of blood loss results in melena. Therefore, if recent bleeding you will find it without a guaiac
- **Admission vs. Outpatient Therapy**[31]
    - **The Glasgow Blatchford score** has the highest accuracy for predicting the need for hospitalization for his gastrointestinal bleed.
        - The pre-endoscopy Glasgow Blatchford bleeding score was more accurate than the pre-endoscopy Rockall and AIMS65 scoring systems as well as the post endoscopy Progetto Nazionale Emorragia Digestiva (PNED) and full Rockall scoring systems in predicting death or the need for in-hospital endoscopic intervention.
        - The Glasgow Blatchford Bleeding Score is determined by **nine factors**:
            - hemoglobin level
            - blood urea nitrogen level
            - initial systolic blood pressure
            - sex
            - heart rate of 100/min or less
            - presence of melena
            - recent syncope
            - history of hepatic disease
            - history of heart failure.
        - The results of this study cannot be applied to inpatients who develop upper gastrointestinal bleeding.
        - Furthermore, the clinical utility for all other outcomes, including the need for endoscopic treatment, rebleeding risk, 30-day mortality, and length of hospital stay, appeared limited for all of the scoring systems.
        - A score of 1 or less on the Glasgow Blatchford bleeding score identified a low-risk patient who could be directed to outpatient management of the upper gastrointestinal bleeding.
    - **Labs**
        - CBC, chemistry panel, type and cross, liver function tests, iron panel, reticulocyte count
        - INR
            - If elevated, consider phytonadione (Vitamin K) 10mg IM daily if INR > 2.0

        - Consider that the patient initially may have a normal Hgb value due to hemoconcentration
        - BUN disproportionately elevated from Cr suggests an upper GI source (30:1)
        - Consider fecal leukocytes/stool culture/C. diff/SSPC if infectious or inflammatory cause suspected
        - TROP if age>45 or hx CAD
        - H. pylori [32]
            - in a patient with a bleeding peptic ulcer, a negative rapid urease test or histology is not sufficient to rule out H. pylori infection, and a second test is warranted such as **H. Pylori serology**
            - The sensitivity of the rapid urease test can be reduced up to 25% in patients who have taken a proton pump inhibitor (PPI) or bismuth within 2 weeks of testing or antibiotic therapy within 4 weeks.
            - The sensitivity of the urea breath test and stool antigen test, like that of the rapid urease test, is reduced by medications that affect urease production. (fecal or urea breath test 2 weeks after cessation of PPI)

- **Imaging**
    - EGD/colonoscopy (timing is uncertain; most recommend within 24 hours of admission)
    - Repeat
    - Small Bowel FT/Pill
    - Nuclear scintigraphy (bleeds < 1cc/min)
    - Angiography (bleeds >1cc/min)
- **Medications**
    - For advanced cirrhosis or variceal bleed, antibiotic prophylaxis with Ceftriaxone (Rocephin)1g IV every 24 hrs
    - Pantoprazole (Protonix) 80mg IV load, then 8mg/hr IV continuous drip x 72 hrs
        - Protonix 40 mg IV daily may be considered
    - Octreotide 0.025-0.05mg continuous infusion for 2-5 days after endoscopy
    - Consider stopping ASA (for 1-7 days; resume after 1 week) unless required for secondary prophylaxis
        - Dual therapy patients should have all except ASA stopped unless catheterization was recent (90 days)
- **Nursing Orders**
    - Type and cross
    - NPO 8 hours before procedure (clears allowed up to 2 hours before procedure)
- **Management**[33]

  Approximately 70-80% of all GI bleeds stop spontaneously.

GI bleed management based on location

Upper GI Bleed

- Initial Management
  - NPO except medications
  - Place NG tube if etiology unclear
  - Do not give the patient sucralfate or antacids until after EGD, as they will interfere with the endoscopy

Threshold	Population
<9	Age>65 ASCAD UA/NSTEMI/STEMI Respiratory Disease Symptomatic
<7	Other

  - Blood transfusions if HGB<7 (restrictive strategy vs 9 showed better outcomes in regard to morbidity and mortality however if patient has underlying unstable CAD, age>65, or respiratory disease goal should be 9)
  - Correct any coagulopathies (FFP if INR > 1.5; keep platelets > 50)
  - Octreotide:
    - If strong suspicion for an ongoing variceal bleed/advanced liver disease
    - Dose at 50 μg IV bolus followed by 50 μg/hr drip.
  - IV PPI drip if high grade lesion x 72 hours post EGD (pantoprazole 80 mg IV × 1 then drip at 8 mg/hr × 72 hours)
  - Can advance to clear liquids within 24 hours

Lower GI Bleed

- Differential:
  - If elderly, consider Angiodysplasia/AVM, diverticulosis, ischemic colitis, malignancy
  - All ages: hemorrhoids (outlet bleeding), fissure, colitis (infectious, radiation), C. diff, IBD, intussusception, vasculitis, NSAID induced
- Correct any coagulopathies (FFP if INR > 1.5; keep platelets > 50)
- NPO except medications for at least 8 hours prior to colonoscopy (fluids are 2 hours prior)
- IV fluids (crystalloid)
- PPI IV/PO b.i.d. (pantoprazole 40 mg IV/PO b.i.d.)
- Colonoscopy prep: 1st choice for initial evaluation of LGIB
  - For colon prep in setting of LGIB, GoLYTELY 800 cc/hour (or Colyte) via NG tube.
  - Start with 4L PM prior to procedure and give additional 4L approximately 5 hrs before planned procedure in AM (4L total)[34]
  - Give 1x dulcolax 10mg the day before procedure
  - Optional magnesium citrate
  - Have versed and fentanyl held at bedside for procedure
  - Reglan 10mg IV 30min prior to and 2 hours after starting the prep.
  - Do not do PO prep when trying to clear bleeding.
- Radiographic Imaging
  - Consider in patients who continue to have significant bleeding despite colonoscopy

- Endoscopy
    - High risk features:
        - Visible vessel
        - Adherent clot
        - Oozing
        - Arterial bleeding
    - 72 hour admission, NPO after endoscopy, IV PPI
    - Clips are most preferred due to lower risk for transmural colonic injury due to contact with thermal therapy
- Discharge
    - Can be discharged same day if no high-risk features (clean ulcer base, no comorbid conditions)
    - Patients that should be monitored for 72 hrs:
        - Comorbid conditions (heart failure, recent cardiovascular or CVA, chronic alcoholism, or active cancer)
        - Hemodynamically unstable
        - Endoscopic finding of high-risk stigmata:
            - Active bleeding
            - NBVV
            - Adherent clot)
    - Home PPI once daily

- Options include CT angiography (preferred method; bleeding as low as 0.3cc/min) and tagged RBC scan (bleeding as low as 0.1 cc/min can be detected)

ACUTE PANCREATITIS

- **Goal**[35,36,37,38]
  - Rest the pancreas and support as necessary.
- **Etiologies**
  - Alcohol
  - Gallstones
  - Blunt trauma
  - Hypertriglyceridemia → in the absence of gallstones +/- hx of EtOH then consider TG (concerning if >1000)
  - Hypercalcemia
  - Family history of pancreatic diseases
  - Autoimmune diseases
  - Medications: pentamidine, azathioprine, 6-mercaptopurine, thiazide diuretics, sulfonamides, valproic acid, estrogens, tetracyclines
  - Malignancy (hypercalcemia)
  - Infections: mumps, CMV, HIV, E. coli
  - Scorpion sting
  - Mechanical: post-ERCP, sphincter of Oddi dysfunction, pancreatic divisum, malignancy, perforated peptic ulcer
  - Miscellaneous: cystic fibrosis, genetic mutations
- **Clinical Signs and Symptoms**
  - **Constant, epigastric tenderness ± radiation to back, nausea/vomiting, relief with** bending forward
  - Gallstone pancreatitis more likely to present as abrupt in onset, with radiation to back
  - Alcoholic pancreatitis more likely to present as dull pain that increases with time
- **Physical Exam**
  - Hypovolemia, abdominal tenderness, guarding, decreased bowel sounds, signs of retroperitoneal hemorrhage (Cullen's and Turner's signs)
- **Diagnosis**
  - **2 of the 3 criteria required:**
    - Clinical Presentation c/w disease (ie. abdominal pain)
    - Imaging evidence on CT, US, or MRI
    - Biochemical lab evidence of amylase or lipase > 3x ULN
  - Diagnostic imaging is reserved for patients in whom the diagnosis is unclear or do not improve clinically with supportive care within 48-72 hrs

Staging of Acute Pancreatitis		
Mild	Moderate	Severe
No organ failure No local complications	Local complications +/- Transient organ failure (<48 hours)	Persistent organ failure (>48 hours) as defined by *Marshal Score*

Local complications include necrosis, peripancreatic fluid collections
Organ failure includes shock (SBP<90), PaO2<60, renal failure (SCr>2 after hydration), GIB (>500cc lost/24 hours)

- **Labs**: amylase, **lipase**, liver function tests, calcium, chemistry panel, C-reactive protein Increase in ALT **to ≥ 3x the baseline** is more specific for pancreatitis but levels <3x cannot be excluded
  - Amylase
    - A sensitive diagnostic method if patient presents within hours of the onset of pain. Returns to normal faster than lipase.

        - Non pancreatic sources of amylase include salivary glands, lung CA, ovaries, fallopian tubes.
        - Amylase levels tend not to be as high in alcoholic pancreatitis as in nonalcoholic forms.
        - Elevated in the first 4-12 hours of diagnosis and returns to normal in 3-5 days
        - **Not favored**
    - Lipase
        - >3x ULN
        - **Is a more sensitive and specific test**. It is made only in the pancreas and stomach.
        - Non pancreatic elevation may be seen if the bowels are inflamed and the lipase is reabsorbed after being properly secreted from the pancreas.
        - *Note that renal insufficiency and inflammation/perforation of small bowel can lead to elevated amylase/lipase levels without active pancreatitis.*
        - Degree of amylase and lipase elevation does not correlate with severity.
    - Others
        - C-RP: >150 @ 48 hours is indicative of severity
        - Procalcitonin
        - Antithrombin III
- **Imaging**
    - Ultrasound
        - Transabdominal US should be performed in all patients in the early assessment period
        - The most sensitive way of evaluating the biliary tract in acute pancreatitis
        - R/o choledocholithiasis and cholelithiasis
    - Contrast-enhanced CT (p.o. and IV) is used to *diagnose* as well as to *determine potential complications*.
        - Indications:
            - 72-92 hours after presentation in patients who are clinically deteriorating or have severe pancreatitis (necrosis, pseudocyst, abscess)
            - If initial diagnosis is in doubt
    - MRCP if you have high suspicion for choledocholithiasis
    - ERCP if concurrent cholangitis present or suspicion for ascending cholangitis
- **Scoring Systems**: *Assessment of severity*
    - APACHE-III (threshold is ≥8)
    - RANSOM (threshold is ≥3)

		SCORING
Age > 55	HCT > 10% decrease	<3 = 1%
BG > 200	Ca < 8	3-4 = 15%
WBC > 16	Base Deficit > 4	5-6 = 40%
LDH > 350	BUN > 5	>7 = 100%
ALT > 250	Fluid sequestration > 6L	
	PPO2a < 60	

    - **BISAP (helps with triage)**

      Presence of three or more of these factors was associated with substantially increased risk for in-hospital mortality among patients with acute pancreatitis. In addition, an elevated hematocrit >44% and admission BUN >22 mg/dL are also associated with more severe acute pancreatitis. Incorporating these indices with the overall patient response to initial fluid resuscitation in the emergency ward can be useful at triaging patients to the appropriate hospital acute care setting.

      In general, patients with lower BISAP scores, hematocrits, and admission BUNs tend to respond to initial management and are triaged to a regular hospital ward for ongoing care. If SIRS is not present at 24 h, the patient is unlikely to develop organ failure or necrosis. Therefore, patients with persistent SIRS at 24 h or underlying comorbid illnesses (e.g., chronic obstructive pulmonary disease, congestive heart failure) should be considered for a step-down unit setting if available. Patients with higher BISAP scores and elevations in hematocrit and admission BUN that do not respond to initial fluid resuscitation and exhibit evidence of respiratory failure, hypotension, or organ failure should be considered for direct admission to an intensive care unit.

        - Within 24 hours of presentation:
            - Factors
                - BUN >25
                - GCS <15
                - Evidence of SIRS
                - Age >60
                - Pleural effusions on CXR
            - Calculation
                - 3 points = 5.3% death
                - 4 points = 12.7% death
                - 5 points = 22.5% death
    - **CT Severity Index**
        - Combination of the sum of the necrosis score and points assigned to five grades of findings on CT. The index ranges from 0 to 10, with higher scores indicating a greater severity of illness
            - <u>CT grade</u>
                - Normal pancreas (grade A) — 0 points
                - Focal or diffuse enlargement (grade B) — 1 point
                - Intrinsic change; fat stranding (grade C) — 2 points
                - Single, ill-defined collection of fluid (grade D) — 3 points
                - Multiple collections of fluid or gas in or adjacent to pancreas (grade E) — 4 points
            - <u>Necrosis score</u>
                - No pancreatic necrosis — 0 points
                - Necrosis of one third of pancreas — 2 points
                - Necrosis of one half of pancreas — 4 points
                - Necrosis of >one half of pancreas — 6 points
- **Management**[39]
    - <u>Risk Stratification:</u>
        - SIRS+/-MODS → ICU; otherwise consider PCU
        - Both the initial BUN level and subsequent change in BUN level during the initial 24 hours of hospitalization are independent predictors of mortality

Figure. Fluid management of acute pancreatitis

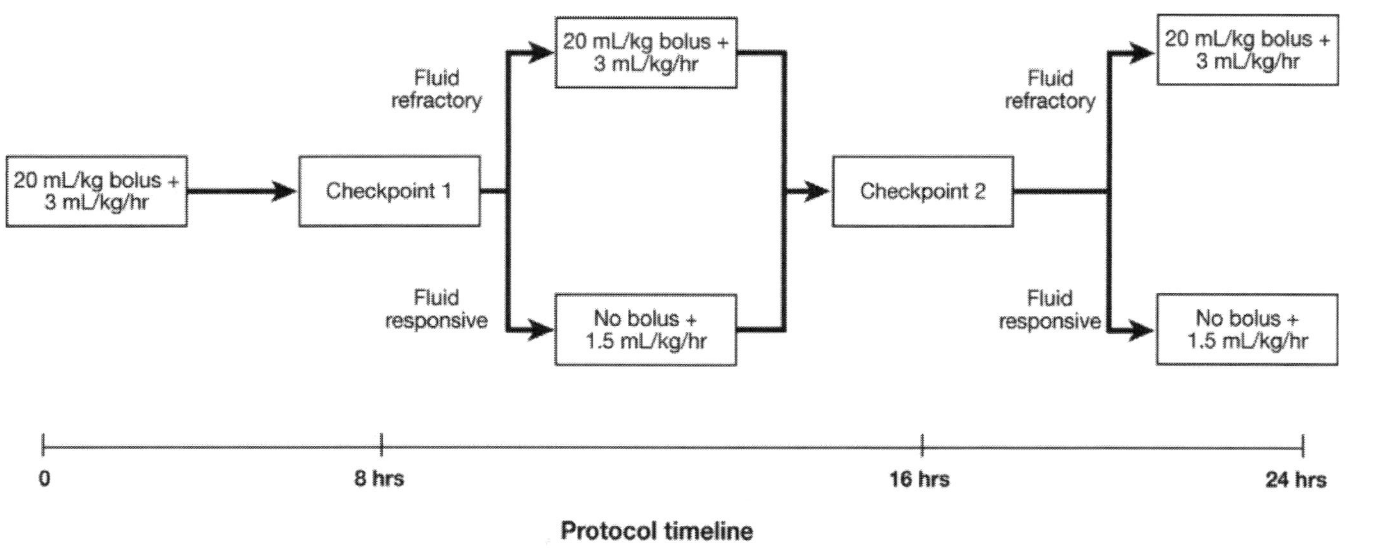

- Fluids[40]
  - *Amounts*
    - **Initial**: 20 cc/kg of **LR** should be given over 30-45 minutes initially
      - infusion of large volumes of NS → development of a hyperchloremic metabolic acidosis→ important factor contributing to pathologic zymogen activation and severity of pancreatitis
      - Monitor the HCT and BUN in the first 12-24 hours, decreases in both are signs that you are giving enough fluids
    - **Maintenance**:
      - First 12-24 hours: 250-500cc/hr of LR
      - Use decreasing BUN as a marker to monitor every 6 hours to determine if hydration is adequate
    - **Total**: 70kg person will often require at least 6L
    - More aggressive based on severity markers below
      - **BUN**: Serial monitoring of BUN to determine fluid resuscitation effectiveness
        - Accurate predictor of in-hospital mortality during first 24 hours
      - HCT (elevation is specifically associated with pancreatic necrosis)
      - ↑SCr as noted below
  - *Type*
    - Crystalloids can be chosen initially however:
      - **New research suggests the use of LR**
      - Colloids (pRBC) if HCT < 25%
      - Albumin if albumin level <2 g/dL
- Monitoring
  - UOP at least 0.5cc/kg/hr → some studies suggest goal of 1 cc/kg/hr in first 24 hours
  - Bladder pressures[41]
    - Intraabdominal hypertension can be worsened by fluid resuscitation. Defined as steady-state pressure within the abdominal cavity which is ≥12 mmHg.
    - Grades:
      - 1: 12-15 mmHg
      - 2: 16-20 mmHg
      - **3: 21-25 mmHg**
      - **4: >25 mmHg**
    - Risks for ICH/ACS:
      - Increased intra-abdominal volume (GI tract dilatation: gastroparesis and gastric distention, ileus, volvulus)
      - Ascites or hemoperitoneum
      - Decreased abdominal wall compliance (2/2 abdominal surgery, especially with tight abdominal closures)
      - Obesity
      - Sepsis, severe sepsis, and septic shock
      - Severe acute pancreatitis
      - Massive fluid resuscitation
      - Major burns (with or without abdominal eschars)
      - Complicated intra-abdominal infection
    - Levels >20 are suggestive of abdominal compartment syndrome
    - Treatment
      - Monitoring (transvesicular technique for at least 4 hours until IAP/IAH/ACS <12 for at least 24 hours)
      - Ultrafiltration
      - Diuretics
      - NG tube if suspecting ileus
      - Endoscopi decompression
      - Limit fluids by using colloids or hypertonic solutions (often in burn patients)
      - Remove any restrictive eschars
      - HOB @ 20 degrees, avoid prone positioning
      - Luminal decompression with rectal tube placement

        - Percutaneous drainage of ascites
        - NM blockade if ventilated to relax abdomen
        - Open abdominal decompression (last resort)
    - Serial ICUP for BUN, SCr, albumin
    - Serial H/H for HCT levels
    - MAP>65
    - Routine CVP not necessary, if present, goal 8-12
  - Feeds
    Data suggest that enteral nutrition helps stimulate the gut and maintain its protective barrier, thus reducing bacterial overgrowth and preventing bacterial translocation and sepsis. Enteral feeding may have benefits that could decrease length of stay, such as reduced intestinal permeability, improved gut motility, and reduced infection of pancreatic necrosis.
    - If mild and patient has no nausea or vomiting, PO is allowed with **low fat diet** (within 24 hours of admission)
    - If symptomatic, NPO until improved (pain-free, hungry)
      - Start NG feeds if ≥ 7 days
      - Enteral nutrition (NG) for necrotizing pancreatitis unless ileus present (then TPN)
        - NJ shows no decreased risk of worsening of condition
  - Repletion of **electrolytes**
  - **NGT** to suction only if protracted nausea and vomiting to prevent aspiration not to help pancreas as previously believed
  - Antibiotics
    - Treat infections if clinically suspected
      - ABx only indicated in infected pancreatitis necrosis (pt presents with fever and ↑WBC)
        - Prior to which a CT guided biopsy for cultures is required
      - No clear studies have shown a benefit to prophylactic ABx however if significant sterile necrosis (>30%) present, some treat with ABx for 14 days
      - ABx to consider: fluoroquinolones, carbapenems, and metronidazole
    - Fevers initially are expected secondary to inflammatory response
    - FNA if suspicious for infection (↑WBC, fevers 10-14d out from dx, tachycardia, **peripancreatic gas on imaging**)
  - **Pain control**: meperidine (morphine in theory causes spasm of sphincter of Oddi; no evidence in humans and most feel clinically safe), or PCA (20-50mcg of fentanyl with 10m lockout)
  - Patients with gallstone-induced pancreatitis who develop cholangitis **require urgent ERCP within 24 hours** and ERCP in 72 hours if no sx of cholangitis are present
- **Complications**
  - If patient is >40 YO, **pancreatic tumor** should be considered as a cause in the DDx
  - Acute fluid collection, pseudocyst, necrosis, cholangitis, abscesses, ARDS, renal failure, sepsis, shock
    - Necrosis is 2/2 to ischemia which is we try to prevent with fluids
      - Percutaneous aspiration of necrosis with Gram stain and culture should be performed if there are ongoing signs of possible pancreatic infection such as sustained leukocytosis, fever, or organ failure.
      - There is no role for *prophylactic antibiotics* in necrotizing pancreatitis. It is reasonable to start broad-spectrum antibiotics in a patient who appears septic while awaiting the results of Gram stain and cultures. If cultures are negative, the antibiotics should be discontinued to minimize the risk of developing opportunistic or fungal superinfection.
      - Repeated fine-needle aspiration and Gram stain with culture of pancreatic necrosis may be done every 5–7 days in the presence of persistent fever. Repeated CT or MRI imaging should also be considered with any change in clinical course to monitor for complications (e.g., thromboses, hemorrhage, abdominal compartment syndrome).
      - Risk of infection (bacterial translocation) based on severity of necrosis

                - <30% necrosis = 22.5% chance of infection
                - >50% necrosis = 46.5% chace of infection
            - SCr of ≥ 1.8 within 48 hours of admission has 35x more likelihood for development of necrosis. Good marker for organ injury
        - Debridement only indicated if evidence of infection, sterile necrosis should not be taken to the OR
    - DIC (PLT<100,000, Fibrinogen <1g/L, ↑aPTT, ↑PT)
    - If suspicion for concurrent cholangitis, obtain ERCP
    - If suspicion for choledocholithiasis, obtain MRCP
- **Prognosis**
    - Outcomes depend on whether disease is interstitial versus necrotizing
        - Interstitial mortality rate < 1%
        - Necrotizing (defined as necrosis of 30% of the gland seen on CT) mortality rate 10-30% mortality risk with a 70% complication risk
    - Scoring systems: Ranson, Glasgow, Apache II (none are completely accurate)

BOWEL OBSTRUCTION

- **Presentation**[42]
    - Abdominal pain, crampy, diffuse, episodic in nature
    - Depending on location → more proximal = vomiting is bilious, more distal = feculent vomiting
- **Etiology**
    - Small
        - Adhesions
        - Hernia
        - IBD
        - GSI
        - Cancer (lymphoma, adenocarcinoma, polyp)
    - Large
        - Cancer
        - Diverticulitis
        - Sigmoid volvulus
- **Types**
    - Complete – passage of neither flatus or stool, more vomiting
    - Partial – can pass flatus; colicky; peristaltic rushes
    - Pseudoobstruction (Ogilvie's)
- **Diagnosis**
    - Capsule imaging
    - KUB
    - CT with oral and IV contrast
- **Treatment**
    - NPO
    - IVF - Provide IV fluids (nothing is being absorbed by the stomach!) → monitor by watching HR and UOP
    - NG if needed: In presence of severe nausea and vomiting, use NG tube with intermittent suctioning to gravity
    - Serial Abdominal Exams
    - If patient does not clinically respond, or, shows signs of ischemia then proceed directly to surgery
        - If surgery required, preoperative ABx:
            - Tazobactam-Piperacillin 3.375g IV q6h
        - Ampicillin-Sulbactam 3g IV q6h

- Avoid medications that ↓ bowel motility:
  - Opioids
  - Anticholinergics
  - CCB
- **Ogilvie's**
  - Most common in hospitalized or institutionalized men >60
  - Symptoms: nausea, vomiting, abdominal distention, CT imaging with dilation without e/o obvious obstruction
  - Treat underlying cause (trauma, electrolytes, infection, post-operative, chemotherapy, neurologic)
  - Replete all electrolytes (look for low K and Mg)
  - Discontinue opiates, anti-Cholinergics, sedatives
  - IV fluids only, NPO, place NG tube, have rectal tube to gravity
  - Serial KUB q12-24h
  - Prone positioning with left and right lateral decubitus positions q1h
  - Neostigmine unless bradycardic or hx of bronchospasm in patients who fail above treatment after **24-48 hours or cecal diameter >12cm**
    - Hold atropine at bedside
    - Keep on telemetry during and 30min after administration
    - **Have bedpan ready**

GERD

- **Definition**: a condition which develops when the reflux of stomach contents causes troublesome symptoms and/or complications.
- **Diagnosis**[43,44]
  - A presumptive diagnosis of GERD can be established in the setting of typical symptoms of heartburn and regurgitation. Empiric medical therapy with a proton pump inhibitor (PPI) is recommended in this setting.
- **Causes of GERD**
  - PUD
  - Motility disorder (achalasia, DES)
  - Reflux Hypersensitivity
  - Nonerosive Reflux Disease
  - Eosinophilic Esophagitis
- **Associated Symptoms**
  - Chronic cough, laryngitis, and asthma have an established association with GERD on the basis of population-based studies.
- **Diagnostics**
  - Barium radiographs - should not be performed to diagnose GERD
  - EGD
    - The principal use of endoscopy in suspected GERD is the evaluation **of treatment failures and risk management.**
    - No direct evidence supports the use of endoscopy **as a screening test** for Barrett's esophagus or esophageal adenocarcinoma in the setting of **chronic** GERD.
    - Regarding the criteria for obtaining mucosal biopsy specimens in the course of performing an endoscopy, there is no basis to advocate doing this routinely but, clearly, biopsy specimens of any areas suspected of being metaplastic obtained and carefully evaluated for dysplasia.

        - Consider in patients with dysphagia, weight loss, family history of GI cancer, odynophagia, unresponsive to therapy trial of BID therapy (4-6 weeks), older than 55 YO
        - Repeat endoscopy is not indicated in patients without Barrett's esophagus in the absence of new symptoms.
    - Manometry – done by GI if patient does not respond to be BID therapy and has no EGD evidence of erosive disease
    - Ambulatory impedance-pH
        - PPI therapy withheld for 7 days
        - to evaluate patients with a suspected esophageal GERD syndrome who have not responded to an empirical trial of PPI therapy, have normal findings on endoscopy, and have no major abnormality on manometry.
        - Wireless pH monitoring has superior sensitivity to catheter studies for detecting pathological esophageal acid exposure because of the extended period of recording (48 hours) and has also shown superior recording accuracy compared with some catheter designs
- **Labs**
    - Screening for *Helicobacter pylori* infection is not recommended in GERD patients.
- **Treatment/Management**
    - Pharmacotherapy
        - Anti-secretory therapy is highly recommended in patients to obtain symptomatic relief and those with evidence of esophagitis
            - *PPI (*An 8-week course of PPIs is the therapy of choice for symptom relief and healing of erosive esophagitis.)
                - Omeprazole 20 mg PO daily
                - Pantoprazole 40 mg PO daily
                - Esomeprazole 20 mg PO daily
            - *H2 therapy*
                - Cimetidine 800 mg PO at bedtime
                - Ranitidine 300 mg PO at bedtime
                - Famotidine 40 mg PO at bedtime
            - PPI>H2 blocker
                - There are no major differences in efficacy between the different PPIs.
                - Understand risks of long term PPI therapy (ie. CKD, osteoporosis, CAP, *C.diff*)
                    - Long term therapy, consider DEXA scan, calcium supplementation, H. pylori screening
                - Traditional delayed release PPIs should be administered 30–60min before meal for maximal pH control.
                - PPI therapy should be initiated at **once a day dosing**, before the first meal of the day.
                    - For patients with partial response to once daily therapy, tailored therapy with adjustment of dose timing and/or twice daily dosing should be considered in patients with night-time symptoms, variable schedules, and/or sleep disturbance.
                    - In patients with partial response to PPI therapy, increasing the dose to **twice daily therapy** or switching to a different PPI may provide additional symptom relief
                - If esophagitis is noted, consider BID therapy
                    - In patients with just symptoms but no pathology, can try PRN therapy or short term use

    - Pharmacokinetics recommend BID dosing however all trials have been with once daily dosing
  - There is no evidence of improved efficacy by adding a nocturnal dose of an H2RA to twice-daily PPI therapy.
  - Side Effects: HA, diarrhea, abdominal pain, CKD, pneumonia, fractures, osteoporosis, ↓Mg, C.diff, ↓VB12, dementia.
    - Chronic PPI therapy may lead to ↑ # of hyperplastic polyps in the gastric fundus
- Non-Pharmacologic
  - Weight loss
  - Elevate head shortly after eating if laying down
  - Avoid late night meals
- Surgery
  - Surgical therapy is a treatment option for long-term therapy in GERD patients.
  - Preoperative ambulatory pH monitoring is mandatory in patients without evidence of erosive esophagitis. All patients should undergo preoperative manometry to rule out achalasia or scleroderma-like esophagus.

- **Duration of Therapy**
  - Subjects not maintained on continuous acid suppressive therapy have high rates of recurrence of erosive disease.
  - Long-term therapy should be titrated down to the lowest effective dose based on symptom control.
  - Consider on-demand therapy for those with no evidence of esophagitis previously; those who did resolve try long term on-demand therapy have high risk for return of erosive disease
  - Chronic PPI therapy ↑ risk for *c.difficile,* PNA, and development of osteoporosis (>7 yrs of PPI use). Theory behind these adverse causes is unknown but suspected to be due to ↓ absorption of Ca by PPI.
    - If you cannot wean them off, consider switching to H2 blocker

HEMORRHOIDS

- **Pearl**[45]
  - Medical management (e.g., stool softeners, topical over-the-counter preparations, topical nitroglycerine), dietary modifications (e.g., increased fiber and water intake), and behavioral therapies (sitz baths) are the mainstays of initial therapy.
  - Hemorrhoidectomy should be reserved for recurrent or higher-grade disease.
- **Differential Diagnosis (rectal pain, bleeding)**
  - Abscess
  - Cancer
  - Condyloma
  - Fistula
  - Fissure
  - Polyps
  - Proctitis
  - IBD
  - Skin Tag
  - Prolapse
- **History**
  - Symptomatic internal hemorrhoids

    - Often present with painless bright red bleeding, prolapse, soiling, bothersome grape-like tissue prolapse, itching, or a combination of symptoms.
    - Bleeding occurs with streaks of blood on stool and rarely causes anemia.
  - External hemorrhoids
    - Can become painful, especially when thrombosed.
    - Patients younger than 40 years with suspected hemorrhoidal bleeding do not require endoscopic evaluation if they do not have red flags (e.g., weight loss, abdominal pain, fever, signs of anemia), do not have a personal or family history of colorectal cancer or inflammatory bowel disease, and respond to medical management.[6]
  - Patients older than 40 years with rectal bleeding and younger patients with risk factors should undergo full colon evaluation by colonoscopy, computed tomographic colonography, or barium enema, unless they have had a normal colon evaluation within the previous 10 years
- **Grading/Treatment**

Grading/Treatment of Hemorrhoids		
Grade	Definition	Treatments
1	Enter the lumen of the bowel but does not extend to the dentate line	1. Rubber band ligation 2. Sclerotherapy 3. Infrared coagulation (IRC) 4. Cryotherapy 5. Sitz bath 6. Topical hydrocortisone 10mg/zinc acetate 10mg rectal suppository 7. Hydrocortisone 25mg rectal 8. Hydrocortisone 2.5% cream 9. Topical nifedipine 0.3% BID x12w 10. Topical lidocaine 1.5% BID x12w 11. Topical mineral oil+Petrolatum+phenylephrine
2	Prolapse past the dentate line with straining but reduce with relaxation.	
3	Prolapse past the dentate line with straining and require manual reduction.	
4	Unable to be reduced	1. Excisional hemorrhoidectomy 2. Stapled hemorrhoidopexy

PEPTIC ULCER DISEASE

- **Pearl**[46]
  - H. pylori important to tx d/t risk for gastric cancer and MALT lymphoma along with it being the most common cause of most ulcers
- **Alarm Symptoms**
  - Weight loss
    - Want to rule out gastric cancer (look for dysphagia as well) or vomiting d/t blockage of the pylorus
  - New onset sx in pt >45 YO
  - Bleeding
  - Anemia
- **Etiology of PUD**

- H. pylori
  - Should test in patients on chronic NSAIDs, unexplained IDA, and ITP via urea breath testing or stool antigen
- NSAIDs
- ZE syndrome

- **Types**
  - Gastric
    - Food ↑pain and not relieved with antacids
  - Duodenal
    - Food relieves pain (worse on empty stomach), is relieved with antacids as well.
- **Symptoms**
  - Symptoms of ulcers are caused by presence of acid without food or other acid buffers
  - Dyspepsia (pain in upper abdomen, fullness, early satiety, bloating, and nausea
    - Nighttime pain may be due to circadian rhythm increasing acid production
  - NUD – upper abdominal IBS, sx are similar to dyspepsia that last for 12+ weeks, likely functional in nature, when EGD done no ulcer is found, patients are often **not** responsive to PPI's
  - GERD – heartburn, mid chest pain, occurs after meals and worse with lying down
- **Diagnosis**
  - Endoscopy reserved for pts not responding to empiric PPI, have red rlag symptoms, or those with new symptoms and $\geq$60
    - R/O H. Pylori: Bx obtained x3 at antrum and incisura angularis, urease testing, CLOtest, fecal antigen
      - Should be done only after off PPI for 2 weeks or 24 hours after H2 blocker
    - May obtain biopsies at duodenum to r/o celiac if necessary
  - For those patients who do not require immediate endoscopy, testing and treating for h.pylori advised along with counseling to avoid smoking, alcohol, and NSAIDs.
    - H.pylori diagnosis via:
      - Urea breath test
        - Best used after tx to confirm eradication as it is only positive in current infections
      - Stool antigen testing
- **Treatment**[47]
  - Pharmacotherapy
    - All four H2 receptor antagonists (cimetidine, ranitidine, famotidine, and nizatidine) are associated with healing rates of 70 to 80 percent for duodenal ulcers after four weeks, and 87 to 94 percent after eight weeks of therapy
    - Split dose, evening, and nighttime therapy are all effective.
    - Cimetidine, ranitidine, and famotidine are approved for gastric ulcer healing in the United States
    - Daily doses of **lansoprazole from 20 to 40 mg** produced better healing results (rabeprazole was the best but cost may be too high to use)
    - Stop all NSAIDs
- **H. pylori Treatment**[48]
  - Traditional triple therapy
    - Lansoprazole 30mg BID, clarithromycin 500mg BID, and amoxicillin 1 g BID) for 10-14 days is reserved for patients with **no** previous history of macrolide exposure who live where clarithromycin resistance among H. pylori isolates is low.
  - Quadruple (14 days)
    - PPI BID (consider lansoprazole)

    - Bismuth (525 mg four times daily)
    - Two antibiotics (eg, metronidazole 250 mg four times daily and tetracycline 500 mg four times daily) given for 14 days.
  - Alternative (14 days)
    - Levothyroxine
    - PPI
    - Amoxicillin
  - Sequential
    - May improve eradication rates, especially with clarithromycin resistant strains.
    - This 14-day regimen involves:
      1) Amoxicillin (1 g twice daily) for five days
      2) PPI (twice daily)
      3) clarithromycin (500 mg twice daily)
      4) metronidazole 500 mg twice daily
  - Confirming Eradication/Treatment
    - After 4 weeks from the last dose, urea breath test or stool antigen testing should be performed to confirm successful treatment
    - If treatment failed, consider testing spouse as infection is transferred via saliva.

ELEVATED LIVER ASSOCIATED ENZYMES

- **General**[49,50]
  - Mild elevation is defined as less than 5x the ULN
  - ALT is more specific than AST
  - The predominant pattern of enzyme alteration (hepatocellular v. cholestatic v mixed)
    - **AST/ALT ratios**
      - Understand that AST>ALT is most common in EtOH associated causes however in cirrhosis this pattern also develops
      - ALT>ALT more common in hepatocellular injuries (non EtOH)
    - "**Hepatocellular**" – AST, ALT (ALT/ALKP > 2.2)
      - See section 2
    - "**Cholestatic**" – ALKPH, GGT (ALT/ALKP < 2.2)
      See next section for full chart
      - ALKP is suggestive of biliary obstruction or intrahepatic cholestasis
      - Liver US to look for bile duct dilatation, r/o chronic liver disease
      - GGT to confirm biliary origin
      - Medications (ACEi) can cause isolated elevations (https://livertox.nih.gov)
      - R/o metastatic malignancy (esp pancreatic cancer)
      - R/o infiltrative diseases
    - "**Biliary**" – TBILI, DBILI, IBILI
      - IBILI – hemolysis
        - Unconjugated or indirect
        - Hemolysis (H/H, smear, LDH, haptoglobin, reticulocyte count)
        - DDx: Gilbert's (clinical dx), Criggler-Najjar
      - DBILI
        - Conjugated or direct
        - Usually sign of liver disease as normally elevated bilirubin can be excreted quickly
        - R/O viral hepatitis, toxic injury, shock liver, AIH (+smooth muscle AB, normal saturation), hemachromatosis (↑iron saturation)
        - Normal AST/ALT but elevations in DBILI and ALKP are suggestive of cholestatic drug reaction, PBC, PSC

- DDx: Dubin-johnson, Rotor's
- Synthetic function – albumin (↓slowly with liver failure), PT/INR

Figure. Etiologies of increased liver associated enzymes by severity

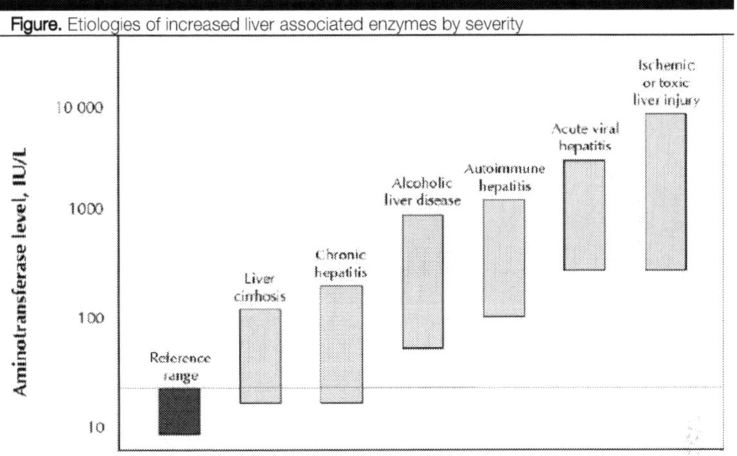

(2) Magnitude of enzyme alteration in the case of aminotransferases

Marked: >10x ULN

- Toxin/Medication
  - EtOH
  - Tylenol
  - Herbal
  - Statin
  - Glucophage
- Ischemia / Shock (TBILI< 34 μmol/L, and ALT/LDH ratio < 1)
- Thrombosis
  - Budd-Chiari
  - Portal vein
- Acute viral hepatitis
  - **A/B**/D/E
  - Less common: CMV**,** EBV**,** HSV
- AIH

Moderate: 5–10x ULN

- Medications
- Chronic viral hepatitis
- **NAFLD** (evidence of metabolic syndrome (increased waist circumference, elevated blood pressure, lipid pattern of high serum triglyceride levels and low serum high-density lipoprotein levels, elevated blood glucose levels or evidence of insulin resistance) See page 77 for more information.
- Wilson's (check ceruloplasmin)
- Alpha-1 antitrypsin (early onset emphysema, family history)
- PBC
- PSC

Mild: < 5x ULN

ALT elevation > than AST is more specific for liver origin (AST elevations can also be caused by thyroid disease, celiac disease, hemolysis, and muscle disorders)

- Hepatitis (anti-HCV and HBsAg)
- Alcohol (AST:ALT >2)
- Hemochromatosis (transferrin saturation, ferritin)
- Autoimmune: ANA, anti-smooth muscle
- Medications
- Celiac' s disease
- NAFLD

(3) Rate of change (increase or decrease over time)

(4) Course of alteration (e.g., mild fluctuation v. progressive increase).

Causes of Liver Enzyme Elevation				
Cause	AST	ALT	ALKP	Bili
NAFLD	ALT>AST (<5x)		Nml	Nml/Direct
Alcoholic Liver Disease	AST>ALT 2:1 (<5x)		Nml	Nml/Direct
Drug-Induced Liver Injury (ie. Tylenol)	↑↑↑ (10x)	↑↑↑ (10x)	Nml	Nml
Chronic Hepatitis B/C	ALT>AST (<5x)		Nml	Nml
Acute Viral Hepatitis	ALT>AST (10x)		Nml	Nml
Hereditary Hemochromatosis	ALT>AST (10x)			
Autoimmune Hepatitis	ALT>AST (10x)		Nml	Nml
Wilson Disease	ALT>AST (10x)		Nml	Nml
Hemolytic	Nml		Nml	Indirect

- **Pathology**
  - Indicates inflammation +/- injury to hepatocytes resulting in leakage of contents into plasma
- **Differential**
  - ***Always rule out:***
    - Viral hepatitis
    - Hemochromatosis (not common in high ALT/AST levels)
    - AIH
    - NAFLD
- **Labs/Work-up**
  - Serial LFTs with GGT
  - Lipid panel (NAFLD)
  - A1c (NAFLD)
  - CBC (MCV>100 more suggestive of thyroid or alcohol cause)
  - Alpha-1
  - Viral panel
    - Hepatitis A: IgM anti-HAV
    - Hepatitis B: HBsAg, IgM anti-HBc, IgG anti-HBc, HBsAg, anti-HBe, HBeAg
    - Hepatitis C: anti-HCV, HCV RNA
    - Hepatitis D: anti-HBs, anti-HDV
    - Hepatitis E: anti-HEV
    - Viral
      - CMV
      - EBV
      - HSV
    - Others to consider

- Anti-smooth muscle (AIH)
- Anti-mitochondrial (PBC)

Hepatitis Panel Evaluation							
	HBsAg	HBeAg	IgM anti-HBc	IgG anti-HBc	Anti-HBs	Anti-HBe	HBV DNA
Early Acute	+	+	+				+++
Late Acute	+	+	+	+			
Window			+				+
Recovery				+	+	+	Likely +
Chronic carrier	+			+			
Acute on chronic	+	Likely +	+	+			
Vaccinated					+		
Immune 2/2 past infection				+	+		

USMLEWorld

The presence of HBeAg is indicative of ongoing infection/viral replication

- RUQ US with Doppler flow
- Toxicology screen
  - APAP
- Consider ceruloplasmin, iron panel (Fe, TIBC, ferritin)
- Anti-smooth muscle AB
- Functional labs:
  - Coagulation panel
  - PLT (CBC)
  - Fractionated bilirubin
  - Albumin

- **Fulminant Hepatic Failure**
  - Encephalopathy (order NH3)
  - Cerebral edema
  - ↑INR, ↑Lactate, PO4
  - Shock
  - Ascites
- **Treatment of statin-induced liver enzyme elevation**[51]
  - Commonly only see elevations 2-3x ULN
  - Direct relationship seen between the dose of statin and elevation of AST/ALT
  - Statins appear to be associated with a very low risk of true and serious liver injury
  - Some cases may see spontaneous resolution without discontinuation of the offending medication (unsure of physiology, could be tolerance vs adaptation)
  - Options include decreasing dose, changing statin, or discontinuing therapy.

NON-ALCOHOLIC FATTY LIVER DISEASE (NAFLD)

- **General**[52]

- Most common cause for mild liver enzyme elevations
- Second most common cause of liver transplant
- It is thought to be the hepatic consequence of **systemic insulin resistance** and the metabolic syndrome characterized by obesity, dyslipidemia, and type 2 diabetes mellitus.
- **Diagnosis of exclusion**, must exlude significant alcohol use or other conditions that could cause liver damage.

- **Subtypes**
  - NAFL (non-alcoholic fatty liver) - steatosis, **without inflammation**, in at least 5% of hepatocytes.
  - NASH (non-alcoholic steatohepatitis) - constellation of features that include steatosis, lobular and portal **inflammation**, and liver cell injury in the form of hepatocyte ballooning. Worse prognosis with development to cirrhosis in 15% of patients.
- **Evaluation**
  - Labs

    Up to 30% of patients have elevated serum ferritin and autoantibodies, including ANA, ASMA, and AMA.
    - Hepatitis panel (2-3x ULN ↑ of AST/ALT)
    - ANA
    - Albumin
    - BMI (from vitals)
    - PLT
    - Anti-smooth muscle AB
    - Anti-mitochondrial AB
    - Iron panel (mild elevations expected due to inflammation)
    - Alpha-1 anti-trypsin
    - Ceruloplasmin
  - Procedures
    - US – the best way to diagnose hepatic steatosis but cannot differentiate between the subtypes (steatosis vs. steatohepatitis)
    - Liver biopsy is the only way to diagnose and stage (assess the degree of steatosis)
    - *Indications*
      - Before starting therapy
      - To confirm diagnosis
  - Non-invasive testing
    - NAFLD fibrosis score / Fibroscan - can be used to identify patients who may have fibrosis or cirrhosis (**without the need for biopsy**) and can help direct the use of liver biopsy in patients who would benefit from prognostication and potential treatment. Based on patient age, body mass index, hyperglycemia, platelet count, albumin, and ratio of aspartate aminotransferase to alanine aminotransferase. Accessed from: http://nafldscore.com
- **Treatment**
  - **It is pivotal to determine which patients are at high risk of progression to advanced disease. The presence of fibrosis on imaging or biopsy is a high risk.**
  - The first step in managing patients who have NAFLD is to treat components of the metabolic syndrome, including obesity, dyslipidemia, and type 2 diabetes.
  - A 2015 meta-analysis concluded that pentoxifylline and obeticholic acid improve fibrosis, while **vitamin E**, thiazolidinediones, and obeticholic acid improve neuroinflammation associated with NASH.

ELEVATED ALKALINE PHOSPHATASE

Figure. Management flow chart for elevated alkaline phosphatase

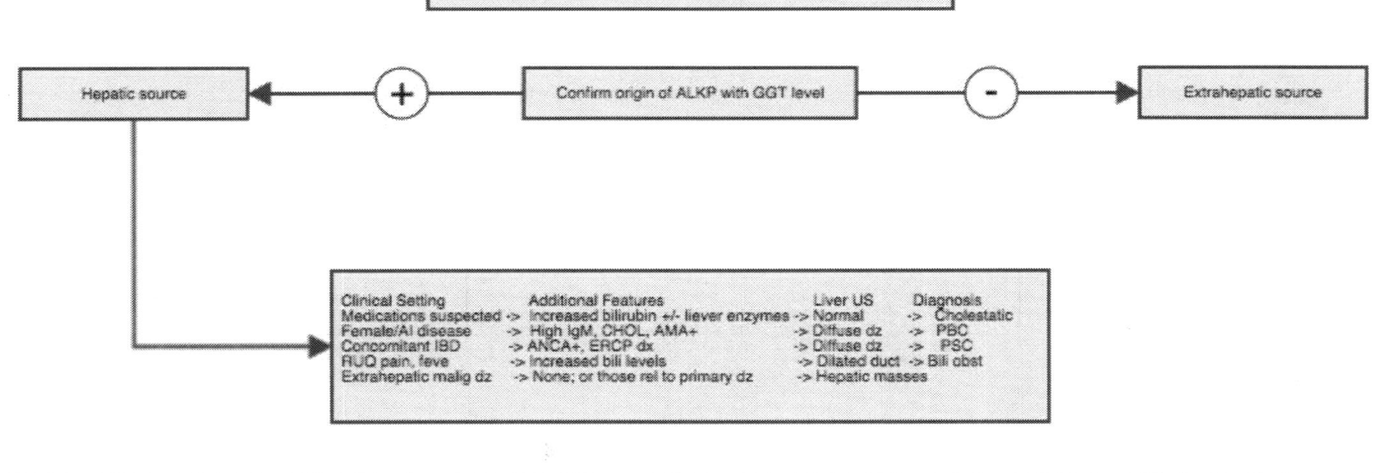

QUICK ACLS

PRIMARY AND SECONDARY ABCD SURVEY

Establish safety net: O2, tele, IV, help

- **Primary ABCD survey**
  - Focus: basic CPR and defibrillation
  - Airway: assess and manage the airway with noninvasive devices.
  - Breathing: assess and manage breathing (look, listen, and feel). If the patient is not breathing, give two slow breaths.
  - Circulation: assess and manage the circulation; if no pulse, start CPR.
  - Defibrillation: assess and manage rhythm/defibrillation; shock VF/VT up to 3 times (200 J, 300 J, 360 J, or equivalent biphasic) if necessary.
- **Secondary ABCD survey**
  - Focus: more advanced assessments and treatments
  - Airway: place airway device as soon as possible.
  - Breathing: assess adequacy of airway device placement and performance; secure airway device; confirm effective oxygenation and ventilation.
  - Circulation: establish IV access; administer drugs appropriate for rhythm and condition.
  - Differential Diagnosis: search for and treat identified reversible causes.
- Potentially reversible causes include: hypoxia, hypovolemia, hyperkalemia, hypokalemia and metabolic disorders, hypothermia, tension pneumothorax, tamponade, toxic/therapeutic disturbances, and thromboembolic/mechanical obstruction

ASYSTOLE

- CPR, obtain IV/IO access, prepare pt for intubation
- Epinephrine 1 mg Q 3-5 minutes up to 3 doses
- Atropine 1 mg Q 3-5 minutes up to 3 doses
- Consider high-dose Epinephrine or continue Epinephrine 1 mg IVP Q 3-5 minutes

BRADYCARDIA

- If possible, in any patient in whom you are worried about symptomatic bradycardia, try to have **atropine** at the bedside before the patient gets unstable. Always ask yourself the following two questions in the bradycardic patient:
  - Is the patient symptomatic or hemodynamically unstable? If so, place the patient in Trendelenburg and follow ACLS protocols (See ACLS: Bradycardia).
  - Does the ECG show either type II 2nd-degree or 3rd-degree AV block? If so, consider trans-cutaneously pacing the patient and prepare for possible transvenous pacer (consult Cardiology).
- If the patient is relatively stable hemodynamically and symptomatically and there is no sign of a dangerous form of AV block, you have some time to do a quick chart biopsy and look for clues from the patient's med list and admitting diagnoses.

Causes of bradycardia:

Category	Examples[53,54]
Meds	ß blockers, calcium channel blockers, digoxin, amiodarone, clonidine (look at the MAR and remember to consider any eye drops–e.g. timolol)
Cardiac	Sick sinus, inferior MI, vasovagal, 2nd or 3rd degree heart block, junctional rhythm
Intrinsic Causes	Idiopathic degeneration (aging), infiltrative diseases (sarcoid, amyloid), collagen vascular disease, surgical trauma, endocarditis
Autonomically Mediated	Neuro cardiogenic syncope, carotid-sinus hypersensitivity, situational: coughing, micturition, defecation, vomiting
Other	Hypothyroidism, hypothermia, increased intracranial pressure (Cushing's reflex), hyperkalemia, hypokalemia, obstructive sleep apnea, normal variant

- In general if the patient is not symptomatic and this is not a significant change from prior days/nights, then an exhaustive workup is unnecessary at night. However, have a low threshold to get an ECG in bradycardic patients and consider ischemia in any patient at risk.
- Take a focused H&P. Focus on signs and symptoms to distinguish the above (chest pain, prior MI, straining or other maneuvers prior to bradycardia, altered mental status, hypothermia, BP, etc.).
- If you believe the bradycardia is secondary to medications, be careful discontinuing them. Remember; treat the patient, not the numbers. Stopping rate control meds could cause a rebound tachycardia and precipitate myocardial ischemia
- Transcutaneous pacing can be quite uncomfortable. If there's time, short-acting analgesics and/or sedatives may be worthwhile considering.
- In asymptomatic patients with bradycardia, the class I indications for pacemakers are as follows:
  - 3rd-degree AV block with asystole lasting > 3 seconds or with escape rates < 40 while awake
  - 3rd-degree or 2nd-degree type II AV block in patients with chronic bifascicular or trifascicular block

- **ASx Bradycardia, AV Block 1 or AV Block Mobitz-type 1**
  - No specific therapy
  - *For AV block Mobitz type 1:* Stop B-blockers, CCBs, Digoxin
- **Symptomatic Bradycardia**

  - Call attending and transfer pt to ICU
  - Put pacer pads on just in case you might need them (bradycardia ACLS)
  - Give 0.5 mg Atropine IV Q 3-5 minutes up to 3mg
  - Transcutaneous pacemaker if no response to Atropine
  - Epinephrine and Dopamine may also be used if no response to Atropine
- **AV block Mobitz-type 2 and AV block 3 degree**
  - Call attending and transfer pt to ICU
  - Put pacer pads on just in case you might need them (bradycardia ACLS)
  - Give 0.5 mg Atropine IV
  - Transcutaneous pacemaker must be placed (even if pt Asx), then arrange for permanent pacemaker

PULSELESS ELECTRICAL ACTIVITY

- Definition: hypotension and absent pulse, but some type of electrical activity on EKG
- Find the cause and treat it
- Treatment: Epinephrine 1 mg Q 3-5 minutes up to 3 doses

V. FIB / PULSELESS V. TACH

- Give 1 shock (or a precordial thump until a defibrillator is available) and resume CPR immediately
- Check for rhythm and pulse; give 1 shock and resume CPR immediately if no pulse present
- Epinephrine 1 mg IV/IO Q 3-5 minutes up to 3 doses
- Give drugs during active CPR
- Give 1 shock after drug administration and resume CPR immediately
- Consider Amiodarone 300mg (second dose is 150mg) or Magnesium (if evidence of Torsades)

Remember: Shock→CPR+drug→shock

TACHYCARDIA

1. **Tachycardia with Pulses**
   - ABCs; give O2
   - Identify reversible causes
   - Obtain IV access
   - Monitor EKG and identify rhythm
   - If pt unstable (altered mental status/signs of shock)→synchronized cardioversion
2. **Ventricular Tachycardia with Pulse**
   - Wide complex tachycardia (QRS >0.12 sec)
     - Use **Brugada Criteria** to differentiate VT from SVT
   - Uniform pattern on EKG; no P waves
   - Amiodarone 150 mg IV over 10 minutes (**may repeat to max dose of 2.2 g/24 hours**)
   - May use Lidocaine or consider cardioversion if no initial response to Amiodarone
3. **Torsades de Pointes**
   - Magnesium initial bolus 1-2 g, then continuous infusion
   - May try IV Lidocaine or Phenytoin
   - Check electrolytes
   - If hemodynamic instability→ immediate electrical cardioversion
4. **Pre-excitation / Wolff-Parkinson-White Syndrome**

- Short PR intervals and wide QRS; Associated with SVT
- Delta waves (slurred upstroke in QRS complex)
- Synchronized cardioversion if unstable
- Procainamide best alternative
- Avoid CCBs, Beta blockers and Adenosine

5. **<u>Narrow Complex Tachycardia</u>**
    - <u>STEP 1: Is the tachycardia regular or irregular?</u>
        - If irregular, the differential is limited to:
            - Atrial fibrillation
            - Atrial flutter with variable block
            - Multifocal atrial tachycardia: defined as tachycardia with 3 or more different p wave morphologies
        - If regular, go to STEP 2
    - <u>STEP 2: Where is the p wave?</u>
        - Look carefully for the presence of p waves- they are often embedded at the end of QRS complexes or within the T wave so always compare the tachycardia ECG to the NSR ECG to look for subtle changes in QRS/T wave morphology (e.g. in cases of atrial tachycardia with 2:1 block, undetected "hidden" p waves may lead to an incorrect diagnosis of sinus tachycardia)
            - If the p wave is identified, measure the RP interval
                - If the RP interval is < ½ the RR interval, this is a SHORT RP tachycardia
                    - Consider AVNRT, orthodromic AVRT, JT
                - If the RP interval is > ½ the RR interval, this is a LONG RP tachycardia
                    - Consider atrial tachycardia, sinus tachycardia, etc.
            - If the p wave is NOT found, one can probably assume that it is embedded within the QRS and is therefore a SHORT RP tachycardia, consider AVNRT

Figure. Management flow chart for narrow QRS tachycardia

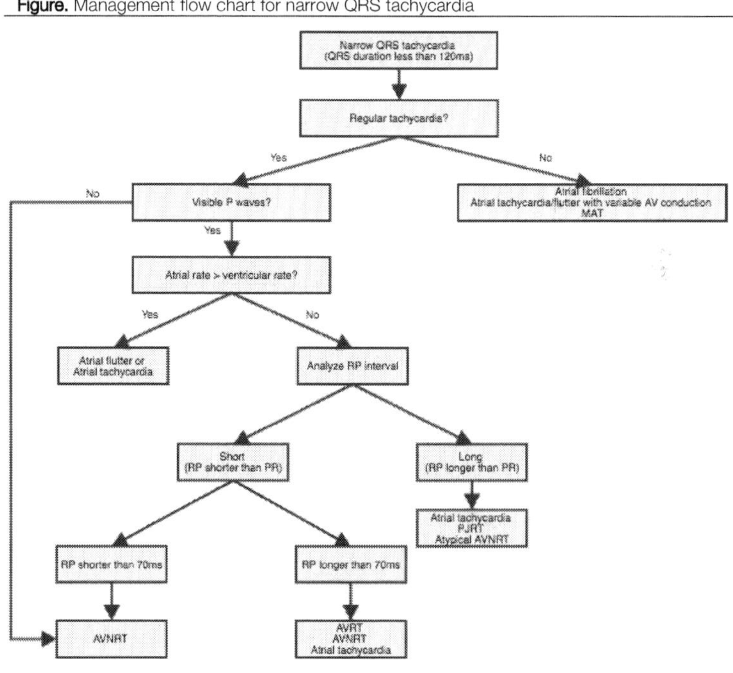

- **Treatment**
    - Adenosine (drug of choice) 6 mg IV **rapid** push initial dose; may give 2nd and 3rd dose of 12 mg IV **rapid** push
        - Warn pts they may feel sense of impending doom or severe pain, which is self-limited and resolves quickly
        - Therapeutic: if AVRT or AVNRT may terminate rhythm
            - AVRT – associated with WPW; look for delta wave
        - Diagnostic: if not the above, will show fibrillation or flutter waves
    - Vagal Maneuvers
        - Carotid sinus massage (R>L in effectiveness), valsalva
    - Radiofrequency Ablation

INFECTIOUS DISEASE

READING MICROBIOLOGY REPORT

Bacterial pathogens from different classes	
Gram-positive cocci [55]	Gram-negative cocci
Aerobic In clusters • Coagulase (+): *Staphylococcus aureus* • Coagulase (-): *Staphylococcus lugdunensis* and other coagulase-negative staphylococci In pairs/chains	Aerobic • Diplococcus: *Neisseria meningitidis, N. gonorrhoeae, Moraxella catarrhalis* • Cocco-bacillus: *Haemophilus influenzae, Acinetobacter* Anaerobic: *Veillonella* spp.
• Optochin sensitive: *Streptococcus pneumoniae* • Alpha-hemolytic: Viridans group *Streptococcus, Enterococcus* • Beta-hemolytic: ○ Group A Strep (*Streptococcus pyogenes)* ○ Group B Strep (*Streptococcus agalactiae)* ○ Group C, D, G Strep	
Anaerobic: *Peptostreptococcus spp.* and many others	
Gram-positive rods	Gram-negative rods

Aerobic • Large: *Bacillus spp* • Cocco-bacillus: *Listeria monocytogenes, Lactobacillus spp* • Small, pleomorphic: *Corynebacterium spp* • Branching filaments: *Nocardia spp, Streptomyces spp* Anaerobic • Large: *Clostridium spp* • Small: *P. acnes; Actinomyces spp*	Aerobic Lactose fermenting (Lactose positive): - *Enterobacter spp, Escherichia coli, Klebsiella spp* - *Citrobacter spp*, Serratia spp** Non lactose-fermenting (Lactose negative): • Oxidase (-): *Acinetobacter* spp, *Burkholderia spp, E. coli, Proteus* spp, *Salmonella* spp, *Shigella spp, Serratia spp*, Stenotrophomonas maltophilia* • Oxidase (+): *P. aeruginosa, Aeromonas* spp. Anaerobic: *Bacteroides spp, Fusobacterium spp, Prevotella spp.*
Mycobacteria	Spirochetes
M. tuberculosis *M. leprae* *M. bovis* *M. abscess* *M. avium* *M. marinum* *M. kansasii*	*Treponema pallidum (syphilis)* *Leptospira* *Borrelia*

SUSCEPTIBILITY INTERPRETATION

One of four interpretations:

- S (susceptible) - isolate is inhibited by the usually achievable concentrations of antimicrobial agent when the dosage recommended to treat the site of infection is used.
- I (intermediate) - isolate is not inhibited by these usually achievable concentrations, OR that the organisms might express a resistance mechanism.
- R (resistant) - the MIA is approaching the usually attainable concentration, but the response rates may be lower than for a susceptible isolate
- NS (non-susceptible) - A "NS" value does not necessarily mean that the isolate has a resistance mechanism, but rather that it has an unusually high MIA.

Figure. Antibiotics with susceptibilities to consider in management of specific organisms

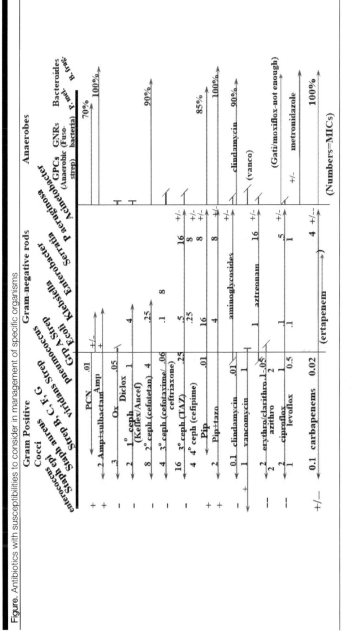

Gram Positive Cocci
Gram-negative rods
Anaerobes

enterococcus
Staph epi
Staph aureus
Strep B, C, F, G
viridans Strep
pneumococcus
Grp A Strep
Ecoli
Klebsiella
Enterobacter
Serratia
P aeruginosa
Acinetobacter
GPCs (Anaerobic strep)
GNRs (Fuso-bacteria)
Bacteroides
P. mel.
B. frag.

+ PCN .01 +/- 70%
+ 2 Amp+sulbactam Amp + 100%
- .3 Ox .05
Diclox
- 2 1° ceph (Keflex/Ancef) 1 4
- 8 2° ceph (cefotetan) 4 .25 90%
- 4 3° ceph (cefotaxime/ceftriaxone) .06 .1 8
- 16 3° ceph (TAZ) .25 .5 16 +/-
4 4° ceph (cefipime) .25 8 +/-
+ Pip .01 16 8 +/- 85%
+ 2 Pip+tazo 4 8 +/- 100%
- 0.1 clindamycin .01 aminoglycosides +/- clindamycin 90%
+ 1 vancomycin 1 (vanco)
1 aztreonam 16 +/-
-- 2 erythro/clarithro .1-.05
2 azithro 2
(Gati/moxiflox-not enough)
-- 2 ciproflox 1 .1 .5 +/-
1 levoflox 0.5 .1 1 +/- metronidazole
+/— 0.1 carbapenems 0.02 4 +/-- 100%
(ertapenem)
(Numbers=MICs)

Figure. Antibiotics with susceptibilities to consider in management of specific organisms

Gram Positive Cocci
Gram-negative rods
Anaerobes
enterococc
Staph epi
Staph aureus
Strep B, C, F, G
viridans Strep
pneumococcus
Grp A Strep
E coli
Klebsiella
Enterobacter
Serratia
P aeruginosa
Acinetobacter
ESBL
GPCs (Anaerobic strep)
GNRs (Fuso-bacteria)
Bacteroides
P. mel.
B. frag.

\+ Dalfopristin/Quinupristin
\+ Linezolid
Colistin
\+ Daptomycin
\+ Tigecycline
+/- +
100%
+/- Telithromycin
\+ 0.1 Doripenem 0.02
1 +/-- +
100%
\+ Telavancin
-- Ceftaroline
\+ Ceftobiprole
100%
-- Faropenem
-- Sitafloxacin ?

Specimen Gram Stains		
When You Know:	Gram Stain Results:	Think:
Meningitis (CSF)	Pleomorphic Gram negative bacilli	*Haemophilus influenzae*
	Gram negative diplococci	*Neisseria meningitidis*
	Gram positive cocci in pairs	*Streptococcus pneumoniae*
Wound infection	Gram positive cocci in clusters	*Staphylococcus aureus*
	Gram positive cocci in pairs	Streptococci
	Gram positive bacilli	*Bacillus, Clostridium*
	Gram negative bacilli	*E coli*, enterics, others
Bacteremia	Gram positive cocci in clusters	*Staphylococcus aureus*
	Gram positive cocci in chains	Streptococci
	Gram positive cocci in pairs	*Streptococcus pneumoniae*
	Gram positive bacilli	*Bacillus, Corynebacterium, Clostridium*
	Gram negative bacilli	*E coli*, enterics, others
	Yeast	*Candida albicans, Cryptococcus neoformans*
Urinary tract infection	Gram positive cocci in clusters	*Staphylococcus aureus*
	Gram positive cocci in chains	Streptococci
	Gram positive cocci in pairs	Enterococci
	Gram negative bacilli	*E coli*, enterics, others
	Yeast	*Candida albicans*

EMPIRIC ANTIBIOTIC MANAGEMENT

1. Site of Infection: drug penetration, common organism
2. Host: immune status, past pathogens, drug-drug interactions, allergies
3. Susceptibility data

Common Antibiotic Classes and Uses						
PCN's	G+	G-	A	MRSA	PsA	Inhibit peptidoglycan cross linking in cell walls
PCN	+					Not staph
Amp/Amox	+	?				
Oxacillin/Diclox	+					Sensitive staph
1st gen Cephalosporins	Less susceptible to B lactamases					
Cefazolin/Cephalexin	+	+				Sensitive staph. Gram - ESBL are resistant
2nd gen Cephalosporins						
Cefuroxime	+	+	+			
3rd gen						
Ceftriaxone	+	+	+			
Cefotaxime	+	+	+			
Cefpodoxime PO	+	+				
Ceftazidime	+	+	?		+	
4th gen						
Cefepime	+	+			+	
5th gen						
Ceftaroline	+	+		+		SSSI CA-PNA

						Good against MRSA
Carbapenems	Highly resistant to B lactamases; Lowers seizure threshold					
Imipenem	+	++	+		+	
Ertapenem	+	++	+			No PsA!
Meropenem	+	++	+		+	
Doripenem	+	++	+		+	Complicated intraabdominal infxn Complicated UTI Best to use against PsA
Combinations	Combo with B lactamase inhibitor					
Amox/Clavulanate (Augmentin)	+	+	+			
Amp/Sulbactam (Unasyn)	+	+	+			
Pip/Tazo (Zosyn)	+	+	+		+	
Aztreonam		+			+	Binds only Gram - penicillin binding proteins
Macrolides	Inhibits bacterial tRNA and ribosome translocation					
Azithromycin	+		+			atypical
Clarithromycin	+		+			
Erythromycin	+?		+			
Quinolones	Inhibit bacterial DNA gyrase and topoisomerase. Watch INR. CDif.					
Levofloxacin	+	++			+	And atypical
Ciprofloxacin	+	++			+	
Moxifloxacin	+	++	+			
Gatifloxacin	+	++	+			
Tetracyclines	Binds ribosome, inhibits tRNA binding. Photosensitivity!					
Doxycycline	+	+	+	+		And most atypical (not Legionella)
Aminoglycosides	Binds ribosome, inhibits protein synthesis. Nephrotoxic, ototoxic					
Gent		+			+	
Tobra		+			+	
Neomycin						Not absorbed
Other	**G+**	**G-**	**A**	**MRSA**	**PsA**	
Vancomycin	++		?	+		Inhibits cell wall synthesis. 15mg/kg bid (less if renal insuff); Redman
Clindamycin	+		+	?		Binds ribosome, inhibits tRNA and ribosomes (like macrolides).
Metronidazole			+			Taken up by anaerobes, forms toxic metabolites. Peripheral neuropathy
Linezolid	++		?	+		Prevents initiation complex of ribosomes. Marrow toxicity
Daptomycin	++			+		Alternative for MRSA SSTI (MRSA) Check CK weekly R side endocarditis No lung penetration
Tigecycline	++	+	+	+		Complicated SSTI (MSSA, MRSA, VSE)

Nitrofurantoin	+	+				Complicated intraabdominal infxn (MSSA, VSE) Toxic metabolites. e. coli only
Rifampin	+			+		Inhibits bacterial RNA polymerase. Neisseria
Trimethoprim/Sulfa	+	+		+		Inhibits successive steps in folate synthesis. Increases Cr but not nephrotoxic

Credit: UNC School of Medicine

Empiric Antibiotic Treatment

Respiratory	Inpatient	Outpatient
CAP (non-ICU)	Ceftriaxone (Rocephin) 1 gm iv q day plus azithromycin (Zithromax) 500 mg po q day 5 dose OR Levofloxacin (Levaquin) 750 mg iv daily Consider addition of steroids in CAP for hospitalized patients	Doxycycline 100 mg po BID OR Augmentin 500 mg po TID OR Levofloxacin (Levaquin) 750 mg po QD
CAP (ICU)	Levofloxacin (Levaquin) 750 mg IV daily PLUS Ceftriaxone (Rocephin) 1 gm IV daily OR Cefepime (Maxipime) 2 gm IV BID PLUS Azithromycin (Zithromax) 500 mg IV daily IF anaphylactic Beta Lactam allergy: Levofloxacin (Levaquin) 750 mg IV daily PLUS Aztreonam (Azactam) 1 gm every 8 hours Consider addition of steroids in CAP for hospitalized patients	Levofloxacin 500 mg po QD Doxycycline 100 mg po BID
Aspiration	Ceftriaxone 1g IV QD + Clindamycin 900mg IV Q8H OR Piperacillin/Tazobactam (Zosyn) 4.5 gm IV Q8H OR Ertapenem (Invanz) 1 gm IV daily	Augmentin 500 mg po TID
Nosocomial/HAP	Piperacillin/tazobactam (Zosyn) 4.5 gm iv every 8 hrs PLUS Levofloxacin (Levaquin) 750 mg iv daily OR Cefepime (Maxipime) 2 gm iv bid PLUS Levofloxacin (Levaquin) 750 mg iv daily plus Tobramycin OR Cefepime (Maxipime) 2 gm iv bid PLUS azithromycin (Zithromax) 500 mg iv / po daily PLUS tobramycin	Levofloxacin (Levaquin) 500 mg po Q day

Abdominal Tract		
Regular	Ceftriaxone (Rocephin) 1 gm IV Q day PLUS Metronidazole (Flagyl) 500 mg IV Q8h OR Piperacillin/Tazobactam (Zosyn) 4.5 gm IV Q8h MAY ADD IF PSEUDOMONAS SUSPECTED: Tobramycin 7 mg/kg IV x1	
C.diff	Flagyl 500 mg po q 8 h x 10 days Vancomycin oral sol'n 125 mg po q 6 h x 10 days Flagyl IV loading dose 1 Gm IVPB, then 500 mg IVPB q 8 h *In severe cases, may combine IV Flagyl with po Vancomycin Consider: Lactobacillus Acidophilus 2 capsules po bid Lactobacillus Acidophilus 2 pkts po bid	
UTI		
Regular	Trimethoprim/Sulfa DS (Septra DS) 1 tab po BID OR Ceftriaxone (Rocephin) 1 gm IV Q day	Trimethoprim/Sulfa DS 1 tab po BID OR Augmentin 500 mg po TID
Nosocomial	Cefepime 2 GM Q 12h	
Urosepsis	Ceftriaxone (Rocephin) 1 gm IV Q day	Levofloxacin (Levaquin) 500 mg po Q day
Soft Tissue		
Cellulitis	Cefazolin (Ancef) 1 gm IV Q8h OR Nafcillin 2 gm IV Q4h MAY ADD: Clindamycin 900 mg IV Q8h for either if not resolving, e.g. toxin-producing strep	Cephalexin (Keflex) 500 mg po QID OR Dicloxacillin (Dynapen) 500 mg po QID
MRSA	Vancomycin 1 gm Q12h per pharmacy protocol OR Linezolid (Zyvox) 600 mg IV Q12h (for MRSA pneumonia)	Trimethoprim/Sulfamethoxazole DS TID OR Minocycline (Dynacin) 100 mg Q12h
Severe	Ceftriaxone (Rocephin) 1 gm IV Q day PLUS Clindamycin (Cleocin) 900 mg 900 mg IV Q8h OR Ertapenem (Invanz) 1 gm IV Q day MAY ADD TO ALL ABOVE REGIMEN: Tobramycin 7 mg/kg IV once, then per pharmacy protocol	Augmentin 500 mg po TID OR Levofloxacin (Levaquin) 500 mg po Q day

Common conditions and treatments

Infection	Bugs	Drugs
Meningitis	S. pneumoniae N. Meningitidis, H. influenzae Listeria	Ceftriaxone + vancomycin ± ampicillin
If post-op	Staphylococcus sp. Gram negative rods (GNR)	Ceftazidime + vancomycin
Ventriculitis due to an infected VP shunt	S. epidermidis S. aureus Coliforms† Diphtheroids P. acnes	Vancomycin + Cefepime
Encephalitis (viral)	Herpes simplex virus Varicella zoster virus West Nile virus	Acyclovir
Sinusitis	S. pneumoniae	Amoxicillin or Augmentin (if prior antibiotic exposure)
Mastoiditis	M. catarrhalis Staphylococcus sp.	Ceftriaxone ± vancomycin
Pharyngitis	Group A, C, G streptococcus	Penicillin
	N. gonorrhoea	Ceftriaxone (IM) + treat for Chlamydia with azithromycin OR doxycycline
Retropharyngeal/neck abscess	Streptococcus sp. Oral anaerobes	Clindamycin
Pneumonia Community-acquired	S. pneumoniae H. influenzae Chlamydia Mycoplasma Legionella *Consider addition of steroids in severe CAP*	Levaquin OR Ceftriaxone + azithromycin
Hospital-acquired (48 hours)	S. pneumoniae S. aureus Enteric GNR (i.e. klebsiella)	Levaquin + Zosyn OR Ceftriaxone/ceftazidime + vancomycin ± gentamicin
Ventilator-associated (48-72 hours)	P. aeruginosa MRSA Acinetobacter Multidrug resistant GNR Stenotrophomonas	Imipenem + levofloxacin ± (vancomycin OR linezolid if suspect MRSA)
Pneumonitis	PCP Cytomegalovirus	High-dose Bactrim OR High-dose Ganciclovir
Endocarditis	S. aureus (MRSA) Viridans streptococcus Enterococcus Coagulase-negative staph Enteric GNR	Blood cultures first! Vancomycin + gentamicin + rifampin (if valve)

FEVER OF UNKNOWN ORIGIN (FUO)

- **Defined** – 100.9F x 3 weeks with no obvious source despite investigation
- **HPI**[56,57]
  - Fevers + NS + chills → infection
  - NS + chills + anorexia + wt loss → neoplasm
  - Myalgias + joint pains → rheumatologic
- **Workup**
  - Travel history
  - Pet exposure
  - Work environment
  - Sick contacts
  - New Medications
- **Full Fever Workup**
  - CBC, ICU panel, CXR, blood cultures x2, UA, Urine culture x1, respiratory (if applicable)
  - Chest X-ray
  - UA
  - Consider cortisol if pt on steroids for ↑period of time
  - Consider lactate +/- proclacitonin (red misc tube) if sepsis is a concern
  - If patient has an indwelling line, culture from that line
  - PE for skin evidence of infection
  - Re-address ABx therapy if applicable

Limited differential diagnosis list for FUO

Infections	Malignancies	Autoimmune	Misc.
Endocarditis Abdominal abscesses TB (extrapulmonary) Pelvic abscesses Dental abscesses Osteomyelitis Sinusitis -------------------- Cytomegalovirus Epstein-Barr virus HIV Lyme disease Prostatitis Sinusitis	Lymphoma Renal cell carcinoma Chronic leukemia Colon carcinoma Metastatic cancers Hepatoma Myelodysplastic syndromes Pancreatic carcinoma Sarcomas	Temporal arteritis Adult Still's disease Systemic lupus erythematosus PAN PMR Rheumatoid arthritis Rheumatoid fever IBD Reiter's syndrome Vasculitides	Drug-induced fever 2/2 cirrhosis Factitious fever Hepatitis (alcoholic, granulomatous, or lupoid) DVT Sarcoidosis Medications

- **Preliminary Evaluation**
  - <u>Labs</u>
    - CBC
    - HFP
    - ESR/CRP
    - UA
    - Cultures
    - HIV
    - 1-step PPD +/- CXR
  - <u>Imaging</u>
    - CXR
    - Abdominal CT
    - PET
    - MRI brain
    - Duplex US
    - TTE

Figure. Diagnosis of Fever of Unknown Origin

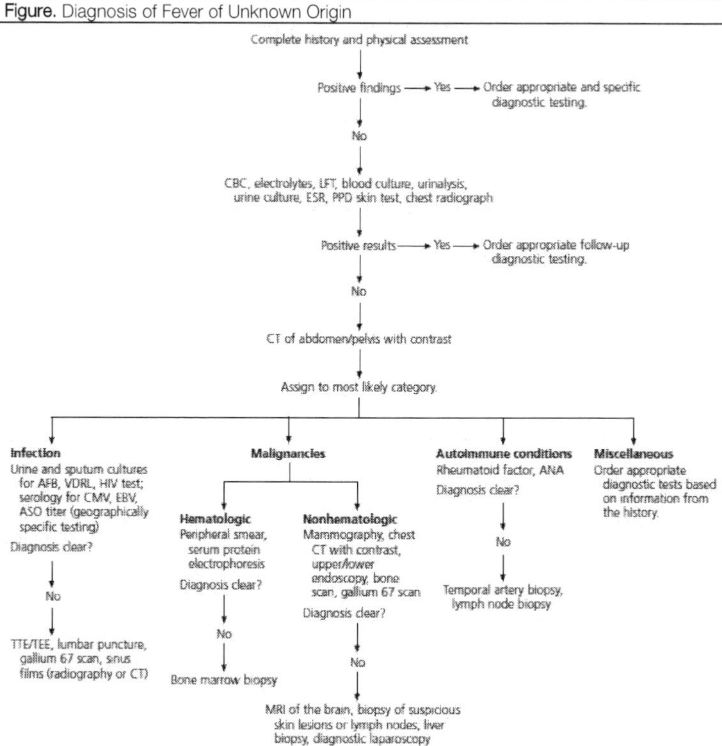

CELLULITIS

- **Overview**[58,59,60]
  - Look for <u>predisposing disease/condition</u> that may cause recurrence:
    - PVD
    - T2DM
    - Onychomycosis
    - Tinea pedis (low involvement → tx with imidazole BID x 2-4w)
    - **Lymphedema**
    - S/P saphenous vein grafting d/t lymphatic vessel disruption
    - S/P mastectomy
  - <u>Causes</u>
    - BHS, S. aureus, GN aerobic bacilli
- **Mimics**
  - <u>Stasis Dermatitis</u>
    - Long-standing, progressive
    - Ill-defined borders, bilateral, nontender, hyperpigmentation (bronzing, hemosiderin deposits), overlying superficial desquamation, serous drainage, no systemic symptoms

        - Due to chronic venous insufficiency → edema → RBA extravasation (↑pigmentation) → ↓O2
        - If chronic, can lead to lipodermatosalerosis
    - Lipodermatosalerosis
        - Sclerosing panniculitis 2/2 chronic venous insufficiency
        - "inverted champagne bottle" appearance to legs
        - Usually involves the lower 1/3 of the leg(s)
        - Known venous insufficiency, hyperpigmentation, lack of systema symptoms, skin is "bound-down", no systema symptoms
        - Chronic course may be associated with scattered ulcerations
    - Contact Dermatitis (ask about new medications, topicals, band aids, adhesives)
    - Lymphedema (high risk in patient's s/p lumpectomy, overweight). Thought to be secondary to compression of lymphatics → ↓O2 distribution → fibrosis. Often no warmth, tenderness, systema symptoms.
- **Risk factors**
    - Trauma
    - Laceration
    - Puncture Wound
    - Post-operative infection at incision site
    - Skin Ulcer
    - Neoplasms
    - Lymphatic Cutaneous metastases from neoplasms
    - Chronic Dependent edema (may progress rapidly)
    - Diabetes Mellitus
- **Diagnosis**
    - Based on clinical manifestations
        - Fever
        - ↑WBC (check for ↑eosinophil count which may be s/o eosinophilic cellulitis)
        - Warmth
        - Erythema
        - Somewhat clear borders (if not clear; and not stasis dermatitis; consider erysipelas)
        - TTP
        - Often associated with puncture wound or ulcer
    - Cultures necessary for suspected systemic toxicity or extensive skin involvement or underlying comorbidities
- **Assessment**
    - Presence of crepitus should lead you to look for *Clostridium* or *Bacteroides*
    - Source
        - Skin – MRSA, GAS
        - Seawater – *Vibrio spp.*
        - Freshwater – *Aeromonas spp.*
- **Treatment**
    - Elevated affected extremity
    - Antibiotics

      PO antibiotics are most often sufficient, IV antibiotics only required if patient has systemic toxicity (fevers, chills) or pressive erythema; switch to PO therapy when pt afebrile and skin findings begin to resolve (often 3-5 days). Coverage should include ***GBS and MRSA***. Total duration of treatment should be 7-10 days.
        - **Erysipelas (Streptococcus coverage)**
            - Mild-Moderate infections (oral, outpatient management)
                - Penicillin VK 500 mg orally four times per day for 7-10 days or

        - Amoxicillin 500 mg orally three times per day for 7-10 days or
        - Cephalexin 500 mg orally four times per day for 7-10 days
      - Penicillin Allergy
        - Azithromycin 500 mg orally on day 1, then 250 mg orally on days 2-5
        - Clindamycin 300 mg orally four times per day for 7-10 days
    - Severe infections (requiring IV antibiotics)
      - Penicillin G 2 million units IV every 6 hours or
      - Cefazolin 1 gram IV every 8 hours or
      - Clindamycin 600 mg IV every 8 hours or
      - Vancomycin 15 mg/kg IV every 12 hours
    - **Empiric**
      - Vancomycin 1-2g IV daily + Cefotaxime/Gentamycin x 7-10 days
      - Cefazolin, 1.0 g intravenously every 6–8 hr
      - Rocephin, 1.0 g intravenously every 6–8 hr
      - Nafcillin, 1.0 or 1.5 g intravenously every 4–6 hr
      - Ceftriaxone, 1.0 g intravenously every 24 hr
      - Linezolid, 0.6 g intravenously every 12 hr
    - **PO Therapy**
      - Dicloxacillin, 0.5 g orally every 6 hr
      - Cephalexin, 0.5 g orally every 6 hr
      - Clindamycin 300mg QID
    - **Purulent (abscess)**
      - Highly suggestive of MRSA
      - Clindamycin, TMP-SMX, Doxycycline/Minocycline, or Linezolid x 5-10 days
    - **Non-Purulent**
      - Targets MSSA and BHS
      - Clindamycin, Amoxicillin+TMP-SMX, Amoxicilin+Doxycycline/Minocycline, Linezolid x 5-10 days
- **Recurrence**
  - Seen in 17% of patients
    - Consider prophylactic therapy if 2 episodes in 3 years with PAN 250mg/d x 1 year[61]

MENINGITIS

- **Overall**[62]
  - Encephalitis (most commonly of viral origin 2/2 HSV esp in older population >70) will present with AMS and focal neurological deficits. These patients require treatment with Acyclovir
  - 95% of patients with meningitis will present with headache, fever, AMS, and neck stiffness
- **Etiology**
  - S. pneumoniae (+latex agglutination) most common cause of bacterial meningitis
  - N. meningitides
  - GNR
  - Listeria monocytogenes
  - H. influenza
  - E. coli
  - S. agalactiae
- **Labs/Diagnostic Testing**
  - CT prior to LP

- Lumbar puncture may be performed without computed tomography of the brain if there are no risk factors for an occult intracranial abnormality. Signs that should warrant CT first prior to LP:
    - Immunocompromised (+HIV, AIDS, s/p chemotherapy)
    - Hx of CNS disease (mass, lesion, stroke, infxn)
    - New seizure (within 1 week of presentation or in post ictal state)
    - Papilledema
    - Abnormal LOC/AMS
    - Focal neurological deficit
- <u>Performing lumbar puncture</u>
    - Measure opening pressure (normal 10-20 cm if average wait, up to 25cm if obese)
        - Measured in the left lateral decubitus position

<table>
<tr><th colspan="3">Labs obtained in lumbar puncture</th></tr>
<tr><td>Tube #</td><td>Amount (cc)</td><td>Studies:</td></tr>
<tr><td>#1</td><td>3cc</td><td>Cell count
Differential</td></tr>
<tr><td>#2</td><td>3cc</td><td>Glucose
Protei</td></tr>
<tr><td>#3</td><td>5-10cc</td><td><table><tr><th>HIV-</th><th>HIV+</th></tr><tr><td>- Gram stain
- Culture
- Cytology

<u>Optional</u>
- India Ink
- VDRL (and serum RPR)
- Cocci serology
- Crypto antigen
- Fungal Culture
- AFB smear/Culture
- Viral culture
- TB PAR
- Bacterial Antigen Panel</td><td>Gram stain
Culture
India Ink
VDRL (and serum RPR)
Cocci serology
Crypto antigen
Fungal Culture
Viral culture
AFB smear/Culture
Toxo serology
Cytology to eval for ANS lymphoma
Consider JA Virus PAR</td></tr></table></td></tr>
<tr><td>#4</td><td>3cc</td><td>Cell count
Differential</td></tr>
</table>

- <u>**Remember however, still give the ABx, then get CT, then LP!**</u>
- Serum: PCT, CRP

- **Treatment**
    - ABx **should not** be delayed in patients suspected of having bacterial meningitis if lumbar puncture cannot be performed in a timely manner
    - A large prospective, randomized, double-blind trial that established the use of adjuvant dexamethasone in adults found that patients who received dexamethasone had a significantly lower risk of an unfavorable outcome than patients who received placebo
        - Most often used in patients with diplococci on GS or culture + *S.pneumoniae* in blood or CSF

    - Dexamethasone 10mg x1 before or w/ first dose of ABx then 10mg q6h x4d
- Vaccination for Streptococcus pneumoniae, Haemophilus influenzae type B, and Neisseria meningitidis is recommended for patients in appropriate risk groups and significantly decreases the incidence of bacterial meningitis.
- Below are treatment regiments, those that are starred (*) are preferred overall

CSF Findings in Meningitis by Etiologic Agent

Agent	Opening Pressure (mm H_2O)	WBC count (cells/μL)	Glucose (mg/dL)	Protein (mg/dL)	Microbiology
Bacterial meningitis	200-300	100-5000; >80% PMNs	< 40	>100	Specific pathogen demonstrated in 60% of Gram stains and 80% of cultures
Viral meningitis	90-200	10-300; lymphocytes with PMN in first 48h	Normal, reduced in LCM and mumps	Normal but may be slightly elevated	Viral isolation, PCR assays
Tuberculous meningitis	180-300	100-500; lymphocytes	Reduced, < 40	Elevated, >100	Acid-fast bacillus stain, culture, PCR
Cryptococcal meningitis	180-300	10-200; lymphocytes	Reduced	50-200	India ink, cryptococcal antigen, culture
Aseptic meningitis	90-200	10-300; lymphocytes	Normal	Normal but may be slightly elevated	Negative findings on workup
Normal values	80-200	0-5; lymphocytes	50-75	15-40	Negative findings on workup

LCM = lymphocytic choriomeningitis; PCR = polymerase chain reaction; PMN = polymorphonuclear leukocyte; WBC = white blood cell.

Common causes of meningitis and treatments

Bacteria	Susceptibility	Antibiotic(s)	Duration (days)
Streptococcus pneumoniae	Penicillin MIC ≤0.06 μg/mL	Recommended: Penicillin G or ampicillin Alternatives: Cefotaxime, ceftriaxone, chloramphenicol	10-14
	Penicillin MIC ≥0.12 μg/mL Cefotaxime or ceftriaxone MIC ≥0.12 μg/mL	Recommended: Cefotaxime or ceftriaxone Alternatives: Cefepime, meropenem	
	Cefotaxime or ceftriaxone MIC ≥1.0 μg/mL	Recommended: Vancomycin plus cefotaxime or ceftriaxone** Alternatives: Vancomycin plus moxifloxacin	
Haemophilus influenzae	Beta-lactamase–negative	Recommended: Ampicillin Alternatives: Cefotaxime, ceftriaxone, cefepime, chloramphenicol, aztreonam, a fluoroquinolone	7
	Beta-lactamase–positive	Recommended: Cefotaxime or ceftriaxone** Alternatives: Cefepime, chloramphenicol, aztreonam, a fluoroquinolone	
	Beta-lactamase–negative, ampicillin-resistant	Recommended: Meropenem Alternatives: Cefepime, chloramphenicol, aztreonam, a fluoroquinolone	
Neisseria meningitidis	Penicillin MIC < 0.1 μg/mL	Recommended: Penicillin G or ampicillin** Alternatives: Cefotaxime, ceftriaxone, chloramphenicol	7
	Penicillin MIC ≥0.1 μg/mL	Recommended: Cefotaxime or ceftriaxone Alternatives: Cefepime, chloramphenicol, a fluoroquinolone, meropenem	
Listeria monocytogenes	...	Recommended: Ampicillin or penicillin G** Alternative: TMP-SMX	14-21
Streptococcus agalactiae	...	Recommended: Ampicillin or penicillin G** Alternatives: Cefotaxime, ceftriaxone, vancomycin	14-21

Enterobacteriaceae	...	Recommended: Cefotaxime or ceftriaxone Alternatives: Aztreonam, a fluoroquinolone, TMP-SMX, meropenem, ampicillin	21
Pseudomonas aeruginosa	...	Recommended: Ceftazidime or cefepime Alternatives: Aztreonam, meropenem, ciprofloxacin	21
Staphylococcus epidermidis		Recommended: Vancomycin Alternative: Linezolid Consider addition of rifampin	

Organisms to consider based on population demographic		
Population	Organism	Treatment
Adults 16-50 YO	*N. meningitidis* *S. pneumoniae* *H. influenzae*	Dexamethasone Ceftriaxone Vancomycin
Adults >50 YO	*N. meningitidis* *S. pneumoniae* *L. monocytogenes* *GNR*	Dexamethasone Ceftriaxone Vancomycin Ampicillin (cover for L. Monocytogenes)
Post-NSurg/Shunt	*S. aureus* *S. pneumoniae* *GNR*	Vancomycin Cefepime
Immunocompromised	*N. meningitidis* *S. pneumoniae* *H. influenzae* *GNR*	Vancomycin Ampicillin Cefepime
Penetrating trauma		Vancomycin Cefepime
HSV Encephalitis	HSV	Acyclovir

URINARY TRACT INFECTIONS

- **General Considerations**
  - Although a urine Gram stain may be useful in guiding therapy, all antibiotics recommended as empiric therapy are effective against Gram-negative bacilli (pyelonephritis is not treated empirically with ampicillin or sulfonamides alone due to E. coli resistance to these antibiotics).
  - In patients with nosocomial pyelonephritis, a history of recurrent UTI, or prior infection with a resistant organism, *initial antimicrobial therapy should cover Pseudomonas aeruginosa* (I.e. cefepime, tobramycin, imipenem, ciprofloxacin, or piperacillin/tazobactam).
  - In all cases, antibiotic therapy should be revised once susceptibility data are available.
  - If bacteriuria persists > 24-48 hours, switch the antibiotic based on susceptibility data.
  - If fever or toxicity persists despite adequate antibiotics, consider perinephric or renal cortical abscess and evaluate with imaging of kidneys.
  - Signs of pyelonephritis (i.e. fever, leukocytosis) may not be present in the elderly.
- **Categories and Empiric Treatment**
  - Acute, uncomplicated cystitis in women
    - Dysuria, urgency, frequency, suprapubic pain
    - No prior urinary symptoms in last 4 weeks
    - No fever or flank pain
    - Treatment:

      First Line Therapy
      - **NSAIDs alone have not been shown to be as beneficial as antibiotic treatment if uncomplicated**
      - Nitrofurantoin monohydrate macrocrystals, 100 mg twice daily for 5 days (with meals),

or TMP-SMX, 160 mg and 800 mg twice daily for 3 days
or Fosfomycin trometamol (Monurol), 3-g sachet in a single dose
or Pivmecillinam, 400 mg twice daily for 3 to 7 days

- DM, >7 days of symptoms, recent UTI, age > 65, or diaphragm use: treat for 7 days with above
- Pregnant: 7 days of oral amoxicillin, nitrofurantoin, cefpodoxime, OR TMP/SMX (do not use near term)

Second Line Therapy (must prove that above options either did not work or are contraindicated)

- Fluoroquinolones: ciprofloxacin, 250 mg twice daily for 3 days; levofloxacin, 250 mg or 500 mg once daily for 3 days

- Acute, uncomplicated pyelonephritis in women
  - Fever, chills, dysuria, urgency, frequency, suprapubic pain, CVA tenderness and/or flank pain
  - No history of urologic abnormalities
  - Treatment:
    - Mild/moderate symptoms without nausea/vomiting: oral FQ x7 days OR amoxicillin/clavulanate or cephalexin or TMP/SMX (DS) x14 days
    - Severe/urosepsis requiring hospitalization: IV FQ OR (ampicillin + gentamicin) OR 3rd generation cephalosporin OR piperacillin/tazobactam until afebrile then oral TMP/SMX (DS) or FQ x14 days
    - Pregnancy: IV ceftizoxime OR gentamicin ± ampicillin OR aztreonam OR TMP/SMX until afebrile then oral amoxicillin OR cephalosporin OR TMP/SMX (DS) x14 days
  - If fever persists beyond 5 days with continued symptoms, US should be obtained to r/o perinephric abscess
- Complicated UTI
  - Any combination of findings in above categories
  - Men or patients with post-void residual > 100 mL, outlet obstruction, calculus, urinary catheter, vesicoureteral reflux, prior renal disease with azotemia
  - Treatment:
    - Mild/moderate symptoms without nausea/vomiting: oral FQ x10-14 days
    - Severe/urosepsis requiring hospitalization: IV ciprofloxacin OR (ampicillin + gentamicin) OR ceftizoxime OR aztreonam OR piperacillin/tazobactam OR imipenem until afebrile then oral TMP/SMX (DS) or FQ x14-21 days
- ESBL UTI
  - Risk factors: hospitalization, catheter placement, CV catheter, feeding tube, prior ABx, ventilator usage, residence in nursing home
  - Treatment: carbapenems (ertapenem, meropenem, and imipenem)
- Recurrent UTI (women)
  - Defined as ≥2 infections in 6 months or ≥3 in one year
  - Postcoital or daily prophylactic ABx are recommended
    - Options include TMP-SMX, Nitrofurantoin, Cephalexin, and Ciprofloxacin

PYELONEPHRITIS

- **Pearls**[63]
  - Fever can last (on average) 3 days in patients
  - After 3 days, consider complications such as abscess
  - Absence of fever is common in the geriatric population
  - Has potential to cause sepsis, shock, and death
- **Symptoms**

- Flank Pain
- Fever>103F common
- Anorexia
- N/V
- Myalgias
- Dysuria, ↑frequency, urgency

- **Diagnosis**
  - CT abd/pelv if suspected sepsis+/-shock, known urolithiasis, pH>7, or ↓GFR to 40 or if symptoms not improving after 24-48h
  - Labs
    - UA: WBC casts, +LE, pyuria (>5 WBCs), +nitrites, WBC cast (renal origin)
    - CBC, BUN/SCr, hCG, GFR
    - UCx: $\geq 10^5$ CFU **cardinal confirmatory diagnostic test
    - CRP
    - Albumin (<3.3 ↑ risk for need to hospitalize)
- **Etiology**
  - E. coli (>80%)
  - Other grame negatives
  - Enterococci
  - Pseudomonas spp.
  - Staph
- **Commonly Associated Conditions**
  - Indwelling catheters
  - Renal calculi
  - BPH
- **Rule out**
  - Complications such as hydronephrosis, concurrent nephrolithiasis, abscess (persistent fevers after 3 days of treatment, hx of DM, flank pain/abdominal pain, bacteremia). Consider re-imaging (or initial imaging) with CT, US, or cystoscopy.
  - Most common causes of failure are abx resistance and nephrolithiasis
- **Treatment**

Triaging patients with pyelonephritis

Triage	Home	Observation	Admission
Symptoms/Hx	Mild; no vomiting No other PMHx	Moderate; +/-vomit None or stable	Sepsis Potential PMHx
Fluids	None/minor	Moderate +/- maintenance fluids	Vigorous
Imaging	None	Only if risk for obstruction, abscess, or emphysematous pyelo	
ABx	IV/Oral/Both Can give single IV dose then continue PO	Start on IV in ER and continue on floor then switch to PO	No PO therapy until stabilized

  - Antibiotics:
    In general, start broad then tailor therapy to culture and sensitivities. PO transition from IV can occur after patient has been afebrile for 24-48 hours. Most Abx require 14 days duration except ciprofloxacin which only requires 7 days.
    - Outpatient
      - Ciprofloxacin, 500 mg given orally twice daily x7d (preg cat C)
      - TMP-SMX 160/800mg BID x14d
      - Levofloxacin, 750 mg given orally once daily for 5 days
      - Cefixime 400mg/d x10-14d (active against many FLQ-res and Bactrim-res GNB

- Inpatient
  - Ampicillin 2g IV q6h + Tobramycin 6mg/kg IV daily x14d
  - Ampicillin 2g IV q6h + gentamycin 1mg/kg IV q8h x14d
  - Ciprofloxacin 400mg Q12H
  - Levaquin 750mg daily
  - Ceftriaxone 1-2g/d
  - Cefotaxme 1g q8-12h up to 2g q4h
  - Ertapenam 1g q24h x7-10d
  - Meropenam 500mg q12h x7-10d
  - Ticarcillin-clavulanate: 3.1g q4-6h
  - Imipenem 500mg IV q6h (covers ESBL but not CRE)
  - Amikacin 15-20 mg/kg q24h x7-10d
- Anesthetic: Phenazopyridine 200mg PO TID x2d after meals unless CKD or ↑LFT
- Analgesic: Tylenol, Opiate
- Anti-emetic: prochlorperazine, Zofran
- Referral Indications
  - UT obstruction and/or high urinary post void residual volumes
  - Nephrolithiasis
  - Itrarenal abscess
  - Perinephric abscess
  - Urology/IR for percutaneous nephrostomy tube if there is concern for pyonephrosis or ureteral obstruction with proximal infection

BACTERIAL ENDOCARDITIS

- **Clinical Manifestations**[64]
  - Signs/Symptoms
  - Fever, chills, sweats, anorexia, weight loss, malaise, myalgias, arthralgias, heart murmur, arterial emboli, splenomegaly, petechiae, peripheral manifestations (Osler's nodes, subungual hemorrhages, Janeway lesions, Roth's spots) and signs of CHF.
- **Risk Factors**
  - Structural heart disease, IVDU, indwelling vasc devices, bacteremia with other infection, prior history of infective endocarditis
- **Laboratory manifestations**
  - Anemia, leukocytosis, microscopic hematuria, elevated ESR, CRP, RF, circulating immune complexes, decreased serum complement
- **Microbiology**
  - S. aureus (30-40%), viridans group strep, enterococci (1%), coagulase-staph, culture negative (2-20%)
- **Work-Up**
  - Blood Cultures
    - If not critically ill: 3 blood cultures over 12-24 hours (can delay treatment)
    - If critically ill: 3 blood cultures over 1 hour (treat)
  - Echo (TTE or TEE)
  - EKG: evaluate for conduction abnormalities, ischemia, infarction
  - CXR: evaluate for septic emboli, valvular calcification, CHF
- **Diagnosis**
  - Modified Duke Criteria (2 major OR 1 major and 3 minor OR 5 minor criteria)
    - Major Criteria
      - Positive blood cultures
        - Typical microorganisms from two separate blood cultures: viridans strep, Strep bovis, HACEK, or community acquired Staph aureus or enterococci in absence of primary focus

        - Persistently positive blood culture: recovery of organism from blood cultures drawn > 12hrs apart OR all of 3 or majority of 4 or more separate blood cultures with first and last > 1hr apart
      - Evidence of endocardial involvement
      - Positive echo: oscillating intracardiac mass or abscess or new partial dehiscence of prosthetic valve
        - TEE recommended as first test in the following patients prosthetic valve endocarditis; or those with at least "possible" endocarditis by clinical criteria; or those with suspected complicated endocarditis, such as perivalvular abscess.
        - TTE recommended as first test in all other patients
        - Definition of positive findings: oscillating intracardiac mass, on valve or supporting structures, or in the path of regurgitant jets, or on implanted material, in the absence of an alternative anatomic explanation or myocardial abscess or new partial dehiscence of prosthetic valve
      - New valvular regurgitation
    - <u>Minor Criteria</u>
      - Predisposing heart condition or injection drug use
      - Fever ≥ 38.0°C
      - Vascular phenomena: major arterial emboli, septic pulmonary infarcts, mycotic aneurysm, intracranial hemorrhage, conjunctival hemorrhages, Janeway lesions
      - Immunologic phenomena: glomerulonephritis, Osler's nodes, Roth's spots, RF
      - Microbiologic evidence: positive blood culture but not meeting above major criteria or serologic evidence of active infection with organism consistent with infective endocarditis

- **Treatment**
  - <u>Empiric</u>
    - For culture-positive endocarditis, use Sanford Guide to determine regimen
      - Unless the pt has a toxic appearance or clinical or echo evidence of progressive valvular regurgitation or CHF, empiric antibiotics should be delayed until blood cultures are drawn. Administration of antibiotics before blood cultures are obtained reduces recovery rate of bacteria by 30-45%.
    - <u>Native valve without IVDU</u>
      - [Penicillin G 20 million units q24h continuous or divided q4h OR ampicillin 12gm IV q24h continuous or divided q4h] AND oxacillin 2 gm IV q4h AND gentamicin 1mg/kg IV q8h
      - Alternative regimen is vancomycin + gentamicin
    - <u>Native valve with IVDU (S. aureus)</u>
      - Vancomycin 1gm IV q12h OR daptomycin 6mg/kg q24h
    - <u>Prosthetic valve</u>
      - Vancomycin 15mg/kg IV q12h + rifampin 600mg PO q24h + gentamicin 1mg/kg IV q8h
      - Prophylaxis (indirect evidence, no randomized trials)
  - <u>Cardiac lesions for which endocarditis prophylaxis is advised:</u>
    - High risk: prosthetic valves, prior bacterial endocarditis, complex cyanotic heart disease (except isolated secundum ASD and completely corrected PDA, VSD or pulmonary stenosis), PDA, coarctation of the aorta, surgically constructed systemic-pulmonary shunts
    - Moderate risk: congenital cardiac malformations, VSD, bicuspid AV, acquired AV and MV, hypertrophic CMY, MVP with valvular regurgitation and/or thickened leaflets

- Procedures for which endocarditis prophylaxis is advised (moderate and high risk patients):
  - Dental procedures: extractions, periodontal procedures, implant placement, root canal, surgery beyond apex, subgingival placement of antibiotic fibers/strips, placement of orthodontic bands but not brackets, intraligamentary injections
- Respiratory procedures: operations involving mucosa, rigid bronchoscopy
- GI procedures: Esophageal variceal sclerotherapy, stricture dilatation, ERCP, biliary tract surgery, bowel surgery involving the mucosa
- Oral cavity, respiratory tract, or esophageal procedures
  - Amoxicillin 2gm orally 1 hour before procedure
  - Unable to take oral medications: ampicillin 2gm IV or IM within 30mins of procedures
- PCN allergy options:
  - Clarithromycin 500mg PO 1h before procedure
  - Cephalexin 2gm PO 1h before procedure
  - Clindamycin 600mg PO 1h before procedure or IV 30mins before procedure
  - Cefazolin 1gm IV/IM 30mins before procedure
- GU/GI procedures
  - High risk: ampicillin 2gm IM/IV and (gentamicin 1.5mg/kg within 30min of procedure); repeat ampicillin 1gm IM/IV or amoxicillin 1g PO 6h later
  - High risk with PCN allergy: vancomycin 1gm IV over 1-2h AND gentamicin 1.5mg/kg IV/IM completed within 30 minutes of procedure
  - Moderate risk: amoxicillin 2g PO 1h before procedure or ampicillin 2g IV/IM within 30min before procedure
  - Moderate risk with PCN allergy: vancomycin 1g IV over 1-2h completed within 30 min of procedure

PNEUMONIA

- **Admission vs. Outpatient therapy**
  - CURB-65 (or PSI) *(level 1 evidence)*
    - Outpatient for scores 0-1
    - Ward for score 2-3
    - ICU for score >3 *(3+ minor criteria)*

Criteria For Severe CAP			
Minor	RR ≥ 30 PaO2/FIO2 < 250 Multilobular infiltrates	Confusion Uremia (≥20) WBC<2000	PLT<100k Temp<36c ↓BP
Major	Mechanical ventilation Vasopressor support		

- **Risk factors associated with increased morbidity and mortality:**
  - Age > 65
  - Coexisting illnesses: dm, renal failure, CHF, chronic lung disease, EtOH, aspiration, recent hospitalization, altered mental status
  - Pe: rr>30, bp<90/60, t≥38.3°c, confusion or lethargy
  - Labs: wbc <4,000 or >30,000, pao2<60, pco2>50, cr>1.2, bun>20, hct<30, coagulopathy; multilobar disease or effusions on CXR
- **Risk factors for MDR pathogens causing HAP, HCAP, and VAP**
  - ABx in preceding 90 d

- Current hospitalization of 5d or more
- High frequency of antibiotic resistance in the community or in the specific hospital unit
- Presence of risk factors for HCAP:
  - Hospitalization for 2 d or more in the preceding 90 d
  - Residence in a nursing home or extended care facility
  - Home infusion therapy (including antibiotics)
  - Chronic dialysis within 30 d
  - Home wound care
  - Family member with multidrug-resistant pathogen
- Immunosuppressive disease and/or therapy

- **Diagnostic Workup**
  - Serum: CBC, LFTs, ICU panel (↓Na may be indicative of legionella), ABG
  - Urine: UA, Urinary antigens to include pneumococcal and legionella
  - CXR (repeat 7-12 weeks after therapy in patients with high risk characteristics such as age>50, and smoking history or with persistent symptoms despite therapy)
  - Cultures (blood, sputum, endotracheal aspirate, viral)
    - Good quality sputum culture
    - <10 epithelial cells
    - >25 PMN
  - QuantiFERON if suspecting TB
  - HIV (if age<55yo, homeless or other risk factors)
  - AFB stain and culture (if cough>1mo, homeless, other risk factors)
  - PCT (may help delineate viral vs bacterial)

Treatment for Pneumonias	
CAP	
Outpatient	Previously Healthy And No Antibiotics In Past 3 Months
	Clarithromycin (500 mg po bid) or azithromycin (500 mg po once, then 250 mg qd)] x 5 days *or* Doxycycline (100 mg po bid) x 5 days
	Comorbidities (CHF, CRF, COPD, DM) Or Antibiotics In Past 3 Months: Select An Alternative From A Different Class
	Moxifloxacin (400 mg po qd) or Levofloxacin (750 mg po qd)] *or* Amoxicillin (1 g tid) + Azithromycin 500mg PO once then 250mg daily
Hospitalized	Medical Ward
	Moxifloxacin (400 mg po or iv daily) or levofloxacin (750 mg po or IV daily) or An antipseudomonal β-lactam [cefotaxime (1-2 g iv q8h), ceftriaxone (1-2 g IV QD), ampicillin-sulbactam (1-2 g iv q4 6h), ertapenem (1 g IV QD in selected patients)] *plus* a macrolide [oral clarithromycin or azithromycin (as listed above for previously healthy patients) or iv azithromycin (1 g once, then 500 mg qd)] ***In patients with severe CAP, consider addition of steroids*

ICU

- An antipseudomonal β-lactam [cefotaxime (1–2 g iv q8h), ceftriaxone (2 g iv qd), ampicillin-sulbactam (2 g iv q8h)]
  plus
  Azithromycin

  or

  Fluoroquinolone (as listed above for inpatients, non-icu)

Special Considerations

- If pseudomonas is a consideration
  - An antipneumococcal, antipseudomonal β-lactam [piperacillin/tazobactam (4.5 g iv q6h), cefepime (1–2 g iv q12h), imipenem (500 mg iv q6h), meropenem (1 g iv q8h)] plus either ciprofloxacin (400 mg iv q12h) or levofloxacin (750 mg iv qd)
- If CA-MRSA is a consideration
  - Add linezolid (600 mg iv q12h) or vancomycin (1 g iv q12h) NOT tigecycline

HAP

Organisms

Staph aureus, strep pneumoniae MRSA, enteric gram negative rods (enterobacter species, e. Coli, klebsiella, proteus species, serratia marcescens), Haemophilus influenzae, anaerobes, pseudomonas aeruginosa, acinetobacter, fungi (candida, aspergillus) in neutropenic patients

No MDR Risk Factors

- Cefepime 2g IV q8h
- Pip-Tazo 4.5g IV q6h
- Levofloxacin 750mg IV daily (same dose po when tolerating oral intake) x 8 days
- Imipenam 500mg IV q6h

If risk factors for MRSA present then add

Vancomycin 15 mg/kg IV q8-12h (goal trough 15-20 mg/mL) -or- Linezolid 600mg IV q12h

MDR Risk Factors (Treat For 7 Days)

Consider using 2 agents (from different classes) that target Pseudomonas aeruginosa and other gram-negative bacteria as well as one agent effective against MRSA

Anti-Pseudomonal Coverage				MRSA Coverage
Beta-lactam/beta-lactam-like		Non-beta-lactams		
piperacillin-tazobactam 4.5 g IV q6h cefepime or ceftazidime 2 g IV q8h imipenem 500 mg IV q6h meropenem 1 g IV q8h aztreonam 2 g IV q8h	+	Levofloxacin 750 mg IV daily Ciprofloxacin 400 mg IV q8h Amikacin 15-20 mg/kg IV daily Tobramycin 5-7 mg/kg IV daily	+	Vancomycin 15 mg/kg IV q8-12h (target trough levels of 15-20 mg/mL) Linezolid 600 mg IV q12h

Legionella

Add macrolide (iv erythromycin or azithromycin)

Aspiration *(See Below For More)*

- Must cover for anaerobic bacteria
- If no infiltrates are present on CXR after 72 hours can stop ABx if they were started empirically
- Clindamycin 600mg iv q8h followed by 300mg po qid (or 450mg po tid) x 7-10 days
- Alternate: amoxicillin-clavulanate 875mg po bid x 7-10 days
- Increase duration if cavitation is present

MSSA

Nafcillin 2 g iv q4h or oxacillin 2 g iv q4h

Fungal Component/Neutropenic

- Add amphotericin b (traditional 1st line agent)
  - Consider alternatives such as itraconazole, voriconazole, caspofungin as less side effects (similar efficacy per RCT)

ESBL

imipenem-cilastatin, ertapenem, meropenem, or doripenem

HIV Positive Patient

- Organisms:
  S. Pneumoniae, h. Influenzae, PCP, m. Tuberculosis, aerobic gnrs (e. Coli, klebsiella), MAI, fungi (cryptococcus, histoplasmosis), CMV, toxoplasmosis

Use therapy for cap and high-dose trimethoprim/sulfamethoxazole to cover PCP (add prednisone for $PaO2<70$) and high-dose ganciclovir to cover CMV

ASPIRATION PNEUMONIA

- **Definition**
  - Infection of lungs caused by inhalation of oropharyngeal material
  - When you inhale steril gastric material, more likely to result in chemical damage rather than infection, thus called pneumonitis
- **Pathogenesis**
  - Most commonly involves GNR rather than anaerobes
  - Biggest risk factors are ↓LOC (alcohol, narcotics, stroke, seizure), dysphagia (malignancy, strictures), GERD, vomiting
- **Presentation**
  - Presentation of true anaerobic pneumonia similar to that of tuberculosis (eg, subacute presentation, low-grade smoldering symptoms, cavitary changes indicated on chest imaging)
  - Patients have vague symptoms of fever, malaise, MS changes, productive cough
  - Look for foul smelling sputum suggestive of anaerobic disease
  - PE shows patients with fever, tachypnea, hypoxemia (new O2 requirement) with diminished breath sounds often on R
- **Imaging**
  - RLL apical segment, RUL inferior segment
  - Look for cavitations and abscesses
- **Labs**
  - CBC, CXR, sputum cultures, swallow study (speech pathology consult; consider modified barium swallow as well)
  - If left shift noted, consider pro-calcitonin
- **Diagnosis**
  - Hypoxemia
  - Fever
  - Leukocytosis
  - CXR infiltrates in the apical RLL and inferior RUL
- **Treatment**
  - if patient not in acute respiratory failure and history of large aspiration event documented, antibiotics not recommended
  - if only gastric contents aspirated, resolution fast (within 24-72 hr) compared with bacterial infection
  - ABx

    ABx with gram-positive coverage usually kill some gram-positive oral anaerobes
    - Fluoroquinolones: Moxifloxacin 400mg qd, Levofloxacin 500mg qd
    - 3rd gen cephalosporins: Ceftriaxone 1-2g IV qd
    - Clindamycin 600mg IV qd
  - Combination therapy
    - Addition of ACEi (ramipril 5mg qd) and amantadine (50mg BID) in patients with dysphagia who are geriatrics may help in recovery

LINE INFECTIONS

- Infected iv catheters are usually due to gram positive cocci, most often coagulase-negative staphylococcus or s. Aureus[65]
- Empirically treat with vancomycin
- If severe sepsis without another obvious source, remove CVC
- Remove CVC if any evidence of infection at catheter site

CARDIOLOGY

HOW TO READ AN EKG

1. **Background**
   - Paper
     - Each small box represents 1mm, and is 0.04 seconds
     - This means that one large box, which is comprised of 5 small boxes, represents 5mm, or 0.2 seconds
     - Each small box is 1mm / 1mV tall
   - Normal ECG Complex
     - P Wave. Caused by depolarization of the atria. With normal sinus rhythm, the P wave is upright in leads I, II, aVF, V4, V5, and V6 and inverted in aVR.
       - Best read in leads II, III → ensure normal morphology
       - AVR should have inverted p wave
       - *Above 3 together = NSR*
     - QRS Complex. Represents ventricular depolarization
     - Q Wave. The first negative deflection of the QRS complex (not always present and, if present, may be pathologic)

        - R Wave. The first positive deflection (R) is the positive deflection that sometimes occurs after the S wave)
        - S Wave. The negative deflection following the R wave
        - T Wave. Caused by repolarization of the ventricles and follows the QRS complex.
        - Normally upright in leads I, II, V3, V4, V5, and V6 and inverted in aVR
    - <u>Axis Deviation</u>
        - The QRS axis is midway between two leads that have QRS complexes of equal amplitude, or the axis is 90 degrees to the lead in which the QRS is isoelectric, that is, the amplitude of the R wave equals the amplitude of the S wave.
        - Normal Axis. QRS positive in I and aVF (0–90 degrees). Normal axis is actually –30 to 105 degrees
        - LAD. QRS positive in I and negative in aVF, –30 to –90 degrees. Seen with LVH, LAHB (–45 to –90 degrees), LBBB, and in some healthy individuals
        - RAD. QRS negative in I and positive in aVF, +105 to +180 degrees. Seen with RVH, RBBB, COPD, and acute PE (a sudden change in axis toward the right), as well as in healthy individuals (occasionally)
        - Extreme Right Axis Deviation. QRS negative in I and negative in aVF, +180 to +270 or –90 to –180 degrees
    - <u>Bipolar Leads</u>
        - Lead I: Left arm to right arm
        - Lead II: Left leg to right arm
        - Lead III: Left leg to left arm
    - <u>Precordial Leads</u>: V1 to V6 across the chest
    - <u>ECG Paper</u>: With the ECG machine set at 25 mm/s, each small box represents 0.04 s and each large box 0.2s. Most ECG machines automatically print a standardization mark.

2. **<u>Introduction</u>**
    - <u>Standardization</u>. With the ECG machine set on 1 mV, a 10-mm standardization mark (0.1 mV/mm) is evident
    - <u>Axis</u>. If the QRS is upright (more positive than negative) in leads I and aVF, the axis is normal. The normal axis range is –30 degrees to +105 degrees.
    - <u>Intervals</u>. Determine the PR, QRS, and QT intervals (Figure 19–2). Intervals are measured in the limb leads.
        - The PR should be 0.12–0.20 s
        - The QRS, <0.12 s.
        - The QT interval increases with decreasing heart rate, usually <0.44 s. The QT interval usually does not exceed one half of the RR interval (the distance between two R waves).
    - <u>Rate</u>. Count the number of QRS cycles in a 6-s strip and multiply it by 10 to roughly estimate the rate. If the rhythm is regular, you can be more exact in determining the rate by dividing 300 by the number of 0.20-s intervals (usually depicted by darker shading) and then extrapolating for any fraction of a 0.20-s segment.
        - *Bradycardia*: Heart rate <60 bpm
        - *Tachycardia*: Heart rate >100 bpm

3. <u>Rhythm</u>. Determine whether each QRS is preceded by a P wave, look for variation in the PR interval and RR interval (the duration between two QRS cycles), and look for ectopic beats.
    - **Sinus Rhythms**
        - *Normal*: P waves (which are positive in II and negative in aVR) with a regular PR and RR interval and a rate between 60 and 100 bpm. There should be one P wave for every QRS wave. Understand that truly "regular" rhythm is ultimately under the influence of the autonomic nervous system therefore variations may exist on the paper due to this, and or the patients respiratory cycle.
        - *Sinus Tachycardia*: Normal sinus rhythm with a heart rate >100 bpm and <180 bpm Clinical Correlations. Anxiety, exertion, pain, fever, hypoxia, hypotension, increased sympathetic tone (secondary to drugs with adrenergic effects [eg, epinephrine]), anticholinergic effect (eg, atropine), PE, COPD, AMI, CHF, hyperthyroidism, and others
        - *Sinus Bradycardia*: Normal sinus rhythm with a heart rate <60 bpm. Clinical Correlations. Well-trained athlete, normal variant, secondary to medications (eg,

beta-blockers, digitalis, clonidine), hypothyroidism, hypothermia, sick sinus syndrome (tachy–brady syndrome), and others

- *Sinus Arrhythmia*: Normal sinus rhythm with a somewhat irregular heart rate. Inspiration causes a slight increase in rate; expiration decreases the rate. Normal variation between inspiration and expiration is 10% or less.
  - **Atrial Arrhythmias**
    - PAC: Ectopic atrial focus firing prematurely followed by a normal QRS. The compensatory pause following the PAC is partial; the RR interval between beats 4 and 6 is less than between beats 1 and 3 or 6 and 8.
      - Clinical Correlations. Usually not of clinical significance; can be caused by stress, caffeine, and myocardial disease
    - PAT: A run of three or more consecutive PACs. The heart rate is usually between 140 and 250 bpm. The P wave may not be visible, but the RR interval is very regular.
      - Clinical Correlations. Can be seen in healthy individuals but also occurs with a variety of heart diseases. Symptoms include palpitations, lightheadedness, and syncope.
      - Treatment: Increase Vagal Tone. Valsalva maneuver or carotid massage.
        - Medical Treatment. Can include adenosine, verapamil, digoxin, edrophonium, or beta-blockers (propranolol, metoprolol, and esmolol). Verapamil and beta-blockers should be used cautiously at the same time because asystole can occur.
        - Cardioversion with Synchronized DC Shock. Particularly in the hemodynamically unstable patient
    - MAT: An atrial arrhythmia that originates from ectopic atrial foci. It is characterized by varying P-wave morphology and PR interval and is irregular.
      - Clinical Correlations. Most commonly associated with COPD, also seen in elderly patients, CHF, diabetes, or use of theophylline. Antiarrhythmics are often ineffective. Treat the underlying disease.
    - AFib: Irregularly irregular rhythm with no discernible P waves. The ventricular rate usually varies between 100 and 180 bpm. The ventricular response is slower with digoxin, verapamil, or beta-blocker therapy and with AV nodal disease.
      - Clinical Correlations. Seen in some healthy individuals but commonly associated with organic heart disease (CAD, hypertensive heart disease, or rheumatic mitral valve disease), thyrotoxicosis, alcohol abuse, pericarditis, PE, and postoperatively.
      - Treatment
        - Pharmacologic Therapy. Intravenous adenosine, verapamil, digoxin, and betablockers (propranolol, metoprolol, and esmolol) can be used to slow down the ventricular response, and quinidine, procainamide, propafenone, ibutilide, and amiodarone can be used to maintain or convert to sinus rhythm.
        - DC-Synchronized Cardioversion. Indicated if associated with increased myocardial ischemia, hypotension, or pulmonary edema
    - Atrial Flutter: Characterized by sawtooth flutter waves with an atrial rate between 250 and 350 bpm; the rate may be regular or irregular depending on whether the atrial impulses are conducted through the AV node at a regular interval or at a variable interval.
      - **Example**: One ventricular contraction (QRS) for every two flutter waves = 2:1 flutter.
      - **Clinical Correlations**. Seen with valvular heart disease, pericarditis, ischemic heart disease, pulmonary disease including PE, and alcohol abuse
      - **Treatment**.
        - Diltiazem is considered drug of choice for rate control (↑AV node refractoriness)
          - Dilt drip (*Diltiazem Atrial Fibrillation/Atrial Flutter Study Group*):

            - IV bolus 0.25 mg/kg over 2 minutes
            - Wait 15 minutes
            - Second bolus of 0.35mg/kg over 2 minutes if first dose tolerated, but inadeq. Response
            - Continuous infusion @ 10-15 mg/h
            - Expect response in 4-5 minutes
          - Monotherapy with PO: 30mg q6h ↑ to max 360 mg/day
            - Calculate monotherapy from drip dose by totaling drip dose over 24 hours then providing that dose through long acting qd Diltiazem (Tiazac)
        - Rate control with BB or CCB.
        - Amiodarone used to slow AV node conduction.
        - Digoxin used to enhance vagal tone.
  - **Nodal Rhythm**
    - AV Junctional or Nodal Rhythm: Rhythm originates in the AV node. Often associated with retrograde P waves that may precede or follow the QRS. If the P wave is present, it is negative in lead II and positive in aVR (just the opposite of normal sinus rhythm). Three or more premature junctional beats in a row constitute a junctional tachycardia, which has the same clinical significance as PAT
    - AVNRT – pseudo R' in V1 or pseudo S in II/III/AVF; commonly presents as SVT with short RP interval.
    - AVRT – ST elevation in AVR; commonly presents as SVT with short RP interval.
  - **Ventricular Arrhythmias**
    - PVC: As implied by the name, a premature beat arising in the ventricle that is caused by **presence of a re-entrant circuit at the level of the Purkinje fibers**. P waves may be present but have no relation to the QRS of the PVC. The QRS is usually >0.12 s with a left bundle branch pattern. A compensatory pause follows a PVC that is usually longer than after a PAC. The RR interval between beats 1 and 3 is equal to that between beats 3 and 5. Thus, the pause following the PVC (the fourth beat) is fully compensatory. The following patterns are recognized:
      - *Bigeminy*. One normal sinus beat followed by one PVC in an alternating fashion
      - *Trigeminy*. Sequence of two normal beats followed by one PVC
      - *Unifocal PVCs*. Arise from one site in the ventricle. Each has the same configuration in a single lead.
      - *Multifocal PVCs*. Arise from different sites; therefore, have different shapes
      - *Clinical Correlations*. PVCs occur in healthy persons and with excessive caffeine ingestion, anemia, anxiety, organic heart disease (ischemic, valvular, or hypertensive), secondary to medications (epinephrine and isoproterenol; from toxic level of digitalis and theophylline), or predisposing metabolic abnormalities (hypoxia, hypokalemia, acidosis, alkalosis, or hypomagnesemia)
      - *Criteria for Treatment*. In the setting of an AMI:
        - >5 PVCs in 1 min (many clinicians would treat any PVC associated with an MI or injury pattern on ECG)
        - PVCs in couplets (two in a row)
        - Numerous multifocal PVCs
        - PVC that falls on the preceding T wave (R on T)
      - *Treatment*
        - Lidocaine. Most commonly used; other antiarrhythmics include procainamide, and amiodarone.
        - Treatment of aggravating cause often sufficient (eg, treat hypoxia, hypokalemia, or acidosis
    - Ventricular Tachycardia:
      - By definition, **three or more beats with QRS>0.12sec at rate of >100 bpm**.
        - Sustained: >30 seconds
      - **Types**
        - Monomorphic – due to circuit through region of old myocardial infarction

    - Polymorphic – active ischemia vs. electrolyte disturbance vs. drugs that prolong QT (torsades)
    - AIVR – wide complex @ 40-100bpm; occur after reperfusion in acute MI or ↑symp tone; no tx necessary
  - **Work up**
    - Check patient's magnesium and potassium levels
    - Hypoxia, hypoventilation
    - Ischemia
  - **Treatment**
    - *Stable*
      - EF<40%
        - Amiodarone 150mg load x1 order (IVPB); Amio gtt AMOUNT: 900; comment: 1.8mg/ml (33.3ml/hr) x 6 hours then decrease to 0.5mg/min (16.6ml/hr)
        - Lidocaine 1-1.5mg/kg IVP then 1-4mg/min maintenance, or cardioversion
      - EF>40%: Procainamide 20-30mg/min IVP then 1-4mg/min maintenance, Amiodarone
    - *Unstable*
      - Rapid defibrillation (up to 3 shocks)
      - If persists, use Epinephrine (1mg IVP q3min) with alternations with vasopressin 40U IVP as single bolus
      - If persists, use Amiodarone, Procainamide, Lidocaine
      - Consider AICD placement in patient that survives for long-term protection from sudden death if repeat TTE in 40 days confirms low EF
- AIVR
  - Benign
  - Not treated successfully with antiarrhythmics
  - Wide-complex, usually has a rate of 60-110bpm vs. 120-250bpm seen with VT
  - *Caused by presence of a ventricular focus that assumes control over the SA node because it is shooting faster; can be sign of early AV block; marker of spontaneous/induced reperfusion of the myocardium*
- Ventricular Fibrillation: Erratic electrical activity from the ventricles, which fibrillate or twitch asynchronously. No cardiac output occurs with this rhythm.
  - *Clinical Correlations*. One of two patterns seen with cardiac arrest (the other would be asystole or flat line)
- Supraventricular Tachycardia-
  - Defined as HR≥100 with short QRS (<120ms)
  - Multiple causes: Atrial fibrillation, Atrial flutter, Multifocal Atrial Tachycardia (MAT), Atrial Tachycardia (AT), AVNRT (AV nodal re-entrant tachycardia), AVRT (AV re-entrant tachycardia), Sinus tachycardia (ST)
    - AVNRT – most common cause; two different pathways exist to the AV node (fast and slow)
    - AVRT – accessory pathway exists which is faster than normal pathway to ventricle (not limited by AV node; thus it bypasses the AV node which would normally slow down and regulate the electrical signal)
      - Two types: orthodromic and antidromic
        - Orthodromic – travels to AV node normally but then returns back to atria via fast path
        - Antidromic – travels to ventricle via fast path and returns to atria via the slow normal path
    - AT and ST – abnormal cells in the atria automatically fire independent of the SA node; this is what differs it from ST where the original source of stimulation is from the SA node.
    - MAT – common in patients with chronic lung conditions causing RA enlargement causing a classic EKG appearance with 3 different P wave morphologies.
    - Afib/AFlutt – defined elsewhere in book

Steps to Identification

Recommended step by step approach to identification of SVT is to (1) first determine if you have a narrow complex tachycardia (NCT) which is suggestive of SVT or a wide complex tachycardia (WCT) which can be SVT with aberrancy due to a BBB or VT/paced/artifact. Next, (2) determine if you have a regular or irregular rhythm and then (3) identify if P waves exist and if they do (4) see if their morphology is the same or if it changes between beats.

- <u>NCT with regular rhythm</u>
  - First determine the RP interval
  - Short RP: AVNRT vs Orthodromic Tachycardia (ORT; may have delta wave)
  - Long RP: AT, ST
- <u>NCT with irregular rhythm</u>
  - No P waves → Afib
  - P waves present
    - Sawtooth: AFlutt
    - 3 Different P waves: MAT

- <u>Management</u>
  - Stable and regular → vagal and consider adenosine 6mg IVP; avoid CCB if WPW
  - Stable and irregular WCT → avoid BB/CCB if AF with pre-excited tachy → instead consider ibutilide
  - Unstable → synchronized cardioversion
  - AVNRT → BB or cardioablation
  - AVRT/ORT → cardioablation; avoid AV nodal blockers

Figure. Regular vs irregular NCT and management

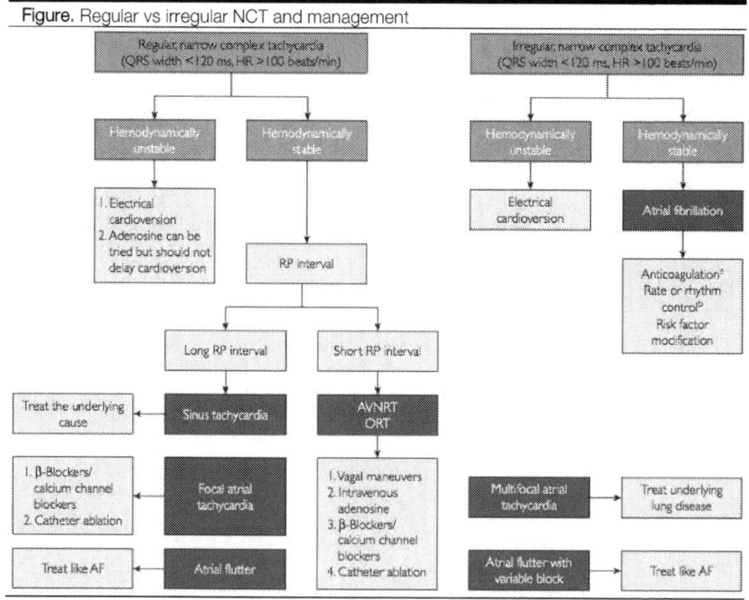

4. <u>Hypertrophy</u>
   - **Atrial hypertrophy:**
     - Right = biphasic P in precordium or > 3 mm in II, III.
     - Left = P duration > 0.12 sec, biphasic in V1 or notched in II, III.

Determining infarct location based on EKG signs				
Leads	Wall Affected	EKG Changes	Artery involved	Reciprocal Lead Changes
II, III, aVF	Inferior	Q, S-T, T	RCA (90%) CIRC (10%)	I, aVL
	With any inferior MI, always consider the following complications: 1) AV node dysfunction 2) Posterior MI 3) RV infarction			
I, aVL	High lateral	Q, S-T, T	Early Diagnosis Circ branch	V1, V3
I, aVL, V5-6	Lateral	Q, S-T, T	Diagonal branch-LAD Circ Early marginal	I, III, aVF
V1-4, I, aVL	Anterior	Q, S-T, T Loss of R progr.	LAD	
V1-2 (more than inferior leads)	Posterior	R>S S-T depression T wave depress.	RCA Circ	
V3-V6	Apical	Q,S-T-T Loss of septal R in V1	LAD RCA	
I, aVL, V5-6	Anterolateral	Q, S-T, T	LAD Circ	I, III, aVF
V1-4	Anteroseptal	Q, S-T, T Loss of septal R in V1	LAD	

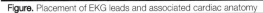

Figure. Placement of EKG leads and associated cardiac anatomy

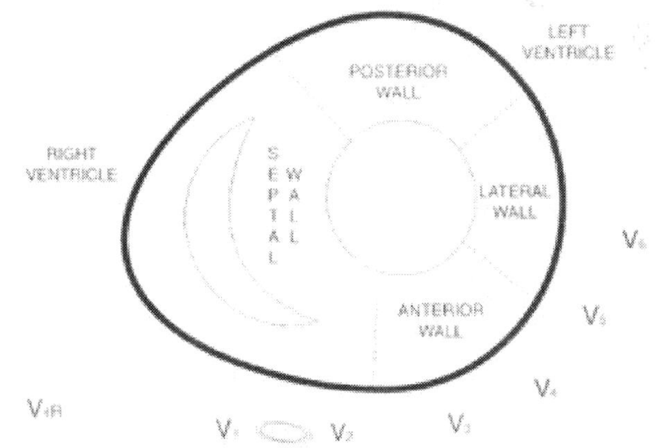

- **Fascicular Block**
  - **LAFB** – LAD in conjunction with negative overall deflection in lead II and III (rS)
  - **LPFB** – RAD in conjunction with positive overall deflection in lead II and III (qR)

- **Ventricular hypertrophy**

Cornell Criteria	
Males	Females
S in V3 + R in AVL > 28mm	S in V3 + R in AVL > 20mm

Sokolow Criteria
S wave in V1 + R wave in V5/V6 > 35mm

5. Infarction or Ischemia. Check for the presence of ST-segment elevation or depression, Q waves, inverted T waves, and poor R-wave progression in the precordial leads.
   - **Inferior infarctions** must be further analyzed to r/o posterior or RV infarction[67, 68]
     - RV Infarction – d/t complication of RCA pts present with hypotension and ↑JVP but **clear lung fields**
       - Indications for RV wall infarction include:
         - ST elevation in inferior leads
         - ST elevation in V1
         - RBBB
         - 2 or 3rd degree AVB
         - Hypotension, clear lung fields
       - EKG Lead Placement:

         1) V1R: 4th ICS at left sternal border
         2) V2R: 4th ICS at right sternal border
         3) V3R: halfway between V2R and V4R on a diagonal line
         4) V4R: 5th ICS, right midclavicular line
         5) V5R: right anterior axillary line, same horizontal line as V4R and V6R
         6) V6R: right mid-axillary line; same horizonal line as V5R and V6R

Figure. EKG lead placement when evaluating for right ventricular infarction

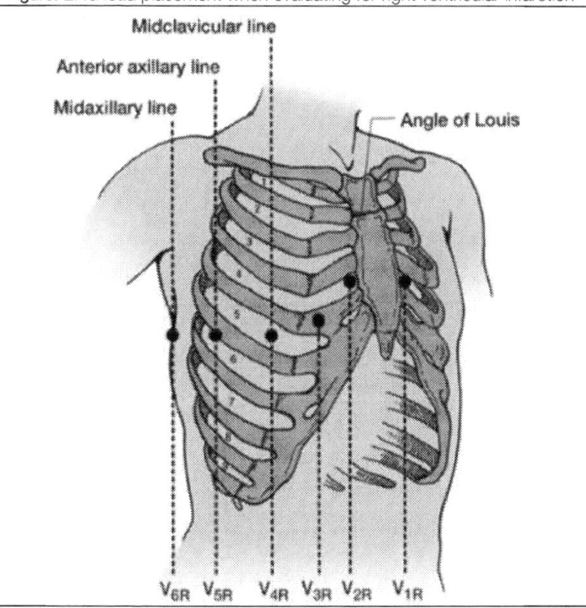

- The ST-segment elevation in **V4R** is a strong independent predictor of major complications and in-hospital mortality.

- Treatment:
  - The initial therapy of a patient with RVI, who has hypotension and no pulmonary congestion, should start with **volume expansion**, often by infusion of isotonic saline to increase the filling of the right ventricle which in turn will increase the filling of the underfilled left ventricle and increase cardiac output. Avoid nitroglycerin!
  - For patients who are unresponsive to initial trial of fluids, hemodynamic monitoring may be necessary, and subsequent volume challenge may be appropriate if the estimated central venous pressure is < 15 mmHg.

- Posterior Infarction[69]
  - In patients presenting with ischemic symptoms, horizontal ST depression in the anteroseptal leads (V1-3) with tall R waves should raise the suspicion of posterior MI.
    - Horizontal ST depression
    - Tall, broad R waves (>30ms)
    - Upright T waves
    - Dominant R wave (R/S ratio > 1) in V2
  - **Posterior infarction is confirmed by the presence of ST elevation and Q waves in the posterior leads (V7-9).**
    - Leads V7-9 are placed on the posterior chest wall in the following positions:
      - V7 – Left posterior axillary line, in the same horizontal plane as V6.
      - V8 – Tip of the left scapula, in the same horizontal plane as V6.
      - V9 – Left paraspinal region, in the same horizontal plane as V6.

Figure. Placement of posterior thoracic EKG leads in suspected posterior infarction

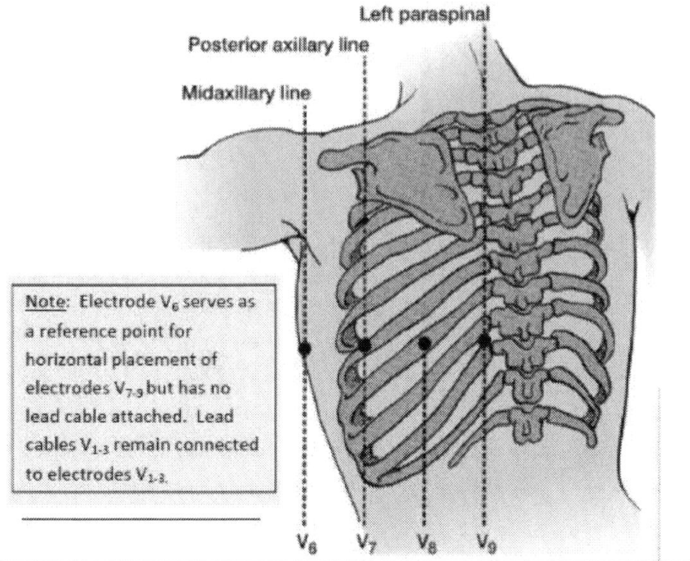
Left paraspinal
Posterior axillary line
Midaxillary line
Note: Electrode V_6 serves as a reference point for horizontal placement of electrodes V_{7-9} but has no lead cable attached. Lead cables V_{1-3} remain connected to electrodes V_{1-3}.
V_6
V_7
V_8
V_9

2. **Bundle Branch Blocks**[70]
    - If the electrical impulse traveling down the bundle of his (BIH) is unable to travel down the right bundle due to a RBBB, then it will go down the intact left bundle.
        - The impulse travels fast down the intact left bundle and then moves slowly up towards the right. This slow depolarization to the right ventricle causes it to contract, but now takes slightly longer than the left and leads to a prolonged QRS. This slow swing of electricity to the right may cause a right axis deviation.
    - If the electrical impulse traveling down the bundle of his (BIH) is unable to travel down the left bundle due to a LBBB, then it will go down the intact right bundle.
        - The impulse travels fast down the intact right bundle and then moves slowly up towards the left. This slow depolarization to the left ventricle causes it to contract, but now takes slightly longer than the right and leads to a prolonged QRS. This slow swing of electricity to the right may cause a left axis deviation.
        - May cause poor R-wave progression

LBBB	RBBB
QRS > 0.12	QRS > 0.12
V1: Q wave or QRS mostly negative	V1: QRS with a RSR pattern or mostly positive
T wave inversion in all or some of the leads over the left : V5, V6, I, and aVL	T wave inversion in all or some of the leads over the right V1, V2, and V3

3. **Poor R-wave progression**[71]
    - Physiology
        - Electrical depolarization from the AV node often moves down through the ventricles in a L→R direction
        - As a result, the initial vector seen is an small R wave in V1-3

      - At V3-4, known as transition zone, the QRS complex changes from a predominantly negative to predominantly positive pattern
        - The R/S ratio becomes >1
        - The R wave should be >2mm by V3, if not 2-4mm tall by V3-4, this is known as **poor r-wave progression**
  - Cause
    - Commonly due to anterior MI, LBBB, or LVH

AORTIC STENOSIS

- **Etiology**
  - Most often caused by bicuspid valve or calcification
  - RF is a rare cause now in the US but can be seen in third world countries
- **Pathogenesis**
  - Atherosclerosis forms on the cusps of valve
- **What it leads to**
  - LVH
  - Heart failure
  - Arrhythmias (→MR→LA dilation)
  - Syncope
- **PE Findings**
  - Crescendo-decrescendo murmur with peak in systole
  - Thrill noted in murmur is seen with advanced disease
- **Diagnosis**
  - TTE (if murmur grade 3/6 or more; or symptomatic)
  - Catherization may be done as well to assess for further coronary artery disease
  - BNP
  - Elevated or serially increasing BNP predicts short-term need for valve replacement in asymptomatic severe aortic stenosis

Degree of Aortic Stenosis			
	Aortic Jet Velocity	Mean Transvalvular Pressure Gradient	Aortic Valve Area
Normal	< 2.5 meters/second	N/A	3-4 cm2
Mild	2.5-2.9 meters/second	< 25 mm Hg	1.5-2 cm2
Moderate	3-4 meters/second	25-40 mm Hg	1-1.5 cm2
Severe	> 4 meters/second	> 40 mm Hg	< 1 cm2

- **Treatment**
  - Medical
    - Options: BB, diuretics, digoxin, AAEi, ARB
    - Chest pain: use beta blockers
    - Avoid aggressive decrease in preload
    - Caution in use of vasodilators due to risk of preload reduction
    - AAE inhibitors associated with hypotension, risk is low
  - Surgical
    - Balloon Valvuloplasty
      - Palliative measure if not surgical candidate for TAVR or as a bridge to TAVR
      - Not a definitive treatment due to ↑ rates of restenosis
      - Consider in: patients refusing surgery, short life expectancy, in severe HF, pregnancy

- AVR improves survival and indicated if:
  - Severe stenosis with symptoms
  - Planned to have CABG
  - LVEF < 50%
  - While mechanical valves require longer anticoagulation, they are associated with ↓ reoperation rates
- TAVI is a new option

- **Prevention**
  - Treat for strep pharyngitis
  - No ABx prophylaxis indicated
  - TTE monitoring if asymptomatic (3-5 if mild; 1-2 if mod; yearly if severe)

CONGESTIVE HEART FAILURE

Contributor: Robert Pangilinan, MD, Jone Flanders, DO, Irena Crook, MD[72,111,73,74,75,76,77]

- **Definition**
  - HF is a clinical syndrome characterized by typical symptoms (e.g. breathlessness, ankle swelling and fatigue) that may be accompanied by signs (e.g. elevated jugular venous pressure, pulmonary crackles and peripheral oedema) caused by a structural and/or functional cardiac abnormality, resulting in either preserved (EF>50%), reduced (EF<40%) or mixed range (EF 40-50%) cardiac output and/or elevated intracardiac pressures at rest or during stress.
    1) Heart failure with reduced ejection fraction, or HFrEF (LVEF<40%, HF-rEF)
    2) Heart failure with preserved ejection fraction, HFpEF (LVEF≥50%, HF-pEF)
    3) Any percentage between 40-50% is classified as mixed range

American Heart Association Stages of Heart Failure[78]	
Stage	Definition
Emphasize development and progression of the disease	
Stage A	At risk (HTN, DM, cardiotoxic rx) for heart failure but without structural heart disease or symptoms
Stage B	Asymptomatic but has structural heart disease (prior MI, valvular dz, LV enlargement, low EF)
Stage C	Structural heart disease is present, AND symptoms have occurred
Stage D	Presence of advanced heart disease (EF <30%) with continued heart failure symptoms at rest (inability to exercise, <300m on 6 min walk) requiring aggressive medical therapy (refractory) often with ≥ 1 hospitalization in past 6 months

New York Heart Association Functional Classification of Congestive Heart Failure		
Focuses on exercise capacity and symptomatic status		
Class I:	None	Patients with cardiac disease but asymptomatic
Class II:	Mild	Patients with cardiac disease that causes symptoms with normal physical activity
Class III:	Moderate	Patients with cardiac disease resulting in symptoms with ADLs; symptoms with moderate activity
Class IV:	Severe	Patients with cardiac disease resulting in symptoms at rest

- **Radiologic Findings**
  - Cardiomegaly

- Bilateral cephalization
- Blunting of the CPA
- ↑lung markings

Characteristics of HFpEF as Compared with HFrEF

Characteristic	HFpEF	HFrEF
Symptoms (dyspnea)	Yes	Yes
Congestive State (LE edema)	Yes	Yes
EF	Normal	↓
LV Mass	↑	↑
Relative Wall Thickness	↑	↓
EDV	Normal	↑
EDP	↑	↑
LA size	↑	↑
Exercise capacity	↓	↓
CO	↓	↓

- **Symptoms**
  - SOB
  - LE edema
  - Cough
  - Orthopnoea
  - ↓exercise tolerance
  - ↑JVP
  - PND
  - Ankle swelling
- **Diagnosis**
  Diagnosis is made based on clinical symptoms (along with radiographic as needed) along with echocardiographic findings
- **Exacerbation Factors**
  - Non-adherence to medical regimen with ↑Na and without fluid restriction
  - ACS
  - HTN (↑140/90)
  - AF and other arrhythmias (commonly leads to HFpEF)
  - Obesity (BMI >35, commonly leads to HFpEF)
  - Recent initiation of negative inotrope (CCB, BB)
  - PE
  - Pacemaker (commonly leads to HFpEF)
  - Initiation of steroids, NSAIDs
  - Illicit drugs (ie. cocaine), EtOH
  - DM, ↑thyroid, ↓thyroid
  - Infections
- **Assessment**
  - Baseline GFR is a better predictor of mortality than NYHA class or EF
    - Renal disease patients with concurrent LVH have accelerated rates of coronary events and uremia
  - Rapid history, vital signs, exam of neck, lungs, heart, extremities.
  - Determine if left-sided, right-sided, or both:

Symptoms in infarction based on infarct location	
Left Sided	Right Sided
Tachypnea	Elevated JVP
Rales	Hepatojugular reflex, RUQ tenderness, congestive hepatopathy
Left-sided S3	Ascites, peripheral edema

  - Sit patient up with legs off bed.
  - IV access
- **Evaluation**
  - <u>Inpatient Setting</u>
    - *Interventions*
      - STAT pulse ox (ABG)
      - EKG (if arrhythmia/ MI suspected).
    - *Imaging*
      - portable CXR
      - TTE to assess valve status and for hypertrophy along with LV cavity size
        - Can help distinguish systolic from diastolic heart failure
      - Can order CCTA if low risk (see page **Error! Bookmark not defined.**)
      - MPS or cardiac catheterization should be performed in patients with new diagnosis of CHF
      - PFTs (presence of COPD or PHTN)
    - *Labs*
      - CMP
        - BUN/SCr (r/o anemia 2/2 renal failure as ↑BUN/SCr may be seen with advanced disease due to cardiorenal syndrome)
        - K
        - Mg
      - CBC (leukocytosis → consider cultures as well, anemia)
      - TSH
      - LFTs
      - Lipid panel
      - Urinalysis
      - Iron panel
        - In patients with NYHA class II and III HF and iron deficiency (ferritin <100 ng/mL or 100 to 300 ng/mL if transferrin saturation is <20%), intravenous iron replacement might be reasonable to improve functional status and QoL.
      - TROP (and trended if initial is positive)
      - If high suspicion for drug use, obtain UDS (r/o cocaine) and EtOH (holiday heart)
      - Lactate – assess for decreased end organ perfusion
      - BNP vs. NT-proBNP (prohormone)
        - <100 excludes cardiac source
        - >400 likely CHF with BNP
        - >900 likely CHF with NT-proBNP
        - Falsely low in patients with elevated BMI
  - <u>Outpatient Setting</u>
    - *Interventions*
      - EKG (if arrhythmia/ MI suspected).

        - *Imaging*
            - PA/LAT CXR
            - TTE to assess valve status and for hypertrophy along with LV cavity size
                - Can help distinguish systolic from diastolic heart failure
            - Can order CCTA if low risk (see page **Error! Bookmark not defined.**)
            - MPS or cardiac catheterization should be performed in patients with new diagnosis of CHF
        - *Labs*
            - CMP
                - BUN/SCr (r/o anemia 2/2 renal failure as ↑BUN/SCr may be seen with advanced disease due to cardiorenal syndrome)
                - K
                - Mg
            - CBC (leukocytosis → consider cultures as well, anemia)
            - TSH
            - LFTs
            - Lipid panel
            - Urinalysis
            - Iron panel
                - In patients with NYHA class II and III HF and iron deficiency (ferritin <100 ng/mL or 100 to 300 ng/mL if transferrin saturation is <20%), intravenous iron replacement might be reasonable to improve functional status and QoL.
            - BNP vs. NT-proBNP (prohormone)
                - <100 excludes cardiac source
                - >400 likely CHF with BNP
                - >900 likely CHF with NT-proBNP
                - Falsely low in patients with elevated BMI

- **Admission Criteria**
    - This varies but patients with new onset CHF maybe considered for inpatient admission or expedited work up
    - Patients who are acutely symptomatic should be admitted
- **Discharge from ER Criteria**
    - Documented history of CHF and mild exacerbation
    - Return to baseline function s/p treatment
    - No evidence of dysrhythmia or infarction
    - Known cause: ie. medication noncompliance
    - Not requiring supplemental oxygen
- **Inpatient nursing interventions**
    - Maintain strict I/Os
    - Daily weights (for more accurate fluid management, weight loss may be seen with cardiac cachexia)
    - Heart healthy 2g Na diet
        - NPO if doing stress test
    - 1.5-2L fluid restriction
    - Frequent electrolyte checks
        - K due to Lasix
        - ↑Na seen with advanced disease
    - VS q4h (SBP <90 is seen with advanced disease)
- **Treatment**[79]
    - <u>Acute Decompensated (both HFpEF and HFrEF)</u>

Diuresis + NTG + Avoidance of antiarrhythmic drugs

- Diuresis
  - Goals of treatment for heart failure due to systolic dysfunction should be diuresis, afterload reduction and inotropy.

SCr x 40 = ### mg of IV Lasix

Jahanmir method

- Blood Pressure Control
  - IV NTG or paste (SBP 160-220 and no severe AS) with gtt if >220
  - Pressors (dobutamine 2 mcg/kg/min or milrinone) if ↑SCr and hypotensive
- Avoid Antiarrythmics
  - Amiodarone okay
- **Medications**
  - *See table on next few pages*
  - Avoid rate controlling CCB such as Diltiazem/verapamil
  - ACEi
  - Sacubitril/ARB should be initiated in the acute setting in patients with acute decompensated heart failure
  - BB (do not start if acute)
  - CAD management drugs
  - Aldactone/Eplerenone
  - Hydralazine+Isordil
- **Others**
  - Oxygen
  - Rx: Morphine, ACEi/ARB (see choices below),
  - Imaging
    - CXR, daily EKG, Stress testing if new diagnosis, TTE to evaluate for valvular disease, LA size for risk of AF, LV hypertrophy

Figure. Treatment for patients with HFrEF and stage C symptoms

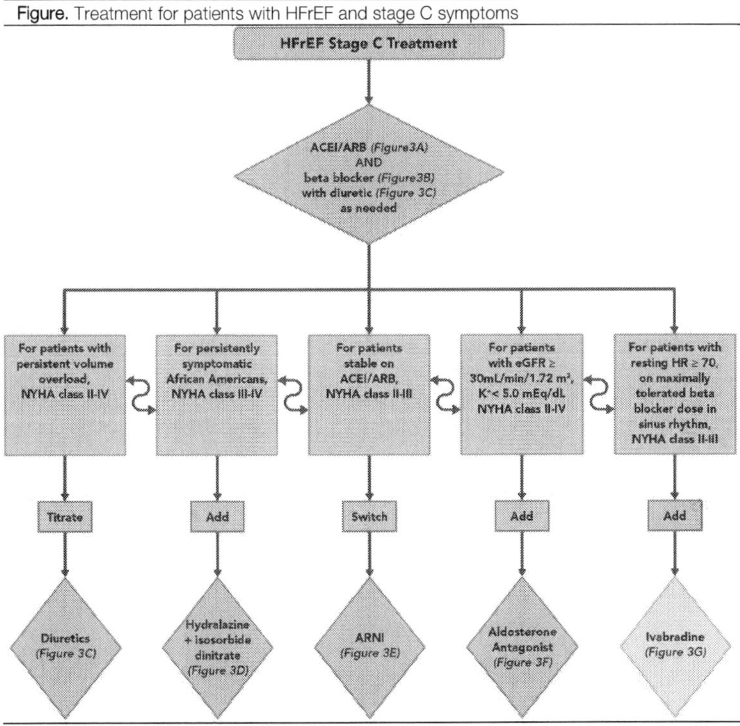

- Chronic
  - Treatment depends on HFrEF vs HFpEF
    - HFrEF has guideline based treatment regimens
    - HFpEF does not have clear guideline based evidence
  - Consults: Referral to cardiac rehab, heart failure clinic
  - **Iron Deficiency**
    - Common in patients with HFrEF (≤45%) and NYHA II-III symptoms
    - Look for ferritin <100 -or- (combination of ferritin 100-300 and saturation <20%) in the setting of HGB<10
    - Treatment
      - IV iron 1g on week 0 with additional 500mg (if wt 35-70kg on week 6) or 1000mg (if wt >70kg)
  - **HFrEF (previously termed 'systolic')**
    - ACEi/ARB
    - Should replace patients already on ACEi or ARB with combination sacubitril/valsartan
    - Start at lowest dose and increase dose every 2 weeks until maximum tolerated dose achieved.
    - If ACE-I not tolerated, can try ARB (angiotensin II receptor blocker) e.g. Losartan.
      - For patients with elevated blood pressure despite maximum ACE inhibitor and β-blocker dosing, consider adding an ARB in non-AA or the **combination of hydralazine and long acting nitrates in AA**-

Figure. When to consider addition of CRT or ICD in patients with HFrEF

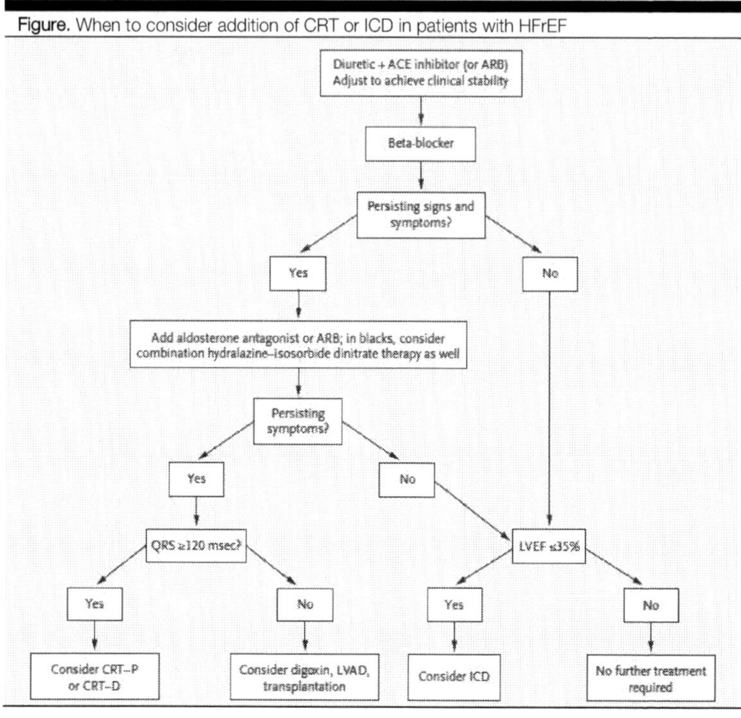

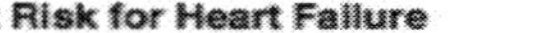

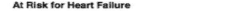

At Risk for Heart Failure

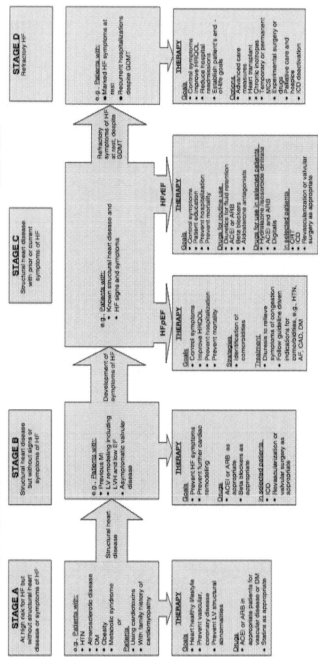

STAGE A
At high risk for HF but without structural heart disease or symptoms of HF

e.g., Patients with:
- HTN
- Atherosclerotic disease
- DM
- Obesity
- Metabolic syndrome

or

Patients
- Using cardiotoxins
- With family history of cardiomyopathy

THERAPY

Goals
- Heart healthy lifestyle
- Prevent vascular, coronary disease
- Prevent LV structural abnormalities

Drugs
- ACEI or ARB in appropriate patients for vascular disease or DM
- Statins as appropriate

→ Structural heart disease →

STAGE B
Structural heart disease but without signs or symptoms of HF

e.g., Patients with:
- Previous MI
- LV remodeling including LVH and low EF
- Asymptomatic valvular disease

THERAPY

Goals
- Prevent HF symptoms
- Prevent further cardiac remodeling

Drugs
- ACEI or ARB as appropriate
- Beta blockers as appropriate

In selected patients
- ICD
- Revascularization or valvular surgery as appropriate

→ Development of symptoms of HF →

Heart Failure

STAGE C
Structural heart disease with prior or current symptoms of HF

e.g., Patients with:
- Known structural heart disease and
- HF signs and symptoms

HFpEF

THERAPY

Goals
- Control symptoms
- Improve HRQOL
- Prevent hospitalization
- Prevent mortality

Strategies
- Identification of comorbidities

Treatment
- Diuresis to relieve symptoms of congestion
- Follow guideline driven indications for comorbidities, e.g., HTN, AF, CAD, DM

HFrEF

THERAPY

Goals
- Control symptoms
- Patient education
- Prevent hospitalization
- Prevent mortality

Drugs for routine use
- Diuretics for fluid retention
- ACEI or ARB
- Beta blockers
- Aldosterone antagonists

Drugs for use in selected patients
- Hydralazine /isosorbide dinitrate
- ACEI and ARB
- Digitalis

In selected patients
- CRT
- ICD
- Revascularization or valvular surgery as appropriate

→ Refractory symptoms of HF at rest, despite GDMT →

STAGE D
Refractory HF

e.g., Patients with:
- Marked HF symptoms at rest
- Recurrent hospitalizations despite GDMT

THERAPY

Goals
- Control symptoms
- Improve HRQOL
- Reduce hospital readmissions
- Establish patient's end - of-life goals

Options
- Advanced care measures
- Heart transplant
- Chronic inotropes
- Temporary or permanent MCS
- Experimental surgery or drugs
- Palliative care and hospice
- ICD deactivation

Pharmacologic therapy in Heart Failure

Type	Trials	Class Restriction	Starting Dose	Target Dose
ACEi	CONSENSUS SOLVD SAVE TRACE	I,II,III,IV	Captopril 6.25mg TID Enalapril 2.5mg BID Lisinopril 2.5-5mg/d Ramipril 1.25mg/d	50mg TID 10-20mg BID 20-40mg/d 10mg/d
First line therapy for afterload reduction in all pts with reduced EF (because heart failure is characterized by systemic vasoconstriction). If cannot be used d/t ↑SCr → use isosorbide denitrate-hydralazine instead. Start lowest dose and increase every 2 weeks until maximum tolerated dose achieved.				
Beta Blocker**	CIBIS-II[%] MERIT-HF[#] COPERNICUS[$] CAPRICORN SAVE REVERT COMET → *carvedilol>lopressor*	I, II, III, iV	Carvedilol[B1] 1.25mg daily (10mg daily) Bisoprolol 1.25mg daily (10mg) Metoprolol succinate[B2] 12.5mg-25mg/d (200mg/d)	10mg 10mg 200mg
Only initiate when patient stable; Help decrease remodeling, ↓mortality, and prevent further adrenergic mediated dysfunction. Offer to patients with LVEF < 40% and no contraindications (dyspneic, signs of congestion, hemodynamically unstable). Target HR<64; titrate up every 2-4 weeks. Carvedilol specifically is good in patients with nonischemic cardiomyopathy.				
Aldosterone Antagonists	RALES EPHESUS EMPHASIS-HF	II-IV and with EF<35% or	Eplerenone 25 mg daily or QOD Aldactone 25 mg	50 mg 100 mg

		Post-STEMI+EF<40% -and- Symptomatic CHF or DM	Metolazone 2.5	10mg
			Spironolactone 12.5-25mg daily (goal K≤5) (↓dose if GFR<50)	25-50mg
Indicated for patients with continued symptomatic HF and LVSD and those who develop LVSD after MI on maximum therapy of ACEi/ARB and BB. Beware ↑K. Spironolactone is 2x as powerful as eplerenone. Often used in combination with loops to increase diuresis. Eplerenone is used for Class II, Spironolactone used for III, or IV.				
Combination ARB+Neprilysin Inhibitor	PARADIGM-HF	II or III with EF<40% and can tolerate ACEi/ARB	Valsartan-sacubitril 24/26mg BID or 49/51mg BID	After 2-4 weeks double the dose to maintenance of 97/103mg PO BID
Indicated to reduce the risk of cardiovascular death and hospitalization for heart failure (HF) in patients with chronic heart failure (CHF) (NYHA class II or III) and reduced ejection fraction ≤40%. Avoid in patients with hypotension or orthostatic symptoms. To convert from patient previously on enalapril (≤10mg) and/or valsartan (≤160mg daily) you can start 24/26mg BID of sacubitril/valsartan (otherwise use 49mg/51mg if enalapril/valsartan dosing was >10/>160mg. Do not use with ACEi – instead, stop ACEi and after 36 hours start on on combo arb/neprilysin inhibitor.				
ARBs	CHARM^ ELITE* Val-HeFT@		Candesartan^ 4-8mg/d Valsartan@ 40 mg BID Losartan* 25-50 mg/d	32 mg daily 160 mg BID 150 mg/d
Isosorbide denitrate/hydralazine *Symptomatic African Americans, NYHA III-IV*	A-HeFT	Selected patients who do not respond to ACEi and BB; beneficial in African Americans	Hydralazine 37.5 mg Isosorbide denitrate 30 mg/d	75 mg TID 30mg TID

Milrinone *Phosphodiesterase-3 Inhibitor; Inotrope that functions by ↑CO, ↓preload + afterload (both inotrope and vasodilator)*	*OPTIME-CHF*	III, IV (with EF <25%); short term therapy; best if combined with B-blocker	Milrinone LD 50 mcg/kg over 10 minutes then gtt based off hemodynamics **often used in patients on maximum therapy with continued symptoms of dyspnea, advanced CHF (stage IV), marginal SBP. Use is associated with ↓BP, ↑arrhythmias, ↑mortality	
Ivabradine *I_f inhibitor*	*SHIFT*	Indicated for patients with symptomatic heart failure, II or III, and LVEF ≤ 35% in NSR with heart rate that persists at 70+ despite maximal beta blocker therapy	Ivabradine 5mg BID for 14 days then increase to 7.5mg/BID	2.5-7.5mg/tablet with a daily dose range of 5-15mg/d
Drugs for Symptomatic Therapy				
Diuretic *NYHA II-IV with volume overload*		Used to manage fluid overload, beware ↓K and ↓Mg. High effectiveness when combined with thiazide (30 min prior)	Furosemide 40mg daily Drip: Bumetanide** 1mg daily Torsemide** 20mg daily HCTZ 25mg daily Metolazone 2.5mg daily	40-400mg daily-TID *Increase 20-40 q6h* start at 5 mg/hr 1-10mg daily-TID 20-100mg daily-TID 25-100mg daily 2.5-10mg daily
Torsemide and Bumetanide are used for patients not responding adequately to furosemide				
Inotrope	DIG	Often utilized in patients with concurrent arrythmia (ie. AF);	Digoxin 0.125mg qhs	0.125-0.375mg nightly (check levels in AM)

		prn (no mortality benefit); use when low output or ↓organ perfusion. Only if EF<30%, SE gallop Keep levels <0.8		
AICD	DINAMIT REVERSE MADIT-CRT	II-IV if EF≤ 35% -or- EF≤30% at least 40 days post MI (or 3 months post CABG/PCI) on optimal therapy	Not to be placed <40 days after MI, <3 months after CABG, survival expected of >1 year	
CRT/Bi-V		II-IV if EF≤ 35%	Best for those with <35% EF and QRS>150ms. Greatest benefit seen in those with LBBB	

        - Avoid NSAIDS as it can worsen acute exacerbation (↓prostaglandin production which aids in vasodilation) leading to decreased renal perfusion leading to fluid retention and worsening symptoms.[83]
    - Diuretics: acutely used to reduce **clinical** symptoms of pulmonary edema and weight loss
        - Choices include furosemide, bumetanide, and torsemide
        - Start with furosemide, and if patient does not respond (no change in weight/symptoms), try other two choices
        - If inadequate diuresis with furosemide alone, try **adding** thiazide (HCTZ 25 mg)
        - Start dosing low!
        - Monitor BUN/SCr for hypoperfusion
        - Watch serum electrolytes (especially K+) carefully and replete as necessary
        - Furosemide 0.5-1.0 mg/kg IV. If inadequate response, double the dose.
        - Outpatient starting dose of 20-40mg is adequate
        - When transitioning to PO, it is double the IV dose
        - Goal is 1 kg/day **weight loss**
    - Digoxin
        - Recommended to be used in patients with LVSDF who have **symptomatic** HF despite the use of triple therapy (BB, ACEi, and diuretic) and have multiple hospitalizations over the past year
        - No survival benefit
        - Best given at night, levels checked in AM (normal 0.5-0.9ng/dL)
        - Optimal level is 0.5-0.8; higher levels are associated with toxicity
    - Nitrates: also useful in acute setting to reduce pulmonary edema by decreasing preload.
        - Sublingual, nitropaste, or IV nitroglycerin (start at 10-20 mcg/min and titrate as BP allows). When stable, can convert to PO nitrate (eg. start with Isordil 10 mg PO tid).
    - Vasodilators: Add hydralazine up to 100mg p.o. QID, Isordil up to 80mg TID if patient's BP remains high despite maximum dose of ACE-I. Also if pt is intolerant to ACEI/ARB due rise in Cr, regimen provides good afterload reduction.
        - Both hydralazine and isosorbide denitrate are **particularly effective in AA** when combined with ACEi and BB → should be considered standard therapy in patients with **symptomatic HF**[84]
    - Spironolactone[85]
        - Demonstrated mortality benefit in Class II-IV CHF
        - Best when used concurrently with ACEi or ARB
        - Start at 12.5-25mg PO QD
            - Consider switching to Eplerenone 25mg x 4 weeks then 50mg/day if pt has side effects as it is associated with less s/e such as **gynecomastia**
        - Must check potassium **after 7 days and every week** until stabile; closely monitor K, BUN, Cr. Goal is ≤5.
        - *Contraindications*: Male Cr > 2.5, Female Cr > 2.0. Only benefit patients with Class III-IV HF (EF <40%), ischemic etiology
    - Intravenous Inotropes
        - Patients presenting with predominantly low output syndrome or combined congestion and low output may be considered for intravenous inotropes (e.g., dopamine, dobutamine, milrinone)
        - May help relieve symptoms caused by poor perfusion and preserve end-organ function in those with severe systolic dysfunction and dilated cardiomyopathy.

- **HFpEF (previously termed 'diastolic')**
  - No proven treatment exists; currently empiric
    - Treat based on causes: treat hypertension, control HR using BB or CCB, ↓sx via diuretics
  - May benefit from cardiac cath (Yusef, Lancet 362: 777-281)
  - Goals of treatment are to "keep 'em dry, keep 'em slow":
    - Reduce congestion
      - Angiotensin II–receptor blockers (Candesartan, 4–**32 mg**, Losartan, 25–100 mg)
        - Candesartan is the only agent studied in a randomized, controlled trial involving patients with diastolic heart failure.
      - Salt restriction (<2g/day)
      - Diuretics (Furosemide, 10–120 mg; Hydrochlorothiazide, 12.5–25 mg)
        - Torsemide 10-40 mg IV or PO dail
        - Furosemide 20-80 mg IV or PO daily
      - ACE Inhibitors (Enalapril, 2.5–40 mg, Lisinopril, 10–40 mg)
    - Decrease incidence of tachycardia, maintain LA contraction
      - Prevent atrial fibrillation, cardioversion if it does occur
      - Beta blockers (Atenolol, 12.5–100 mg, Metoprolol, 25–100 mg)
      - CCB (Verapamil, 120–360 mg, Diltiazem, 120–540 mg)
    - Prevent myocardial ischemia
      - Nitrates (Isosorbide dinitrate, 30–180 mg, Isosorbide mononitrate, 30–90 mg)
      - BB (see above)
      - CCB (see above)
      - CABG vs. PCI
    - Control high blood pressure (<130/80)
      - Chlorthalidone, 12.5–25 mg
      - Hydrochlorothiazide, 12.5–50 mg
      - Atenolol, 12.5–100 mg
      - Metoprolol, 12.5–200 mg
      - Amlodipine, 2.5–10 mg
      - Felodipine, 2.5–20 mg
      - Enalapril, 2.5–40 mg
      - Lisinopril, 10–40 mg
      - Candesartan, 4–32 mg
      - Losartan, 50–100 mg

- **Other things to consider**
  - Alternating leg tourniquets, phlebotomy if truly desperate.
  - Check electrolytes and replace K+ early, especially if heavy diuresis.
  - New diagnosis of heart failure warrants MPS or cardiac catheterization
  - Swan- Ganz line may be helpful if hemodynamically unstable. Remember: CHF and bilateral pneumonia can be hard to differentiate. PCWP helps.
  - Intra-aortic balloon pump for cardiogenic shock from acute MI.

	Ten Commandments of HF Treatment
1	Maintain patient on 2-3 g sodium diet. Follow daily weight. Monitor standing blood pressure in the office, as these patients are prone to orthostasis. Determine target/ideal weight, which is not the dry weight. In order to prevent worsening azotemia, some patients will need to have some edema. Achieving target weight should mean no orthopnea or paroxysmal nocturnal dyspnea. Consider home health teaching.
2	Avoid all nonsteroidal anti-inflammatory drugs because they block the effect of ACE inhibitors and diuretics. The only proven sale calcium channel in heart failure is amlodipine.
3	Use ACE inhibitors in all heart failure patients unless they have an absolute contraindication or intolerance. Use doses proven to improve survival and back off if they are orthostatic. In those patient who cannot take an ACE inhibitor, use an angiotensin receptor blocker.
4	Use loop diuretics in most NYHA class II-IV patients in dosages adequate to relieve pulmonary congestive symptoms. Double the dosage (instead of giving twice daily) if there is no response or if the serum creatinine level is > 2.0 mg/dL.
5	For patients who respond poorly to large dosages of loop diuretics, consider adding 5-10 mg of Zaroxolyn one hour before the dose of furosemide once or twice a week as tolerated.
6	Consider adding 25 mg spironolactone in most class III-IV patients. Do not start if the serum creatinine level is 2.5 mg/dL. Has controversial effect in diastolic heart failure.
7	Use metoprolol, carvedilol, or bisoprolol in all class II-III heart failure patients unless there is a contraindication. Start with low doses and work up. Do not start if the patient is decompensated.
8	Use digoxin in most symptomatic systolic heart failure patients.
9	Encourage a graded exercise program.
10	Considerer a cardiology consultation in patients who fail to improve.

- **Consequences**
  - Cardiorenal Syndrome
    - Defined as a state in which therapy to relieve HF is limited by worsening RF; each organ has the ability to initiate and perpetuate disease in the other organ
    - *Pathophysiology*
      - Not due to impaired renal flow from depressed EF but instead a multitude of factors interacting to include: CV congestion, anemia, oxidative stress (HGB is an antioxidant), renal sympathetic activity
      - Low-Flow-State: old hypothesis was that depressed EF (CO) resulted in inadequate renal perfusion prompting RAS to ↑renin release. This is true however is not the sole mechanism at play
      - Another hypothesis is based off that patients with HF have ↑CV congestion which leads to ↑gradient across the glomerular capillary network → ↑renal venous pressure
    - *Treatment*
      - Fluid removal – no diuretic superior over another; limited by ↑SCr, azotemia, contraction alkalosis
      - Inotropes – mixed reviews on efficacy
    - *Discharge* - Do not hold ACEi on discharge
- **Primary Prevention**
  - HF clinic for frequent monitoring
    - 6 minute walk test – document distance each time to look for worsening function
      - Formal exercise or pharmacologic stress testing
  - Hyperlipidemia[86]
  - Hypertension

- Hyperglycemia
- Check of OSA
- Tobacco Cessation
- Sodium restriction
- Daily Weights

- **Secondary Prevention**
  - Implantable aardioverter-defibrilltor (AIAD)[87]
    - Placement of an IAD is recommended in patients with:
      Assuming patients are on optimal medical therapy with an expected life span of >1 year
    - With LVEF ≤ 35% due to prior MI who are at least 40 days post-MI and are in NYHA Functional Class II or III
    - With LV dysfunction due to prior MI who are at least 40 days post-MI, have an LVEF ≤ 30%, and are in NYHA Functional Class I
    - As secondary prevention to prolong survival in patients with current or prior symptoms of HF and reduced LVEF who have a history of cardiac arrest, ventricular fibrillation, or hemodynamically destabilizing ventricular tachycardia (Level of evidence A).
  - Cardiac Resynchronization Therapy
    - *Indications*
      - QRS>150
      - NYHA Class II, III, or IV with LBBB with QRS>150
      - EF<35%
  - Heart Transplant
    - Refractory NYHA Class IV, 65% 5-year survival and 55% 10 year survival

CORONARY ARTERY DISEASE OVERVIEW[88]

- Atherosclerosis with superimposed thrombosis is the main cause of myocardial infarction, coronary death, heart failure, and large-artery stroke
- The plaques that have overlying thrombus are at risk for thrombosis and are thus called "high-risk" plaques when they are present in the coronary or carotid vessels
- It is important to find patients at risk for ASCVD because the first indicator of its presence often is an MI leading to unexpected death and thus we can do our best to ↓ their risks for further progression of the disease if present
- ASCVD is any of the following: CHD such as MI, angina, or known stenosis >50%, CVD, TIA, ischemic stroke, and carotid stenosis >50%, PAD, Aortic disease

- **Risk**
  Moderate risk is ASCVD % between 7.5-19.9%
  - ASCVD % Levels
    - High: ≥ 20%
    - **Intermediate**: 7.5-19.9%
    - Low: <7.5%
  - Factors
    - HLD (LDL>100 and CHOL>240)
      - Goal is LDL<100; high risk patients should have LDL<70
    - HTN (SBP>140, DBP>90)
      - ACEi + CCB is first line treatment (ACCOMPLISH trial)
    - Smoking
    - HDL<40
    - DM (FS>126x2, random>200, HbA1c>6.5)

    - Age (45/55 for male/female)
    - Family Age of MI (55/65 for male/female)
  - High Risk Defined
    - **Four groups most likely to benefit from statin therapy are identified:**
      1. Patients with any form of clinical ASCVD
      2. Patients with primary LDL-C levels of 190 mg per dL or greater
      3. Patients with diabetes mellitus, 40 to 75 years of age, with LDL-C levels of 70 to 189 mg per dL (high dose for those with risk score ≥ 7.5%)
      4. Patients without diabetes, 40 to 75 years of age, with an estimated 10-year ASCVD risk ≥7.5%
  - Screening Calculators (generally for those ≥40)
    - **ACC ASCVD Calculator** http://tools.acc.org/ASCVD-Risk-Estimator-Plus/
    - QRISK2
    - Framingham/ATP III Risk Score
    - SCORE
  - Screening Algorithm
    - *SHAPE guidelines*
      - It's a risk assessment algorithm based on patients who are asymptomatic to determine which cardiovascular screening they need (non-invasive testing) to detect subclinical atherosclerosis
      - Healthy Population: cholesterol level >200 mg/dL (5.18 mmol/L), blood pressure >120/80 mm Hg, diabetes mellitus, smoking, family history of coronary heart disease, or metabolic syndrome
        - Low risk: Must not have any of the following: total cholesterol level >200 mg/dL (5.18 mmol/L), blood pressure >120/80 mm Hg, diabetes mellitus, smoking, family history of coronary heart disease, or the metabolic syndrome
        - Intermediate: everything in between
        - High Risk: Population >75 years old is considered high risk and must receive therapy without testing for atherosclerosis
- **Labs/Assessment**
  - Screening tool as above
  - Cholesterol panel (start at 40 unless major CV risk factor present such as DM, HTN, smoking, or +fam hx)
  - hsCRP (if at moderate risk)
  - A1c
  - Coronary CTA
  - LFTs
  - TSH
  - SCr/GFR
- **Imaging/**
  - Stress Testing
    - EKG/Treadmill
    - Nuclear
    - TTE
  - Coronary Cath
  - Coronary CTA[90,91]
    - Risk stratification tool used in patients at **intermediate** risk of CAD based on ACC ASCVD risk calculator to look for subclinical CAD. In this population, found to be noninferior to functional stress testing (*PROMISE*).

        - The imaging allows for one to calculate a coronary calcium score (CAC) by measuring density and extent of calcifications in coronary artery walls.
            - High negative predictive value
            - The amount of calcium deposits correlates to the risk of future cardiac events, it does NOT tell you about the severity of luminal obstruction
                - Provides information on coronary plaque morphology and stenosis
            - With the CaC score, you can then use the MeSA calculator to determine the 10 year CHD risk score which determines statin eligibility
                - Consider starting a statin in patients with a score >0
                - Consider starting ASA in patients with a score >100

Score	Category
0	No CAD
1-99	Mild CAD
100-399	Moderate CAD
$\geq$ 400	Severe CAD

        - Who To Test

          HR should be at $\leq$ 55; otherwise if >60 BPM then give 100mg metoprolol 30min/1hr prior to procedure; if >55 then give 50mg metoprolol
            - *2016 ACC/AHA guidelines recommend:*
                - **Asymptomatic** patients at **intermediate** risk
                - Known family history of premature CAD (male <55; female <65) and 10 year risk < 5%
            - *2010 ACC/AHA guidelines recommend:*
                - Any patient with an intermediate risk score
        - Who NOT to test
            - Patients at high risk for CAD (consider proceeding straight to cath)
- **Treatment**
    - Primary Prevention - the prevention of cardiac events and mortality in patients **without** a history of previous major adverse cardiac events (MACE).
        - Maximum dose high-intensity statin in those at high risk (see page 146 for medication dosing)
            - Atorvastatin 40-80mg
            - Rosuvastatin 20-40mg
            - Add ezetimibe (*IMPROVE-IT*) if LDL is not at goal of $\geq$50% reduction despite high dose statin
        - Add PCSK9 inhibitors (alirocumab 75mg SQ q2w and evolocumab) in those who are not at an "LDL goal" (*ODYSSEY LONG TERM*) defined as patients **with ASCVD with LDL 70-189mg/dl on maxium statin+ezetimibe**[92]
            - Other indication for starting therapy include stable ASCVD, HDL>190, and statin intolerance (*GLAGOV, FOURIER*)
        - ASA not indicated in primary prevention due to ↑ bleed risk.
    - Secondary Prevention – prevention of recurrent cardiac events or mortality in patients **with** a previous history of MACE.
        - Complete smoking cessation (see page 664)
        - Blood pressure control (see page 179)
        - Appropriate lipid management (see page 145)
        - Physical activity goal of at least 30 minutes, 7 days per week
        - Prevention of metabolic syndrome and weight control
        - Antiplatelet agents

  - ASA 81mg/d indicated in secondary prevention of CAD (Plavix is an alternative in patients with ASA allergy)
    - ASA should be started within 6 hours post CABG started at 100-325mg/d for 1 year then 81mg/d thereafter
  - Concurrent ASA+P2Y12 indicated in patients with stent placed for maximum of 12 months.
- Diabetes mellitus management (see page 217)
  - Focus on agents that have known benefits in patients with CVD (ie. SGLT-2 inhibitors and GLP-1 agonists)
- ACEi/ARB
  - Should be implemented in patients with known ↓EF, DM, CKD, and HTN (unless AA)
  - ARB should be considered in patients intolerant to ACEi
- β-Blockers
  - Similar to ACEi/ARB, indicated in patients with ↓EF or prior ACS limited to metoprolol succinate, carvedilol, bisoprolol. See page 160 for more information.
  - If patients have normal EF, then only use for 3 years and re-assess thereafter if continued use is indicated
- Keep patients up to date on all vaccines
- Consider cardiac rehab consultation

Figure. How to asses recommended interventions based on atherosclerosis test results

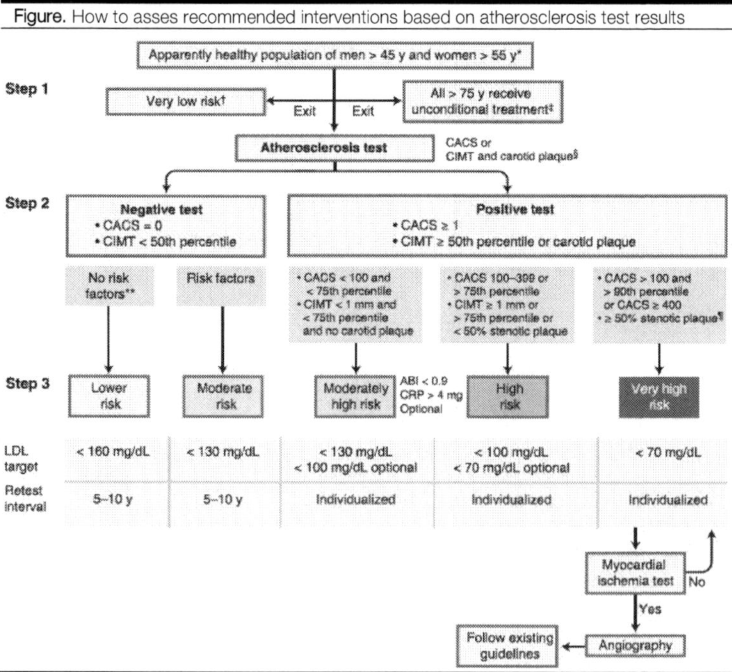

METABOLIC SYNDROME

The diagnosis is made by the presence of three or more of the following five criteria: [93]

1) Waist circumference >40 in (102 am) in men and >35 in (88 am) in women
2) Systolic blood pressure ≥130 mm Hg or diastolic blood pressure ≥85 mm Hg
3) HDL cholesterol level <40 mg/dL (1.04 mmol/L) in men and <50 mg/dL (1.30 mmol/L) in women
4) Triglyceride level ≥150 mg/dL (1.70 mmol/L)
5) Fasting plasma glucose level ≥110 mg/dL (6.1 mmol/L)

HYPERLIPIDEMIA

- **Goals / Risk Stratification**[94,95,96]
  - Framingham Calculator for those with 2+ risk factors but no evidence of CAD
  - Intermediate risk patients that are asymptomatic with no history of CAD should have either (1) coronary artery calcium scoring or (2) hsC-RP done to determine level of risk factor modification

Goal LDL based on risk factors			
Risk Category	LDL goal	LDL to start TLC	Non-HDL Goal
CAD or risk equivalents (10-year risk >20%) • Male > 45YO or Female > 55YO • Smoker • HTN • HDL < 35 • DM • Family hx of CAD	<100	≥ 100	<130
2+ Risk Factors	<130	≥ 130	<160
0-1 Risk Factors	<160	≥ 160	<190

Non-HDL is calculated by subtracting total cholesterol from HDL

Management of Elevated TG		
Classification	Serum TG	Additional Treatments
Normal	<150	
Borderline High	150-199	↓Weight, ↑activity
High	200-499	Intensify LDL therapy or add nicotinic acid or fibrate
Very High	>500	Prevent pancreatitis by lowering TG; low fat diet, ↓weight, ↑activity, and TG lowering drug (fibrate or nicotinic acid). Once level <500, focus on LDL

- **Statins**
  - Types
    - *Hydrophilic*
      - Atorvastatin (liver metabolized → avoid if pt on mult meds; used if high-dose statin therapy req'd)
      - Fluvastatin (liver metabolized → avoid with concurrent warfarin use)

- Rosuvastatin (liver metabolized → avoid with concurrent warfarin use; used if high-dose statin therapy req' d)
- Pravastatin (renally metabolized → good if pt taking multiple medications but not considered 'high' dose statin therapy)
- Pitavastatin

- *Lipophilic*
  - Lovastatin (liver metabolized → avoid if pt on mult meds)
  - Simvastatin (liver metabolized → avoid if pt on mult meds)

- Choosing Intensity

Choosing Statin Intensity	
High Intensity	Moderate Intensity
• Clinical ASCVD and Age≤75 • LDL≥190 • DM + Age 40-75+10 year risk ≥ 7.5% • 10 year risk ≥ 7.5%**	• Clinical ASCVD and Age>75 • Type 1 or Type 2 Diabetes Mellitus (10 year risk <7.5%) • Any patient with 10 year risk 5-7.5%

**or moderate-intensity

Newer researchers are suggesting higher thresholds feeling that ASCVD risk calculator is inappropriately starting statins in patients at low risk without a longterm CVD benefit (suggest threshold of >14% in men 40-49 and 21% if 70-75, and >17% in women of any age)[97]

(see flow chart on following page)

Statin Therapy Options (dose in parenthesis was used in RCTs)		
High Intensity	Medium Intensity	Low Intensity
Daily dosage lowers LDL-C by approximately ≥ 50% on average	Daily dosage lowers LDL-C by approximately 30% to 50% on average	Daily dosage lowers LDL-C by < 30% average
Atorvastatin 40-80 mg Rosuvastatin 20(40) mg	Atorvastatin, 10 (20) mg Rosuvastatin (5) 10 mg Simvastatin 20-40 mg Pravastatin 40 (80) mg Lovastatin 40 mg Fluvastatin XL 80 mg Fluvastatin 40 mg BID Pitavastatin 2-4 mg	Simvastatin, 10 mg Pravastatin, 10-20 mg Lovastatin, 20 mg Fluvastatin, 20-40 mg Pitavastatin, 1 mg

- Effects
  - ↓LDL
    - Lovastatin
    - Pravastatin
  - Normal LDL and underlying CAD
    - Simvastatin
  - ↓LDL with underlying CAD
    - Atorvastatin

Management of Elevated TG			
Genetic Name and Dosage	Avg Expected LDL ↓	Clinical Studied Dosages	Starting mg
Rosuvastatin 10,20, 40mg	55-60%	20mg	10mg
Atorvastatin 20,40, 80mg	42-54%	10mg	20mg
Simvastatin 20, 40, 80	30-50%		40mg
Lovastatin 20, 40, 80, 60ER	39-40%	40mg	40mg
Pravastatin 20, 40, 80mg	30-37%	40mg	40mg
Fluvastatin SR80mg	35%		

Figure. Statin implementation based on risk factors

Heart-healthy lifestyle habits are the foundation of ASCVD prevention
(See 2013 AHA/ACC Lifestyle Management Guideline)

Age ≥21 y and a candidate for statin therapy

Definitions of High- and Moderate-Intensity Statin Therapy*

Moderate	**High**
Daily dose lowers LDL-C by approx. 30% to <50%	Daily dose lowers LDL-C by approx. ≥50%

Clinical ASCVD
- Yes → Age ≤75 y **High-intensity statin** (Moderate-intensity statin if not candidate for high-intensity statin)
- Yes → Age >75 y **OR** if not candidate for high-intensity statin **Moderate-intensity statin**
- No ↓

LDL-C ≥190 mg/dL
- Yes → **High-intensity statin** (Moderate-intensity statin if not candidate for high-intensity statin)
- No ↓

Diabetes Type 1 or 2 Age 40-75 y
- Yes → **Moderate-intensity statin**
- Yes → Estimated 10-y ASCVD risk ≥7.5%† **High-intensity statin**
- No ↓

DM age <40 or >75 y

Primary prevention
(No diabetes, LDL-C 70-189 mg/dL, and not receiving statin therapy)
Estimate 10-y ASCVD risk every 4-6 years
Pooled Cohort Equations†

- **<5% 10-y ASCVD risk**‡
- **Age <40 or >75 y and LDL-C <190 mg/dL**‡
- **≥7.5% 10-y ASCVD risk** (Moderate- or high-intensity statin)
- **5% to <7.5% 10-y ASCVD risk** (Moderate-intensity statin)

In selected individuals, additional factors may be considered to inform treatment decision making§

Clinician-Patient Discussion
Prior to initiating statin therapy, it is important to discuss:

1. Potential for ASCVD risk-reduction benefits||
2. Potential for adverse effects and drug-drug interactions¶
3. Heart-healthy lifestyle
4. Management of other risk factors
5. Patient preferences
6. If decision is unclear, consider primary LDL-C ≥160 mg/dL, family history of premature ASCVD, lifetime ASCVD risk, abnormal CAC score or ABI, or hs-CRP ≥2 mg/L§

No to statin ↓
Emphasize adherence to lifestyle
Manage other risk factors
Monitor adherence

Yes to statin ↓
Encourage adherence to lifestyle
Initiate statin at appropriate intensity
Manage other risk factors
Monitor adherence*

Regularly monitor adherence to lifestyle and drug therapy with lipid and safety assessments

Classes of Cholesterol-Lowering Drugs					
Drug class	Cholesterol	LDL	HDL	Triglycerides	Side effects
Bile acid-binding resins	↓20%	↓10% to 20%	↑3% to 5%	Neutral or ↑	Unpalatability, bloating, constipation, heartburn
Nicotinic acid	↓25%	↓10% to 25%	↑15% to 35%	↓20% to 50%	Flushing, nausea, glucose intolerance, abnormal liver function test
Fibric acid analogs	↓15%	↓5% to 15%	↑14% to 20%	↓20% to 50%	Nausea, skin rash
HMG-CoA reductase Inhibitors	↓15% to 30%	↓20% to 60%	↑5% to 15%	↓10% to 40%	Myositis, myalgia, elevated hepatic transaminases
Omega-3-Fatty Acids	--	--	--	↓ (unknown %)	Low but large amount (4g/d) required

Combination Therapies If Single-Agent Not Effective in Reducing Lipid Levels	
Lipid levels	First drug → drug to add
Elevated LDL level and triglyceride level <200 mg per dL	Statin → bile acid-binding resin
	Nicotinic acid* → statin*
	Bile acid-binding resin → nicotinic acid
Elevated LDL level and triglyceride level 200 to 400 mg per dL	Statin* → nicotinic acid*
	Statin * → gemfibrozil (Lopid)†
	Nicotinic acid‡→ statin‡
	Nicotinic acid → gemfibrozil

- **Side Effects**
  - Myalgias
    - Tx by switching to lipophilic, changing to QOD dosing, trying pitavastatin, adding coenzyme Q10 or vitamin D98
  - Assessing and treating low vitamin D levels (25-hydroxyvitamin D; less than 32 ng/mL) may be worth considering before starting or restarting a statin in patients who develop muscle pain while taking a statin. Supplementation with vitamin D2 (ergocalciferol) supplements (from 50,000 units to 100,000 units per week) advised for Vitamin D levels <10 mg/mL, can use cholecalciferol for levels between 20-30 mg/mL at 400mg U daily.
    - A retrospective chart review found that replenishing vitamin D before a statin rechallenge in previously intolerant patients increases statin tolerability and adherence.
  - Elevated LFTs
  - GI intolerance
  - Monitoring
  - Obtain lipid panel 6 weeks after starting therapy
  - Then obtain every 6-12 months from then on out

CHEST PAIN / ACS

- **Define** – can be defined as any type of pain in the central chest region, this is **not** the same as angina.
- There are only about four important causes of chest pain, which should be diagnosed/treated at night; the other causes can wait until morning.
- The five:

1. **Cardiac**[99]
   - Determine risk categorization: TIMI or HEART criteria see page 191
   - Typical angina (definite):
     - Substernal chest discomfort with a characteristic quality and duration that is (ii) provoked by exertion or emotional stress and (iii) relieved by rest or nitroglycerin
       - **Angina/MI** -- most common cause and takes many forms: chest, arm, back, jaw pains, sometimes dizziness, nausea and vomiting
       - Determine if stable or unstable
         - Unstable
           - Rx with sublingual NTG q 2-4 minutes. Keep checking BPs to be sure SBP > 90 before the next dose!
           - Use dilaudid 0.5 to 1 mg IV if NTG unsuccessful. (Can also try Maalox 30 cc p.o.) Be aware that Procardia can cause a reflex tachycardia. Unrelieved angina or recurrent/prolonged angina in a post-MI patient should go to the PCU. Don't wait. Call the upper year resident.
           - Acute ST elevations require IV nitro, heparin, TPA or streptokinase, lopressor if no contraindications (low BP, HR, CHF, RAD hx). For IV nitro, use Tridil 50/250 D5W, titrate to pain free and SBP > 100.
           - Heparin 5000 u bolus, then run at 18 unit/kg/hour and check PTT in 6 hours. You should call the attending (cardiology) to start TPA/strepto, notify ICU/PCU for transfers to the respective unit.
         - Stable
           - Stress testing and outpatient management (ASA, BB, statin, CCB, long acting nitrate, prn NTG)
   - Atypical angina (probable): *Meets 2 of the above criteria.*
     - Determine risk factors present and do stress test if necessary (see page 141)
   - Non-cardiac chest pain: *Meets 1 or none of the above criteria.* MSK, GI, psychogenic, continued below
2. **Pericarditis** -- sharp or dull ache, patient wants to sit up, friction rub, pulsus paradoxus. Only two of the symptoms are required for diagnosis (typical chest pain, rub, ECG changes with diffuse ST elevation and PR depression in AVR, effusion). Consider myocarditis if the previous symptoms are present along with ↑CK-MB/TROP, ↓EF on TTE, or MRI showing myocarditis. Treatment first with NSAIDs (ie. indomethacin, ibuprofen) + colchicine. Only use steroids if refractory symptoms or allergies to former as they can actually ↑ relapse rates otherwise. ASA should be used if post-MI pericarditis is the diagnosis.
3. **Aortic aneurysm** -- "tearing pain," asymmetric pulses suspicious especially with pain to back or right side
   - Stat EKG and CXR; if still suspicious, CT of chest. Try to lower the BP (nitro or lopressor).
4. **Pulmonary embolus** -- sudden onset, often pain more peripheral, suspect especially with tachypnea and tachycardia, pO2<80
   - Risk factors: inactivity, venous stasis, post-op (esp ortho and urology), hx of DVT, cancer, pre or post-partum, OCP's, HRT, CHF, COPD.

- Signs/symptoms: tachypnea, dyspnea, pleuritic chest pain, sinus tachycardia (or bradycardia, esp w/ β-Blocker), anxiety, S1/Q3T3, new RBBB, RAD.
- Tests
  - Stat ABG – resp. alkalosis with normal/↓ pO2 (and poor response to O2) (90% with PE have low pO2; therefore, 10% of PE presents with nml O2).
  - CXR (need to r/o pneumothorax, CHF, pneumonia).
  - TTE
  - U/S for DVT
- Treatment:
  - Hemodynamically stable: UFH
  - Hemodynamically unstable: alteplase
  - Contraindication to AC or thrombolytics - IVC filter

5. **Esophageal reflux/PUD/pancreatitis** -- can masquerade as substernal chest pain; need to belch, burning sensation in throat
6. **Others** – see table below

When called, check sign-out sheets, ask for vitals and for an EKG. Go to see patient. Is there IV access?

On arrival: BE CALM. Look at the patient. Check vitals, pulses. Ask about the pain. Is it positional? Pleuritic?

Palpable? Radiation? Any Associated Symptoms? Get an EKG; major changes should go to the PCU.

People with pacers or pre-existing LBBB have unreadable EKG's with respect to ST-T changes and you will have to judge clinically. EKGs are still useful for rhythm changes in these people.

Brief differential of chest pain	
Cardiac Related	GI Related
o ACS/Myocardial infarction must always be ruled, see below o Aortic dissection o Pericarditis	o GERD o Esophageal spasm o Mallory-Weiss o Peptic ulcer disease
Pulmonary Related	Others
o Pneumothorax (PTX) o Pneumonia o Pleuritis o PE	o MSK (costochondritis) o Anxiety o Zoster

- **Approach**
  - History
    - Characterize the pain (site, severity, time/duration, stabbing/gripping, radiation, precipitating and relieving factors, previous history of similar sx
    - Associated symptoms (SOB, n/v, palpitations, dizziness)
    - Drug history, ECGs
    - Cardiac history in self or family
  - Exam
    - VS, cardiac exam, reproducible, lung exam, edema
  - Diagnostics
    - CXR

- EKG (w/i 10 minutes of symptoms; serially thereafter)
  - Remember to get posterior EKG if ST↓ noted in V1-V3
- Pulse ox
- Labs: CBC,, d-dimer if indicated, CMP, BNP if indicated
  - TROP: 2 sets separated by 6-8h unless the onset of sx was >8-12 hours ago, then a single TROP is appropriate

- Follow angina pathway on following pages if necessary, otherwise for other specific conditions see their respective sections in this book.
- Risk Score - after performing your exam, obtaining biomarkers, and getting an EKG, now determine the risk score (TIMI and HEART) which will predict the risk of adverse short-term outcomes in 30 days.
- Based on the risk score, then go down appropriate management (early invasive, delayed, stress testing).

Figure. Algorithim for patients presenting with anginal symptoms

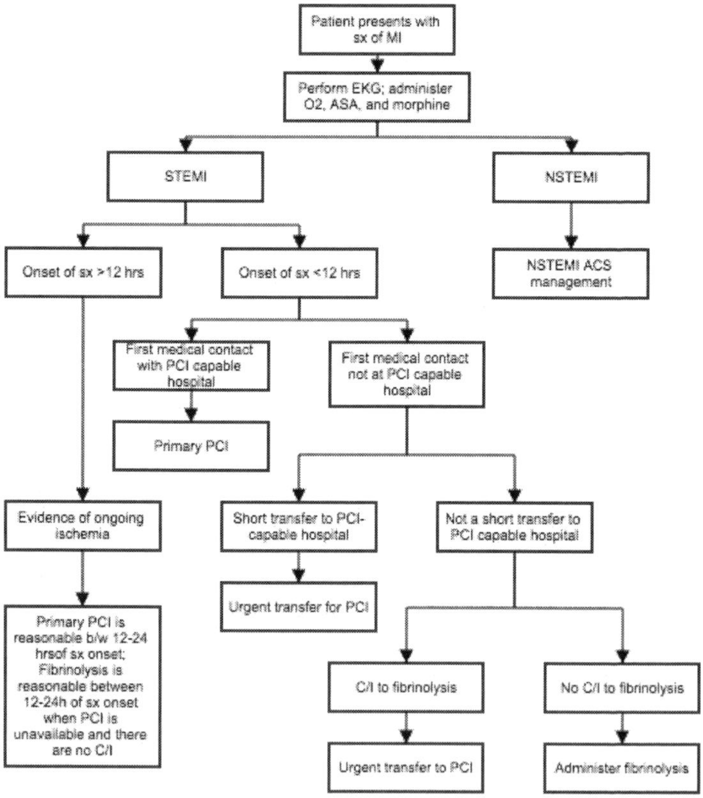

Patient presents with sx of MI
Perform EKG; administer O2, ASA, and morphine
STEMI
NSTEMI
Onset of sx >12 hrs
Onset of sx <12 hrs
NSTEMI ACS management
First medical contact with PCI capable hospital
First medical contact not at PCI capable hospital
Primary PCI
Evidence of ongoing ischemia
Short transfer to PCI-capable hospital
Not a short transfer to PCI capable hospital
Urgent transfer for PCI
Primary PCI is reasonable b/w 12-24 hrsof sx onset; Fibrinolysis is reasonable between 12-24h of sx onset when PCI is unavailable and there are no C/I
C/I to fibrinolysis
No C/I to fibrinolysis
Urgent transfer to PCI
Administer fibrinolysis

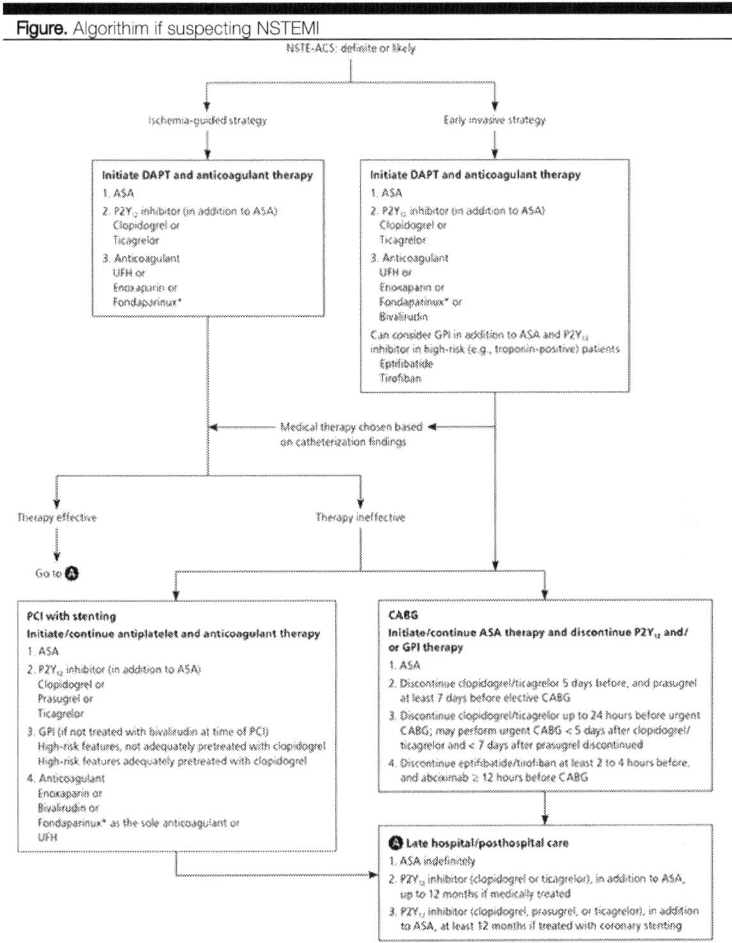

Figure. Algorithim if suspecting NSTEMI

*—*In patients who have been treated with fondaparinux (as up-front therapy) who are undergoing PCI, an additional anticoagulant with anti-II activity should be administered at the time of PCI because of the risk of catheter thrombosis.*

IS THIS ACUTE CORONARY SYNDROME?

	STEMI	NSTEMI	USA	Atypical Chest pain
	MYOCARDIAL INFARCTION: typical rise and fall in troponin in the setting of either: (1) anginal symptoms (2) EKG changes or (3) Echo changes			
Symptoms	Chest pressure +/- with NTG Dyspnea Diaphoresis Nausea, Vomiting Dizziness Fatigue Symptoms at rest/↑frequency/Δ from normal pattern			Atypical
EKG	ST elevation	ST depression TWI	Normal or ST depression/TWI	Normal
Cardiac Enzymes	+	+	-	Normal
	1) Type 1 MI - ischemia due to primary ACS (plaque rupture, erosion) **2)** Type 2 MI - ischemia related to demand/supply mismatch; likely unmasking underlying CAD **3)** Type 3 MI - sudden unexpected cardiac death **4)** Type 4A MI - ACS secondary to PCI **5)** Type 4B MI - documented stent thrombosis **6)** Type 5 MI - related to CABG			
Classification	***Canadian Cardiovascular Society Grading System*** Grade I - Angina with strenuous, rapid, or prolonged exertion; ordinary physical activity, such as climbing stairs, does not provoke angina			

		Grade II – Slight limitation of ordinary activity; angina occurs with postprandial, uphill, or rapid walking; when walking more than 2 blocks of level ground or climbing more than 1 flight of stairs; during emotional stress; or in the early hours after awakening Grade III – Marked limitation of ordinary activity; angina occurs with walking 1-2 blocks or climbing a flight of stairs at a normal pace Grade IV – Inability to carry on any physical activity without discomfort; rest pain occurs	

HOW DANGEROUS IS THIS?

Risk Assessment

AAS Risk Assessment

High	*Intermed*	*Low*
Prev MI	*Age>70*	*Atypical AP*
Hx AAD	*Male*	*Reproducibility*
EKG Δ w/ sx	*DM*	*TWI <1mm*
Symm TWIs	*PVD*	øEKG
EF<40	*ST↓<1mm*	
Elev TROP	*TWI >1mm w/ ↑R*	
VT or VF		
Prior CABG		

- Angina: mismatch of myocardial oxygen supply and demand often described as pressure sensation with increased work. Often lasts 10 sec - 30 min.
  - Stable: due to concentric plaques
  - Unstable: due to ruptured plaque[12]

STEP 1	STEP 2	STEP 3	
Ask 3 questions:	**Total the number of "yes" answers to identify symptom pattern:**	**Find the cell in the matrix (below) where age, gender, and symptom pattern converge:**	
• Is chest pain substernal?	0 of 3=Asymptomatic	High probability	>90%
• Is chest pain brought on by exertion?	1 of 3=Non anginal chest pain	Intermediate	10%-90%
	2 of 3=Atypical angina	Low	<10%
• Is chest pain relieved within 10 minutes by rest or nitroglycerin?	3 of 3=Typical angina	Very low	<5%

PRETEST PROBABILITY OF CORONARY ARTERY DISEASE[100]

AGE (YRS)	SYMPTOMS					
	NON ANGINAL CP		ATYPICAL ANGINA		TYPICAL ANGINA	
	MEN	WOMEN	MEN	WOMEN	MEN	WOMEN
30-39	17.7	5.3	28.9	9.6	59.1	27.5
40-49	24.8	8.0	38.4	14.0	68.9	36.7
50-59	33.6	11.7	**48.9**	20.0	77.3	**47.1**
60-69	43.7	16.9	**59.4**	27.7	83.9	**57.7**

Adapted from Diamond GA, T.S.S. Genders

Online model: http://rcc.simpal.com/RCEval.cgi?Owner=tgenders&RCName=CAD%20consortium

Management	*See STEMI on page 166*	*Calculate TIMI to determine invasive vs conservative. See NSTEMI management on page 160*	ACS rule out to include either stress test or coronary AT

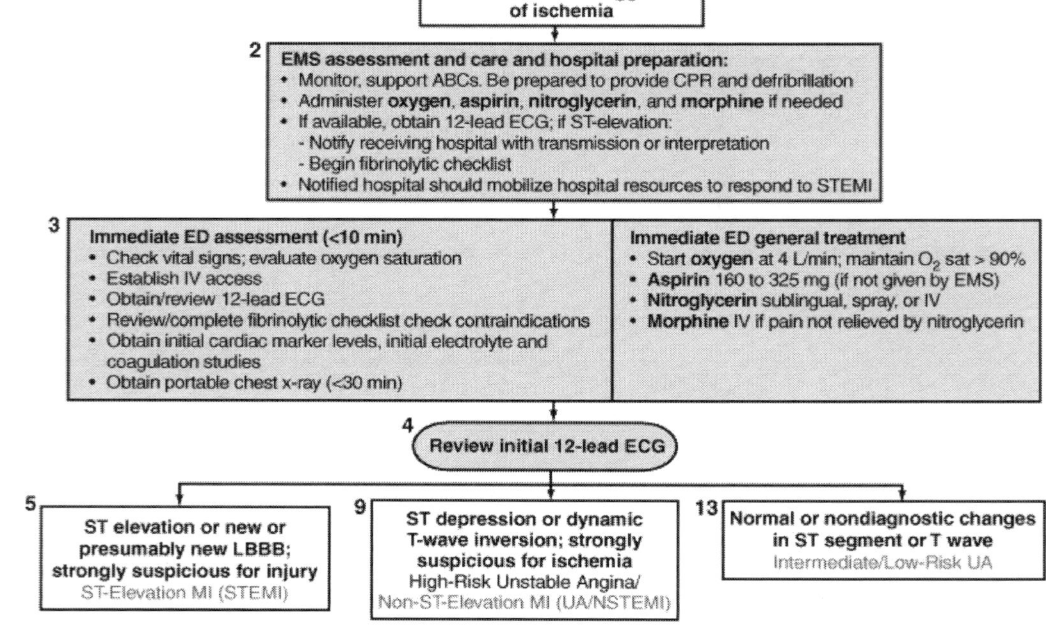
1
Chest discomfort suggestive of ischemia
2
EMS assessment and care and hospital preparation:
• Monitor, support ABCs. Be prepared to provide CPR and defribrillation
• Administer oxygen, aspirin, nitroglycerin, and morphine if needed
• If available, obtain 12-lead ECG; if ST-elevation:
- Notify receiving hospital with transmission or interpretation
- Begin fibrinolytic checklist
• Notified hospital should mobilize hospital resources to respond to STEMI
3
Immediate ED assessment (<10 min)
• Check vital signs; evaluate oxygen saturation
• Establish IV access
• Obtain/review 12-lead ECG
• Review/complete fibrinolytic checklist check contraindications
• Obtain initial cardiac marker levels, initial electrolyte and coagulation studies
• Obtain portable chest x-ray (<30 min)
Immediate ED general treatment
• Start oxygen at 4 L/min; maintain O_2 sat > 90%
• Aspirin 160 to 325 mg (if not given by EMS)
• Nitroglycerin sublingual, spray, or IV
• Morphine IV if pain not relieved by nitroglycerin
4
Review initial 12-lead ECG
5
ST elevation or new or presumably new LBBB; strongly suspicious for injury
ST-Elevation MI (STEMI)
9
ST depression or dynamic T-wave inversion; strongly suspicious for ischemia
High-Risk Unstable Angina/ Non-ST-Elevation MI (UA/NSTEMI)
13
Normal or nondiagnostic changes in ST segment or T wave
Intermediate/Low-Risk UA

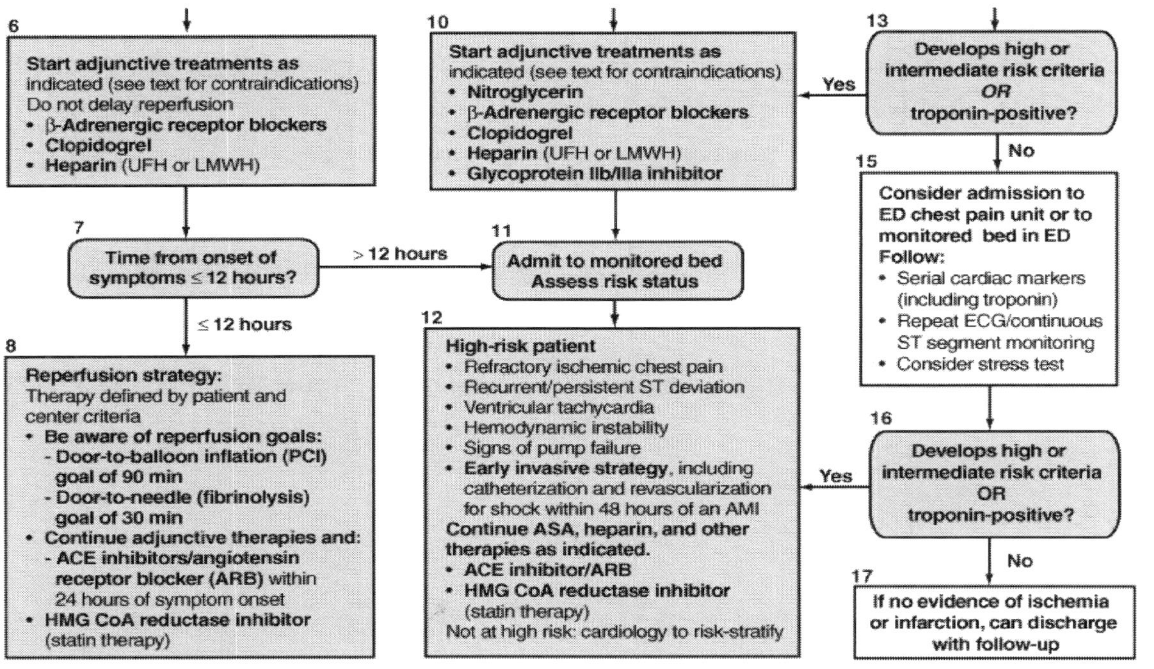
6
Start adjunctive treatments as indicated (see text for contraindications)
Do not delay reperfusion
• β-Adrenergic receptor blockers
• Clopidogrel
• Heparin (UFH or LMWH)
7
Time from onset of symptoms ≤ 12 hours?
> 12 hours
≤ 12 hours
8
Reperfusion strategy:
Therapy defined by patient and center criteria
• Be aware of reperfusion goals:
- Door-to-balloon inflation (PCI) goal of 90 min
- Door-to-needle (fibrinolysis) goal of 30 min
• Continue adjunctive therapies and:
- ACE inhibitors/angiotensin receptor blocker (ARB) within 24 hours of symptom onset
• HMG CoA reductase inhibitor (statin therapy)
10
Start adjunctive treatments as indicated (see text for contraindications)
• Nitroglycerin
• β-Adrenergic receptor blockers
• Clopidogrel
• Heparin (UFH or LMWH)
• Glycoprotein IIb/IIIa inhibitor
11
Admit to monitored bed
Assess risk status
12
High-risk patient
• Refractory ischemic chest pain
• Recurrent/persistent ST deviation
• Ventricular tachycardia
• Hemodynamic instability
• Signs of pump failure
• Early invasive strategy, including catheterization and revascularization for shock within 48 hours of an AMI
Continue ASA, heparin, and other therapies as indicated.
• ACE inhibitor/ARB
• HMG CoA reductase inhibitor (statin therapy)
Not at high risk: cardiology to risk-stratify
13
Develops high or intermediate risk criteria OR troponin-positive?
Yes
No
15
Consider admission to ED chest pain unit or to monitored bed in ED
Follow:
• Serial cardiac markers (including troponin)
• Repeat ECG/continuous ST segment monitoring
• Consider stress test
16
Develops high or intermediate risk criteria OR troponin-positive?
Yes
No
17
If no evidence of ischemia or infarction, can discharge with follow-up

UA/NSTEMI

	IMMEDIATE INVASIVE	*DELAYED INVASIVE*	*EARLY INVASIVE (TIMACS trial)*	*ISCHEMIA-GUIDED / CONSERVATIVE*
TIME	*Within 2 hours*	*24-72 hours*	*<24 hours*	*N/A*
SCORE	*TIMI ≥ 3* *GRACE > 140* *ACCF/AHA: intermediate/high* *HEARTS3: 35.3%*	*TIMI ≥ 2* *GRACE 109-140* *ACCF/AHA: intermediate/high* *HEARTS3: 35.3%*	*GRACE > 140* *ACCF/AHA: intermediate/high* *HEARTS3: 4.6%*	*TIMI 0-1* *GRACE < 109* *ACCF/AHA: low* *HEARTS3: 0%*
SYMPTOMS /INDICATIONS	• Refractory angina • Sustained VT/VF • Hemodynamic instability • Electrical instability • New signs of heart failure	• PMHx of DM, CHF, Hx PCI<6mo ago, prior CABG • +MPS • EF<40% • Hx of PCI in last 6 months or prior CABG • Not at high/intermediate risk • GRACE 109-140. TIMI ≥ 2	• Temporal change in Troponin • New or presumably new ST depression • GRACE > 140 • High risk for clinical events	• Patient or clinician preference in the absence of high-risk features • Low TIMI (0 or 1) or GRACE (<109) • Patient/Physician preference
ORDERS	• Admit directly to cath unit or "step-down" unit			• Admit to telemetry (call MD for > 6 PVC/min, A-fib, V-fib, > 3 beat run of VT, R on T). • Bed rest until ruled out
MEDS	1. ASA 325mg chewed 2. Beta Blocker - only if no active HF, PR prolongation, or RAD	1. ASA 325mg chewed and continued daily until discharge then 81mg/d 2. Beta Blocker - only if no active HF, PR prolongation, or RAD		1. ASA 325mg then ASA 81mg/d indefinitely (coronary CTA score of >100 suggests initiation of ASA; primary prevention

	- Metoprolol 5mg IVP q5min x 3 OR Metoprolol 25-50mg PO to target HR<60 (other options include carvedilol or bisoprolol) 3. P2Y12 Inhibitor with Ticagrelor 180mg loading f/b 90mg BID or Plavix (300-600mg loading f/b 75mg daily) 4. Statin (atorvastatin 80mg/day) even if LDL is known to be <70 5. ACEi (Captopril 6.25mg PO TID) for HF; EF<40%, or STEMI in anterior location 6. Supplemental Oxygen[101] - only if SaO2 is <90%	- Metoprolol 5mg IVP q5min x 3 OR Metoprolol 25-50mg PO to target HR<60 (other options include carvedilol or bisoprolol) 3. P2Y12 Inhibitor with Ticagrelor 180mg loading f/b 90mg BID or Plavix (300-600mg loading f/b 75mg daily) 4. Statin (simvastatin 80mg/day) even if LDL is known to be <70. Can also be considered if coronary CTA is >0. 5. ACEi (Lisinopril 5mg/d titrated to 10mg/d; Captopril 6.25mg → 12.5mg after 2 hrs → 25mg 12 hours later → 50mg BID; Ramipril 1.25mg BID titrated to 5mg BID) 6. Supplemental Oxygen - only if SaO2 is <90%	recommended only if 10 year risk score ≥ 10%) 2. Morphine 3. Oxygen via NC at 2 L/min if SpO2 <90% 4. Metoprolol 25 mg **PO** BID • If this IV dose is tolerated you can usually start 25 mg PO bid but be sure to write hold parameters. • Can consider statin however can also use coronary CTA results to guide initiation (score > 0 should have statin initiated) • If C/I (active wheezing, allergy) then give Diltiazem • NTG • Lipitor 80mg/day or Crestor 20mg/d • ACEi indicated if patient has evidence of LVD/CHF
P2Y12	• In patients going to the cath lab, give the following **before** cath: o Clopidogrel 300/600mg load then 75mg/d (if fibrinolysis then use 75mg/d dose) o Ticagrelor 180mg load (recommended over Plavix if early invasive strategy used) then 90mg BID		
ANTICOAG	• Enoxaparin 30mg IV load then 1mg/kg SC q12h (reduce to 1mg/kg SC daily if CrCl < 30cc/min) and continue until PCI or for duration of hospitalization (max 8 days) • Heparin (UFH) 60 IU/kg (maximum 4000 IU) loading dose with initial infusion of 12 IU/kg per hour (maximum 1000 IU/h) adjusted per APTT to maintaint herapuetic anticoagulation according to the specific hospital protocol, continued for 48 hours or until PCI is performed *Alternatives*		

	• Bivalirudin 0.1mg/kg loading dose followed by 0.25mg/kg per hour (**only if early invasive strategy**)	
RADS/PROC	Angiography	*Stress testing should be done within 72 hours of presentation.* MPS (if no ischemia sx in 24 hours) • ECG with ischemic change (ST depression >1mm) → exercise echo test • Uninterpretable ECG (LBBB, paced, LVH) - stress echo • ECG without changes → exercise ECG • Patients with COPD, obesity, chest wall deformities → MPS • Patients unable to exercise → MPS • For more detailed information, see page 190 TTE (look at LV function) ECG - avoid in women (high false +) CORONARY CTA (see page 142)
LABS	• Troponin q3-6h x 2 (or further if sx develop) • PT/PTT • Cholesterol panel if no previous workup • HgA1C if diabetic	• Troponin q6-12h x 2 • PT/PTT • Cholesterol panel if no previous workup • HgA1C if diabetic.
OUTCOME	1. CABG • Continue ASA 81mg/d • Discontinue clopidogrel 5 to 7 d prior to elective CABG or 24 hour before urgent CABG • Discontinue IV GP IIb/IIIa 2-4 h prior to CABG	If patient classified as low risk after stress test, then: • No angiography is indicated • ASA 81mg, BB, statin, CCB, nitrate indefinitely

	• Continue UFH; discontinue enoxaparin 12 to 24 h prior to CABG; • Treat exacerbations of chest pain with NTG prn → Nitro paste (1" removed daily) → nitro gtt • Cardiac rehab referral • Avoid concurrent NSAIDs 2. <u>PCI</u> • DAPT required (ASA+P2y12) for minimum 12 months then calculate DAPT score and if ≥ 2 then continue dual therapy for 30 months. o Continue ASA 81g/d o Loading dose of clopidogrel (600mg) if not given pre angio, maintained at 75mg after o Consider GPI if not treated with bivalirudin at time of PCI • Discontinue anticoagulant after PCI for uncomplicated cases • Cardiac rehab referral • Avoid concurrent NSAIDs 3. <u>Medical Therapy</u> • No significant obstruction → ASA and Plavix • CAD → continue ASA, continue UFH x 48 hours or Lovenox for hospitalization • P2y12 inhibitor (clopidogrel 75mg/d or ticagrelor 90mg BID) up to 12 months • Consider PPI if patient on triple therapy (+warfarin) or h/o GIB • If Warfarin required, consider lower INR goal of 2.0-2.5. Calculate HAS-BLED score • Cardiac rehab referral • Avoid concurrent NSAIDs	• Ticagrelor 90mg BID x 12 month *(PLATO)* • Stop GP2B3A if already started • Continue heparin x 48 hours or Lovenox x 8 days • Cardiac rehab referral

DECISION: SELECT MANAGEMENT STRATEGY

Favors Invasive Strategy:
Recurrent chest pain despite maximal medical therapy
Elevated cardiac biomarkers
New ST-segment depression
Signs of heart failure
New or worsening mitral regurgitation
Hemodynamic instability
Sustained ventricular tachycardia
Prior CABG
High risk score (e.g., TIMI 5–7)
PCI within 6 months
Reduced LV ejection fraction

Favors Conservative Strategy:
Low risk score (e.g., TIMI 0–2)
Patient or physician preference
Risk of revascularization outweighs benefits

Calculated TIMI Score	14-day Risk of MACE
0 or 1	5%
2	8%
3	13%
4	20%
5	28%
6 or 7	41%

INVASIVE STRATEGY
(i.e., Diagnostic catheterization with intent to perform PCI)

Early invasive strategy (i.e., requiring immediate catheterization) should be considered in patients with:
- Refractory chest discomfort despite vigorous medical therapy
- Hemodynamic or rhythm instability

CONSERVATIVE STRATEGY

DRUGS—Unless contraindicated, all patients should receive the following regardless of the strategy:
- Anticoagulant therapy:
  Unfractionated heparin: 60 U/kg IV bolus, max 4000 U; then 12 U/kg/hr, max 1000 U/hr
  OR,
  Enoxaparin (Lovenox): If <75 years, then 30 mg IV bolus followed 15 min later with 1 mg/kg SQ q12h (or q24h if CrCl < 30); If >75 years, then omit IV bolus and inject 0.75 mg/kg SQ avoid if Cr > 2.0
  OR,
  Fondaparinux (Arixtra): 2.5 mg SQ daily (avoid if CrCl < 30)
  OR,
  Bivalirudin (Angiomax): 0.1 mg/kg IV bolus; then 0.25 mg/kg/h
- Dual antiplatelet therapy:
  For the invasive strategy, If there is a high suspicion for CAD that may require CABG (i.e., diabetes or known multi-vessel CAD) then consider withholding therapy and starting a GP IIb/IIIa inhibitor until the anatomy is defined:
  Clopidogrel (Plavix) 300–600 mg PO loading dose then 75 mg daily
  For patients undergo PCI, you may consider Prasugrel (Effient) 60 mg PO loading dose at the time of PCI then 10 mg daily (see Algorithm 19.1 for contraindications)

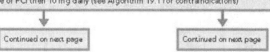

Continued on next page

Continued on next page

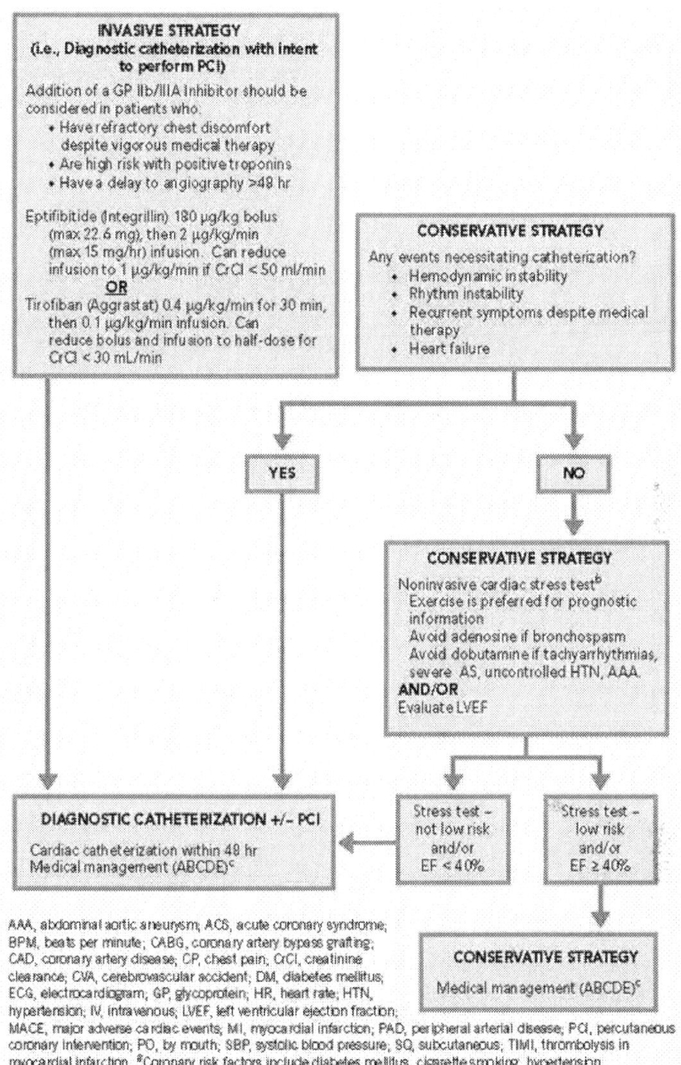

INVASIVE STRATEGY
(i.e., Diagnostic catheterization with intent to perform PCI)
Addition of a GP IIb/IIIA Inhibitor should be considered in patients who:
• Have refractory chest discomfort despite vigorous medical therapy
• Are high risk with positive troponins
• Have a delay to angiography >48 hr
Eptifibitide (Integrillin) 180 μg/kg bolus (max 22.6 mg), then 2 μg/kg/min (max 15 mg/hr) infusion. Can reduce infusion to 1 μg/kg/min if CrCl < 50 ml/min
OR
Tirofiban (Aggrastat) 0.4 μg/kg/min for 30 min, then 0.1 μg/kg/min infusion. Can reduce bolus and infusion to half-dose for CrCl < 30 mL/min
CONSERVATIVE STRATEGY
Any events necessitating catheterization?
• Hemodynamic instability
• Rhythm instability
• Recurrent symptoms despite medical therapy
• Heart failure
YES
NO
CONSERVATIVE STRATEGY
Noninvasive cardiac stress test[b]
Exercise is preferred for prognostic information
Avoid adenosine if bronchospasm
Avoid dobutamine if tachyarrhythmias, severe AS, uncontrolled HTN, AAA
AND/OR
Evaluate LVEF
DIAGNOSTIC CATHETERIZATION +/– PCI
Cardiac catheterization within 48 hr
Medical management (ABCDE)[c]
Stress test – not low risk and/or EF < 40%
Stress test – low risk and/or EF ≥ 40%
CONSERVATIVE STRATEGY
Medical management (ABCDE)[c]

AAA, abdominal aortic aneurysm; ACS, acute coronary syndrome; BPM, beats per minute; CABG, coronary artery bypass grafting; CAD, coronary artery disease; CP, chest pain; CrCl, creatinine clearance; CVA, cerebrovascular accident; DM, diabetes mellitus; ECG, electrocardiogram; GP, glycoprotein; HR, heart rate; HTN, hypertension; IV, intravenous; LVEF, left ventricular ejection fraction; MACE, major adverse cardiac events; MI, myocardial infarction; PAD, peripheral arterial disease; PCI, percutaneous coronary intervention; PO, by mouth; SBP, systolic blood pressure; SQ, subcutaneous; TIMI, thrombolysis in myocardial infarction. [a]Coronary risk factors include diabetes mellitus, cigarette smoking, hypertension (>140/90 mm Hg or on antihypertensive medication), low HDL cholesterol (<40 mg/dL), family history of premature CAD (male first-degree relative ≤55 years old or female first-degree relative ≤65 years old), and age (men ≥45 years old; women ≥55 years old). [b]Diagnostic accuracy of various stress tests are exercise treadmill: men—68% sensitive, 77% specific, women—61% sensitive, 70% specific; exercise, adenosine thallium—88% sensitive, 77% specific; exercise or dobutamine echo—76% sensitive, 88% specific. [c]See Table 19.2

STEMI

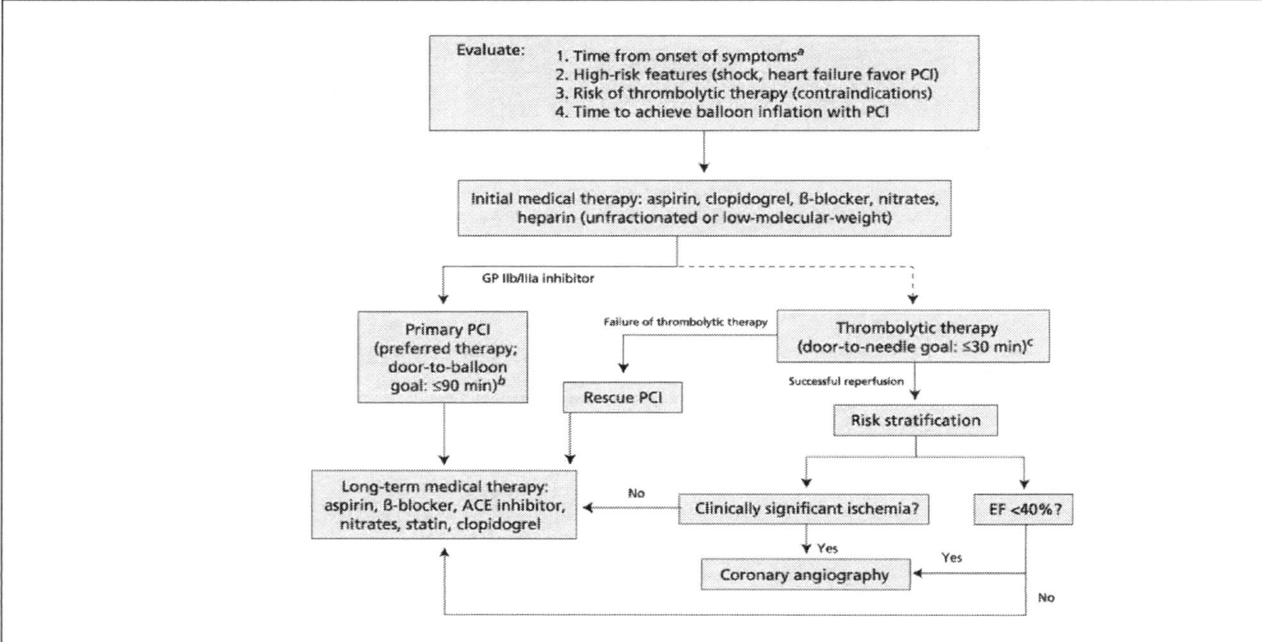

Evaluate:
1. Time from onset of symptoms[a]
2. High-risk features (shock, heart failure favor PCI)
3. Risk of thrombolytic therapy (contraindications)
4. Time to achieve balloon inflation with PCI
Initial medical therapy: aspirin, clopidogrel, ß-blocker, nitrates, heparin (unfractionated or low-molecular-weight)
GP IIb/IIIa inhibitor
Primary PCI (preferred therapy; door-to-balloon goal: ≤90 min)[b]
Failure of thrombolytic therapy
Thrombolytic therapy (door-to-needle goal: ≤30 min)[c]
Rescue PCI
Successful reperfusion
Risk stratification
Long-term medical therapy: aspirin, ß-blocker, ACE inhibitor, nitrates, statin, clopidogrel
No
Clinically significant ischemia?
EF <40%?
Yes
Yes
Coronary angiography
No

- **Definition**[102,111,103,104,105,106]
  - **Acute ST elevation MI requires two of the following:**
    - Chest pain or chest pain-equivalent (indigestion, SOB, dizziness, etc.)
    - EKG with ≥ 1mm ST elevation in ≥ 2 contiguous leads
      - Inverted T waves
      - Elevated ST segment (area of injury)
        - Leads V1-V4 → anterior wall → LAD
        - Leads V1-V2 → anteroseptal → Proximal LAD
        - Leads V2-V3 → anteroapical → LAD or branches
        - Leads I and aVL → lateral → CFX
        - Leads II, III, or aVF → inferior wall → RCA
        - Leads V1 R>S, Q in V6 → posterior wall → PDA
        - **Asymmetric ST depression is associated with strain not ischemia**
      - Q waves (area of infarction, usually develop during 12-36 hr)
    - Left bundle branch block, not known to be old (*Scarbossa criteria*)
      - ST-segment elevation at least 1mm concordant with a predominantly positive QRS complex in at least one lead
      - ST depression at least 1mm in leads V1, V2 or V3
      - ST elevation at least 5mm discordant (in the opposite direction) from a predominantly negative QRS complex
  - Patients with sustained symptoms in absence of diagnostic EKG should have repeat EKG in 30mins
  - Patients who have symptoms associated with an EKG showing ST depression unrelieved within 30 minutes of initiating medical therapy should be considered to have refractory unstable angina.
  - As the resident, call cardiology immediately if suspected AMI patient (meeting above criteria); perform a brief evaluation of all chest pain/rule out MI patients and review EKG within 10 minutes of being informed of admission; call MOD if any question on EKG.
- **Assessment**
  - **Rapid** assessment is key → should receive an EKG within 10 minutes of symptoms:
  - **Focused H&P**:
    - Current symptoms: onset, duration, and quality; exacerbating/alleviating factors; associated symptoms.
    - Prior ischemic disease? CHF? Arrhythmia? Other cardiac disease?
    - Cardiac risk factors: Age, HTN, DM, PVD, CVD, hyperlipidemia, family history of premature CAD, smoking
    - Other medical problems: renal failure, bleeding disorders, GI bleeds
    - Assess vital signs—look for signs of cardiogenic shock or CHF; BP in both arms, JVP, murmurs (MR, VSD, etc)
  - **Diagnostic tests:**

- EKG: (with rapid interpretation) call resident with any questions; repeat EKG in 6 hrs, or if any recurrent symptoms, then QD x 2d and on day prior to discharge; in reperfusion patients, check an end of therapy and repeat in 4-6hrs, then as above
- Labs: CBC with platelets, Chem 7, PT/PTT, non-fasting lipid panel; others as indicated (ABG for respiratory insufficiency, hypoxia, etc.).
  - Cardiac enzymes:
    - Measure troponin I or T at presentation and 3—6 h after symptom onset in all patients with suspected ACS to identify pattern of values
    - Obtain additional troponin levels beyond 6 h in patients with initial normal serial troponins with electrocardiographic changes and/or intermediate/high risk clinical features
- CXR
- Echocardiography: indicated acutely if you suspect pericarditis, aortic dissection (TEE), tamponade, acute MR; also, useful to assess LV dysfunction, size, location and severity of regional wall motion abnormalities, valvular abnormalities. Otherwise, obtained after thrombolytics provided for risk stratification.
- Acute coronary angiography: for urgent reperfusion by angioplasty or CABG, or localization of lesions for further management
- Right heart catheterization: for complicated MI—hypotension, oliguria, CHF, cardiogenic shock. Considered if you have inferior wall infarction (II, III, aVF) with V3R and V4R ST elevation.

Initial Therapy for planned PCI[102]

- Access: IV: 2 lines, large bore; Foley catheterization
- Oxygen: ≥90%
- ASA: 325mg chewed immediately → 81mg afterwards if received Ticagrelor otherwise continue 325mg/d
  - If ASA allergy, use Plavix
- Thienopyridine
  - **Plavix**: 600mg loading dose then 75mg for one year (with ASA 81mg)
  - **Prasugrel**: 60mg loading dose then 10mg daily
  - **Ticagrelor**: 180mg loading dose then 90mg BID
- GP2B3A
  - *Only ordered by cardiology!*
  - *For expected PCI intervention*
  - Eptifibatide dosing 180mcg/kg IV bolus over 1-2min then cont infusion 2mcg/kg/min as long as SCr <2 *6 hours before PCI* and for *18-24 hours after*
    - If SCr 2-4 then cont infusion ↓ to 1 mcg/kg/min.
    - If SCr >4 then use abciximab instead
    - After first bolus, give second bolus after 10 minutes.
- Metoprolol[107]
  - Oral β-Blockers should be initiated in the first 24 hours in patients with STEMI who do not have any of the following: signs of HF, evidence of a low output state, AVB, increased risk for cardiogenic shock (age>70, BP<120, ST at 110bpm)

        - **Newer research is suggesting that if patients do not have evidence of depressed EF (nml TTE) beta blockers may not be as beneficial as once thought (this is controversial).**[108]
    - *Contraindicated if in HF, bradycardic, or SBP<90*
    - *Generally, only given if HR>90*
    - *If allergy, then use CCB such as verapamil or diltiazem*
    - Reduce oxygen demand via contractility, HR, and pressure
    - Metoprolol 5mg x 3 IV then 50mg q6h PO x 24 hours → 100mg BID thereafter with target HR <60
    - Other options include carvedilol and bisoprolol
- ACEi
    - To all patients with STEMI with anterior location, HF, or ejection fraction (EF) less than or equal to 0.40, unless contraindicated
        - Contraindicated: CKD (SCr > 2.5), RAS, ↓BP
    - ↓workload and post-MI remodeling
    - Start within 24 hours of symptoms
    - Lisinopril 5mg daily titrated to 10mg/day[109]
    - Captopril 6.25mg → 12.5mg after 2 hrs → 25mg 12 hours later → 50mg BID
    - Ramipril 1.25mg BID titrated to 5mg BID
- Heparin/Lovenox
    - Patients with STEMI undergoing reperfusion with fibrinolytic therapy should receive anticoagulant therapy for a minimum of 48 hours, and preferably for the duration of the index hospitalization, up to 8 days or until revascularization if performed
    - Depending on renal function (heparin preferred if SCr elevated)
        - UFH: Bolus of 60 units/kg (maximum, 5000 units) followed by infusion of 12 units/kg/h (maximum, 1000 units/h) *titrated to an APTT time 50-70 sec (1.5-2x control) for 48 hours*.
            - Check PT/PTT every 6 hours
            - Stop when patient about to go to cath lab
            - Continue **48 hours after PCI** if *large thrombus found, afib, or EF<30%*
        - Enoxaparin: 1mg/kg milligrams IV bolus followed by 1 milligram/kg SC every 12 h until discharge
            - Hold 6 hours prior to PCI
        - Fondaparinux: <50kg: 5mg SC once daily; 50-100kg: 7.5mg SC once daily; >100kg: 10mg SC once daily
- NTG
    - Contraindications: R heart failure, dehydration, ↓BP (SBP>90)
    - Sublingual
    - Consider drip if recurrent unresolved CP
- Statin:

- Check lipid profile
- Goal LDL <70 mg/dL
- Start atorvastatin 80mg

FIBRINOLYSIS / NON-PCI

1. Invasive strategy is not an option (e.g., lack of access to skilled PCI facility or difficult vascular access) or would be delayed
2. **Goal fibrinolysis initiated within 30 minutes** if patient cannot be transported to PCI capable hospital within **120 minutes**
3. No contraindications to fibrinolysis (*see table below)*
4. For patients with STEMI, fibrinolytic therapy should be simultaneously accompanied by antithrombotic (eg, heparin 4-5k IU and then titrated to reach aPTT 1.5-2x normal values ie. 75-80s) and antiplatelet (aspirin plus clopidogrel 300mg load if <75yo or 75mg if >75 and then 75mg/d thereafter) therapies.
5. Urgent angiography with a view toward "rescue PCI" should be pursued if there is less than 50% resolution of ST-segment elevation 90 minutes after administration.
6. Resolution of chest pain and the presence or absence of reperfusion arrhythmias are also useful markers of successful reperfusion. Importantly, patients should be given a full 90 minutes after fibrinolytic therapy before being taken to the catheterization laboratory because percutaneous intervention immediately after fibrinolysis (ie, so-called facilitated PCI) has been shown to worsen outcomes. Moreover, patients who receive fibrinolytic should be routinely transferred to a PCI-capable hospital for planned angiography (3-16 hours after receiving fibrinolytic) regardless of clinical status as part of the delayed-invasive strategy of care (class IIa recommendation).

PCI

1. Late presentation (sx onset >3 hr ago)
2. **Medical contact-to-balloon / door-balloon <90 min**
3. Outside transfer from non-PCI center to PCI center time <120 min
4. Contraindications to fibrinolysis, including ↑ risk of bleeding and ICH
5. High risk from STEMI (CHF, Killip class is ≥3)
6. Dx in doubt

Glycoprotein IIb/IIIa Inhibitors	
Abciximab	0.25 milligram/kg bolus followed by infusion of 0.125 microgram/kg/min (maximum, 10 micrograms/min) for 12-24 h.
Eptifibatide	180 micrograms/kg bolus followed by infusion of 2.0 micrograms/kg/min for 72-96 h.
Tirofiban	0.4 micrograms/kg/min for 30 min followed by infusion of 0.1 microgram/kg/min for 48-96 h.

$P2Y_{12}$ Inhibitors	
Clopidogrel	Load: 600mg Daily: 75mg Onset: 2-6h depending on loading dose Duration: 3-10d W/d before surgery: 5d
Prasugrel	Load: 60mg Daily: 10mg

Door-to-needle goal (initiation of therapy): $\leq$ 30 min

Fibrinolytic Agents	
Tenecteplase	Weight / Dose: <60 kg — 30 milligrams >60 but <70 kg — 35 milligrams >70 but <80 kg — 40 milligrams >80 but <90 — 45 milligrams >90 — 50 milligrams
Streptokinase	1.5 million units over 60 min.
Anistreplase	30 units IV over 2-5 min.
Alteplase	Body weight >67 kg: 15 milligrams initial IV bolus; 50 milligrams infused over next 30 min; 35 milligrams infused over next 60 min.
	Body weight <67 kg: 15 milligrams initial IV bolus; 0.75 milligrams/kg infused over next 30 min; 0.5 milligram/kg infused over next 60 min.
Reteplase	10 units IV over 2 min followed by 10 unit's IV bolus 30 min later.

	Onset: 30min Duration: 7-10d W/d before surgery: 7d
Ticagrelor	Load: 180mg Tiwce a Day: 90mg Onset: 60min Duration: 3-5d W/d before surgery: 5d

Contraindications to fibrinolytic therapy	
Absolute	Relative
Active internal bleeding	BP > 180/110
History of CNS hemorrhage	Recent internal bleeding
Ischemic stroke within 3 mo	Prolonged CPR (<10m)
Head trauma within 3 mo	Pregnancy
CNS neoplasm	Surgery in past 3 weeks
Known AVM	
Suspected AD	

- **Post Catheterization/PCI**
  - Care
    - Check groin for oozing, bleeding, hematoma, or bruit.
    - Oozing: direct pressure for at least 10 minutes, pressure bandage.
    - Bleeding: manual compression ASAP and contact cath team. Consider FemoStop®.
    - Hematoma: check Hct, platelets, type and cross. Outline borders in ink, document lower limb neuro exam, follow size, ensure blood bank sample and IV access.
  - Procedures
    - TTE
    - Medications
      - **ASA** 325mg for 1 month then 81mg/d indefinitely
      - **ACEi (*GISSI-3; ISIS-4)***
        - Indicated if CHF or LV dysfxn present
        - Titrate to maximal dose
        - Zofenopril+ASA combination was found to be superior than Ramipril+ASA combination in patients post MI with LVEF<40% (*SMILE-4*)
      - **β-Blocker**
        - Expert opinion is to continue **for 3 years if normal EF**, no clear benefit after (*Reduction of Atherothrombosis for Continued Health (REACH) registry*)
        - In patients with LV dysfunction, long term treatment recommended
        - Most evidence supports use of propranolol, timolol, and metoprolol.
      - **Aldosterone Antagonists**
        - *Eplerenone* (if concurrent HF with EF<40% that is symptomatic or concurrent DM)[110]
      - **Heparin/Lovenox**
        - Continued for DVT prophylaxis
        - Lovenox 40mg SQ daily
        - Heparin 5000U TID
      - **Statin**
        - Lipitor 80mg daily
      - **GB2B3A**
        - Decided by cardiology
        - Abciximab: 0.25-mg/kg IV bolus, then 0.125 mcg/kg/min (maximum 10 mcg/min)
        - Tirofiban: (high-bolus dose): 25-mcg/kg IV bolus, then 0.15 mcg/kg/min
        - Eptifibatide: 180-mcg/kg IV bolus, then 2 mcg/kg/min; a second 180-mcg/kg bolus is administered 10 min after the first bolus
      - **P2Y12 Inhibitors**
        - Plavix is the only P2Y12 inhibitor approved for triple therapy use (when treating for Afib)
      - **Anticoagulation for Stents**
        - Overview[111] - The risk of coronary stent thrombosis is approximately 0.7% and is increased with early discontinuation of dual antiplatelet therapy (aspirin and clopidogrel).
        - Choosing
          - *DES* has a lower rate of repeat target vessel revascularization but requires longer-term platelet blocker therapy to prevent stent thrombosis. As a result, the risk of major bleeding on long term dual antiplatelet therapy is higher

- *BMS* should be used when:
    - Patients are not a candidate for DES for technical reasons.
    - Patient is not likely to comply with recommended 12 months of dual antiplatelet therapy
    - Patient will require surgery (requiring cessation of dual antiplatelet therapy) in the coming year.
    - Patient is a high risk of bleeding

Anticoagulation Management in ACS		
Indication	Recommended loading and maintenance dose	Recommended duration of therapy
Medical Management	Plavix 75mg/day Prasugrel 10mg daily Ticagrelor 90mg BID Cangrelor 4 mcg/kg/m	Depends on type of intervention 12 months 12 months 2h or duration of PCI
BMS	Plavix 600 mg load / 75 mg po daily Prasugrel 60mg load / 10mg daily Ticagrelor 180mg load / 90mg BID Cangrelor 30 mcg/kg load	ACS: minimum 1 year; may extend to 30 months if tolerated 12 months Non-ACS: Preferably 1 year; minimum 1 month; extend to 30 months if DAPT score ≥2
DES	Plavix 600 mg load / 75 mg po daily	ACS: minimum 1 year; extend to 30 months if DAPT score ≥2 Non-ACS: Preferably 1 year; minimum 6 months

The John H. Stroger, Jr. Hospital Intern Survival Guide

- **PCSK9 Inhibitor**
    - Patients with angiographic evidence of nonobstructive coronary artery disease (20% to 50% stenosis in a target vessel) treated with statin and evolocumab after 76 weeks of treatment had significantly greater reduction in percent atheroma volume, as measured by serial intravascular ultrasound (*GLAGOV* trial)

- Bleeding
    - Treat as medically indicated. For groin bleeding, apply direct pressure
    - CBC, platelets, and type and cross STAT to monitor HCT and to rule-out immune mediated thrombocytopenia
    - Transfuse PRBC, FFP, and platelets as indicated. For abciximab (ReoPro\) consider platelet transfusions even if platelet count is normal; for eptifibatide (Integrilin□) consider platelets only if patient thrombocytopenic
- Lipid Management
    - All ACS patients should have a fasting lipid profile during the hospitalization, preferably within 24 hours of presentation.
    - Patients with a LDL cholesterol > 100 and a HDL cholesterol > 40 should be started on statin therapy unless known drug allergy to statins is present.
    - Such patients who are already taking a statin should have the dose increased appropriately
    - Patients with a LDL cholesterol < 100 (drawn within 24 hours of presentation) and HDL cholesterol < 40 who are not already taking a statin should be started on gemfibrozil 600 mg bid or niacin.
- Cardiac Rehab[112]

- **Post Fibrinolysis**

- ASA 81mg indefinitely
- Plavix 75mg (at least 14 days, ideal 1 year)

- **Post-Discharge Care**
  - Medications
    - ASA 81mg indefinitely (*OASIS 7 trial)* or consider 10 year ASCVD risk score (≥10% → start ASA) and/or coronary CTA (≥100 suggests starting).
    - P2Y12 Inhibitor (12 months minimum for DES; 1 month for BMS)
      - Plavix 75mg daily or Ticagrelor 90mg BID if ischemia driven NSTEMI or ACS for 12 months
      - Plavix 75mg/d, Prasugrel 10mg daily or Ticagrelor 90mg BID x12m in those receiving BMS or DES
    - Statin: consider initiation based on 10 year ASCVD risk (≥7.5% for high/mod dose) and/or coronary CTA score >0
  - Risk Factor Modification
    - Smoking: all ACS patients who smoke should be counseled to quit smoking. Document this in the medical record.
    - Diet: all ACS patients should be counseled on a diet low in saturated fat and cholesterol.
      - Provide the patient with educational materials if available.
    - Lipid management:
      - All ACS patients should have a fasting lipid panel within 24 hours of presentation.
      - Patients with an LDL > 100 mg/dl should be started on a statin. If they are already on a statin, the dose should be increased.

ORTHOSTATIC HYPOTENSION

- **Pathophysiology**[113]
  - The autonomic nervous system responds to changes in position by constricting veins and arteries and increasing heart rate and cardiac contractility. When these mechanisms are faulty or if the patient is hypovolemic, orthostatic hypotension may occur. In persons with orthostatic hypotension, gravitational opposition to venous return causes a decrease in blood pressure and threatens cerebral ischemia.
- **Differential Diagnosis**
  - Medications
  - Non-neurogenic causes such as impaired venous return, hypovolemia, and cardiac insufficiency
  - Neurogenic causes such as multisystem atrophy and diabetic neuropathy
- **Exam**
  - BP and heart rate are measured with the patient supine, seated, and standing
    - A 1-min interval is needed between each change in position.
- **Diagnosis**
  - SBD decrease of at least 20 mm Hg –or–
  - DBP decrease of at least 10 mm Hg
  - Symptoms of cerebral hypoperfusion, such as dizziness
  - Within 2-5min of standing
- **Treatment**
  - Medications
    - Increasing salt and fluid intake often is an initial step
    - Nonsteroidal anti-inflammatory drugs can be used to increase intravascular volume

- Fludrocortisone (Florinef) may be used in some patients to expand intravascular volume
- Midodrine (ProAmatine), a vasoconstrictor, is effective in some cases of orthostatic hypotension

- Non-Medication
  - Dorsiflex feet several times before standing
  - Increase salt and fluid intake
  - Elevate head of bed 5 to 20 degrees
  - Wear compression stockings

MURMURS

Differential of Murmurs

Cause[111]	Characteristics	Location	Radiation	Findings	Serial Evaluation
Systolic					
AS	Crescendo-Decrescendo midsystolic	Base	Carotids	<u>Accentuation</u> Valsalva release Sudden squatting Passive leg raising <u>Decrease</u> Handgrip Valsalva Standing	Mild (Vmax <3 m/s, AVA >1.5 cm2) → yearly clinical exam Mod (Vmax 3-4 m/s, AVA 1-1.5 cm^2) → echo 1-2 year Severe (Vmax >4 m/s, AVA <1.0 cm^2) → echo every year
Pulmonic stenosis	Crescendo-decrescendo, midsystolic	Base	None	Valve opening click, right-sided S4	
HOCM	Crescendo, mid-or late systolic	Base	Carotids	<u>Accentuation</u> Valsalva strain Standing <u>Decrease</u> **Handgrip** Squatting Leg elevation	
Mitral Regurgitation	Holo- or late Systolic	Apex	Axilla or Back	<u>Accentuation</u> Sudden squatting **Isometric handgrip** <u>Decrease</u> Valsalva Standing	Mild (VC <0.3 cm, ROA <0.10 cm2, RV <30 mL/beat); normal EF mL/beat); EF normal; LV size normal → echo if sx Severe (VC _0.7 cm, ROA _0.4 cm2, RV _60 mL/beat, RF >50%) → echo q6-12mo

Tricuspid Regurgitation	Holosystolic	LLSB	LRSB	Accentuation Inspiration Passive leg raising Decrease Expiration	
Diastolic					
Aortic Regurgitation	Decrescendo	LLSB	None	Increase Sudden squatting Isometric handgrip	Mild (VC <0.3 cm, ROA <0.10 cm2, RV <30 mL/beat) →echo q2-3y Severe (VC >0.6 cm, ROA _0.3 cm2, RV _60 mL/beat, RF >50%) EF >50%; LV size normal → echo yearly EF >50%; LV size increased → echo q6-12mo
Mitral stenosis	Low-pitched Rumble	Apex	None	Increase Exercise Left lateral position Isometric handgrip Coughing	
Tricuspid Regurgitation	Mid-diastolic Loud S2	LLSB	None	Increase Inspiration Passive leg raising Decrease Expiration	

CARDIOMYOPATHY

- **Definition**: disease of the myocardium resulting in ventricular dysfunction and clinical heart failure
- **Types**
  - Ischemic – due to myocardial ischemia and infarction related CAD
  - Non-ischemic –
    - *Genetic* – HOCM, ARVD
    - *Mixed* – idiopathic dilated, restrictive
    - *Acquired* – inflammatory (myocarditis), peripartum, 2/2 ↑HR
    - *Secondary* – infiltrative (amyloid, hemochromatosis), toxin (EtOH, chemo), endocrine (↓thyroid), inflammatory (sarcoid), autoimmune (SLE, RA)
- **Evaluation**
  - TTE - Ejection fraction and functional capacity are frequently used markers of disease severity
- **Management**
  - The same as that for heart failure (*see page 126*)
  - RX:
    - BB – carvedilol>metoprolol (*COMET trial*)
    - ACEi/ARB
      - Hydralazine+nitrate for those unable to take ACEi/ARB +/- AA descent (*A-HeFT trial*)
    - Aldosterone antagonist if NYHA>3
  - ICD (ventricular arrythmia, HF<35%+QRS prolonged, cardiac arrest)

HYPOTENSION

- **Causes**[115]
  - Hypovolemia: hemorrhage (internal or external), vascular dissection, GI losses, over-diuresis, post-dialysis, third spacing
  - Cardiogenic: MI, valvular dysfunction, arrhythmia
  - Obstructive: PE, tamponade, tension pneumothorax, atrial myxoma
  - Distributive: sepsis, anaphylaxis, medications, neurogenic, adrenal insufficiency
- **Evaluation**
  - Any signs or symptoms of hypoperfusion or shock? (i.e. altered mental status, cool, clammy skin, diaphoresis, chest pain, decreased urine output, decreased peripheral pulses) If so, call for back up and begin initial management listed below.
  - Hypovolemia: volume status (mucous membranes, low JVP, skin turgor), post cath bleed, GI bleed, aortic dissection, LV free wall rupture s/p MI.
  - Cardiac ischemia: chest pain, SOB, history of CAD, EKG
  - Arrhythmia: pulse rate & rhythm, rhythm strip
  - Tamponade: pulsus paradoxus, distant heart sounds, JVD, electrical alternans on EKG
  - Pneumothorax: tracheal deviation, JVD, unequal breath sounds, hyperresonance
  - Pulmonary Embolism: dyspnea, hypoxia, JVD, loud P2, RV strain/S1Q3T3 pattern on EKG (sinus tachycardia occurs in 80% of the time)
  - Hemorrhage: GI, retroperitoneum, thigh, abdomen, pancreas, adrenal, hip or pelvic fracture
  - Anaphylaxis: stridor, wheezing, urticaria, flushed skin, pruritus, angioedema
  - Sepsis: fever or hypothermia, leukocytosis or leukopenia
  - Adrenal insufficiency: history of steroid use, hypopituitarism, adrenal hemorrhage/infection/trauma
- **Specific Management**

- Cardiac ischemia: see acute MI protocol.
- Tamponade: call resident/cardiology fellow for emergent echo and pericardiocentesis
- Pneumothorax
  - SOB and or rim of air >2cm on CXR?
    - f yes then place 14 or 16 gauge needle into second intercostal space at midclavicular line ASAP. Call pulmonary fellow for chest tube placement/drain if aspiration does not relieve symptoms.
    - If not, then discharge and outpatient review in 2-4 weeks
- Pulmonary Embolism: Start warfarin on the first or second treatment day and continue **fondaparinux** until INR is ≥2 for at least 24 hours (usually 5-7 days); <50 kg: 5 mg once daily; 50-100 kg: 7.5 mg once daily; >100 kg: 10 mg once daily. Usual duration: 5-9 days
- Bleeding: large bore IV, NS, blood product repletion, reverse any coagulopathy,
- Anaphylaxis: (see page 430)
- Sepsis: start broad spectrum ABx emergently (always double gram negative, and don't be afraid to give aminoglycosides) and pressors (Levophed > dopamine > vasopressin > Neo-Synephrine) as needed
- Adrenal insufficiency[116]: suspect in patients with ↑K, ↓Na, NAGMA who do not respond to multiple fluid boluses; hydrocortisone 100mg IV bolus then 200mg over 24 hours (50mg q6h), after attaining ACTH and random cortisol (levels higher than 15-18 mcg/dL helps rule out condition). If need to later do adrenal testing, must withhold hydrocortisone for 24 hours. After patient is stable, obtain abdominal CT to evaluate for adrenal hemorrhage. Formal diagnosis requires ACTH stimulation test (determine primary cortisol deficiency, secondary low ACTH, or tertiary low CRH).
  - *ACTH stim test*: Starting at any time of the day, provide IM or IV injection of high dose 250 μg cosyntropin and measuring total serum cortisol at baseline, 30 minutes, and 60 minutes to assess the response of the adrenal glands.
    - If the cosyntropin is IV, any value > than 18 to 20 μg/dL indicates normal adrenal function and excludes adrenal insufficiency.
    - If IM is used, any value > than 16 to 18 μg/dL at 30 minutes post-cosyntropin excludes adrenal insufficiency.
    - The ACTH stimulation test may not exclude acute secondary or tertiary adrenal insufficiency.
  - Patients who have the diagnosis require chronic treatment with oral hydrocortisone and fludrocortisone.

HYPERTENSION

- **Diagnosis** – high measurements on two or more occasions separated by time (1-2 min apart). Confirm stage 1 within 1-4 weeks but can start prescription medication immediately if patient presents in stage 2. Masked hypertension can be evaluated with ambulatory blood pressure testing.

Classifying BP		
Category	SBP	DBP
Normal	<120	<80
Elevated	120-129	<80
Stage 1 HTN	130-139	80-89
Stage 2 HTN	≥140	≥90
Ambulatory BP Monitor (ABPM)		
Daytime (awake)	140	90

Night time (sleep)	125	75
24 hour average	135	85
Non-dipper	Does not fall >10% at night	

*based on average of ≥2 careful readings obtained on ≥2 occasions

Etiologies

- Essential: 30% of adults; only ½ may achieve target BP
- Secondary: should consider in patients <30 (that are nonobese, nonblack, without family history) or sudden onset HTN or refractory (see page 189)

Conditions to consider in secondary hypertension

	Conditions	Examination	Workup
Renal	Parenchymal (2-3%) Renovascular (1-2%) -Atherosclerosis -Fibromuscular dys -Polyarteritis nodosa -Scleroderma	DM history PCKD GN	UA SCr UCx Urine albumin/protein Evaluate for RAS only if ↓GFR also noted
Endocrine	Hyperaldosteronism (1-5%) Cushings (1-5%) Pheochromocytoma (<1%) Myxederna (<1%) Hypercalcemia (<1%) Thyroid dyfunction	ARF secondary to ACEi/ARB Flash pulm edema Renal bruit ↓K	MRA w/ gad CT angio TSH Renal artery duplex US 24-hr urinary free cortisol 24-hr urinary frx metneph Angio Aldosterone:renin ratio
Other	Obstructive sleep apnea Alcohol Supplements (ginsing, ephedra, ma huang) Medications (OCP, steroids, NSAIDs, buspar, lithum, SNRI, decongestants) Psych (SSRI, clozapine) Aortic coarctation PCV		

- **Labs** – lipids, sodium, potassium, calcium, TSH, uric acid, SCr, H/H, UA, ECG
- **High Risk Patients**
  - AA ethnicity
  - LVH by electrocardiography (without critical coronary stenosis)
  - DM without orthostatic hypotension
  - Prior stroke or TIA
  - Prior heart failure admissions
- **Goals**[118]
  - For most individuals <130/90 mm Hg.
  - In elderly individuals, ≥60 years, <150/90 mm Hg.
  - In individuals with DM, CKD, and CAD OR have a family history of cardiac events, <130/80 mm Hg.

Hypertension Goals Based on Demographics		
Past Medical History Based Guidelines		
CHF, LVSD	<120/80	
CAD, AAA, PAD	<130/80	
18-60 CKD DM	<140/90	
60+	<150/90 (<140/90 if comorbid dz)	
Age		
<50	<120 (130 if high risk)	*SPRINT* >50 with h/o or high risk of CVD but no DM or TIA → restrictive to <120 goal
50-74	<130 (140 if DM)	
≥75	<140	
Patient Characteristics		
Nonblack	Thiazide CCB ACEi ARB	Level B
Black	Thiazide CCB	Level B
CKD	ACEi ARB	

- **Treatment**
  - Initial treatment should be based on 10 year risk assessment (www.cvriskcalculator.com) → if ≥10% -or- known CVD then treat with medication, if less than 10% and no h/o CVD can trial lifestyle modifications for 3-6 months assuming no CKD, DM, and <65 YO
  - Goal: <130/80

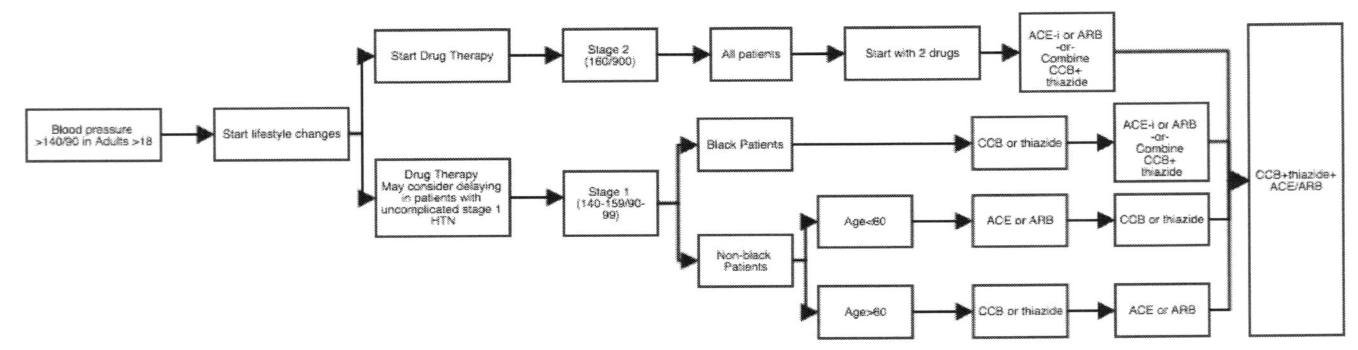

Treatment Decision				
Category	SBP	DBP	CVD Risk	Treatment
Normal	<120	<80	N/A	Healthy Lifestyle
Elevated BP	120-129	<80	N/A	Nonpharm Tx
Stage 1 HTN	130-139	80-89	ASCVD <10%	Nonpharm Tx
	130-139	80-89	ASCVD ≥10% -or- h/o CVD	Anti-HTN Tx (two medications recommended if Stage ≥2)
	130-139	80-89	DM, CKD, Age≥65	
Stage 2 HTN	≥140	≥90	N/A	

- Treatment on Wards (IV Therapy)
  - ↑BP ↑HR
    - Labetalol 10 mg IV prn Q4hours
    - Lopressor (Metoprolol) 2.5-5 mg IV Q 6 hours OR 25 mg PO x1
    - IV Lasix
  - ↑BP ↓HR: Hydralazine 10 mg IV Q6H prn
  - Other Options
    - Furosemide 20mg PO daily
    - Clonidine 0.2mg/week
    - Captopril 6.25 mg PO tid (if normal K+ and Creatinine)
- Diet Changes
  - Encourage healthy lifestyles for all individuals.
  - Prescribe lifestyle modifications for all patients with prehypertension and hypertension.
  - Components of lifestyle modifications include weight reduction, DASH eating plan, dietary sodium reduction, aerobic physical activity, and moderation of alcohol consumption
- Essential/Benign[119]
  - See table on next page
- Combination hypertension treatments
  - *Preferred combinations*
    - ACEI + thiazide
    - ACEI + dihydropyridine CCB
    - ARB + thiazide
    - ARB + dihydropyridine CCB
  - *Acceptable combinations*
    - CCB + thiazide
    - Thiazide + K+-sparing diuretic
    - Aliskiren + thiazide or CCB
    - β-blocker + diuretic or dihydropyridine CCB

Pharmacologic Treatment of Essential Hypertension

Drug Class	Usual Dose	Indications	Side Effects
Thiazide			
Chlorthalidone	12.5-25mg/d	First-line or add-on High quality evidence showed ↓mortality, cardiac events, stroke, and CAD	Hyponatremia, hypokalemia, orthostasis; not effective if GFR<30
HCTZ	12.5-50mg/d		
Indapamide	1.25-2.5mg/d		
Metolazone	2.5–5 mg once daily		
ACE Inhibitors			
Benazepril	5-80mg/d in one or two doses	First line or add on; CKD with albuminuria, CHF, post MI ACEI specific: Low to moderate quality evidence showed ↓mortality, stroke, CAD ARB specific: good choice for gout patients and those intolerant to ACE inhibitors	Hyperkalemia Angioedema
Enalapril	10-15mg/d		
Fosinopril	10-80mg/d in one or two doses		
Lisinopril	5-40mg/d		
Moexipril	7.5-30mg/d in one or two doses		
Perindopril	4-16mg/d in one or two doses		
Ramipril	2.5-20mg/d in one or two doses		
ARBs			
Candesartan	8-32mg/d in one or two doses		
Irbesartan	150-300mg/d		
Losartan	50-100mg/d in one or two doses		
Telmisartan	20-80mg/d		
Valsartan	80-320mg/d		
Loop			
Bumetanide	0.5-2 mg/day in 2 divided doses		

Furosemide	20-80 mg/day in 2 divided doses	
Torsemide	2.5-10 mg once daily	
Combination medications		
ACE+thiazide		
Captopril/HCTZ	25/15 25/25 50/15 50/25	Take 1hr before meals. Adjust at 6wk intervals. Usual max 150mg captopril, 50mg HCTZ daily.
Benazepril/HCTZ	10/12.5 20/12.5 20/25	Switching from monotherapy with either component: initially 10/12.5mg once daily; may increase after 2-3wks as needed up to max 20/25mg daily.
Lisinopril/HCTZ	10/12.5 20/12.5	Not for initial therapy. Initially 10mg/12.5mg or 20mg/12.5mg; increase HCTZ dose 2–3wks after. Max 80mg/50mg daily. CrCl <30mL/min: not recommended.
ARB+thiazide		
Losartan/HCTZ *(Hyzaar)*	50/12.5 100/12.5 100/25	May increase after 3wks as needed to max 100/25mg daily
Telmisartan/HCTZ *(Micardis HCT)*	40/12.5 80/12.5 80/25	Not for initial therapy. May titrate up to 160mg/25mg after 2-4wks. Severe renal or hepatic impairment: not recommended.
Valsartan/HCTZ	80/12.5 160/12.5 160/25 320/12.5 320/25	Add-on or initial therapy and not volume-depleted: initially 160mg/12.5mg once daily; may increase after 1-2wks up to max 320mg/25mg daily.
CCB+ACEi		

Amlodipine/benazepril	2.5/10 5/10 5/20 5/40 10/20 10/40	Unable to achieve BP control with amlodipine without developing edema: Initially 2.5mg/10mg once daily; may titrate up to 10mg/40mg once daily if BP remains uncontrolled. CrCl ≤30mL/min: not recommended.	
CCB			
Dihydropyridine			
Amlodipine	5-10mg/d	First line or add on therapy; minimal effect on CO	Edema of the legs, may worsen proteinuria
Felodipine	2.5-10mg/d		
Nicardipine ER	5-20mg/d		
Nifedipine ER	30-120mg/d in one or two doses		
Non dihydropyridine			
Diltiazem SR	180-360mg/d in one or two doses	Tachycardia; LVOT obstruction, migraine prophylaxis	Constipation, heart block if used with BB
Verapamil SR	120-480mg/d in one or two doses		
BB with sympathomimetic activity			
Acebutolol	200-1200mg 1-2 doses	Indications - myocardial infarction, angina	Contraindications - asthma, chronic obstructive pulmonary disease (COPD) however cardioselective are okay such as atenolol, bisoprolol, metoprolol, heart block
Penbutolol	10-80mg/d		
Pindolol	10-60mg/d		
BB without intrinsic sympathomimetic activity			
Atenolol	50-100mg/d	Cardioselective	
Betaxolol	5-20mg/d		
Bisoprolol	5-20mg/d		
Toprol XL	25-400mg/d		
Lopressor	25-200mg in 1-2 doses		

Nadolol	20-320mg/d	Not cardioselective	
Propranolol	40-240mg/d in 2 doses	Not cardioselective	
Potassium-sparing diuretics			
Amiloride	5-10mg/d in 1-2 doses		
Triamterene	50-100mg in 1-2 doses		
Aldosterone antagonists			
Eplerenone	50-100mg/d	May increase to 50 mg twice daily if needed after 4 weeks; initial dose 25 mg once daily if concomitant weak CYP3A4 inhibitors (erythromycin, verapamil, saquinavir, fluconazole)	
Spironolactone	25-50mg/d		
Others			
Clonidine	0.1mg BID-0.2mg BID or 0.1mg patch qweek		
Minoxidil	5-10mg/d		
Hydralazine	25-100mg BID		

- Hypertensive Urgency
  - Exists when BP>220/120 without evidence of end-organ damage
  - Decrease dose over the following days to 25-30% of the baseline
  - Management (usually treated with short acting oral medications):
    - **Clonidine**: 0.2mg orally, followed by 0.1mg q hour to total of 0.8mg. Watch for sedation, bradycardia with AV nodal blockers. Onset in 30-60 minutes. Rebound hypertension if abruptly stopped.
    - **Captopril** 12.5-25mg orally works in 15-30 minutes with variable episodes of excessive response. May increase to 50-100mg q90-120min
    - **Metoprolol** 12.5-100mg PO BID (ok to start titrating 25 mg p.o. q6hrs x 48 hrs -> then convert to BID). Try to avoid IV MTP as it lasts a short time. (2.5 mg PO MTP = 1 mg IV MTP)
    - **Labetalol PO 200-400mg**
    - **Topical Nitropaste** 1-2 inches to chest wall q6hr; wipe off for BP < (your parameter)
- Hypertensive Emergency
  - Exists when elevated BP (usually DBP>120) is associated *with end-organ damage*
  - Signs/Symptoms
    - CNS: headache, mental status changes, seizure, stroke, irritability
    - Eyes: blurred vision, papilledema, exudates, flame hemorrhages
    - Cardiac: chest pain, EKG strain or ischemic changes, pulmonary edema
    - Vascular: aortic dissection
    - Renal: low urine output, edema, hematuria, azotemia
  - Management
    - Hypertensive emergencies require admission to ICU with arterial line and reduction of BP, usually with IV medications, to reduce permanent organ dysfunction and death
    - Reduce mean blood pressure by 25% in first hour → goal SBP 160-180

Pharmacologic management of hypertensive emergency

Drug	Dose	Information
IV Labetalol	20mg IV bolus over 2 minutes, then 2mg/min or 20-80mg q10min prn	• ($\alpha 1$, $\beta 1$, $\beta 2$ antagonist) • First choice agent for patients with myocardial ischemia, acute aortic dissection, pregnancy, CVA • Most potent adrenergic blocker. • Favorable response in hypertension associated with pregnancy. • Do not lower BP too abruptly as sudden drop in BP may lead to cerebral and other organ hypoperfusion; goal is 25% reduction in mean arterial pressure or to reduce DBP to no lower than 100-110mmHg in first 12-24 hrs. • Onset: 2-5min • Duration: 2-4h

IV Nitroprusside	0.25-.5 mcg/kg/min IV titrated to 8-10mcg/min	• 1st line in most patients • Arteriolar and venous dilation • Toxicity with thiocyanate and cyanide metabolite must be considered with several days of therapy and with renal and hepatic insufficiency • Beware of cytotoxicity! • Onset: Seconds • Duration: 1-2 min
IV Esmolol	0.5-1 mg/kg loading over 1 minute, then continue infusion at 50-200 mcg/kg/min	• Short acting • Titratable • Good for aortic dissection • Onset: 1 min • Duration: 20 min
IV Hydralazine	10-40mg q15-30m with a drip rate of1.5-5 mcg/kg/min if necessary	Good for pregnancy
IV Nicardipine	5mg/hr increased by 2.5mg/hr q5min up to max 15 mg/hr	Great for SAH, CVA (ischemic)
IV Nitroglycerin	5mcg/min titrated up to 100mcg/min	• First choice agent for patients with myocardial ischemia • Venous dilation
IV Clevidipine	1mg/hour titrate to 21 mg/hour	

- Hypertensive Crisis
  - Treat only if signs of end organ damage are present.
  - **Do not** reduce MAP > 20–25% over 30–60 min.
  - **Meds**
    - Labetalol 20 mg IV bolus then 2 mg/min IV to target BP
    - Sodium Nitroprusside 0.5 mcg/kg/min to max (10 mcg/kg/min)

RESISTANT HYPERTENSION

- **Define**
  - JNC 7 and AHA define resistant hypertension as the failure to reach target BP despite treatment with 3 concurrent antihypertensive medications.
  - Both JNC 7 and AHA require that each medication should be from a different class of antihypertensive medications, with 1 medication from the diuretic class, and that all medications should have been optimally dosed.
    - Data from large clinical trials of antihypertensive therapy place the prevalence at 13% to 54%
- **Population** - Patients have higher risk for stroke, MI, CHF, and CKD
- **Causes**
  - Nonadherence to prescribed medications and the white coat syndrome are the 2 main reasons for failure to control BP.

    - White coat syndrome can be ruled out by performing 24-hour ambulatory BP monitoring (ABPM) or home BP monitoring.
    - Officially diagnosed if office blood pressure is ≥ 140/90 and 24 hour average of ABPM is ≤ 130/80
  - Excessive dietary salt and alcohol consumption as well as nonsteroidal anti-inflammatory drugs (NSAIDs), sympathomimetic agents (eg, decongestants, diet pills, and cocaine), and stimulants (eg, methylphenidate, dexmethylphenidate, dextroamphetamine, amphetamine, methamphetamine, and modafinil) can all elevate BP.
  - Some forms of secondary hypertension, are more common in individuals with resistant hypertension, including **obstructive sleep apnea, chronic kidney disease, primary aldosteronism, and renal artery stenosis**.
- **Treatment**
  - The first 3 agents recommended by treatment guidelines for the management of hypertension include a diuretic, a CCB, and an ACE inhibitor or an ARB, either as monotherapy or as combination therapy.
  - At equivalent doses, chlorthalidone is a more effective BP-reducing agent than hydrochlorothiazide.
    - It also has a longer duration of action.
  - **Beta-blockers or alpha blockers** may be used as fourth agents after inadequate BP control on CCB + ACE inhibitor + diuretic combination therapy. **Mineralocorticoid receptor antagonists (MRAs), spironolactone** or eplerenone, are also often recommended as the fourth agent in individuals with resistant hypertension. They are especially helpful in patients with concurrent **OSA**. Eplerenone may be a better option as it **does not** have the gynecomastia effects like spironolactone.

STRESS TESTING

- **Indication**[120,121,122,148,123]
  - Exercise stress testing is used to:
    - Detect inducible cardiac ischemia in symptomatic intermediate-risk patients who can exercise and who have interpretable electrocardiography results
    - Detection of CAD in patients with CP
    - Evaluation of anatomic and functional severity of CAD
    - Assessment of response to medical interventions
    - Atypical symptoms but risk factors for CAD
    - Coronary Calcium score >100 in patients with ↑RF but **asymptomatic**
    - Evaluation post PCTA @ 2 years or CABG @ 5 years
- **Pretest Probability**
  - Estimate pretest probability of CAD in patients with chest pain on the basis of age, sex, pain characteristics, and cardiovascular risk factors (Bayes theorem)
- **Physiology**
  - 80% maximum predicted HR relates to a sensitivity of ability to detect a stenosis of >50% (↑ sensitivity)
- **Definitions**
  - Typical angina is defined as having all of the following: substernal chest pain or discomfort, provocation by exertion or emotional stress, and relief with rest or nitroglycerin.
  - Atypical angina has two of the three characteristics.
  - Non anginal chest pain may have one or none.

Evaluation of chest pain to determine anginal etiology			
STEP 1	STEP 2	STEP 3	
Ask 3 questions:	Total the number of "yes" answers to identify symptom pattern:	Find the cell in the matrix (below) where age, gender, and symptom pattern converge:	
Is chest pain substernal?	0 of 3=Asymptomatic	High probability	>90%
Is chest pain brought on by exertion?	1 of 3=Non anginal chest pain	Intermediate	10%-90%
	2 of 3=Atypical angina	Low	<10%
Is chest pain relieved within 10 minutes by rest or nitroglycerin?	3 of 3=Typical angina	Very low	<5%

Diamond/Forrester classification of chest pain and risk for cardiac event						
AGE (YRS)	SYMPTOMS					
	NON ANGINAL CHEST PAIN		ATYPICAL ANGINA		TYPICAL ANGINA	
	MEN	WOMEN	MEN	WOMEN	MEN	WOMEN
<39	Low	Very low	Intermed	Very low	Intermed	Intermed
40-49	Intermed	Very low	Intermed	Low	High	Intermed
50-59	Intermed	Low	Intermed	Intermed	High	Intermed
≥60	Intermed	Intermed	Intermed	Intermed	High	High

Adapted from Diamond GA
High = > 90% pretest probability
Intermediate = 10% to 90
Low = 5% to 10%
Very low = < 5%.

HEART Score (for use in ER; total possible score 10)[124]		
Variable	Score	
Hx	2	History highly suspicious for coronary syndrome
	1	History moderately suspicious for coronary syndrome
	0	History slightly suspicious for coronary syndrome
EKG	2	EKG with Significant ST Depression
	1	EKG with Non-specific repolarization disturbance
	0	EKG Normal
Age	2	65+
	1	45-64
	0	<45
RF	2	Three or more risk factors for or history of atherosclerotic disease
	1	One to 2 risk factors for atherosclerotic disease
	0	No risk factors for atherosclerotic disease
Troponin	2	More than twice the normal Troponin upper limit
	1	One to 2 times the normal Troponin upper limit
	0	Within normal limits for Troponin levels
Scoring		
0-3	Adverse outcome risk: 2.5% (very low) Supports early discharge with appropriate f/u	
4-6	Adverse outcome risk: 20.3% (moderate risk) Supports admission with standard rule-out management (serial TROP) and stress testing	
7-10	Adverse outcome risk: 72.7% (high to very high) Risk in first 30 days >50%	

	Supports early aggressive management and typically with cardiac cath

- **Getting a stress test?**
  - Very low pretest probability patients should not have an exercise test, since they have a high risk of false-positive results. Evaluate and treat them for non-cardiac causes of chest pain and begin primary prevention of CAD
  - Low pretest probability patients should undergo **exercise treadmill testing alone** since negative results carry a high negative predictive value in both men and women, but positive test results may be false and can be evaluated by more studies.
  - **Intermediate pretest probability** patients, including those with complete right bundle branch block or less than 1 mm ST depression at rest should have an exercise treadmill test without imaging modality. However, intermediate pretest probability patients with baseline ECG abnormalities such as electronically paced ventricular rhythm or left bundle-branch block will **require myocardial perfusion imaging**.
    - MPS is also best in patients with chest wall deformities, COPD, or are obese
  - High pretest probability patients should have coronary angiography as an initial strategy for diagnosis of CAD.

Figure. How to determine which type of stress test to order

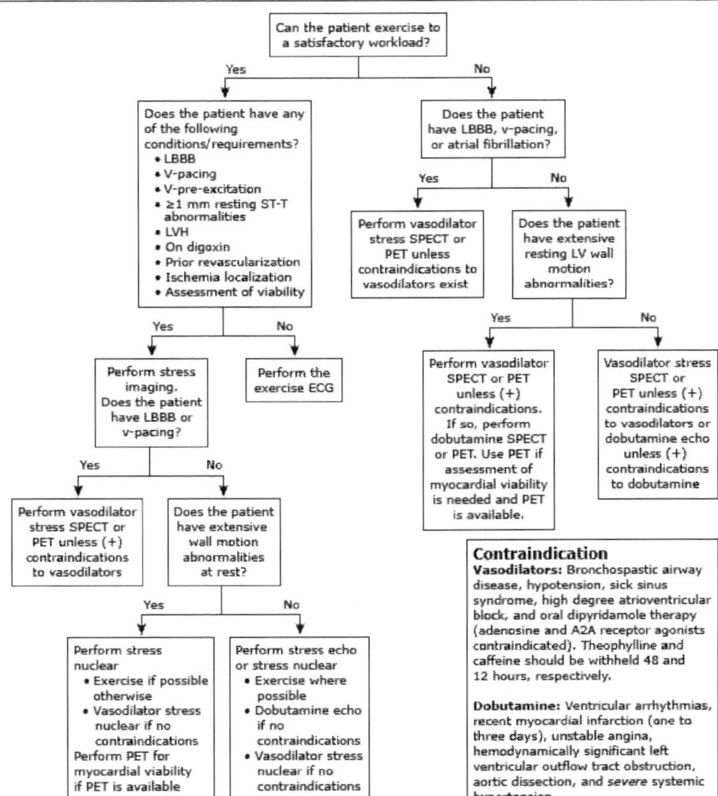

What type of test to get

Type of stress	Purpose	Mechanism	Best for	Not for
Exercise EKG		↑HR, ↑BP	Patients able to reach target HR of (85% x 220-age), men *inexpensive but many limitations	LBBB Pacer Cannot reach HR ST elevations/deviations at baseline WPW
Pharmacologic stress testing with adenosine, etc.	Assess myocardial function	Dilates coronary arteries without ↑HR or BP	LBBB Pacer Cannot reach HR H/O PCI or CABG Obesity	Reactive airway dz Taking theophylline

			SENS: 87-90% SPEC: 73-89% *most sens/spec*	
Dobutamine stress echo	Assess myocardial perfusion	↑HR + BP	Cannot reach HR Reactive airway dz SENS: 68-98% SPEC: 44-100% *no radiation but quicker results	Tachyarrhythmias Significant obesity LBBB (↑ false +)

- **With and Without Imaging**
  - Imaging is often added to exercise testing if there is one of the following:
  - Baseline abnormality on EKG that may make interpretation difficult
  - Symptoms at rest or poor exercise tolerance that may limit their ability to achieve full BRUCE protocol
  - Anatomic abnormalities expected
- **Preoperative Use**
  - Preoperative exercise stress testing is not indicated for risk stratification before non-cardiac surgery in patients who are able to achieve a minimum of 4 METs (e.g., walking up one flight of stairs) without cardiac symptoms, even if they have a history of CAD.
  - Exercise stress testing is helpful for risk stratification in patients undergoing vascular surgery and in those who have active cardiac symptoms before undergoing non emergent non cardiac surgery.
  - Patients with poor functional capacity (unable to achieve 4 METs) should undergo stress echocardiography or exercise single-photon emission computed tomography (SPECT) before undergoing vascular surgery or a kidney or liver transplant.
- **Exercise**
  - Treadmill testing
    - Sensitivity varies from 45% to 67% and specificity 72% to 90% with operator and patient variables. An abnormal test in a man at a heart rate of 85% of predicted maximum for age has a sensitivity of about 65% and a specificity of 85% for CAD. In women, one meta-analysis demonstrated a sensitivity of only 61% and a specificity of only 70%.
  - Echocardiography
    - Overall sensitivity for exercise echocardiography was about 85% and for dobutamine stress echocardiography 82%. Dobutamine has a higher sensitivity than vasodilator echocardiography. No difference in efficacy between echo and nuclear.
  - Pharmacologic
    - Pharmacologic stress myocardial imaging is similar to exercise treadmill testing. Dipyridamole and adenosine PSMI with thallium T1 201 or technetium Tc 99m have a similar sensitivity of 90%, and specificity of 70% for detection of CAD.
      - *Regadenoson* - Avoid any caffeine 12 hours prior to testing.
      - *Adenosine*

- A potent vasodilator, this endogenous nucleoside is rapidly cleared (half-life, <10 seconds) along with its side effects of flushing, headache, and nausea. **Contraindicated in patients with asthma or baseline 2nd degree HB.**

- *Dipyridamole*
  - This coronary vasodilator inhibits the uptake of adenosine. The same side effects as adenosine—flushing, headache, nausea—may last longer with dipyridamole (half-life,13 hours) but they are more common with adenosine and are relieved by administering theophylline. Avoid both adenosine and dipyridamole in patients with **asthma, severe COPD** (FEV<30%), second- or third-degree heart block, hypotension, or those who are on oral dipyridamole.
- *Dobutamine*
  - This synthetic catecholamine increases heart rate, systolic blood pressure, and myocardial contractility, thereby provoking ischemia. It is preferred in patients who are unable to use adenosine or dipyridamole. If patient is taking a beta blocker it should be stopped prior to the exam. Contraindication is in patients with **hypertension or hx of arrhythmias.** Echo vs. Nuclear perfusion is based off the quality of images expected (larger/obese patients may put out poor quality images). **Best for patients with any asthma, COPD, or reactive airway disease.**

- **Results**
  - Low Risk: medical management with ASA, BB, CCB, statin, and long acting nitrate
  - Moderate/High Risk: referral to cardiology
- **Findings associated with poor outcomes**
  - Poor exercise capacity (<5 METS)
  - Exercise-induced angina during minimal exercise
  - Inability to achieve 85% of age-predicted maxium HR
  - Fall in SBP during exercise from baseline
  - ST elevation
  - ≥2mm ST depression during minimal expenditure
  - Early onset or prolonged duration of ST depression during exercise test
  - ST depression in multiple leads
  - Ventricular couplets or tachycardia during recovery
- **Contraindications**
  - Absolute Contraindications
    - Severe/Symptomatic AS
    - Acute MI (within 2 days)
    - Unstable Angina
    - Decompensated HF
    - Unstable Arrhythmias
    - Acute PE
    - Suspected Aortic Dissection
  - Relative Contraindications
    - Left Main CAD
    - Moderate AS
    - HOCM
    - Electrolyte Abnormalities
    - Afib with RVR
    - 3rd degree AV block
    - Resting BP > 200/110
- **Imaging**

  - Indication: high pretest probability for CAD, abnormal baseline EKG (BBB), previous myocardial damage or revascularization procedure
  - Add echocardiography if you want to analyze wall motion function and to determine the physiologic significance of a lesion that is presence and the probable success of an intervention
- **Scoring/Risk**
  - If your patient had a positive or negative exercise treadmill test, consider calculating his **Duke Treadmill Score (DTS)**, which is predictive of 5-year survival and significant severe CAD for patients who are younger than 75 years
    - DTS helps you to exclude low-risk patients from further invasive testing and ensure high-risk patients receive further evaluation and appropriate treatment. DTS appears to be more useful in women with an intermediate pretest score but not with a low pretest score.
    - DUKE Treadmill Score:
      - Duration of Exercise – 5 X max ST deviation – 4 X treadmill angina index (0, none till 2, limiting angina)
      - Scores
        - Low-risk — score ≥+5 (99% 4 yr survival)
        - Moderate-risk — score from -10 to +4 (95% 4 yr survival)
        - High-risk — score ≤-11 (79% 4 yr survival)
- **EKG Changes During Test**
  - ST Depression – 2mm; downsloping, horizontal; represents subendocardial ischemia (1mm at least); the greater the depression, more likely occlusion present on angiography
  - ST Elevation – >1mm; rare; indicates transmural ischemia; represents high grade stenosis

ATRIAL FIBRILLATION

- **Diagnosis:**
  - Irregular ventricular rate in the absence of P waves or well-defined flutter waves in all leads
  - Check chemistry panel, thyroid function tests, cardiac enzymes in patients with known heart disease, echo to help determine cause and risk stratify
- **Cause (PIRATES):**
  - Pulmonary disease
  - Idiopathic (common cause)/Ischemia (rarely causes Afib acutely)
  - Rheumatic heart disease (valvular disease)
  - Atrial myxoma (very rare cause of Afib)
  - Ethanol
  - Metabolic (stress, infection, post-operative, pheochromocytoma), thyrotoxicosis
  - Sepsis (uncommon cause of Afib)
  - Hypertension (#1 cause)/CHF
  - WPW (consider if HR>200)
- **Terminology**
  - Paroxysmal AF - recurrent AF (≥2 episodes) that terminates spontaneously within 7 days
  - Persistent AF - sustained beyond 7 days or lasts less than 7 days but requires pharmacologic or electrical cardioversion.

- Long-standing persistent AF - patient presents with continuous AF for more than 1 year.
- Permanent AF - AF in which cardioversion either has failed or has not been attempted because the patient has decided not to pursue restoration of sinus rhythm by any means.

- **Work-up**
  - History: EtOH, caffeine, stimulants, supplements, family history, recent surgery, medications
  - Lab: TSH, Mg
  - Imaging: TTE

Immediate treatment of Atrial fibrillation with RVR in the inpatient setting	
Scenario	Treatment
Unstable (ie. ↓BP, ↓mentation, angina)	Direct Current Cardioversion ▪ Synchronized DC (100J, 200J, 300J, 360J) ▪ Requires 1 month of anticoagulation no matter the CHA2DS2-VASc score
Stable (goal HR<110)	No active COPD or CHF
	Rate Control Method **Metoprolol/Lopressor** 5mg IV over 2 min q5min x3 (contraindicated in COPD and low EF) with IV magnesium 4.5mg[125] • If initial stabilization is achieved with this, consider starting Lopressor PO 25-100mg PO BID or TID • IV maintenance dose: 60-200 mcg/kg/min *Rhythm Control Method* **Amiodarone** • IV: 150mg load x1 order (IVPB); Amio gtt AMOUNT: 900; comment: 1.8mg/ml (33.3ml/hr) x 6 hours then decrease to 0.5mg/min (16.6ml/hr) for 18 hours • PO: o 800 mg daily for 1 wk, orally o 600 mg daily for 1 wk, orally o 400 mg daily for 4 to 6 wk, orally o 200-400mg daily thereafter
	Cardioversion • Consider elective electrical synchronized cardioversion 100 joules, then 200 then 360 • Pretreatment with amiodarone, flecainide, ibutilide, propafenone, or sotalol can be useful to enhance direct current cardioversion and prevent recurrent AF • For patients with AF of 48-h duration or longer, or when the duration of AF is unknown, anti-coagulation (INR 2.0 to 3.0) is recommended for at least 3 wks. prior to and 4 wks. after cardioversion • Heparin should be administered concurrently by an initial intravenous injection followed by a continuous infusion (aPTT

	1.5 to 2 times control). Thereafter, oral anticoagulation (INR 2.0 to 3.0) should be provided for at least 4 wks., as for elective cardioversion. • For patients with AF of less than 48-h duration associated with hemodynamic instability, cardioversion should be performed immediately without anticoagulation. • Contraindicated if patient is hypokalemic!
	Active COPD or CHF
	Calcium Channel Blocker • Can pretreat with calcium chloride 200mg if worried about hypotension • **Diltiazem** 0.25 mg/kg IV (over 2 min) with IV magnesium 4.5mg. o If no response after 15 minutes → give 5-15mg/h infusion o If response: ▪ PO: Diltiazem 120-360mg PO in divided doses ▪ Drip: 5-15 mg/hr if unable to control rate then transfer to ICU • **Verapamil** 5-10mg IV over 2 min (can repeat in 30m) o PO: 120-360 mg/d in divided doses
	Low blood pressure or Heart Failure
	Digoxin • Can combine with Lopressor • Load 0.25 mg IV q2h up to 1.5mg/24h, then 0.125mg-0.375mg PO/IV daily; check level after 3-4d in AM; slow onset of action; adjust dose in renal failure, with amiodarone, etc. • Should be added to CCB or BB, NEVER used alone! • Not considered effective rate control with atrial fibrillation (only provides control at rest)

- **Treatment**
  - Rate control:
    Goal is to achieve HR<110; rate vs rhythm not important (AFFIRM trial)
    - Beta-blocker: Metoprolol/Lopressor 5mg IV q5min x3 (contraindicated in COPD and low EF)
      - If initial stabilization is achieved with this, consider starting Lopressor PO 12.5-25mg PO q6h
    - Ca-channel blockers:
      - Can pretreat with calcium chloride 200mg if worried about hypotension
      - Diltiazem 15-20mg IV (0.25mg/kg IV over 2 min)
        - If no response after 15 minutes → give 0.35mg/kg IV x1 or gtt (2.5mg/min for max 50mg
        - If response:
          - PO: Diltiazem 30mg PO q6h
          - Drip: 5-15 mg/hr if unable to control rate then transfer to ICU
    - Digoxin:
      - Good for patients that are **hypotensive**
      - **Can combine with Lopressor**
      - Load 0.25 mg IV x 1 (10mcg/kg), then 0.25mg IV q6h x 2, then 0.125mg PO/IV qd; check level; slow onset of action; adjust dose in renal failure, with amiodarone, etc.
      - Should be **added** to CCB or BB, NEVER used alone!

- Not considered effective rate control with atrial fibrillation (only provides control at rest)

Antiarrhythmics for Atrial Fibrillation				
Factors	Medication	Conversion Dose	Maintenance Dose	Pearls
HTN with LVH Known CAD Known CHF	Amiodarone	5-7 mg/kg IV over 30-60m → 1 mg/min, 10g load	200-400 mg daily	↑QT, can lead to pulm, liver, and thyroid dz. ↑INR if taking warfarin
Known CAD	Dronedarone	N/A	400mg BID	↓s/e compared to amio; ↑liver tox
	Ibutilide	1 mg IV over 10 min; may repeat once	N/A	C/I if ↓K or ↑QT interval
Known CAD Known CHF	Dofetilide	500mcg PO BID	500 mcg BID	↑QT interval
Known CAD	Sotalol	N/A	80-160 mg BID	May ↓HR, ↑QT interval
No HTN, LVH, or ischemic heart dz	Flecanide	300mg PO once	100-150 mg BID	
	Propafenone	600mg PO once	150-300mg TID	
Nml BP	Procainamide	10-15 mg/kg IV over 1 h	N/A	May ↓BP, ↑QT interval

- Antiarrythmics (see table above also)
  - Known structural heart disease +/- CAD
    - *Amiodarone* 150mg load x1 order (IVPB); Amio gtt AMOUNT: 900; comment: 1.8mg/ml (33.3ml/hr) x 6 hours then decrease to 0.5mg/min (16.6ml/hr) for 18 hours
      - <1 week – 800 – 1600mg PO/day
      - 1-3 weeks – 600-800mg PO/day
      - >3 weeks – 400mg PO/day
      - S/e include hypotension, bradycardia, QT prolongation, torsades de pointes (rare), GI upset, constipation, phlebitis (IV)
    - Ibutilide—risk of torsades; use with guidance of Cardiology
  - No structural heart disease or CAD
    - *Flecainide*[126]: pill in the pocket approach (300mg if wt >70kg and 200mg if <70kg); studied in patients who suffer from infrequent paroxysms, few symptoms, without known structural dz, arrhythmias, and hemodynamically stable when in AF
      - IV dosing: 1.5-3.0 mg/kg over 10-20 min
    - *Procainamide*: 1gm IV over 1 hour, then Procan SR 750mg PO QID; check for QT prolongation, QRS prolongation, hypotension; follow procainamide and NAPA (toxic metabolite) levels (total level of 10-20 is therapeutic); be sure to give AV nodal blocking agent (e.g. Digoxin) first
    - *Dofetilide*: Must renal dose but can start at 500mcg BID (contraindicated if GFR<20). S/e include QT prolongation.
- Cardioversion
  - Indications: hemodynamic instability, angina, decompensated heart failure
  - Can also be considered in patients nonresponsive to pharmacotherapy
  - AF onset within 48 hours (+/- low risk for stroke):
    - Cardioversion with anticoagulation x 4 weeks
  - AF onset after 48 hours (+/- high risk for stroke):

- Can perform TEE and if no thrombus then cardiovert with 4 weeks of anticoagulation. If thrombus noted then perform below:
  or
- Empiric oral anticoagulation for 3 weeks then perform cardioversion with 4 weeks of post cardioversion anticoagulation as well.

- Synchronized DC (100J, 200J, 300J, 360J)
- Requires 1 month of anticoagulation no matter the CHA2DS2-VASc score

Scoring Risk of Stroke in AFib	
CHA_2DS_2-VASc Risk Criteria	Score
Congestive Heart Failure	1
Hypertension	1
Age > 75	2
DM	1
Prior stroke or TIA	2
Vascular Disease (prior MI, PAD, aortic plaque)	1
Age > 65-74	1
Gender (F)	1
MAX SCORE	9

- Anticoagulation:
  - **Chosing VKA vs DOAC**
    - Warfarin remains the standard of care for the management of patients with valvular AF or mechanical heart valves[127,128]
    - Patients with hepatic dysfunction or associated coagulopathies or impaired renal function (CrCl <30 mL/min per 1.73 m2) are not good candidates for NOACs owing to their hepatic metabolism and renal excretion.
    - If compliance is an issue, rivaroxaban, with its once-daily administration, might be a better choice than dabigatran or apixaban.
    - Dabigatran is best avoided in patients with ulcer/non ulcer dyspepsia given its tartaric acid core and described associations with GI adverse effects.
      - Reversal available with Idarucizumab (*REVERSE AD*)
    - In patients with a recent history of GI bleeding, apixaban may be a better choice as it has a lower incidence of GI bleeding than dabigatran and rivaroxaban.
    - Given the recent association of dabigatran with a trend toward an increase in the incidence of myocardial infarction, rivaroxaban or apixaban should possibly be considered when selecting an NOA in this subset of patients.
      - On the other hand, in patients with a history of ischemic strokes while taking warfarin, dabigatran and apixaban may be suitable alternatives as they are the only NOACs with a lower rate of ischemic stroke than warfarin.
  - Any pt with Afib>48hours (or unknown) duration should be anticoagulated if no definitive contraindication (active hemorrhage, recent neurosurgery, recent hemorrhagic CVA, etc.) to prevent risk of thrombo embolization
    - Start with Heparin drip (see protocol under Hematology), then Coumadin
    - Pt must be therapeutic (INR 2-3) for 3 weeks prior to attempt at cardioversion and must remain on anticoagulation for 1 month subsequent to successful cardioversion
    - Patients requiring DAPT in combination with anticoagulation should be started on low dose ASA (100mg) and Plavix (75mg)
    - Alternatively get TEE to r/o atrial appendage clot and proceed with earlier cardioversion, still need to anticoagulate for **4 or more weeks post cardioversion**

- Direct Oral Anti-Coagulants (DOAC)
  - Avoid in: (1) mechanical heart valve (2) rheumatic heart disease with mitral stenosis (3) significant mitral stenosis and (4) decompensated valvular heart disease with expected surgery in the near term.
    - These patients should Warfarin; patients with a mechanical valve require INR goal of 2.5-3.5
  - Okay in: (1) non-valvular disease (2) native valvular heart disease (3) bioprosthetic heart valve (4) non-mitral stenosis AF
    - Valvular disease causing mild MS, MR, AR, AS, and TR

FDA indications for DOAC

	VTE prevention	VTE treatment	Non-valvular AF	Mechanical HV
Apixaban	Hip+knee	Yes	Yes	No
Dabigatran	Hip	Yes	Yes	No
Edoxaban	No	Yes	Yes	No
Rivaroxiban	Hip+knee	Yes	Yes	No
Warfarin	Hip+knee	Yes	Yes	Yes

DOAC Options

	Nonvalv Afib	VTE/PE	VTE prophy	Trans from VKA	Best population	Preoperative Interruption
Dabigatran *Pradaxa*	RE-LY	RE-COVER	RE-MODEL RE-NOVATE I	When INR<2	Hx of TIA or CVA (superior to warfarin) For stroke while on Warfarin: 150mg BID	High Risk Procedure: stop 3 days prior (4 if SCr≤50cc and 6 days if <30) Low Risk Procedure: stop 2 days prior (3 if SCr≤50cc and 4 days if <30)
	SCr<30: 75mg BID SCr>30: 150mg BID	150mg BID	Hip surgery prophylaxis: 110mg day 1 then 220mg daily for 28-35 days			
Apixaban *Eliquis*	AVERROES ARISTOTLE		ADVANCE	When INR<2	Hx of MI Hx of TIA or CVA (superior to warfarin; also ↓ systemic embolization) Hx of PUD or GI bleed	High Risk Procedure: stop 3 days prior (4 if SCr≤30cc) Low Risk Procedure: stop 2 days prior
	5mg BID (or 2.5mg BID if any of the 2: age>80, BW<60kg or SCr≥1.5	10mg BID x 7d then 5mg BID	2.5mg BID -Knee: x12 days -Hip: x35 days			
Rivaroxaban *Xarelto*	ROCKET-AF	EINSTEIN EINSTEIN-PE	10 mg daily -Knee: x12 days -Hip: x35 days	When INR<3	Hx of MI Hx of PUD Wants a once-daily dosing option	High Risk Procedure: stop 3 days prior (4 if SCr≤30cc) Low Risk Procedure: stop 2 days prior (3 if SCr≤30cc)
	SCr>50: 20mg/d SCr 30-50: 15mg/d	15mg BID x 3w then 20mg/d for 3-6m				
Edoxaban	60mg daily	10 days IV Lovenox then 60mg daily		When INR<2.5	High overall bleed risk Dyspepsia Wants a once-daily dosing option	High Risk Procedure: stop 3 days prior (4 if SCr≤30cc) Low Risk Procedure: stop 2 days prior (3 if SCr≤30cc)

Low Risk Procedure: Colonoscopy, breast bx, minor orthopedic, cardiac cath
High Risk Procedure: Abdominal, Cardiac, Kidney, Neuro, Prostate, Spinal, and Vascular

- Risk factors for thromboembolism:
  - **CHA2DS2VASc (score 2+ requires anticoagulation)**
    - CHF
    - HTN
    - Age (65-74: 1pt; 75+ 2pts)
    - Diabetes
    - Stroke/TIA
    - Vascular disease history (previous MI, peripheral artery disease, aortic plaque
    - Gender (female gets point)

Rates of Stroke in Patients With Atrial Fibrillation Not Undergoing Anticoagulation

CHA_2DS_2VASc	Annual stroke risk		Annual thromboembolism risk in the CHA2DS2-VASc cohort
	Lower-risk cohort	Higher-risk cohort	
0	0.49	1.9	0.8
1	1.52	2.8	2.0
2	2.50	4.0	3.7
3	5.27	5.9	5.9
4	6.02	8.5	9.3
5	6.88	12.5	15.3
6	6.88	18.2	19.7
7	NA	NA	21.5
8	NA	NA	22.4
9	NA	NA	23.6

Bundrick et al. Clinical Pearls in General Internal Medicine 2012. Mayo Clinic Proceedings January 2013;88(1):106-112

- Risk factors for major bleed
  - **HAS-BLED**[129]
    Low:0; Moderate:1-2; High≥3
    - Hypertension
    - Abnormal Liver/Renal Function
    - Stroke History
    - Bleeding Predisposition
    - Labile INRs
    - "Elderly" (Age >65)
    - Drugs/Alcohol Usage
- *Treat underlying cause:*
  - Rarely possible (e.g. thyrotoxicosis)
- *Maintenance of sinus rhythm:*
  - Complex problem! Choice of antiarrhythmic is dependent on pt's other medical problems (i.e. amiodarone is safest drug in patients with ischemic disease and/or low EF). Involve cardiology!

Figure. Determing best anti-arrythmic for treatment of Atrial Fibrillation

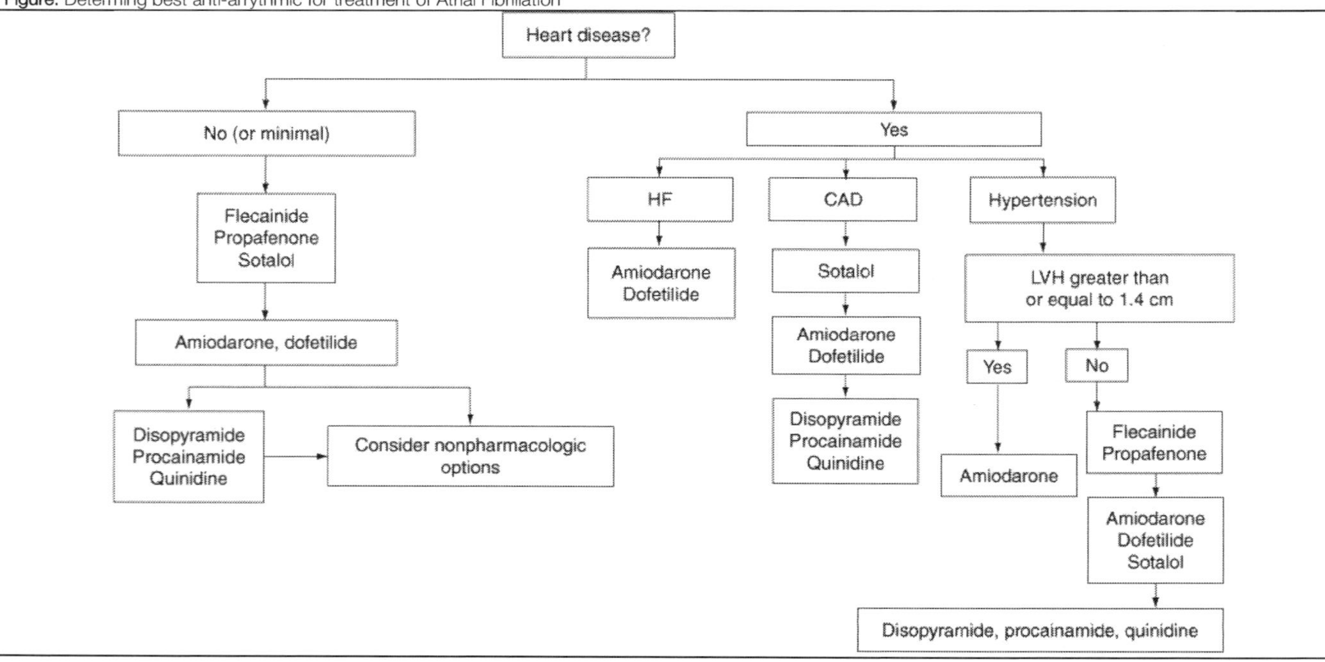

PACEMAKER BASICS

- **Indications for Permanent Pacemaker**[130]
    - Guidelines for implantation of cardiac pacemakers have been established by a task force formed jointly by the American College of Cardiology, the American Heart Association, and the Heart Rhythm Society (ACC/AHA/HRS).
    - Symptoms
        - Dizziness, lightheadedness, syncope, fatigue, poor exercise tolerance all which may be due to bradyarrhythmias (SA node dysfunction)
        - AV node dysfunction may lead to PR prolongation, AV blocks
    - Sinus Node Dysfunction Indications
        - *Class I* — The following conditions are considered class I indications for pacemaker placement:
            - Sinus bradycardia in which symptoms are clearly related to the bradycardia (usually in patients with a heart rate below 40 beats/min or frequent sinus pauses).
            - Symptomatic chronotropic incompetence.
        - *Class II* — The following are considered to be class II, or possible, indications for pacemaker placement in patients with sinus node dysfunction:
            - Sinus bradycardia (heart rate <40 beats/min) in a patient with symptoms suggestive of bradycardia, but without a clearly demonstrated association between bradycardia and symptoms.
            - Sinus node dysfunction in a patient with unexplained syncope.
            - Chronic heart rates <40 beats/min while awake in a minimally symptomatic patient.
            - A less distinct group of patients with sinus bradycardia of lesser severity (heart rate >40 beats/min) who complain of dizziness or confusion that correlates with the slower rates.

- AV Node Block Indications
  - AV block is the second most common indication for permanent pacemaker placement. Causes include the following: fibrosis and sclerosis of the conduction system, ischemic heart disease, digitalis, calcium channel blockers, beta blockers, amiodarone, increased vagal tone, valvular disease, congenital heart disease, cardiomyopathies, myocarditis, hyperkalemia, and infiltrating malignancies
  - *Class I Indications* — The following conditions represent severe conduction disease and are generally considered to be class I indications for pacing, regardless of associated symptoms:
    - Complete (third-degree) AV block*
    - Advanced second-degree AV block (block of two or more consecutive P-waves)
    - Symptomatic Mobitz I or Mobitz II second-degree AV block
    - Mobitz II second-degree AV block with a widened QRS or chronic bifascicular block, regardless of symptoms
    - Exercise-induced second or third degree AV block (in the absence of myocardial ischemia)
  - Current ACC/AHA/HRS guidelines classify asymptomatic third-degree AV block with average awake ventricular rates ≥ 40 beats/min, in a patient with normal left ventricular size and function, as a class IIA indication for permanent pacemaker implantation. Yet many cardiologists consider this condition a definite indication for pacemaker placement. The ACC/AHA/HRS guidelines consider asymptomatic complete AV block in the setting of cardiomegaly or left ventricular dysfunction to be a class I indication
  - *Class II Indications* — Patients with less severe forms of acquired AV block may still benefit from pacemaker placement. In such patients, determinations are often based upon correlation of bradycardia with symptoms, exclusion of other causes of symptoms, and/or results of electrophysiology (EP) testing.
- Other indications for possible pacemaker implantation:
  - Asymptomatic Mobitz II second-degree AV block with a narrow QRS interval; patients with associated symptoms or a widened QRS interval have a class I indication for pacemaker placement.
  - First-degree AV block when there is hemodynamic compromise because of effective AV dissociation secondary to a very long PR interval.
  - Bifascicular or trifascicular block associated with syncope that can be attributed to transient complete heart block, based upon the exclusion of other plausible causes of syncope (specifically ventricular tachycardia)
  - Patients that meet Class I indications for pacing after myocardial infarction, regardless of symptoms:
    - Third-degree AV block within or below the His-Purkinje system.
    - Persistent second-degree AV block in the His-Purkinje system, with bilateral bundle branch block.
    - Transient advanced infranodal AV block with associated bundle branch block.
  - Patients that meet class I indications in patients with neurocardiogenic syncope:
    - Significant carotid sinus hypersensitivity, defined by syncope and >3 seconds of asystole following minimal carotid sinus massage

Pacemaker Modes

1st letter Chamber Paced	2nd Letter Chamber Sensed	3rd letter Response to sensed beat	4th letter Program features	Antitachycardia Function
A	A	T	P	P (pacing)
V	V	I	M	S (shock)
D	D	D	C	D (dual shock+pace)
O	O	O	R	
			O	

A = atrium
V = ventricle
D = dual (both chambers)
O = none
T = triggered I = inhibited
R = rate adaptable available

Mode	Description
AAI	Demand atrial pacing; output inhibited by sensed atrial signals
AAIR	Demand atrial pacing; output inhibited by sensed atrial signals Atrial pacing rates ↓ and ↑ in response to sensor input up to the programmed sensor-based upper rate
VVI	Demand ventricular pacing; output inhibited by sensed ventricular signals
VVIR	Demand ventricular pacing; output inhibited by sensed ventricular signals. Ventricular paced rates ↓ and ↑ in response to to sensor input up to the programmed sensor-based upper rate
VDD	Paces ventricle, senses in both atrium and ventricle Synchronizes w/atrial activity and paces ventricle after a preset AV interval up to the programmed upper rate
VDDR	Paces ventricle, senses in both atrium and ventricle Synchronizes w/atrial activity and paces ventricle after a preset AV interval up to the programmed upper rate; in absense of spontaneous atrial activity, functions as VVIR
DDD	Paces and sense in both atrium and ventricle Paces ventricle in response to sensed atrial activity up to the programmed upper rate
DDDR	Atrial and ventricular paced rates can both ↑ and ↓ in response to sensor input up to the programmed sensor-based upper rate

- The first 3 letters are used most commonly. More modern pacemakers have multiple functions. A pacemaker in VVI mode denotes that it paces and senses the ventricle and is inhibited by a sensed ventricular event.
- Alternatively, AAT mode represents pacing and sensing in the atrium, and each sensed event triggers the generator to fire within the P wave.
- The DDD mode denotes that both chambers are capable of being sensed and paced. This requires two functioning leads, one in the atrium and the other in the ventricle. In the ECG, each QRS is preceded by two spikes. One indicating the atrial depolarization and the other indicating the initiation of the QRS complex. Given that one of the leads is in the right ventricle, a left bundle branch pattern may also be

evident upon the ECG. Note that a two-wired system need not necessarily be in DDD mode, since the atrial or ventricular leads can be programmed off. Additionally, single tripolar lead systems are available that can sense atrial impulses and either sense or pace the ventricle.
  - Thus, this system provides for atrial tracking without the capability for atrial pacing and can be used in patients with atrioventricular block and normal sinus node function.
- **Early Pacemaker Complications**
  - Pneumothorax (check CXR)
  - Hematoma formation (especially if patient on anticoagulation)
  - Lead perforation of RA or RV (suspect if hemodynamically unstable)
  - Lead dislodgment or pacemaker failure (suspect if failure to sense or capture)

ENDOCRINOLOGY

ADRENAL INCIDENTALOMA

- The objective in devaluating an adrenal incidentaloma is to determine the risk of malignancy and assess for subclinical endocrine activity.
    - Must first determine if it is secreting hormones!
- **Imaging**
    - Imaging cannot distinguish functioning from nonfunctioning (need for hormonal evaluation)
    - After initial diagnosis on CT, follow up with triphasic scan (10-15min delay)
        - Benign lesions enhance up to 80-90HU with wash out up to 50% on delay
        - Metastatic/CA/Pheo will show enhancement to >100HU
- **Differential Diagnosis**[131]
    - <u>Benign</u>
        - If surgical resection is not recommended, then follow-up every 3-6 months and then every 1-2 years
        - Hormonal evaluation at time of diagnosis and every annually for 5 years
        - If during this time, it grows > 1cm consider surgical resection
    - <u>Malignant Characteristics</u>
        - Adenoma > 4 cm
        - Irregular borders
        - >50% contrast retention after 10 minutes
        - Unilateral
        - Calcifications/heterogenous
        - HU>10
        - ↑ growth over short time period
    - <u>Pheochromocytoma</u>
        - *Labs*: plasma/24-hour urine fractionated metanephrine and normetanephrine with fractionated catecholamines (urine or plasma), aldosterone:renin ratio (+ if >20:1), dexamethasone suppression test
        - Prescribe alpha-adrenergic blocker prior to surgery
        - Should have surgical resection with long term follow-up afterwards due to ↑ rate of reoccurrence
    - <u>Cushing's Disease</u>
        - Look for elevated 24 hr urine cortisol (normal < 90 mcg/day) in setting of patient with obesity, diabetes, osteoporosis, and HTN
        - If elevated, follow up with either:
            - Midnight salivary cortisol
            - 1mg-dexamethasone suppression test which will show serum cortisol level > 5 (lack of suppression). Performed by:
                - 1mg given at 11-pm to midnight
                - 0800 cortisol checked the following AM, should be low (<5mcg/dl)
                    - A value >10 mcg/dl suggests Cushing's Syndrome
        - If (+) and surgical resection done, f/u with exogenous glucocortoids until HPA axis recovers
    - <u>Aldosterone secreting tumor</u>
        - Look for Aldosterone:Renin ratio > 20 with absolute aldosterone level > 15
        - If above are positive, follow up with 24 hour urine study to look for **lack of** suppression after salt load (saline infusion or oral sodium) which confirms diagnosis if persistent aldosterone production exists despite this load.
- **Workup**

- Labs
  - 24 Hour Urine Metanephrine
  - 24 Hour Urine Catecholamines
  - Serum aldosterone (if hypertensive)
  - Serum renin activity factor (if hypertensive)
  - Urine cortisol

Figure. Algorithm for management of adrenal incidentaloma

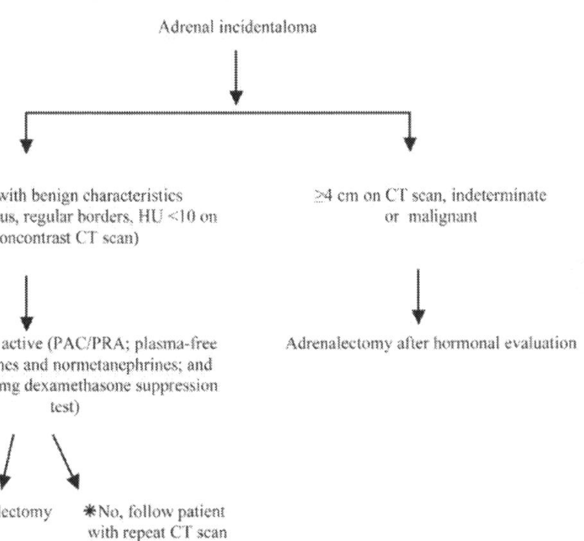

- **Follow-up**
  - Optimal follow up strategy is not clear
  - Can consider repeat in 6 months and then annual imaging for 4-5 years

OSTEOPOROSIS

- **Risk Factors**
  - Low BMI (<21)
  - Alcohol use (>3 drinks/d)
  - ↓Vitamin D or Ca
  - Smoking
  - Female
  - Parenteral history of hip fracture
  - ↑age (>65)
  - Chronic steroids
- **Screening**[132,133]
  - Women: ≥65 or >50 with ≤10 year risk of fracture of >9.3% based on FRAX tool
  - Men: >70 or at increased risk

Intervals of Screening	
15 years	For those with normal BMD (T-score ≥−1.0) or mild osteopenia (T-score <−1.0 and >−1.5)
5 years	For those with moderate osteopenia (T-score <−1.5 and >−2.0)
1 year	For those with advanced osteopenia (T-score <−2.0 and >−2.5)

- **Risk Factors**
  - Family history
  - Low body weight (<127#)
  - Systemic steroids, diuretics, SSRI, depo-provera
  - Low BMI
- **Imaging**
  - DEXA scan q5y (or q10y) of the lumbar hip and spine for screening
  - DEXA scan q1-2y if osteopenia/porosis
- **Labs**

  Current evidence is insufficient to support routine laboratory testing in patients with osteoporosis to identify possible secondary causes.
  - CBC
  - 25-OHD (goal >30 ng/mL) but conflicting data regarding utility of testing for this
  - TSH
  - PTH
  - CMP
    - Serum calcium
    - Serum creatinine
  - *Specialized labs*
    - Iron, ferritin (r/o hemochromatosis)
    - Testosterone (men; r/o hypogonadism)
    - SPEP/UPEP (r/o MM)
    - Urine free cortisol (r/o Cushings)
    - Transglutaminase (r/o Celiac)

Diagnosis/Interpretation	
Diagnosis	T-score
Normal	>−1.0
Osteopenia	−1.0 to −2.5
Osteoporosis	<−2.5 -or- osteopenia+fragility fracture
Severe osteoporosis	<−2.5 plus fragility fractures

- BMD gives your bone mineral density - the number of grams per centimeter of bone.
- Numbers of +1.0 or above are good.
- T score shows how your bone mineral density compares with women in their 30's, the peak bone density years.
- Calculated using the formula: (patient's BMD − young normal mean)/SD of young normal.
- Scores between -1 and -2.5 indicate Osteopenia (thin bones).
- Several large studies have shown an unacceptably high risk of fracture in postmenopausal women who have T-scores of −2.5 and below.
- Z score compares your bone mineral density with others of your own age.
- Are calculated similarly to the T-score, except the patient's BMD is compared with an age-matched (and race- and gender-matched) mean, and the result expressed as a SD score.

- In premenopausal women, a low Z-score (below −2.0) indicates that bone density is lower than expected and should trigger a search for an underlying cause.

- **Treatment**
  The goal of treatment is to prevent disabling fractures.
  - **<u>Osteopenia</u>**
    - <u>FRAX</u>
      - In patients not meeting diagnostic criteria for osteoporosis, use the http://www.shef.ac.uk/FRAX/tool.jsp to determine who would benefit still due to increased risk
      - FRAX was developed by the WHO to be applicable to both postmenopausal women and men aged 40 to 90 years;
      - It is validated to be used in **untreated** patients only.
      - NOF recommends **treating patients** with FRAX 10-year risk scores of <u>>3% for hip fracture or >20% for major osteoporotic fracture</u>, to reduce their fracture risk.
        - T-score of <-2.5 –or- osteopenia (-1 to -2.4) with **FRAX risk of at least 20% for major osteoporotic fracture of hip fracture of 3%**
  - **<u>Known Osteoporosis (T<-2.5)</u>**
    - Offer pharmacologic treatment to women with <u>known</u> osteoporosis to reduce the risk for hip and vertebral fractures
      - Alendronate, risedronate, zoledronic acid, or denosumab may be used. See table for more information.
    - Avoid alcohol, tobacco, excessive caffeine
    - Weight-bearing Exercise
      - Jogging, walking, stair climbing can ↑ BMD by more than 5% from baseline
      - Duration has to be 30-60 min at least 3x/week
    - <u>Medications</u>
      - *ERT*
        - All women with decreased bone density should be offered estrogen replacement therapy (ERT) unless contraindications exist.
        - Not used to treat, but can help progression
        - Best within 5 years of menopause for 10+ years
        - Conjugated estrogens in dosages of 0.625 and 1.25 mg per day and transdermal estrogen (a weekly patch containing 0.05 mg) are equally effective in reducing bone loss in postmenopausal and oophorectomized women
      - *Calcium/Vitamin D Supplementation*
        - Combined calcium and vitamin D supplementation at prudent doses should be recommended in older institutionalized patients and community-dwelling older adults with inadequate dietary intake.
        - Elemental Ca (1g/d if <50; 1.2g/d >50) and Vitamin D (600IU if <70; 800-1000IU if >70)
          - Or have patient take one MVI (400U Vitamin D) with two tablets of calcium/vitamin D (600mg calcium and 200IU vitamin D)
          - Goal vitamin D (25-OHD) is ≥75 nmol/L
      - *Bisphosphonates*
        - Indicated for women with osteoporosis, osteopenia (if FRAX major osteoporotic fracture probability is ≥20%, or if hip fracture probability is ≥3%), and low bone mass with fragility fracture.
        - Take 30 minutes prior to laying down/eating/taking other medications with plenty of water

- Therapy for known osteoporosis should last 5 years (if PO) or 3 years (if IV); **no need** to monitor BMD during this time. After this time period, re-evaluate fracture risk.
    - High risk: continue PO for total of 10 years or IV for total of 6 years.
    - Low risk: a drug holiday of 2-3 years can be considered after 3 to 5 years of PO treatment.
- In women aged ≥65 with osteopenia and at high fracture risk, treatment initiation is based on patient preference, fracture-risk profile, benefits, harms, and price of medications.

Therapy Options (trial in parentheses)		
Alendronic Acid *FIT*	10mg/d or 70mg/w (unless GFR<35) for 5 years (mild risk) or 6-10 years (high risk) 5mg/d for prevention purposes in patients only 7.5mg/d of prednisone for >3 months	Primary option for Osteoporosis
Risedronate *VERT-NA, VERT-MN*	35mg/w or 150mg/m	Alternative option if patient cannot tolerate Alendronic Acid
Ibandronate	PO 150mg/month or IV 3mg q3m	Once a month dosing or every 3 months
Zoledronic acid *HORIZON-PFT*	IV 5mg/year	Good for those who do not want to take PO medications
Denosumab *FREEDOM*	SQ 60mg q6m	Good to prevent vertebral and hip fx (unlike bisphosphonate and zoledronic acid)
Raloxifine	PO 60mg/d	SERM that acts similarly to ERT, lower breast cancer risk than ERT; It can be considered in the treatment and prevention of osteoporosis in postmenopausal women with high risk for invasive breast cancer. Due to the risk of DVT, PE, or stroke (especially in postmenopausal women at risk for coronary heart disease), it must be weighed against the benefits
Teriparatide *FPT*	SQ 20mcg/d for <2 years	Recombinant PTH; useful for those who suffer from fragility fractures despite tx

- **Follow-up**
    - <u>At each yearly exam, determine...</u>

      (1) Continuing bisphosphonate treatment
        - Total of 3 years if low risk; *BMD<-2; no risk factors*
        - Total of 5 years if mild-moderate risk; *BMD≥2-2.5 but stable, famhx of hip fx*

- Up to 10 years if on PO tx; 6 years if IV) in patients at high risk; *see below*)

(2) Starting drug holiday[134]

- No clear data regarding this, based on *FLEX* and *HORIZON-PFT* trials
- Goal is to maintain fracture risk at a low level while avoiding therapy as some data has suggested no benefit of bisphosphonate therapy >5 years and bisphosphonates themselves are associated with long-term safety risks.
- Re-assess fracture risk (see next section for specific variables to monitor) after pre-defined ranges above in patients who:
    - Have had no hip, spine, or multiple or other osteoporotic fx
    - BMD in the osteopenic or normal range
    - Not at high fx risk (BMD≥-2.5; history of recent hip or spine fx, ongoing high-dose steroid tx
- Reasonable to stop therapy in patients at low-moderate risk for fracture who have been on therapy for 3-5 years and meet criteria above. Patients at high risk should continue therapy or change treatments and have re-assessment in another 2-3 years.

(3) Changing pharmacologic treatment

- If decrease in BMD≥4% in the spine or hip noted or new fracture occurs during holiday
- Consider switching to Raloxifine

- Monitoring Drug Holiday
    - Obtain DEXA (to calculate FRAX), vitamin D, and calcium levels
    - Ask about history of recent fratures
    - Ask about high dose steroid use
    - A treatment-induced BMD increase can only be detected in general after 2 years; goal is for stability or increase in T-score
        - Can ↓ to 1 year if patient on long-term steroids
        - Decline ≤3% is considered stable
    - Expressed as SDD, a BMD change should exceed 0.02 g/cm2 at the total hip (3.56%) and 0.04 g/cm2 at the spine (5.60%) before it can be considered a significant change.
- Referral Criteria
    - If there is uncertainty regarding whether a patient will benefit from pharmacotherapy for fracture prevention
    - when to resume medication after a drug holiday
    - Which medication should be used after a drug holiday
    - In patients with intolerance to standard drug treatments or those in whom treatment failure is suspected.
    - Consultation with orthopedic or physical medicine and rehabilitation specialists is often required for management of patients presenting with an acute fracture.

- **Other Helpful Factors**
    - ↑Exercise
    - HRT not indicated unless patient has moderate to severe post-menopausal symptom

SEXUAL DYSFUNCTION

- **Types**[135]
    - Libido
    - Ejaculation
    - Erectile function - inability to achieve or maintain an erection of sufficient duration and firmness to complete satisfactory intercourse through vaginal penetration

- Combination of the above
- **Symptoms**
  - Osteoporosis
  - Anemia
  - Muscle weakness
  - Depression
  - Sexual dysfunction
- **Causes**
  - Psychologic – underlying depression, anxiety, fear of sexual failure (often sudden onset ED is a clue to this)
  - Primary Hypogonadism
  - OSA
  - Hyperprolactinemia
  - Social – tobacco, EtOH
  - Systemic illness
  - Post-Surgical – colon, radiation therapy to prostate
  - Vascular – irradiation, peripheral vascular disease, T2DM, HTN
  - Neurologic – TBI, stroke, seizure d/o, dysmyelinating disease, T2DM c/b neuropathy, RLS
  - Hormonal - ↑prolactin or ↓testosterone; hypothyroidism, adrenal insufficiency, Cushing's
  - Medications (SSRI), antihistamines, decongestants, BB, spironolactone
- **History**
  - Loss of AM erections may be a sign of no REM sleep, not necessarily organic pathology
    - Presence of AM erections almost always points to psychologic causes
  - Longer duration of symptoms may mean that psychologic issues may cause persistence of symptoms even if pharmacologic therapy is initiated
- **Physical Exam**
  - BP
  - Secondary Sexual Characteristics
    - Gynecomastia
  - Thyroid
  - Scrotal formation, size, consistency, nodules
  - DRE
- **Screening neurologic exam**
  - <u>Labs</u>
    - CBC (HCT>52% is relative contraindication to testosterone replacement therapy)
    - CMP (evaluate kidney function)
    - TSH
    - Lipid Panel
    - Fasting Glucose
    - PSA (if likely to start testosterone therapy)
    - Testosterone → if low on 2 measurements then obtain LH/FSH to determine Primary or Secondary
      - [19–39 years] 264 to 916 ng/dL
      - [40-49 years] 208 to 902 ng/dL
      - [50-59 years] 192 to 902 ng/dL
      - [60-79 years] 190 to 902 ng/dL
      - [80-99 years] 119 to 902 ng/dL
    - Prolactin
- **Treatment**

- CBT
- If applicable, optimization of glucose and blood pressure
- Tobacco cessation
- Treatment of hyperlipidemia
- Decreased EtOH
- Testosterone Replacement Therapy
  - Before initiating therapy, evaluate for OSA, BPH (do a DRE), prostate cancer (DRE), and PCV (obtain a CBC as above)
  - Evaluate within **1 to 3 months** after starting therapy, then every **6-12 months** thereafter.
  - Improvement should be seen in 3 months, if not, consider alternative diagnosis
  - **Options**
    - Patch (Androderm) – placed on the scrotal skin with peak levels in 3-5 hours; apply in evening
    - Gel (1%)

DIABETES MELLITUS

- **Diagnosis**[136,137,138]

Glucose Testing and Interpretation			
	Normal	High Risk	Diabetes
Fasting	<100 mg/dL	100-125 mg/dL	≥126 mg/dL
Post-Prandial	<140 mg/dL	140-199 mg/dL	≥ 200 mg/dL
A1c	<5.5%	5-6-6.4%	≥ 6.5%

- Symptoms of DM (polyuria, polydipsia, unexplained weight loss with glucosuria and ketonuria) plus a random plasma glucose > 200 mg/dL or 2H post prandial 75g load of >200. (Whole blood values are lower by 10-15 mg/dL). Of note, symptoms are most commonly absent.
- **A second test is always required if patients do not present with classic symptoms and >200mg on glucose level (ie. fasting >126, A1c>6.5 require confirmatory test)**
- Prediabetes
  - Also called "high-risk"
  - A1c between 5-6.4%
- The diagnostic cutoff point for diabetes is a fasting plasma glucose level of **126** mg per deciliter (7.0 mmol per liter); the diagnosis requires confirmation by the same or the other test.
  - Impaired fasting glucose (pre-diabetes) is 100-125 mg/dL; higher risk was considered to be A1c between **5.7-6.4%**
    - Preventative metformin should be considered if patients are in this range and obese (BMI >35) and <60 YO and fail to respond to decrease their risk through lifestyle change (150 min activity/week and 5-7% weight loss)
  - Fasting value determined in the morning after absence of caloric intake at least 8 hours.
- Additional Labs
  - Type 1 or 2: CMP, TSH, lipids, C-peptide can help differentiate between DM1 and DM2 (<5 microU/mL suggests type 1 whereas >1 ng/dL suggestive of Type 2)
  - Type 1: anti-insulin, glutamic acid decarboxylase antibodies (GAD) and anti-islet antibodies (ICA) within 6 months of diagnosis
    - May suggest earlier need for insulin therapy if positive

    - DKA: ABG, urine ketones, beta-hydroxybutyrate, CMP for HCO3
  - Gestational
    - Overt: ≥ 126 mg/dL
    - Gestational: Fasting 92-125 mg/dL | 1-h post load ≥ 180 mg/dL | 2-h post load 153-199 mg/dL

Comparison between Type 1 and 2	
Type 1	Type 2
Presenting at young age (prior to puberty) Thin +FHx of T1DM or autoimmune disease AB positive (ICA, insulin, GAD) C-peptide < 5 ↑↑ glucose Abrupt onset DKA	Overweight Negative AB Older age Gradual onset HHS

- **Treatment**
  - Hypertension: debates, but ADA recommends a goal of <140/90
  - Prediabetes
    - Primary goal is weight loss
    - No medications are FDA approved solely for pre-diabetes use; metformin and acarbose can ↓ risk of overt diabetes by up to 30%
  - Outpatient
    - Type 2
      - Lifestyle modification
      - A1c
        - <7.5%: Metformin 500-1000mg BID
        - 7.5-8.9%: combination therapy with metformin and medication in table below
        - ≥ 9.0%: Insulin+metformin
        - Insulin should always be used for **symptomatic** hyperglycemia, A1C≥10, and/or BG ≥300 mg/dL.
      - Sulfonylureas
        - Not recommended unless patient preference (cost)
        - Glimepiride has longer half-life (once daily dosing) while Glyburide and Glipizide are BID dosing and thus have ↓ onset of hypoglycemia
        - See page 220 for oral medication options.
      - Insulin
        - See next section
        - Consider after 2 oral medications on board and A1c remaining above 8
    - **Targets**[139]
      - Reasonable glycemic targets would be:
        - <6.5% in healthy older adults with long life expectancy
        - <7.0% in patients with concurrent illness and at risk for hypoglycemia
      - Nonpregnant adults
        - <7%

- <6.5% if can be obtained safely without risk for hypoglycemia or significant comorbidities; see below for more information under *Preventive Medicine*)
- Fasting/Pre-prandial 80-130 mg/dL
- Post-prandial <180 mg/dL
- Monitoring can be done with random glucose, post-prandial, and A1c (q3m)

Figure. Algorithm for management of T2DM that is poorly controlled on PO medications

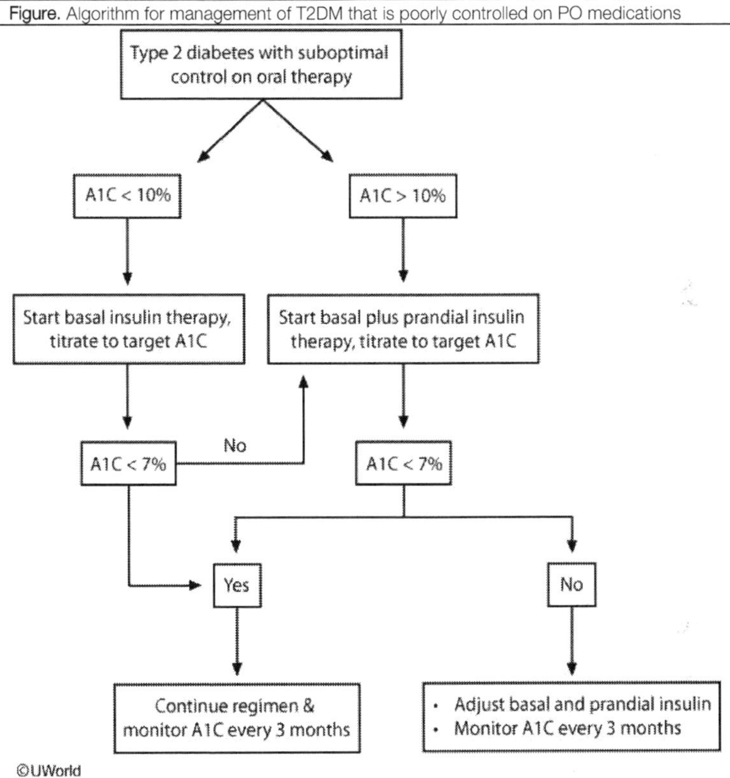

Pharmacologic Options in the treatment of T2DM

Order of Initiation	Class /A1c↓	Dose	Pathophysiology	S/E	Points of Consideration
Non-insulin injectables					
- If after 3 months patient's glucose is not at goal with therapy started, add second/third agent. - Consider dual-therapy if A1c > 7.5% (understand a third agent is unlikely to help with A1c of 8 or more) - Consider injectable (insulin, GLP-1) if A1c > 9% - Initial therapy is always lifestyle modification with activity goal of 150 min/week and weight loss of 7% body fat					
1	**Biguanide** 1% to 2%	**Metformin/Metformin ER** INITIAL: 500 to 2,000 mg in divided doses INITIAL ER: 1,000 to 2,000 mg every evening MAX INITIAL: 2,500 mg/day MAX ER: 2000mg/d	Inhibits hepatic glycogenolysis, gluconeogenesis and enhances insulin sensitivity in muscle and fat. Decreases the sugar that comes from the liver.	**Nausea**, diarrhea, abdominal pain. Lactic acidosis but GFR lower limits have been relaxed: must be **at least 30** cc/min Add B12 if neuropathy develops If patient received IV contrast, restart after **48** hours	• Promotes modest weight loss. • Newer data suggests it is okay to use even in the face of CHF, LF, CRF[140] • Do not start in patients with eGFR<45 but can be maintained if eGFR>30 • Do NOT stop use even if patient is now on insulin. It has been shown to decrease MACE, can lead to overall decrease in insulin requirements (6.6U/d) • Monitor B12 levels in patients with anemia

					or peripheral neuropathy
2	**GLP-1 receptor agonist** 0.5-1%	**Liraglutide** *(Victoza)* INITIAL: 0.6 mg **SC** once daily x 1 week, then increase to 1.2 mg SC daily. MAX: 1.8 mg/day Exenatide *(Byetta)* INITIAL: 5 mcg SC BID within 60 min of a meal with 6h b/w meals. ↑ to max dose after 1 month. MAX: 10 mcg SC BID Exenatide extended-release *(Bydureon)* INITIAL: 2 mg SC once weekly MAX: 2 mg SC once weekly Albiglutide *(Tanzeum)* INITIAL: 30mg/week MAX: 50mg/week Dulaglutide *(Trulicity)* INITIAL: 0.75mg/week MAX: 1.5mg/week	Stimulates GLP-1 receptors which increases production of insulin in response to high blood glucose levels, inhibits postprandial glucagon release, slows gastric emptying. (GLP-1 is an incretin hormone.)	Headache, **nausea**, diarrhea. May be associated with pancreatitis. May be associated with renal insufficiency.	• Transient n/v • **Continue in patients on insulin** • Causes weight loss • Injectable that sometimes is considered last line in combination **with insulin** especially if fasting levels are controlled by A1c remains high • **Contraindicated if severe kidney disease present (GFR<30) or FHx of medullary thyroid cancer** • Greater glucose reduction in daily preparations vs. weekly however those patients also had more s/e • Liraglutide had greater glucose reduction than exenatide

					• **Significantly lower risk of cardiovascular death, nonfatal MI, or nonfatal stroke than placebo in *LEADER* trial** • ↓BP, no hypoglycemia
3	**SGLT2 inhibitor**[141] 0.7% to 1%	**Empagliflozin *(Jardiance)*** <u>INITIAL</u>: 10-25g/d <u>MAX</u>: Canagliflozin *(Invokana)* <u>INITIAL</u>: 100 mg PO once daily <u>MAX</u>: 300 mg/day Dapagliflozin *(Farxiga)* <u>INITIAL</u>: 5 mg PO once daily <u>MAX</u>: 10 mg/day	Sodium-glucose co-transporter 2 inhibitor reduces reabsorption of filtered glucose and lowers the renal threshold for glucose, resulting in increased urinary glucose excretion.	**Genital fungal infections** (male and female), urinary tract infection, increased urination, hypo-tension, ketoacidosis ↑risk for DKA when combined with insulin in T1DM patients Canaglifozin had ↑ risk for amputations	• Causes weight loss. • **Good option in ↓ CVD in those with pre-existing dz, ↓** hospitalization in HF patients, and those with CKD (*EMPA-REG OUTCOME)* • Causes slight reduction of BP. • May increase LDL. • Stop 24 hours prior to surgery • Can cause positive urinary glucose test. • Can help decrease overall insulin required if concurrent insulin is used

DPP-4 0.5% to 1%	**Sitagliptin *(Januvia)*** INITIAL: 100 mg PO once daily Alogliptin *(Nesina)* INITIAL: 25 mg PO once daily Linagliptin *(Tradjenta)* INITIAL: 5 mg PO once daily *Saxagliptin (Onglyza)*: INITIAL: 2.5 mg/day MAX: 5 mg/day	Inhibits degradation of endogenous incretins which increases insulin secretion, decreases glucagon secretion (glucose-dependent).	May be associated with pancreatitis. Alogliptin and saxagliptin are associated with heart failure, but sitagliptin is likely not.	• Weight neutral. • Should not be used in patients with history of cardiac disease as it may increase risk of heart failure (alogliptin and saxagliptin only) • Contraindicated in **severe** kidney disease (GFR<50) but can reduce dose. • Low risk of hypoglycemia. • Dosage modification with renal impairment needed with sitagliptin, saxagliptin, and alogliptin. • Combination with metformin showed lower risk for all-cause death, MACE, stroke, and hypoglycemia[142]
Meglitinide 0.7-1.1%	**Repaglinide *(Prandin)*** INITIAL: 0.5mg TID/meals or 1-2mg TID if already on	Simulate insulin secretion	Avoid in patients with liver dysfunction	• Good option if patient is (1) intolerant to metformin +/-

		hypoglycemic med MAX: 4mg TID/meals Nateglinide *(Starlix)* INITIAL: 120mg TID/meals but can start at 60mg if close to A1c goal MAX: 120mg TID/meals Exenatide INITIAL: IR-5mcg BID within 60 min of AM or PM meal; ↑ to 10mcg BID p̄ 1 month ER-2mg/week with or without foods			sulfonylurea and have CKD or (2) need add-on therapy to metformin • Rapid onset, short duration • ↑weight • Risk of hypoglycemia • Great for patients who have erratic eating schedules (you only take it with meals) or late postprandial hypoglycemia on sulfonylurea
4	**Sulfonylurea** 0.7-1.5%	Glimepiride *(Amaryl)* INITIAL: 8mg/d Glyburide *(DiaBeta)* INITIAL: 5mg/d Glipizide *(Glucotrol)* INITIAL: 10mg/d	Stimulates the pancreas to put out more insulin over several hours.	Hypoglycemia ↑Weight	• Higher risk for hypoglycemia • Patients cannot skip meals • Avoid in patients with known sulfa allergies

Name/Generic/A1c	Class	Dose	Pathophysiology	S/E	Points of Consideration
Combination Oral Medications					
Glucovance Glyburide+Metformin **Metaglip** Glipizide+Metformin 0.7-1.3%	Sulfonylurea +Biguanide	INITIAL: 5/500mg/BID INITIAL: 20/2000mg/BID	Stimulates pancreatic insulin secretion	Hypoglycemia ↑weight Nausea Abdominal pain Diarrhea	• Hypoglycemia • ↑Weight
Actoplus Met Pioglitazone+Metformin 0.8-0.9%	Thiazolidine +Biguanide	INITIAL IR: 15/500mg BID 15/850mg daily ER: 15/1000mg daily 45/2000mg daily	Increases insulin sensitivity in muscle and fat	Edema ↑weight Nausea Abdominal pain Diarrhea CHF risk ↑ risk of bladder CA	• ↑weight • Edema • Decreased dosing if CHF
Janumet Sitagliptin+Metformin 0.5-0.7%	DPP-4 inhibitor +Biguanide	Already on Metformin: 100/(daily metformin) Not on Metformin: 100/1000mg daily	Increases insulin secretion in response to elevated blood glucose, decreases glucagon secretion, increases sense of fullness, and slows gastric emptying	Hives (if allergi) Nausea GI upset Diarrhea	• Risk of hives • Pancreatitis • Weight neutral • May ↑ risk for CHF • May ↑ joint pains

Invokamet Canaglifozin+Metformin **Glyxambi** Empaglifozin+Linagliptin 0.4-0.7%	SGLT-2 inhibitor +Biguanide	<u>INITIAL</u>: 100/1000mg daily (divide total BID if IR formulation) <u>MAX</u> 300/2000mg daily max <u>INITIAL</u>: 10/5mg daily <u>MAX</u>: 25/5mg daily	Blocks glucose reabsorption in the kidney, and increases urinary excretion of glucose	Nausea Abdominal pain UTI Yeast infections Dehydration	• Risk of UTIs higher • Dehydration risk • Empagliflozin use in patients with CVD for about three years may reduce CV disease

Antidiabetic Medication Profiles

	Metformin	GLP-1	SGLT-2	DPP-4	Metaglinide	Insulin
↑ Hypolycemia	Neutral	Neutral	Neutral	Neutral	Mild	Moderate/Severe
Weight	↓	↓↓	↓↓	Neutral	↑	↑
Renal or GU dz	C/I if GFR<30	Exenatide C/I Liraglutide a benefit	Avoid if GFR<45 ↑genital mycotic infxn Empaglifozin a benefit	Dose adjustment ↓albuminuria	Higher hypoglycemia	Higher hypoglycemia
GI Sx	Moderate	Moderate	Neutral	Neutral	Neutral	Neutral
Cardiac						
-CHF	Neutral	Liraglutide ↓MACE	Empaglifozin ↓CV mortality Canaglifozin ↓ MACE	↑hospitalization in CHF	Neutral	↑CHF risk
-ASCVD					↑ASCVD risk	Neutral
Bone	Neutral	Neutral	↑ fx risk	Neutral	Neutral	Neutral

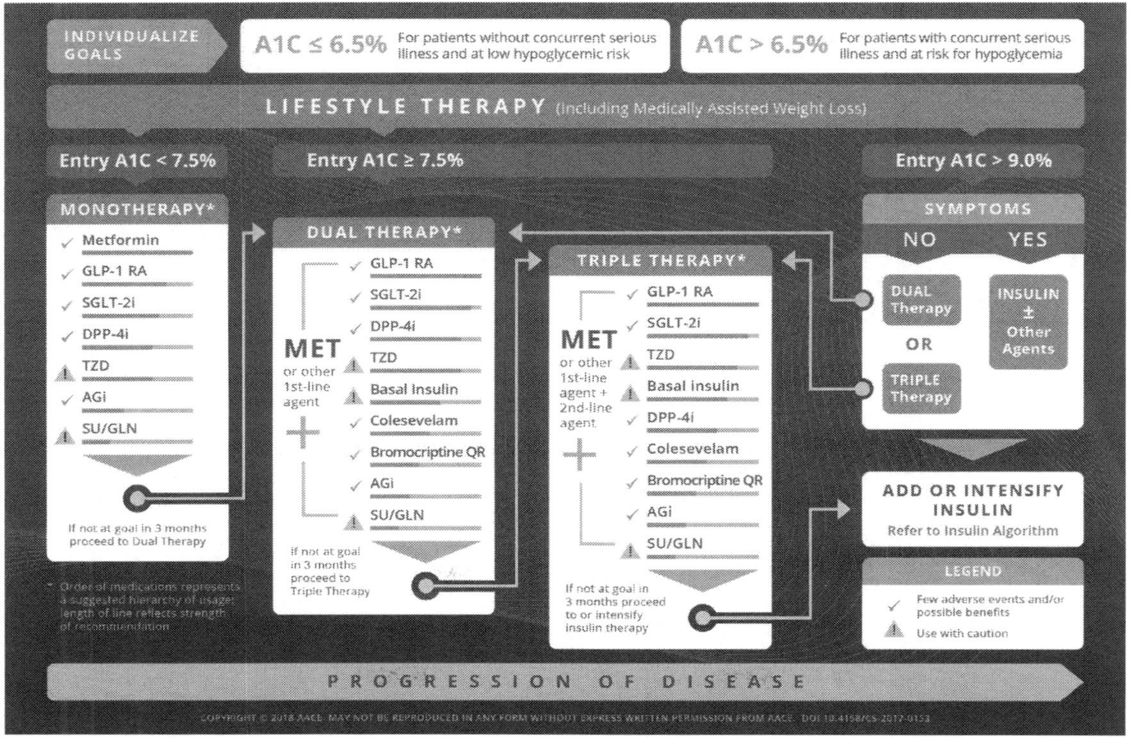

INDIVIDUALIZE GOALS

A1C ≤ 6.5% For patients without concurrent serious illness and at low hypoglycemic risk

A1C > 6.5% For patients with concurrent serious illness and at risk for hypoglycemia

LIFESTYLE THERAPY (Including Medically Assisted Weight Loss)

Entry A1C < 7.5%

MONOTHERAPY*

- ✓ Metformin
- ✓ GLP-1 RA
- ✓ SGLT-2i
- ✓ DPP-4i
- ⚠ TZD
- ✓ AGi
- ⚠ SU/GLN

If not at goal in 3 months proceed to Dual Therapy

* Order of medications represents a suggested hierarchy of usage; length of line reflects strength of recommendation

Entry A1C ≥ 7.5%

DUAL THERAPY*

MET or other 1st-line agent +

- ✓ GLP-1 RA
- ✓ SGLT-2i
- ✓ DPP-4i
- ⚠ TZD
- ⚠ Basal insulin
- ✓ Colesevelam
- ✓ Bromocriptine QR
- ✓ AGi
- ⚠ SU/GLN

If not at goal in 3 months proceed to Triple Therapy

TRIPLE THERAPY*

MET or other 1st-line agent + 2nd-line agent +

- ✓ GLP-1 RA
- ✓ SGLT-2i
- ⚠ TZD
- ⚠ Basal insulin
- ✓ DPP-4i
- ✓ Colesevelam
- ✓ Bromocriptine QR
- ✓ AGi
- ⚠ SU/GLN

If not at goal in 3 months proceed to or intensify insulin therapy

Entry A1C > 9.0%

SYMPTOMS

NO: DUAL Therapy OR TRIPLE Therapy

YES: INSULIN ± Other Agents

ADD OR INTENSIFY INSULIN

Refer to Insulin Algorithm

LEGEND

✓ Few adverse events and/or possible benefits

⚠ Use with caution

PROGRESSION OF DISEASE

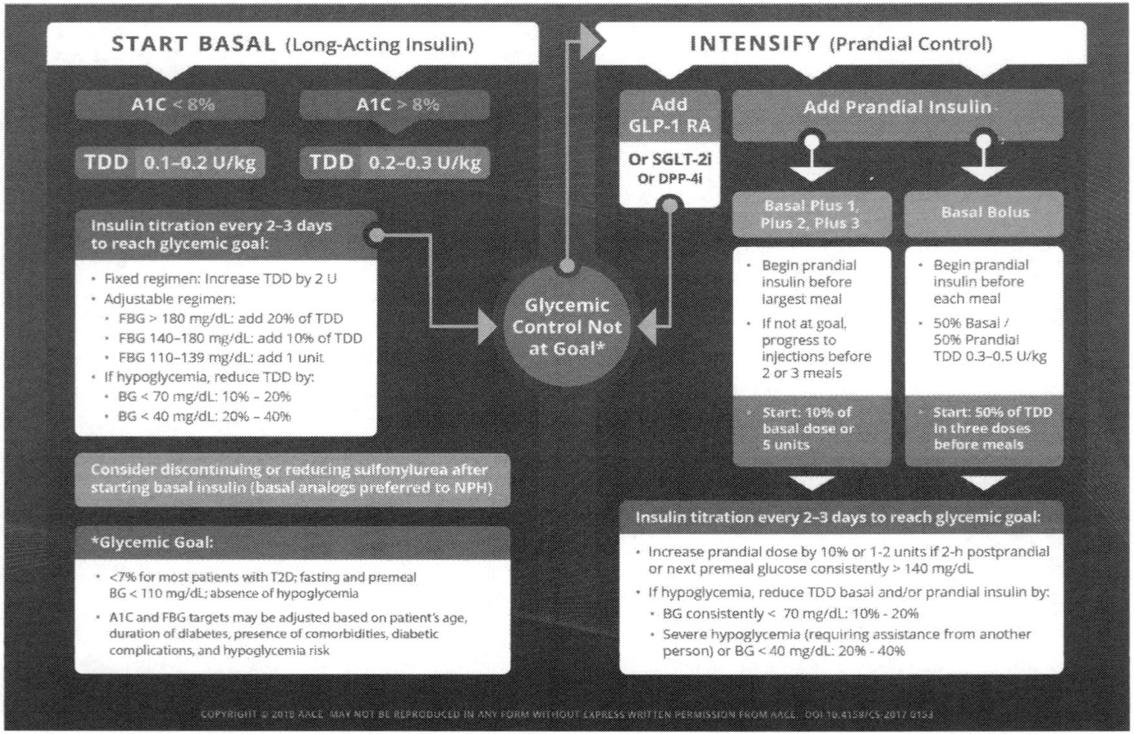
START BASAL (Long-Acting Insulin)
A1C < 8%
A1C > 8%
TDD 0.1–0.2 U/kg
TDD 0.2–0.3 U/kg
Insulin titration every 2–3 days to reach glycemic goal:
• Fixed regimen: Increase TDD by 2 U
• Adjustable regimen:
• FBG > 180 mg/dL: add 20% of TDD
• FBG 140–180 mg/dL: add 10% of TDD
• FBG 110–139 mg/dL: add 1 unit
• If hypoglycemia, reduce TDD by:
• BG < 70 mg/dL: 10% – 20%
• BG < 40 mg/dL: 20% – 40%
Consider discontinuing or reducing sulfonylurea after starting basal insulin (basal analogs preferred to NPH)
*Glycemic Goal:
• <7% for most patients with T2D; fasting and premeal BG < 110 mg/dL; absence of hypoglycemia
• A1C and FBG targets may be adjusted based on patient's age, duration of diabetes, presence of comorbidities, diabetic complications, and hypoglycemia risk
Glycemic Control Not at Goal*
INTENSIFY (Prandial Control)
Add GLP-1 RA
Or SGLT-2i
Or DPP-4i
Add Prandial Insulin
Basal Plus 1, Plus 2, Plus 3
• Begin prandial insulin before largest meal
• If not at goal, progress to injections before 2 or 3 meals
• Start: 10% of basal dose or 5 units
Basal Bolus
• Begin prandial insulin before each meal
• 50% Basal / 50% Prandial TDD 0.3–0.5 U/kg
• Start: 50% of TDD in three doses before meals
Insulin titration every 2–3 days to reach glycemic goal:
• Increase prandial dose by 10% or 1-2 units if 2-h postprandial or next premeal glucose consistently > 140 mg/dL
• If hypoglycemia, reduce TDD basal and/or prandial insulin by:
• BG consistently < 70 mg/dL: 10% - 20%
• Severe hypoglycemia (requiring assistance from another person) or BG < 40 mg/dL: 20% - 40%
COPYRIGHT © 2018 AACE. MAY NOT BE REPRODUCED IN ANY FORM WITHOUT EXPRESS WRITTEN PERMISSION FROM AACE. DOI 10.4158/CS-2017-0153

Feeding Options	
Feeding Method	Plan
PO/ Bolus Tube Feeds	Check BS AC and HS Basal: 50% of TDD during each feeding Premeal: 1/3 of ½ of TDD
Enteral/Continuous Tube	Check BS q4h Basal: 20% of TDD Premeal: 80% of TDD divided into 6 doses given equally q4h Hold if TF interrupted for >2 hours or if BS<100 mg/dL
Fasting/Clear Liquid/TPN	Check BS q4h Basal: 40-80% of TDD q4h Premeal: none

- Inpatient
  - See feeding options above
  - **Target**:
    - In critically ill patients - aiming for a target range of 140-180 mg/dL
    - Non critically ill patients - goals of pre meal glucose < 140 mg/dL and random < 180 mg/dL
    - Preoperative - ≤ 200 mg/dL
- **Gestational Diabetes**[143]
  - Preconception
    - Women already on insulin should be treated with multiple daily doses of insulin or continuous sc insulin infusion in preference to split-dose, premixed insulin therapy
    - Women with diabetes successfully using the long-acting insulin analogs insulin detemir or insulin glargine preconceptionally may continue with this therapy before and then during pregnancy.
    - Beginning 3 months before withdrawing contraceptive measures or otherwise trying to conceive, a woman with diabetes take a daily folic acid supplement to reduce the risk of neural tube defects
  - Treatment
    - Target values as close to normal as possible
      - Preprandial Goal: ≤ 95 mg/dL
      - 1 h after meal: ≤ 140 mg/dL
      - 2 h afer meal: ≤ 120 mg/dL
    - Initial treatment will always be dietary, however insulin (lispro, aspart as rapid acting along with long acting detemir or glargine) or glyburide are the only approved pharmacologic therapies in pregnancy (metformin can be added after first trimester)
  - All women should track glucose via 1 or 2 hour post prandial, bedtime, and 3am levels

- **Treatment in Hospital**
  - Discharge Orders
    - If newly diagnosed diabetic, needs glucometer, oral medications, and close follow-up
    - Consider the following regimen in newly diagnosed patients:

        - Begin low-dose metformin (500 mg) once or BID w/meals (breakfast and/or dinner)
        - After 5–7 days, if GI s/e have not occurred, ↑ dose to 850–1,000 mg before breakfast and dinner.
        - If gastrointestinal side effects appear as doses advance, decrease dose to the previous lower dose and try to advance at a later time.
        - The typical therapeutic dose is 850 mg twice daily. Higher doses, up to 2,550 mg daily, can be used but tend to be associated with more significant side effects and are not recommended as starting doses.

- **Preventive Medicine**
    - Microvascular Disease
        - The Diabetes Control and Complications Trial (DCCT), a prospective randomized controlled trial of intensive versus standard glycemic control in patients with relatively recently diagnosed type 1 diabetes, showed definitively that improved glycemic control is associated with significantly decreased rates of microvascular (retinopathy and diabetic kidney disease) and neuropathic complications.
            - Follow-up of the DCCT cohorts in the Epidemiology of Diabetes Interventions and Complications (EDIC) study demonstrated persistence of these microvascular benefits in previously intensively treated subjects, even though their glycemic control approximated that of previous standard arm subjects during follow-up.
            - Achieving glycemic control of **A1C targets of <7%** has been shown to **reduce microvascular** complications of diabetes and, in patients with type 1 diabetes, mortality. If implemented soon after the diagnosis of diabetes, this target is associated with long-term reduction in macrovascular disease.
                - Retinopathy: annual exam (q2y if no evidence of retinopathy is found)
                - Nephropathy: Annual assessment of SCr, eGFR, and albumin/creatinine ratio
                    - UACR < 30 normal
                    - UACR 30-299 is an early predictor for kidney complications
                    - UACR $\geq$ 300 mg/g are likely to develop ESRD
                - Hypertension: <130/80
                    - PM administration of losartan (vs daytime) has found to be beneficial in preventing onset of new type 2 diabetes[144]
    - Vaccinations
        - Hepatitis B vaccination if 19+ YO and no prior vaccination on record
        - Pneumococcal (13+23V) if >65
    - Lipids: <100 if no ASCVD, if ASCVD also present then target <70
    - Neuropathy: 5 years after diagnosis then annual assessment thereafter with 10g monofilament testing
    - Smoking cessation
    - Labs: LFT, spot urine protein/creatinine, SCr, GFR
    - Podiatry visits annually
    - Nutrition consultation (target 7% loss in body fat)
        - Patients who are obese (BMI$\geq$30) that had **pre**diabetes (FS 100-125 mg/dL; A1c 5.7-6.4%) were found to have lower progression to overt diabetes if they took Liraglutide (Saxenda) at 3mg/d (SQ) for 160 weeks.
        - Bariatric surgery for adults with BMI >35 kg/m and T2DM
        - FDA approved medications for weight loss: orlistat 60-120mg TID, Belviq 10mg BID

INSULIN MANAGEMENT

- **Considering Initiation**

Figure. Algorithm for initation of insulin therapy

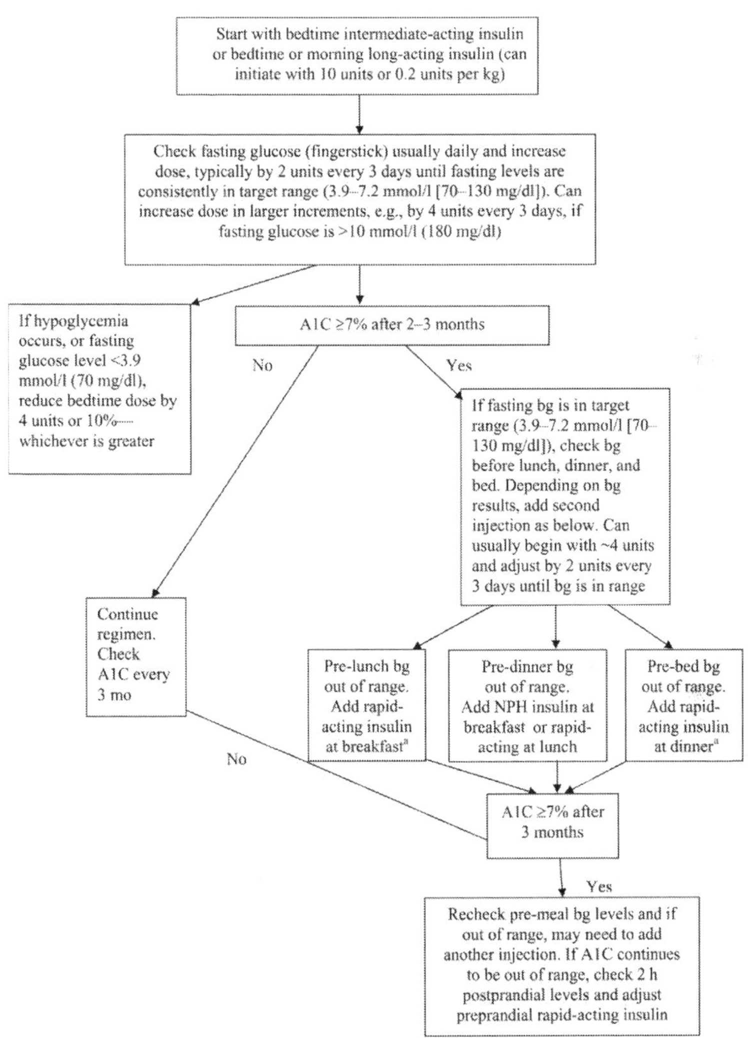

- **Calculating dose to start**

Managing Insulin in Diabetes

Unknown TDD	Known TDD	Known TDD (Premix)
1. Use medical history / body type to determine the TDD: <u>Malnourished/No h/o DM/Elderly/Frail</u> TDD = weight (kg) x (0.2 or 0.4) *Understand in insulin-naïve patients, you will likely have to work up to 0.6-0.7U/kg/d)* <u>Lean (BMI <25) T2DM, T1DM, 2/2 steroids</u> TDD = weight (kg) x 0.4 <u>Overweight (BMI 25-30)</u> TDD = weight (kg) x 0.5 <u>Obese (BMI>30), T2DM+steroids</u> TDD = weight (kg) x 0.6 *Renal impairment: Reduce total daily dose by 50% if creatinine clearance of <30ml/min* 2. Divide this # by 2 (or by 3 if you are doing pure short acting replacement before each meal) a. Half will be given as Lantus qhs and another half will be given pre-prandial as NovoLog b. Or consider 4U/d as a starting point 3. Now fine-tune your rapid acting	• TDD = o Total # units during 24 hour period -or- o (Avg hourly insulin drip rate over 6 hrs) x 20 which comes out to be about 80% of the daily infusion dose *Renal impairment: Reduce total daily dose by 50% if creatinine clearance of <30ml/min* • Consider TDD of 10U as a starting point for basal insulin • Divide this # by 2 (or by 3 if you are doing pure short acting replacement before each meal) o Half will be given as Lantus qhs and another half will be given pre-prandial as NovoLog (consider 4U/d as a starting point) o Patients on TF should have this dose split into 4 and given as regular insulin q6h o Add sliding scale on top of this to determine how much correction was needed • The following day, make changes as necessary to your regiment • Use the fasting AM glucose (0500-0700) to determine changes needed to **basal** insulin	1. Add up all doses of premix given in 24 hours 2. Give half as basal 3. Divide pre meals by 1/3

<u>MDI regimen (basal + rapid)</u>
• Basal, long-acting insulin once or twice a day
• Prandial, short-acting insulin based on:
  o # of carbohydrate portions (e.g., 1:10, meaning 1 U of insulin for every 10 g of carbohydrate to be eaten)
  o Correctional short-acting mealtime insulin based on premeal blood glucose level (subtract target blood glucose level and divided by sensitivity factor)
  o Preset sliding scale utilized which you then add to prandial dosing the following day based on totals: If your patient required 15U total of SSI throughout the day then add this to your TDD and repeat step (2)
 	
<u>CSII regimin (insulin pump)</u>
• May use regular insulin or rapid-acting insulin analogues
• Insulin is infused continuously at a preset rate, and bolus doses are given with meals as above.
	• Post meal insulin should then be used to adjust the **pre meal** insulin	

- Guidelines to starting insulin glargine (Lantus)
  - Multiple methods are utilized to convert to long-acting insulin after insulin requirements stabilize
  - Recommend giving 0.1-0.2 units/kg if A1c is <8% (0.2-0.3 U/kg if A1c 8-10%) with 50% of dose as Lantus and 50% as nutritional dose divided qAC. Then titrate dose as needed.
    - Starting points:
      - Basal: 10U
      - Prandial: 4U/day
  - Goals: A1c<7% (<6.5% if very healthy)
    - Fasting and Preprandial: 90-130 mg/dL
    - Postprandial (2 hrs): <180 mg/dL
    - Bedtime/overnight: 90-150 mg/dL

- **Options**

Insulin Adjuncts					
Type	Onset	Peak	Duration	Timing of Dose	Dosing
Rapid Acting					
Lispro *(Humalog)*	5-15min	30-90min	3-5h	15 min before meal	N/A
Aspart *(Novolog)*	5-15min	30-90min	4-6h	15 min before meal	N/A
Glulisine *(Apidra)*	5-15min	30-90min	5.3h	15 min before meal	N/A
Short Acting					
Regular *(Novolin R or Humulin R)*	30-60min	2-4h	6-10h	30-45min before meal	N/A
Intermediate					
NPH *(Humulin or Novolin)*	2-4h	4-10h	13-16h	Twice a day	N/A
Basal/Long					
Degludec *(Tresiba)* (U100/U200) (lower risk for hypoglycemia)	2h	9h	42h	Once a day	Type 1: 0.2-0.4 U/kg Type 2: 10U SC/d
Glargine *(Lantus)* (U300) (higher risk for hypoglycemia)	2h	None	24 hours	Once a day	
Detemir *(Levemir)*	2h	None	12-24 hours	Once or twice/day	

Figure. Duration of action of popular long acting insulin medications

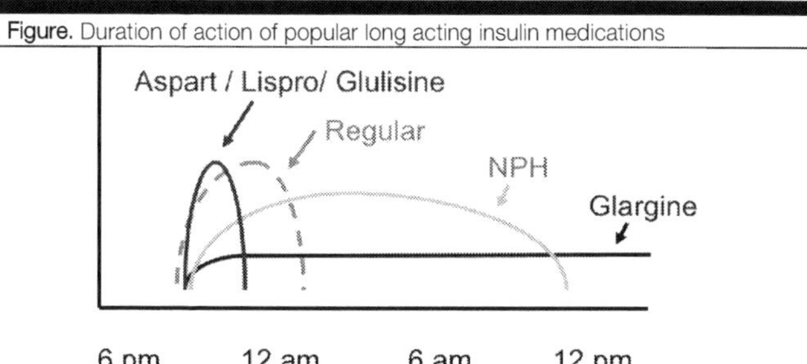

Styner, Maya. "Management of diabetes in Non-ICU hospitalized patients" PPT presentation

- **Titration of Insulin**

Insulin Titration		
Fasting Glucose (mg/dL)	AACE/ACE	ADA
>180	↑20% TDD	Increase dose 10-15% or by 2-4U
140-180	↑10% of TDD	
110-139	↑1U	
<70	↓10-20%	Determine cause, if not clear, ↓ by 10-20% or 2-4U
<40	↓20-40%	

  - Insulin Sensitivity Ratio (ISF) estimates the point drop in mmol/L per unit of rapid- or short-acting insulin.

1700* / Total Daily Dose of Insulin = ISF →amount 1U of insulin will drop BS

  - Now you know how much insulin to add to the pre meal insulin dose

    or

  - To use the insulin sensitivity factor calculate the difference between the current blood sugar (glucose) and the desired blood sugar. Then divide the result by the sensitivity factor. The result is the amount of insulin that needs to be added or subtracted from the pre meal insulin dose.

(CURRENT BG – IDEAL BG) = X

X / ISF = INSULIN ADDED TO PREMEAL DOSE

- **Insulin Sliding Scale**
  - Check patients' blood glucose qAM and qHS if NPO
  - **Type 1**: type 1 patients require less insulin than type 2's. They need basal insulin (even when NPO) to prevent DKA and extra insulin with each meal. If patients are

carbohydrate counting, allow patient to help determine meal insulin bolus. Sample type 1 pre-meal scale along with basal insulin (e.g. NPH 8 U SQ BID). Again, this scale is not intended for bedtime insulin coverage or patients that are not eating.
  - **Type 2**: for an average type 2 patient on orals meds as an outpatient consider the following sliding scale pre-meals (do not use these levels of insulin at bedtime) along with 5-10 units NPH qhs
- **Insulin Drip**
  - Indications
    - DKA
    - Hyperosmolar hyperglycemic state
    - Very poorly controlled diabetes despite Sub-Q insulin (BG >300-350 x 2 over 6-12 hr)
    - TPN
    - Type I DM who are NPO, periop, or in L & D
    - Post-MI with hyperglycemia
    - ICU pt with hyperglycemia
    - Suspect poor subQ absorption of insulin
  - Transition
    - When put back on Sub-Q insulin, give lispro 1-2 hr or long acting insulin 2-3 hr prior to stopping drip

PREOPERATIVE INSULIN DOSAGE

- *Preoperative glucose levels of <200 mg/dL on the day of surgery is ideal for elective surgery (also a goal of HgA1c of <8% is ideal)*

Perioperative Management[146]	
Situation	Changes Recommended
Basal QHS + Premeals = 50/50 with no hypoglycemic episodes	Full basal dose given (75% dose if experiencing hypoglycemic episodes)
Basal QAM + Premeals = 50/50 with no hypoglycemic episodes	75% of basal dose in AM
Premixed insulins	Two Options 1. Switch to regimen of long acting and short acting independent of one another and follow above instructions 2. Take half of normal morning dose and give concurrent D5W and routine BS checks
Preprandial insulin	Stop doses on the AM of surgery
Oral hypoglycemic for T2DM	1. Hold sulfonylurea or secretagogue on day of procedure and resume when tolerates NL diet 2. Hold metformin for safety concern the day of procedure and resume 48 hr post-op if renal fxn normal or near normal 3. Can continue TZDs
Sliding scale insulin	Used to correct for BS>200 mg/dL
Fluids	D5W with 1/2NS @ 50cc/hr

- **Perioperative insulin management**

- Maintain BG **100-180 mg/dL** to prevent dehydration/ketosis, promote wound healing, optimize leukocyte function, avoid hypoglycemia.
- Start 5 gm/hr glucose infusion (i.e. D51/2NS + 20 mEq KCl @ 100 mL/h).
- Can start IV insulin (1 unit/h) and adjust for goal or, if surgery is minor and patient's glucose is well-controlled, give 50% of usual SC insulin (if NPH) in the AM of surgery and supplement with regular insulin q4-6 hr to achieve goal.

OSTEOMYELITIS

- **Clinical Features**[147]
- High risk patients (ie. DM) with ulcer >2cm lasting >2 weeks with potentially visualized bone and elevated ESR
- **Diagnosis**
  - Labs - ↑ESR
  - Bone biopsy is the gold standard
  - Imaging
    - Plain film is first test to obtain
      - Only show changes 2-4 weeks into infection
      - Look for **periosteal reaction** and osseous lucency
      - Cannot distinguish from Charcot osteoarthropathy (disruption in foot architecture due to trauma repeatedly sustained due to poor sensation)
    - MRI
      - If strong suspicion of OM and negative plain film, then obtain MRI
      - Has high false positive rate
      - Focal areas of decreased marrow signal intensity on **T1-weighted** images
      - Focally increased signal intensity on fat-suppressed **T2-weighted** images
    - CT
      - Good to obtain if patient cannot obtain MRI
      - Lacks specificity
    - WBC scanning (triple phase bone scan)
      - Ordered if CT nor MRI available
      - Obtained with indium In 111
      - Cannot differentiate between osteomyelitis and fracture or charcot joint
- **Management**
  - Bone biopsy
  - Surgical debridgement of necrotic material
  - ABx

DIABETIC KETOACIDOSIS (DKA)

Diagnosis of HHS and DKA

	Plasma Glucose	Venous or Arterial pH	Serum Bicarb	Urine or Serum Ketones	Effective Serum Osmolarity	Anion gap	Mental Status
Mild DKA	>250	7.25-.7.30	15-18	+	Variable	>10	Alert
Mod. DKA	>250	7.00-<7.24	10-15	+	Variable	>12	Alert/Drowsy
Severe DKA	>250	<7.00	<10	+	Variable	>12	Stupor Coma
HHS	>600	>7.3	>18	Small	>320	Variable	Stupor Coma

- **Pearl**[148,149,151]

  - Mainstay of treatment is **insulin** rather than fluids (HHS)
- **Diagnosis**
  - Glucose > 250
  - pH < 7.30
  - low HCO3- (<18)
  - high anion gap (>12)
  - positive ketones
- **Useful calculations**
  - Anion gap = Na - (Cl + HCO3) –or– ALBUMIN x 3
  - Corrected Na = Na + [(glucose - 100)/100] x 1.6
  - Effective osmolality = {2 [Na + K]}/18 + glucose/2.8 + BUN
  - Evaluation for pure metabolic acidosis:
    - pCO2 = the last two numbers of pH
    - pCO2 = 1.5 [serum HCO3] + 8
- **Monitoring**
  - Daily EKG (↑K)
  - Vitals
  - Q1H glucose
  - Can follow anion gap to ensure resolution (do not follow ketones)
  - Q2-4H CMP alternating with glucose checks
- **Labs**
  - ICU panel q2h to monitor glucose, K, PO4, AG
    - Increase to Q4H when BS <200
  - FS q1hour
  - Serum and urine ketones one time
  - ABG x 1
  - Diet: NPO, but advance as tolerated

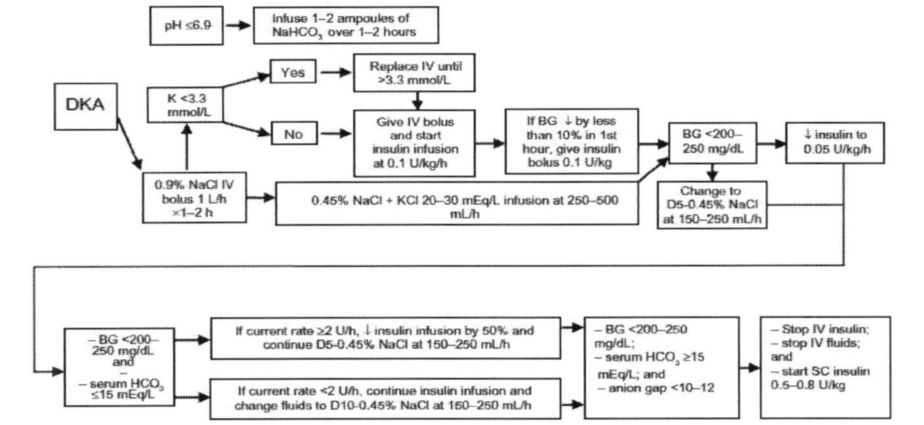
pH ≤6.9
Infuse 1–2 ampoules of NaHCO3 over 1–2 hours
DKA
K <3.3 mmol/L
Yes
Replace IV until >3.3 mmol/L
No
Give IV bolus and start insulin infusion at 0.1 U/kg/h
If BG ↓ by less than 10% in 1st hour, give insulin bolus 0.1 U/kg
BG <200–250 mg/dL
↓ insulin to 0.05 U/kg/h
0.9% NaCl IV bolus 1 L/h ×1–2 h
0.45% NaCl + KCl 20–30 mEq/L infusion at 250–500 mL/h
Change to D5-0.45% NaCl at 150–250 mL/h
– BG <200–250 mg/dL and – serum HCO3 ≤15 mEq/L
If current rate ≥2 U/h, ↓ insulin infusion by 50% and continue D5-0.45% NaCl at 150–250 mL/h
If current rate <2 U/h, continue insulin infusion and change fluids to D10-0.45% NaCl at 150–250 mL/h
– BG <200–250 mg/dL; – serum HCO3 ≥15 mEq/L; and – anion gap <10–12
– Stop IV insulin; – stop IV fluids; and – start SC insulin 0.5–0.8 U/kg

Phase 1 (0-6 hours)	Phase 2 (6-12 hours)	Phase 3 (12-24 hours)
❑ Perform history and physical ❑ Order labs ❑ Monitor plan for clinical sx and labs ❑ Give 1L 0.9NS with potential K ❑ Start insulin after above fluids have finished and K > 3.3 mEq/L ❑ Consult diabetic team (if app)	❑ Continue monitoring labs and clinical sx ❑ Change to D51/2NS if glucose <200 ❑ Adjust insulin drip as needed ❑ Maintain K at 3.3-5.3 mmol/L	❑ Continue monitoring labs and clinical sx ❑ Start SQ insulin if glucose < 200 and tolerating PO intake with 4-6 hour overlap with drip

- **Treatment**
  - Fluids/Electrolytes
    - **Fluids**: assume about 10% dehydration (100 ml/kg) with deficit of 5-10L to be corrected over 36-48 hours
      - *If hypotensive – 1L 0.9NS over 5-10 minutes (bolus) then 500 cc/hour (7.5 cc/kg/hr) for the next 2-4 hours →100-250 cc/hour*
      - *If normotensive – 1L 0.9NS over 60 minutes then 500 cc/hour (7.5 cc/kg/hr) for the next 2-4 hours →100-250 cc/hour*
      - Change to D5NS or D51/2NS when BG < 200 mg/dl
        - During therapy, hyperchloremic non-gap acidosis may develop as ketones cleared and bicarbonate deficit replaced with chloride ions from saline.

Hours	Volume
30min-1 hour	1L
2nd hour	1L
3rd hour	500cc-1L
4th hour	500cc-1L
5th hour	500cc-1L
Total 1-5hrs	3.5-5L
6-12th hours	200-500cc/hr

    - **Potassium** replacement: potassium will initially be falsely elevated due to acidosis and hypovolemia, but can drop quickly (deficit usually 200-1000 mEQ)
      - Wait until potassium is <5.3 mEq/L, then begin replacement aggressively:
        - Potassium < 3.3
          - Consider holding insulin drip until K at least 3.3
          - *Peripheral access:*
            - KCl 40mEq in 500mL over 4 hours
            - KPhos 30 mmol in 500 mL over 4 hours (consider if phos is <2.5)
          - *Central access:*
            - KCl 40mEq in 100mL over 1-4 hours (recommend 1-4 hour infusion)
            - KPhos 30 mmol in 250 mL over 1-4 hours
        - Potassium 3.3 – 4, add KCL 40 mEq / L to maintenance IVF
          - 0.45% NS 1L + potassium chloride 40mEq IV
          - 0.9% NS 1L + potassium chloride 40mEq IV
        - Potassium 4.1 – 5, add KCL 20 mEq / L to maintenance IVF
          - 0.45% NS 1L + potassium chloride 20mEq IV
          - 0.9% NS 1L + potassium chloride 20mEq IV
      - Max KCl administration rate: central line – 20 mEq/hour, peripheral line – 10 mEq/hour.
    - **Phosphate** replacement: generally replacement not recommended despite anticipated fall during days 1 and 2.
      - may administer only if serum PO4 < 1.5 mg/dL
        - Use sodium phosphate (3 mmol PO4/cc; 4 mEq Na/cc)
        - Or KPO at 0.5cc/hr

        - Give 0.3-0.6 mmol PO4/kg/day. Give phosphate ordered in millimole over 6 hours.
          Do not use if patient has hypercalcemia or renal failure. Monitor Ca, PO4, and Na.
      - **Magnesium**: administer only if serum Mg < 1.8 mg/dL or if patient has tetany.
      - **Bicarbonate**: generally replacement not recommended.
        - For pH 6.9 - 7: Sodium Bicarbonate 50mEq IV in 0.45% NS 250mL IV over 1 hr
        - For pH < 6.9: Sodium Bicarbonate 100mEq IV in 0.45% NS 500mL IV over 2 hr
        - The non-gap acidosis that occurs in the recovery phase of DKA generally does not require management (2/2 to ↑Cl)
  - **Insulin**
    - Initialization ONLY if K > 3.3 mEq/L and 1L has already been given!
      - 0.1u/kg regular insulin, single bolus IV push *then*
      - 0.1 u/kg/hr regular insulin continuous IV drip (usually 5 – 7 u/hr)
    - If glucose does not fall by 10% in the first hour, rebolus with insulin 0.14U/kg IV then continue previous infusion rate
    - BS<=200 and tolerating PO intake, AG<12, HCO3>15
      - Switch to SQ insulin when BS reaches 200-250 and resolution of anion gap, patient tolerating PO inake, HCO3 >15, serum/urine ketones are low or absent
      - Either be sure acidosis has resolved on repeat ABG or check that there are no urine ketones.
      - Begin subcutaneous insulin appx 1-2 hrs before stopping IV insulin. There are no guidelines for this, here are some options:

> Average insulin drip rate over previous 6 hours x 24 = TDD
>
> TDD x 60% = Basal insulin dose
>
> TDD x 10% = Preprandial dose
> Usually 0.5-1.3 u/kg/d divided 2/3 AM and 1/3PM with each dose divided 2/3 NPH and 1/3 R
>
> -or-
> Restart home dosage
> -or-
> Lantus (.1U/kg x ½)

    - Keep IV insulin on board (1/2 normal rate or appx 0.02-0.05U/kg/hr) for 4 hours if you started Lantus, 2 hours if NPH
      - Start either prior dose of insulin or if starting on insulin then calculate long acting + short acting based on dose of 0.5-0.8 U/kg/d.
        - Add SSI for correction as needed
      - Fluids should be changed to D51/2NS from 0.9NS and maintain at 150-250 cc/hr
      - Maintain glucose at 150-200

Management of DKA			
Glucose	Insulin Drip	IV Fluids	Potassium Repletion
<u>To begin:</u> - Fluids: Administer 0.9NS or 0.45NS at 500-1000cc/hr during the first 1-2 hrs depending on serum Na level - First give insulin bolus at 0.1 U/kg of regular insulin - Start IV insulin gtt at 0.1 U/kg/hr and check glucose levels q1-2h			
>500	Increase drip by 4 units/hr (or 25 %, which ever increase is less)	Na >135: 0.45NS Na <135: 0.9NS	K > 5: none K 4.1 - 5: add 20 mEq/L K 3.3 - 4: add 40 mEq/L K <3.3: use an IVPB
251-500	Do not adjust rate if blood glucose is decreasing by 50-75 mg/dL/hr If blood glucose is NOT decreasing by 50-75 mg/dL/hr, then increase the drip rate by 2 units/hr	Na >135: 0.45NS Na <135: 0.9NS	K > 5: none K 4.1 - 5: add 20 mEq/L K 3.3 - 4: add 40 mEq/L K <3.3: use an IVPB
151-250	When the plasma glucose reaches **200** mg/dl in DKA, decrease the insulin infusion rate to 0.05 - 0.1 unit/kg/h (or 3-6 units/h) to maintain serum glucose of 150-200 mg/dl	Change to Na >135: D5W-0.45NS Na<135: D5W-0.9 NS	K > 5: none K 4.1 - 5: add 20 mEq/L K 3.3 - 4: add 40 mEq/L K <3.3: use an IVPB
101-150	Decrease insulin drip by 50%	Na >135: D5-0.45NS Na<135: D5-0.9 NS	K > 5: none K 4.1 - 5: add 20 mEq/L K 3.3 - 4: add 40 mEq/L K <3.3: use an IVPB
71-100	Hold insulin drip for 1 hour	Na >135: D5-0.45NS Na<135: D5-0.9 NS	K > 5: none K 4.1 - 5: add 20 mEq/L K 3.3 - 4: add 40 mEq/L K <3.3: use an IVPB
<70	Hold insulin drip (if not already held). Give D50, 12.5 IV Recheck FS in 15 minutes	Change to D10W	K > 5: none K 4.1 - 5: add 20 mEq/L K 3.3 - 4: add 40 mEq/L K <3.3: use an IVPB

- **Resolution**
  - Glucose <200-250
  - Anion Gap <12
  - Serum Bicarb at least 19
  - Patient tolerating PO intake
  - Absent or low serum/urine ketones but not absolutely necessary as they can often be falsely elevated

Figure. Algorithm for management of adult patient with DKA

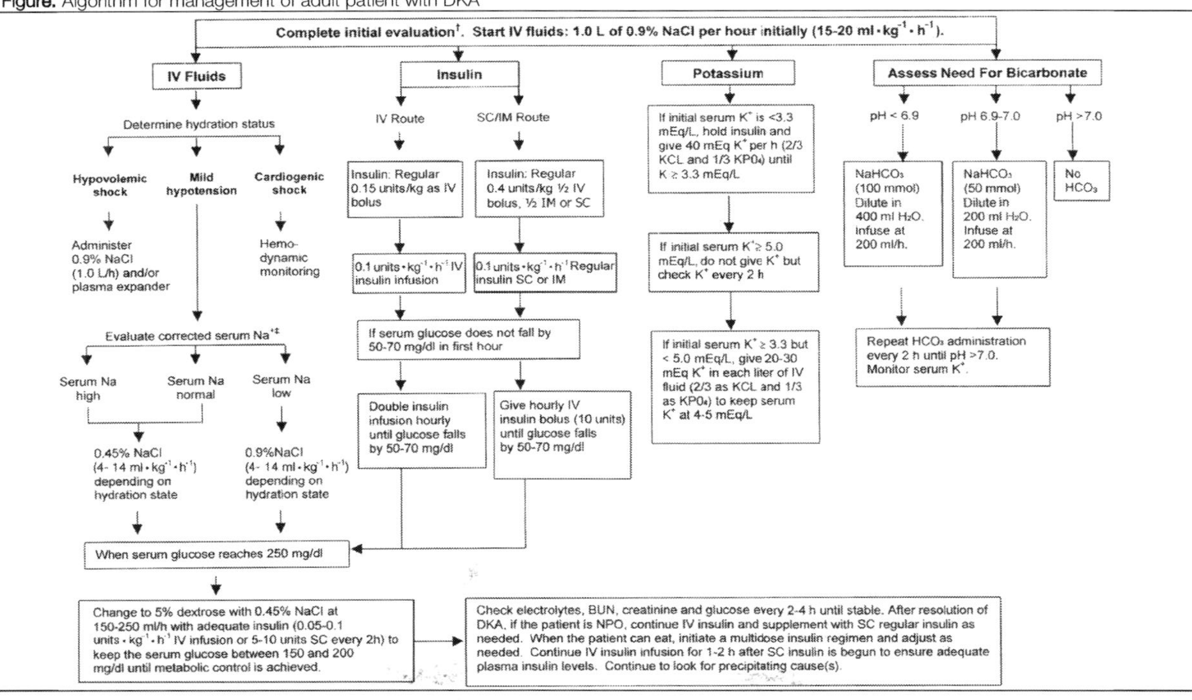

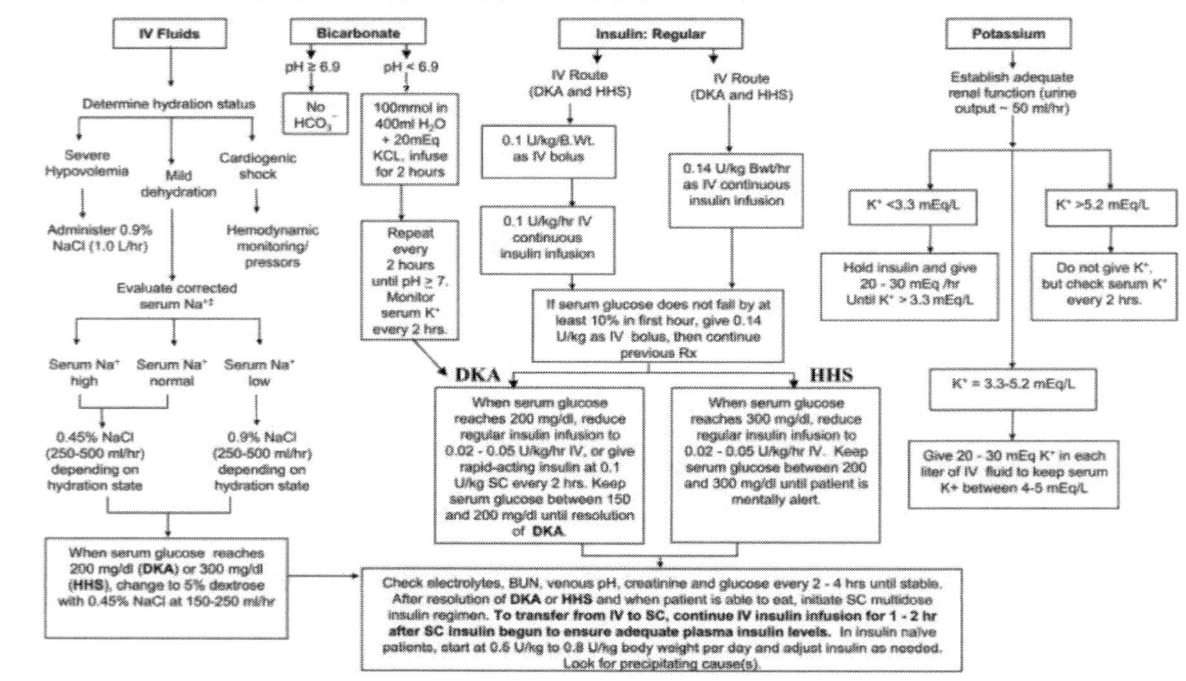
Complete initial evaluation. Check capillary glucose and serum/urine ketones to confirm hyperglycemia and ketonemia/ketonuria. Obtain blood for metabolic profile. Start IV fluids: 1.0 L of 0.9% NaCl per hour.†
IV Fluids
Determine hydration status
Severe Hypovolemia
Mild dehydration
Cardiogenic shock
Administer 0.9% NaCl (1.0 L/hr)
Hemodynamic monitoring/ pressors
Evaluate corrected serum Na+‡
Serum Na+ high
Serum Na+ normal
Serum Na+ low
0.45% NaCl (250-500 ml/hr) depending on hydration state
0.9% NaCl (250-500 ml/hr) depending on hydration state
When serum glucose reaches 200 mg/dl (DKA) or 300 mg/dl (HHS), change to 5% dextrose with 0.45% NaCl at 150-250 ml/hr
Bicarbonate
pH ≥ 6.9
pH < 6.9
No HCO3−
100mmol in 400ml H2O + 20mEq KCL, infuse for 2 hours
Repeat every 2 hours until pH ≥ 7. Monitor serum K+ every 2 hrs.
Insulin: Regular
IV Route (DKA and HHS)
IV Route (DKA and HHS)
0.1 U/kg/B.Wt. as IV bolus
0.1 U/kg/hr IV continuous insulin infusion
0.14 U/kg Bwt/hr as IV continuous insulin infusion
If serum glucose does not fall by at least 10% in first hour, give 0.14 U/kg as IV bolus, then continue previous Rx
DKA
HHS
When serum glucose reaches 200 mg/dl, reduce regular insulin infusion to 0.02 - 0.05 U/kg/hr IV, or give rapid-acting insulin at 0.1 U/kg SC every 2 hrs. Keep serum glucose between 150 and 200 mg/dl until resolution of DKA.
When serum glucose reaches 300 mg/dl, reduce regular insulin infusion to 0.02 - 0.05 U/kg/hr IV. Keep serum glucose between 200 and 300 mg/dl until patient is mentally alert.
Potassium
Establish adequate renal function (urine output ~ 50 ml/hr)
K+ <3.3 mEq/L
K+ >5.2 mEq/L
Hold insulin and give 20 - 30 mEq /hr Until K+ > 3.3 mEq/L
Do not give K+, but check serum K+ every 2 hrs.
K+ = 3.3-5.2 mEq/L
Give 20 - 30 mEq K+ in each liter of IV fluid to keep serum K+ between 4-5 mEq/L
Check electrolytes, BUN, venous pH, creatinine and glucose every 2 - 4 hrs until stable. After resolution of DKA or HHS and when patient is able to eat, initiate SC multidose insulin regimen. To transfer from IV to SC, continue IV insulin infusion for 1 - 2 hr after SC insulin begun to ensure adequate plasma insulin levels. In insulin naïve patients, start at 0.5 U/kg to 0.8 U/kg body weight per day and adjust insulin as needed. Look for precipitating cause(s).

HYPEROSMOLAR NONKETOTIC COMA (HONC/HHS)

- **Pearls**[151]
  - Mainstay of treatment is fluids rather than insulin (DKA); fluid deficit can be up to 10L
  - Often will have hyponatremia; need to correct for hyperglycemia!
- **Pathogenesis**: decreased insulin, increased stress hormones, usually precipitating event
- **Characteristics**: hyperglycemia, water deficit, hyperosmolarity, mental status changes
- **Diagnosis**: serum glucose > 600-800, Osm > 350, mental status changes, absent to low ketones, no acidosis
- **Symptoms**: polyuria, polydipsia, fatigue, weakness, lethargy, drowsiness, anorexia, mental status changes, seizures, aphasia, hemiplegia
- **Precipitants**: infection, CVA, pneumonia, MI, acute pancreatitis, drugs (phenytoin, diuretics, steroids, immunosuppressants)
- **Physical Exam**: orthostasis, tachycardia, tachypnea (shallow), fever, dry skin, myoclonus, hyperreflexia, positive Babinski sign, altered mental status/coma, sensory deficits, volume contraction, no Kussmaul breathing
- **Labs**: CBC, chemistry panel, glucose, serum/urine ketones, RUA, ABG, CXR, EKG, blood cultures
- **Treatment**:
  - <u>**IV fluids**</u>: start with rapid repletion NS 2-3 liters, replete 1/2 estimated deficit within 6 hours (usual total deficit is 8-10 L), then change to 0.45NS. Given the large amount of fluid administered, very careful monitoring of fluid status is imperative.
  - <u>Insulin</u>:
    - Initial loading dose of Regular Insulin 0.1U/kg (max 10U) f/b infusion at 0.1U/kg/hr
    - Titrate to decrease glucose 100 mg/dL/hour, use regimen described above for DKA
    - **Only give insulin after fluid deficit is starting to be replete** and potassium level normalized
      - Low K can precipitate arrhythmias
      - Often patient's glucose will normalize with fluids alone
  - Consider antibiotics if infection suspected

Figure. Algorithm for management of adult patients with HHS/HNK

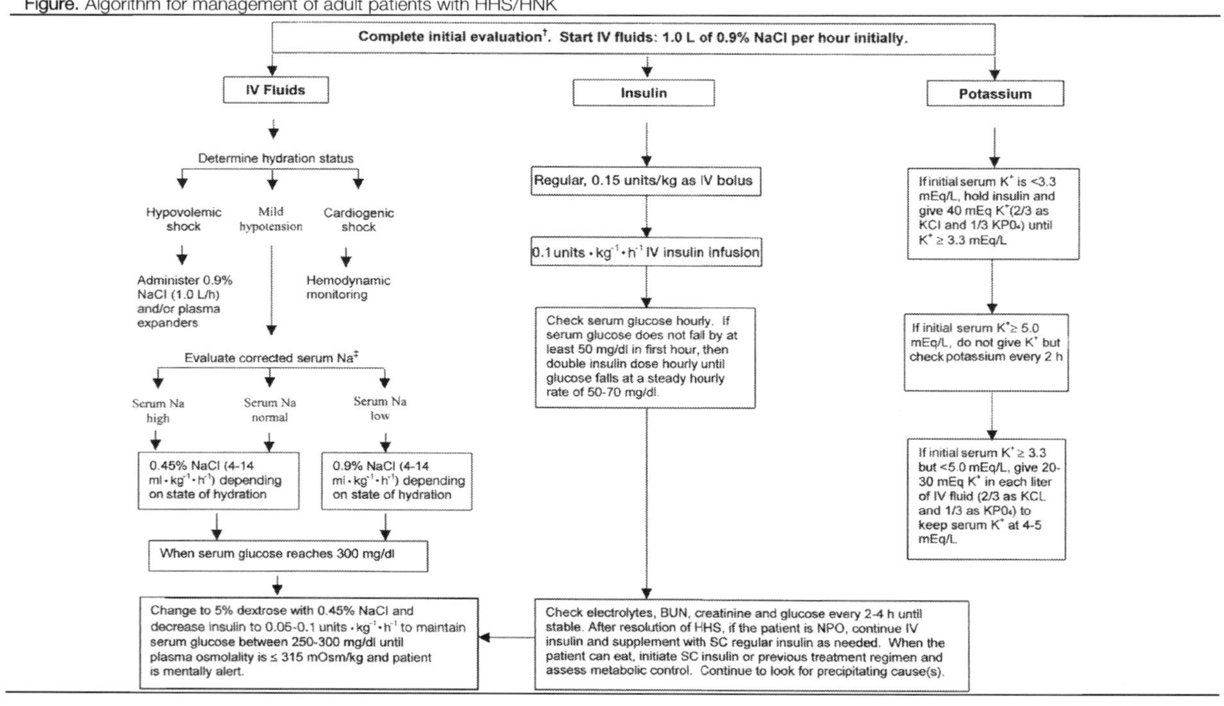

Complete initial evaluation†. Start IV fluids: 1.0 L of 0.9% NaCl per hour initially.
IV Fluids
Insulin
Potassium
Determine hydration status
Hypovolemic shock
Mild hypotension
Cardiogenic shock
Administer 0.9% NaCl (1.0 L/h) and/or plasma expanders
Hemodynamic monitoring
Evaluate corrected serum Na‡
Serum Na high
Serum Na normal
Serum Na low
0.45% NaCl (4-14 ml·kg⁻¹·h⁻¹) depending on state of hydration
0.9% NaCl (4-14 ml·kg⁻¹·h⁻¹) depending on state of hydration
When serum glucose reaches 300 mg/dl
Change to 5% dextrose with 0.45% NaCl and decrease insulin to 0.05-0.1 units·kg⁻¹·h⁻¹ to maintain serum glucose between 250-300 mg/dl until plasma osmolality is ≤ 315 mOsm/kg and patient is mentally alert.
Regular, 0.15 units/kg as IV bolus
0.1 units·kg⁻¹·h⁻¹ IV insulin infusion
Check serum glucose hourly. If serum glucose does not fall by at least 50 mg/dl in first hour, then double insulin dose hourly until glucose falls at a steady hourly rate of 50-70 mg/dl.
Check electrolytes, BUN, creatinine and glucose every 2-4 h until stable. After resolution of HHS, if the patient is NPO, continue IV insulin and supplement with SC regular insulin as needed. When the patient can eat, initiate SC insulin or previous treatment regimen and assess metabolic control. Continue to look for precipitating cause(s).
If initial serum K⁺ is <3.3 mEq/L, hold insulin and give 40 mEq K⁺(2/3 as KCl and 1/3 KPO₄) until K⁺ ≥ 3.3 mEq/L
If initial serum K⁺≥ 5.0 mEq/L, do not give K⁺ but check potassium every 2 h
If initial serum K⁺ ≥ 3.3 but <5.0 mEq/L, give 20-30 mEq K⁺ in each liter of IV fluid (2/3 as KCL and 1/3 as KPO₄) to keep serum K⁺ at 4-5 mEq/L

HYPOGLYCEMIA

Hormone levels in Hypoglycemia				
	C-Peptide	Proinsulin	Serum Insulin	Circul. PO Hypoglycemic Agent
Exogenous Insulin	↓	↓	↑	Negative
PO Hypoglycemic agents	↑	↑	↑	Present
Insulinoma	↑	↑	↑	Negative

Interpretation of Labs				
Test	Normal	Insulinoma	Factitious (insulin injection)	Factitious (oral hypoglycemic)
Insulin	<3	Norm-High	Very High	Norm to High
C-peptide	<0.2	Norm-High	Low	Norm to High
Oral hypoglycemic screen	Negative	Negative	Negative	Positive
Proinsulin	<5	High	Low	High

- **Pearls**[151]
  - Sulfonylureas and meglitinide increase insulin secretion/activity and can cause hypoglycemia unlike metformin
    - ½ life often 14-16 hours
  - Consider naloxone and thiamine for patients with AMS and concern for need for intubation
    - Dosing:
      - IV/SQ: Narcan 0.4mg (can do 0.2mg initially if patient is opiate naïve) repeated q3-5 minutes
      - Intranasal: 4.0mg intranasal repeated q3-5 minutes until effect.
      - Drip: often done in patients on methadone; use 2/3 of total effective dose of naloxone per hour (typically 0.25-6.25mg/hr) and provide ½ of that bolus dose about 15 minutes after starting the drip to prevent a drop in naloxone levels
- **Treatment**
  - Check BS q20m
- **Treatment**
  - If pt alert
    - Give 15-30g carbs via:
      - 8 oz juice/soda = 30 g carbs
      - ½ cup of juice
      - ½ cup of regular soft drink
      - 2 graham cracker squares = 10 g carbs
      - 3-4 glucose tablets
    - 15 g carbs will increase BG by 25-50 mg/dL
  - Non-alert pt
    - Give 25 g dextrose IV (1 amp D50) or 1 mg glucagon IM if no IV access and recheck BG after 5-10 min
    - If severe or recurrent hypoglycemia
      - Use D5 or D10 drip

- When BG>90: Wait 1 hour, Recheck BG
- If BG still >90: Restart infusion at 50% of most recent rate

HEMOCHROMATOSIS

- **Pathophysiology**[152]
  - Excess iron stimulates oxidative DNA damage and free radical activity due to *HFE* protein defect
  - HFE is responsible for regulating hepcidin a protein that regulates iron deposition which becomes unable to regulate iron levels (cannot respond in face of ↑iron in serum)
- **Symptoms/Diagnosis**
  - Weakness, lethargy, impotence, joint pain
  - Bronze diabetes (diabetes, cirrhosis, and bronze pigmentation)
  - Cardiac abnormalities (heart failure 2/2 restrictive cardiomyopathy)
  - Cirrhosis (iron deposition in hepatocytes)
  - Joint pains (r/o pseudogout which will present in knees, wrists, ankles and present as chondrocalcinosis on plain films)
- **Testing**
  - Serum **ferritin**, **transferrin saturation**, and **iron**
    - **Ferritin** is used as a marker of disease severity, elevation may be secondary to inflammation
    - **TS** is calculated by dividing IRON serum/TIBC
  - **Elevated TS>45% is highly sensitive** but also look for ↑ferritin and ↑Fe
    - To differentiate from ACD, TS is ↓
    - If ferritin normal, not hemochromatosis
  - Liver biopsy used to determine degree of fibrosis
  - Can consider genetic testing (C282Y) via HFE
- **Treatment**
  - Phlebotomy; frequency is guided by severity of **ferritin**
- **Prevention/Screening**
  - No indication for HFE screening unless first degree relative with +HFE, active liver disease, or abnormal iron serology
  - No indication to alter one's diet

HAIR LOSS

- **Differential**[153,154]
  - Alopecia Areata – rapid loss with sharply defined border; "clumps of hair falling out"; often have h/o autoimmune disease. Treat with intralesional steroids.
  - Androgenic Alopecia – also known as male or female pattern baldness;
  - Telogen effluvium – sudden diffuse hair loss d/t stressor; no specific treatment other than ↓stress
  - *Less Common*
    - Trichotillomania – recurrent hair pulling; req psychotherapy
    - Tinea Capitus – fungal infection with multiple small areas of alopecia; dx with KOH prep; treatment with topical selenium sulfide or PO antifungals
    - Syphilis (secondary→RPR or VDRL and consider dilution to r/o false negative)
- **Labs**
  - TSH
  - CBC (evaluate for anemia)
  - Consider testosterone and DHEA if androgenic alopecia

- **Treatment**
  - Androgenic Alopecia[155]:
    - Females: Topical minoxidil 2%, Spironolactone 100/200mg/d, Flutamide 250mg/d
    - Males: Propecia 1mg/d, topical minoxidil 5% or 2% 1cc/BID
    - Either Gender
      - Intralesional Corticosteroids (triamcinolone acetate 5mg/cc to the scalp and 2.5mg/cc to the face every 4-6 weeks) Stop treatment if no improvement after 6 months.
      - Topical Steroids – helpful if you combine clobetasol propionate foam 0.05% with minoxidil 5%
  - Telogen
    - Consider minoxidil; no established tx options
  - Alopecia Areata
    - Intralesional steroids

HYPOMAGNESEMIA

- **Etiology** – m/c due to renal or GI losses
  - Increased excretion - Alcoholism, DM, renal tubular disorders, hypercalcemia/hypercalciuria, hyperaldosteronism, Bartter's syndrome, excessive lactation, marked diaphoresis, diarrhea/vomiting
  - Reduced intake/malabsorption - starvation, bowel bypass/resection, TPN w/o Mg, chronic diarrhea
  - Medications: thiazides & loop diuretics, aminoglycosides, amphoterecin B, cisplatin, pentamidine, Fl poisoning, cyclosporin.
  - Other - acute pancreatitis, low Albumin, Vit D therapy
- **Symptoms**
  - Lethargy, weakness, decreased mentation, nausea, vomiting, tachyarrhythmias, hypocalcemia, and hypokalemia.
- **Diagnostics**
  - Labs: CMP w/Mg, 24hr urine Mg, consider Mg retention test, LFTs, amylase/lipase if suspect pancreatitis
  - EKG/tele: prolong PR, QT, QRS and arhythmias
  - Consider calculating functional excretion of Mg:

$$FE_{Mg} = \frac{U_{Mg} \times P_{SCr}}{(0.7 \times S_{Mg}) \times U_{SCr}} \times 100$$

    $Fe_{Mg} > 2\%$ drugs such as diuretics, aminoglycosides, or cisplatin.

    $Fe_{Mg} < 2\%$ extrarenal causes
- **Treatment**
  - Goal: >2
    - *Mg 1.8- 2.0*: give 1gm IV MgSO4 or 400mg PO TID of MgOH
    - *Mg 1.4-1.8*: MgSO4 2gm IV or 800mg PO MgOH
    - *Mg 1.0-1.3 or if Sx*: MgSO4 4gm IV over 4h and recheck
      - Caution in patients with reduced kidney function.
  - Beware, SE Oral magnesium = Diarrhea (can be used to your advantage if pt constipated…)
  - If pt has chronic Mg deficiency, give daily supplement

HYPERCALCEMIA

- **Symptoms**[156,157,158]
  - Neuromuscular - somnolence, confusion, depression, psychosis, coma, muscle weakness
  - Gastrointestinal - constipation, anorexia, nausea, abdominal pain, peptic ulcer disease, pancreatitis
  - Renal- decreased ability to maximally concentrate urine, polyuria, polydipsia, nephrolithiasis, nephrocalcinosis, renal failure
  - Cardiovascular - hypertension, short QT interval, arrhythmias, digitalis sensitivity
  - Skeletal - osteoporosis, fracture, bone pain
- **Differential**
  - Vitamin A/D overdose
  - Iatrogenic
  - Thyroid (bone turnover)
  - Addison's (adrenal failure)
  - Milk alkali syndrome
  - Immobilization / Infection (think TB, histoplasmosis)
  - Neoplastic (think lymphoma, leukemia, SCC)
  - Medications (thiazides, lithium, theophylline)
  - Rhabdomyolysis
  - AIDS
  - Hyperparathyroidism
  - Sarcoidosis
  - Pagets
- **Orders**
  - Restrict dietary Calcium to 400 mg/day, push PO fluids
  - Vitals Q 4 hours; Seizure precautions; I&Os
- **Imaging**
  - CXR, EKG, mammogram
- **Labs**
  - Total and ionized Calcium, PTH, CMP, Phosphate, Mg level, PSA, CEA, 24 hour urine Calcium and Phosphate
- **Classifications**
  - Asymptomatic (Calcium < 12 mg/dL)
    - No immediate therapy required
    - Hold any diuretics
    - Avoid volume depletion
    - ↑activity
  - Moderate (calcium 12-14 mg/dL)
    - No immediate treatment unless symptomatic
    - *See below*
  - Severe (>14; symptomatic)
    - Aggressive IVF (NS) and more as below

Figure. Differential diagnosis of hypercalcemia

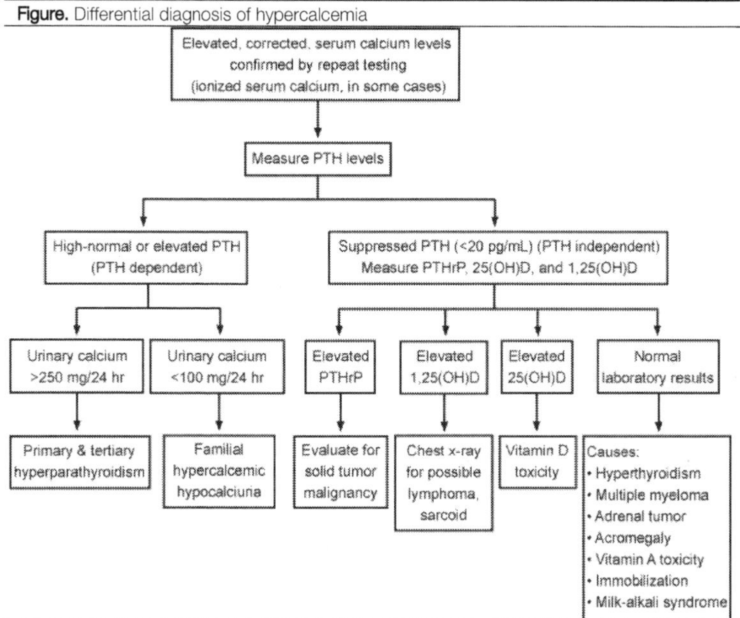

- **Treatment**[159]
  - Immediate
    - Fluids first
      - 1-2 L of 0.9% saline over 1-4 hours until no longer hypotensive, then saline diuresis with 0.9% saline infused at 200-500 cc/hr **AND**
    - Calcitonin (Calcimar) 4-8 IU/kg IM Q 12 hr **OR** 2-4 IU/kg SQ Q 6-12 hours (effective only for 48 hrs)
    - Lasix 20-100 mg IV Q 4-12 hours
      - *Only if patient does not respond initially to fluids above and concern for **hypervolemia (CHF)***
      - Maintain urine output of 200ml/hr; Monitor serum Na, K, Mg
    - Pamidronate 60-90 mg IV over 2-24 hrs in patients with hypercalcemia 2/2 malignancy
    - Prednisone 50-100mg/d can be considered
    - Dialysis is employed if cannot safely give fluids due to severe renal failure or HF
  - Long-Term
    - Bisphosphonate (take 2-4 days for full effect) and act to inhibit osteoclast function and bone resorption **but can worsen renal function**.
      - Zoledronic Acid 3-4mg over 15-30 minutes – has the best efficacy compared to other bisphosphonates but is usually **reserved for malignancy** with **renal insufficiency (Cr Cl <35)**
      - Etidronate (Didronel) 7.5 mg/kg/day in 250 ml of normal saline IV infusion over 2 hours. May repeat in 3 days
      - Pamidronate (Aredia) 60 mg in 500 ml of NS infused over 4 hours **OR** 90 mg in 1 L of NS infused over 24 hours x 1 dose
      - Denosumab is used for patients who do not respond to above bisphosphonates

- Surgery – asymptomatic hypercalcemia is treated if patients have a serum level > 1mg/dL over normal, osteoporosis, GFR<60, and are less than 50 years old

HYPOCALCEMIA

- **Etiology** – either due to deficiency in parathyroid hormone or vitamin D
- **Differential**
  - Hypoparathyroidism
  - Parathyroid hormone resistence
  - Vitamin D defiency or resistence
  - CRF
  - Hungry bone syndrome
  - Pancreatitis
  - Multiple blood transfusions (due to citrate)
  - ↑PO4
  - Osteoblastic metastasis
  - Bisphosphonates
  - Calcitonin
- **Symptoms**
  - Parasthesias, Chovstek's sign, laryngospasm, bronchospasm, carppedal spasm, tetany, seizures, ↑ICP
  - Bradycardia, ↑QT
- **Confirmation**
  - Check serum albumin
    - Serum Ca decreases by 0.2 mmol/L or 0.4mEq/L for every 1 g/dL decrease in serum albumin

> Corrected Ca= (Measured Ca)+{(4.0-albumin) x 0.8}

  - Check Mg to ensure concurrent ↓Mg not present
- **Treatment**
  - Goals: >8.5 or ionized 1
  - Replacement:
    - **Ca Gluconate 1-2 amps in 100cc 1-2 h** (1 amp =1g = 4.65 mEq)
    - Calcium Chloride in Central IV only (3x stronger)
    - PO: Ca carbonate/citrate 500-1000mg PO TID plus daily supplement of Ca+Vit D (600mg/400IU) BID
  - Symptomatic Hypocalcemia
    - CaCl 10% (270 mg Ca/ 10 ml vial) give 5-10 ml slowly (or skin will slough) over 10 min or dilute in 50-100 ml of D5W and infuse over 20 min, repeat Q 20-30 min if symptomatic, or hourly if asymptomatic. Correct hyperphosphatemia before hypocalcemia **OR**
    - Calcium Gluconate 20 ml of 10% solution IV (2 vials) (90mg elemental Ca/10 ml vial) infused over 10-15 minutes, followed by infusion of 60 ml of Ca gluconate in 500cc of D5W (1 mg/ml) at 0.5-2.0 mg/kg/hour
    - Common in **blood transfusions** in patients with renal or hepatic impairment. *See page 297*.
- **Chronic Hypocalcemia:**
  - Ca Carbonate with Vitamin D (Oscal-D) 1-2 tab PO tid OR
  - Ca Carbonate (Oscal) 1-2 tabs PO tid OR
  - Ca Citrate (Citracal) 1 tab PO Q 8 hour or Extra Strength Tums 1-2 tabs PO with meals
  - Vitamin D2 (Ergocalciferol) 1 tab PO daily
  - Calcitriol (Rocaltrol) 0.25mcg PO daily, titrate up to 0.5-2.0 mcg

HYPERKALEMIA

- **Etiology**[160]
  - Consider hemolysis, sepsis (metabolic acidosis), hypoaldosteronism
- **IV Fluids:** D5NS at 125 cc/hr

Treatment options for Hyperkalemia

Agent	Mechanism	Dosage	OOA	Duration
Calcium gluconate (10%)	Direct antagonism Membrane stabilization	30cc (or 10cc of calcium chloride 30%)	1-3min	30-60min
Hypertonic Saline* *(if ↓Na)*	Membrane stabilization	50-250cc	5-10min	2 hours
Sodium Bicarbonate *(consideration if pH≤7.1)*	Redistribution	50 mEq IV over 1-5min 150 cc/hr; at least 3 amps HCO3;	5-10min	2 hours
Glucose/Insulin	Redistribution	50 cc (50g) D50W with 10U regular insulin IV then D10W 1L with regular insulin 25-50U @ 250cc/hr	30min	4-6 hours
Albuterol/Xopenex	Redistribution	2U neb over 5 min	30min	2 hours
Kayexalate	↑ Elimination	30-45g PO now and Q3-4h prn	2-3 hours	6-8 hours
Lasix	↑ Elimination	40-80mg IV repeat prn	Varies with start of diuresis	Until diuresis present
Fludrocortisone* *(known aldosterone deficiency)*	↑ Elimination	0.1mg or higher (up to 0.4-1mg/d for chronic use)	N/A	N/A

- **Identification:**
  - Earliest sign is an EKG with peaked T waves with a narrow base best seen in leads II, III, V2-V4
    - *Don't be fooled: other causes for peaked T waves include acute myocardial infarction, early repolarization, and LVH*
  - Other signs include a shortened QT interval and ST depression
  - PR interval widening and QRS widening will later be seen
  - The last sign is often a disappearance of the P wave with QRS widening into a sinusoidal pattern
- **Labs:** CBC, CMP, Mg
  - UA, Urine SpG, Urine Na and Cr, 24 hour Urine K

- Monitor ICU panel q2h
- **Other Source:**
  - STAT EKG, recheck BMP; consider holding ACEI/ARB
  - Immediate Tx for EKG changes with measures that work quickly by shifting K+ into cells:
    - Calcium gluconate 1 amp
    - 2 amps D50 + 10 unit's regular insulin IV over 15 mins
    - Albuterol nebs (20 mg neb over 15 min)
    - HCO3 gtt 150cc/hr
  - Give additional agents to decrease total body store of K+:
    - Kayexalate 30 g PO (repeat Q 2 hours until BM) or retention enema **this is not an FDA approved use**
  - Dialysis if necessary- contact nephrology, consider placing trialysis catheter or mahuker

HYPOKALEMIA

- **Work-up**
  1) TTKG = $\frac{Urine_K}{Plasma_K} / \frac{Urine_{osm}}{Plasma_{osm}}$ (Urine K)(PlasmaOsm)UrineOsm(Plasma K)
     - TTKG > 4 = renal or endocrine defect
     - TTKG < 2 = extrarenal cause
  2) Check 24 hr urine K
     - UK > 30 mmol/day suggests renal losses
     - UK < 25 mmol/day suggests extrarenal losses
- **Guide**
  - Estimated mEq KCl needed = $\frac{\text{Desired K-Measured K}}{\text{Serum SCr}}$ DesiredK-MeasuredKSerumSCr x 100
  - If SCr < 1, then assume SCr = 1
- **Acute Therapy**
  - K Lyte 50 mEq Po x 1
  - K flash: 40 mEq KCl with 25 cc Lidocaine 1% in NS at 125 cc/hr
  - KCl 20-40 mEq in 100 cc saline infused IVPB over 2-4 hours
    - **OR** Add 40-80 mEq to 1 L of IV fluid and infuse over 4-8 hours
  - KCl elixir 40 mEq PO tid (in addition to IV)
    - Max total dose 100-200 mEq/day (3mEq/kg/day)
- **Chronic Therapy:**
  - Micro-K 10 mEq tabs 2-3 tabs PO tid after meals (40-100 mEq/day) **OR**
  - K-Dur 20 mEq tabs 1 PO bid-tid
- **Hypokalemia with Metabolic Acidosis:**
  - Potassium citrate 15-30 ml in juice PO QID after meals (1 mEq/ml)
  - Potassium gluconate 15 ml in juice PO QID after meals (20 mEq/15 ml)
- **Extras:** EKG, dietetics consult
- **Labs:** CBC, Mg, CMP
  - UA, Urine Na and Cr, 24 hour urine K+
- **Other Source**
  - Preferred to do PO replacement up to 40 mEq as more can cause GI upset
  - Preferred to do IV replacement if patient sx or has EKG changes
    - Max IV rate
      - Peripheral line = 10 mEq/hr

        - Central line = 20 mEq/hr
    - Add 10 mEq K+ for every 0.1 mEq K+ above 3.0
    - Add 20 mEq K+ for every 0.2 mEq K+ below 3.0
        - Ex: if K is 2.8 and want to correct to 4.0, you need (20x1)+(10x10)=120 mEq
    - For urgent replacement give PO liquid or IV
    - If pt has renal failure, cut dose by 1/2
    - If pt extremely low, most K+ you can give at one time is "40mEq PO and 40 mEq IV over 4 hours"

Sliding Scale	
Potassium Level	IV or PO Replacement
3.7-3.8	20 mEq KCl
3.5-3.6	40 mEq KCl
3.3-3.4	60 mEq KCl
3.1-3.2	80 mEq KCl
<3.0	100 mEq KCl

- **Immediate Treatment Indications**
    - Hepatic Encephalopathy (often 2/2 use of loop diuretics)
    - Cardiac arrythmia (stabilize with calcium gluconate first)
    - Ventilatory failure

HYPONATREMIA

- **Pathophysiology**[161,162,163]
    - Based on volume status:
        - Hypovolemic (decreased total body water with greater decrease in sodium level)
        - Euvolemic (increased total body water with normal sodium level)
        - Hypervolemic (increased total body water compared with sodium).11
    - Osmolality refers to the total concentration of solutes in water.
        - Effective osmolality is the osmotic gradient created by solutes that do not cross the cell membrane.
        - Plasma osmolality is maintained by strict regulation of ADH and thirst.
            - If plasma osmolality increases, ADH is secreted and water is retained by the kidneys
            - If plasma osmolality decreases, ADH also decreases, resulting in diuresis of free water and a return to homeostasis.
- **Step by Step Approach**
  (also see flow chart at end of section)
    - Must get labs
        - Serum osmolarity
            - Hyper: >295
            - Iso: 285-295
            - Hypo: <280
        - Urine Na (under Random Urine Electrolytes)
        - Urine Osmolarity
        - Serum Uric Acid
        - FE_{Uric} to rule out reset osmostat
        - ICUP to look at glucose and albumin
        - UA to look for excess protein

    - Consider
        - Lipid panel
        - Cortisol
        - TSH
  - Rule out pseudohyponatremia
    - ↑Lipids → often seen with PBC; tx with statin
    - ↑Protein → tx with chemo (r/o MM)
    - ↑Glucose (DKA, Gluc>400) → tx with fluids, IV insulin
    - ↑TG
  - Determine fluid status
    - *Hypervolemic* – hx of CHF, cirrhosis, or nephrotic syndrome. Significant edema, JVD. S3 gallop auscultated.
    - *Euvolemia* – no evidence of fluid overload of dehydration. U_{Na}>30, $U_{Osmolarity}$>300
    - *Hypovolemia* – recent or chronic use of diuretics, UA with ↑SG, orthostatic hypotension/tachycardia, poor cap. refill, MM dry. U_{Na}<20, $U_{Osmoloarity}$>500
- **Lab assistance**
  - 3 most accurate tests are
    (1) spot urine sodium
    (2) FENa
    (3) FEUrea / FECr
  - Spot Urine Na
    - U_{Na} > 30: euvolemia/SIADH
    - U_{Na} < 10: hypovolemia (elevated if ARF present)
    - Most hypovolemic patients avidly reabsorb sodium resulting in decreased urine sodium concentration.
    - Helps differentiate SIADH from CSW as well
    - Average urinary sodium in hypovolemic patients: 18.4 mEq/L, compared with 72 mEq/L in euvolemic patients
  - FE_{Na} and FE_{Urea} – see below
    - Recent diuretics? Yes, then do FE_{Urea}, if not do FE_{Na}
    - FE_{Urea} <=35% - prerenal (hypovolemia)
    - FE_{Na} <= 1% - prerenal (hypovolemia)
  - Urine Osmolarity
    - Determine the kidneys capacity to dilute urine
    - U_{osm} < 100 : dilute urine due to appropriate suppression of ADH; hypervolemic state

Evaluation of Hypotonic (S_{OSM}<275 mOsm/kg) Hyponatremia based on Volume Status

	Definition	Differential	Labs/Management	Treatment
Hypervolemia	*U_{Osm} >100* U_{Na}>20 mmol/Lthen think renal failure U_{Na}<20 mmol/Lthen nephrotic syndrome, cirrhosis, CHF	• Heart failure (HF) • Cirrhosis • Nephrotic syndrome • Renal failure (glomerular filtration rate [GFR] < 5 mL/min)	• Serum albumin, UA, BUN, SCr, spot Prot/SCr ratio, PT/PTT, LFTs • Imaging: CXR, TTE	• Fluid restriction (1-1.5L), treat as below • Sodium restriction of 40mEq/day • Optional: Furosemide 40-80 mg IV/PO daily-BID

Euvolemia	*U_{Osm} <100 (PP, Beer potomania)*
	***Urine Na>20**,*
	U_{Osm}>100: SIADH, diuretic induced, rest osm
		• Syndrome of inappropriate **antidiuretic hormone** (SIADH)
		  ○ Most common cause, 40%
		  ○ Must rule out thyroid or adrenal source with normal cortisol and TSH
		  ○ CNS: trauma, hemorrhage, CVA, infection, vasculitis
		  ○ Pulmonary: TB, pneumonia, empyema, COPD
		  ○ Malignancy: small cell, pancreatic, lymphoma, thymoma
		  ○ Drugs: Chlorpropamide, vincristine, vinblastine, cyclophosphamide,
			• Check urine osmolarity (estimate = 35 x last 2 digits of SG on UA), TSH, EtOH, K, cortisol
			• Primary adrenal insufficiency
			  ○ ↓Na /↑K/↑Ca/↓cortisol
			• Beer potomania/ Psychogenic polydypsia
			  ○ Urine osmolarity <= 100 mOsm/L
			• SIADH or Cerebral Salt Wasting
			  ○ Urine osmolarity >= 300 mOsm/L with ↑FENa
				• Fluid restriction (1-1.5L), treat as below
				• Oral NaCl tablets (TID)
				• Optional: Conivaptan (Vaprisol) 20 mg IV over 30 minutes once, followed by a continuous infusion of 20 mg over 24 hours
				• If response is inefficient, increase dose to 40 mg/24 hours; Max 4 days; ADH inhibitor

		carbamazepine, morphine, SSRI, TCAs, HCTZ o Cancers (eg, pancreas, lung) o CNS disease (eg, cerebrovascular accident, trauma, infection, hemorrhage, mass) o Pulmonary diseases (eg, infections, respiratory failure) o Drugs o Thiazides o Vasopressin o Chlorpropamide o Carbamazepine o NSAIDs o TCAs o Opiates • Hypothyroidism • Psychogenic polydipsia • Beer Potomania (↓protein to allow for adequate H_2O excretion; normal kidney function) • Secondary adrenal insufficiency • Exercise-associated hyponatremia • Psychogenic Polydypsia o U_{Na}<30	• SIADH: o U_{Na}>20 o S_{UA}<4mg/dL o ↑FE_{Na} o Uric acid low o Low anion gap o Low urea	
Hypovolemia	*U_{Osm}>100*	• Salt and water loss with free water replacement		• **Concept is that with vessels contracted d/t**

	Urine Na<10: *vomiting, diarrhea, 3rd space/resp/skin loss* *Osm <280,* ***Urine Na>20***: *Diuretics,* ***CSW****, RTA, Adrenal insufficiency, Partial obstruction*	• Severe diarrhea with free water ingestion • Large burns with free water replacement • Third-spacing with free water replacement • Primary adrenal insufficiency • Renal disease • Diuretics • Salt-wasting nephropathy		**↓BP, ADH is released causing dilution. With resuscitation, vessels expand and no ADH is released often resulting in large diuresis.** • Give 0.5-2 L of **0.9% NS** over 1-2 hours until no longer hypotensive, then 0.9% NS at 125 ml/hr **OR** 100-500 ml of 3% hypertonic saline over first 4 hours and titrate to avoid ↑ of more than 12 mEq/L/day • Urinary Na < 20

Comparison of Laboratory Findings in SIADH with CSW		
	SIADH	CSW
Intravascular volume contraction	No	Yes
Serum sodium	↓	↓
Urine sodium	↑	↑↑
Urine volume	N or ↓	↑
Endocrine		
Plasma ADH	↑	N or ↑
Plasma aldosterone	↓	N or ↑
Plasma renin	↓	N or–↓
Plasma ANP	↑	↑
Urea nitrogen, serum	N or ↓	↑
Serum uric acid	↓	N or ↑

- **Pearls**
  - Diuretics on board – consider diuretic induced hyponatremia (hypovolemic)
  - Hyperkalemia with Hypocalcemia and Hypoglycemia – think adrenal insufficiency
  - Urine osmolarity <= 100 consider PP
  - Patient glucose or lipids highly elevated consider pseudohyponatremia
  - General labs: urine lytes, serum osmolarity, TSH, AM cortisol, urine osmolarity

- **Replacing Sodium**
  1. First correct sodium for any hyperglycemia present

     Corrected = Measured sodium + 0.024 * (Serum glucose - 100)

  2. Determine the speed of correction
     http://www.mdcalc.com/sodium-correction-rate-in-hyponatremia/
     - **Acute**[164]
       - *No established guidelines*
       - 6-8 mmol/L in 24 hours
       - 12-14 mmol/L in 48 hours
       - 14-16 mmol/L in 72 hours
     - **Chronic**
       - ≤12 mmol/L in first 24 hours
       - ≤18 mmol/L in first 48 hours
     - **Asymptomatic**
       - Increase PNa @ 0.5 mEq/hr and/or 10 mEq/day or desired Na x wt in kg
     - **Symptomatic**
       - Mild symptoms (n/v, HA, abd pain) – ↑ PNa up to 1.0 mEq/L/hr for 3-4 hours then decrease rate to ↑ PNa 10 mEq/day
       - Severe symptoms (seizure, coma) - ↑ PNa 1.5-2 mEq/L/hr for 3-4 hours then ↓ rate to achieve 12 mEq/L/day
  3. Order ICU Panel Q2H for first 24 hours
  4. Goal correction is for Na to be 120-130 mEq/L
  5. Calculate the sodium deficit

Na deficit = Weight x 0.6 (target S_{Na} – current S_{Na})

** correct 6 units over a 3 hour period, then correct final 3 units over remaining 9 hours

6. <u>Volume of Saline needed to correct Na deficit</u>

Volume Req = (Na deficit / 512) x 1000

7. <u>Infusion Rate</u>

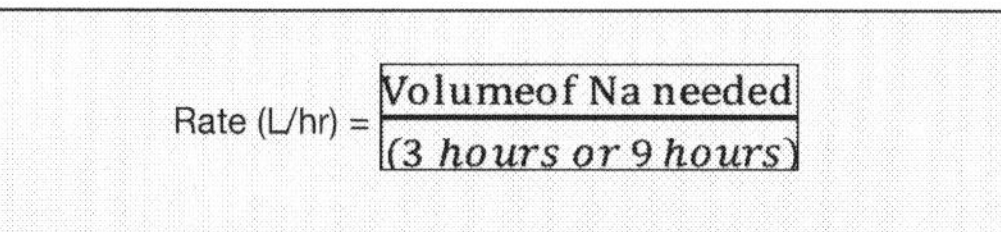

- <u>Determine the best fluid replacement and amount to give:</u>

Fluid	Na+	K+	Cl-	HCO_3	Other	Osmolality
Plasma	142	4	104	27	29	306
NS	154	-	154	-	-	308
D_5W	-	-	-	-	-	278
$D_5$1/2NS	77	-	77	-	-	421
1 amp $NaHCO_3$	50	-	-	50	-	100
20 mEq KCl	-	20	20	-	-	40

Ex. If patient is 504 mmol down of Na, then take 504 / 154 (if you want to give 0.9NS) and you need to then give a little over 3L to correct their Na

- Start with 0.9NS at 85cc/hr and obtain ICU panel q2h
- After first returned lab, compare to see if you corrected too much
  - If too high of correction, switch to D5W and after you are able to then correct, then turn off fluids
    - If want to reverse, add DDAVP
  - If right rate, keep going

- **Severe Symptomatic Hyponatremia**
  - Seizure, neurologic sequelae
  - If volume depleted, give 1-2 L of 0.9% NS (154 mEq/L) over 1-2 hours until no longer orthostatic
  - Determine volume of 3% hypertonic saline (513 mEq/L) to be infused:
  - Na (mEq) deficit= 0.6 x (wt kg) x (desired Na-actual Na)

$$\frac{\text{Volume of Solution (L)}}{\text{Number of Hours}} = \frac{\text{Sodium to be infused (mEq)}}{\text{(mEq/L in solution) x Number of hours}}$$

- Correct half of Na deficit intravenously over 24 hours until serum Na is 120 mEq/L; Increase Na by 12-20 mEq/L over 24 hours **(1 mEq/L/hr)**
- **Alternative method:** 3% saline for first 3 hours then titrate to avoid increasing by more than 12 mEq/L/day

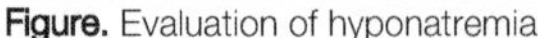

Figure. Evaluation of hyponatremia

Hyponatremia
Serum sodium <135 mEq/L
Symptomatic (ie. confusion, ataxia, seizures, obtundation, coma, resp depression)
Severe hyponatremia (treat appropriately)
Asymptomatic or mild symptoms (ie HA, lethargy, dizziness)
Determine serum osmolarity
Normal
280-285 mOsm/kg
Isotonic Hyponatremia (pseudohyponatremia)
Assess for hyperlipidemia or hyperproteinemia
Low
<280 mOsm/kg
Hypotonic Hyponatremia
Assess volume status
Evaluate VS, orthostatics, jugular venous pressure, skin turgor, mucous membranes, peripheral edema, BUN, Uric Acid
High
>285 mOsm/kg
Hypertonic Hyponatremia
Assess for hyperglycemia, check for mannitol or sorbitol use, or recent administration of radiocontrast media
Hypovolemic (decreased TBW and Na level)
Urinary Sodium >20 mEq/L
Renal loss (ie. diuretics, mineralocorticoid deficiency)
Isotonic saline
Urinary Sodium <20 mEq/L
Extrarenal loss (ie. vomiting, diarrhea, third spacing, or bowel obstruction)
Isotonic saline
Euvolemic (increased TBW, normal total body sodium level)
Urinary sodium usually >20 mEq/L
Urine osmolarity >100 mOsm/kg
SIADH, Hypothyroidism, Adrenal insufficiency, Stress, Drug use
Fluid restriction
Urine osmolarity <100 mOsm/kg
PP, low solute intake (beer potomania)
Fluid restriction
Variable urine osmolarity
Reset osmostat
Fluid restriction
Hypervolemic (increased TBW)
Urinary Sodium <20 mEq/L
CHF, Cirrhosis, Nephrosis, Hypoalbuminemia
Diuresis, fluid and sodium restriction
Urinary Sodium >20 mEq/L
Renal failure
Fluid + sodium restriction, dialysis

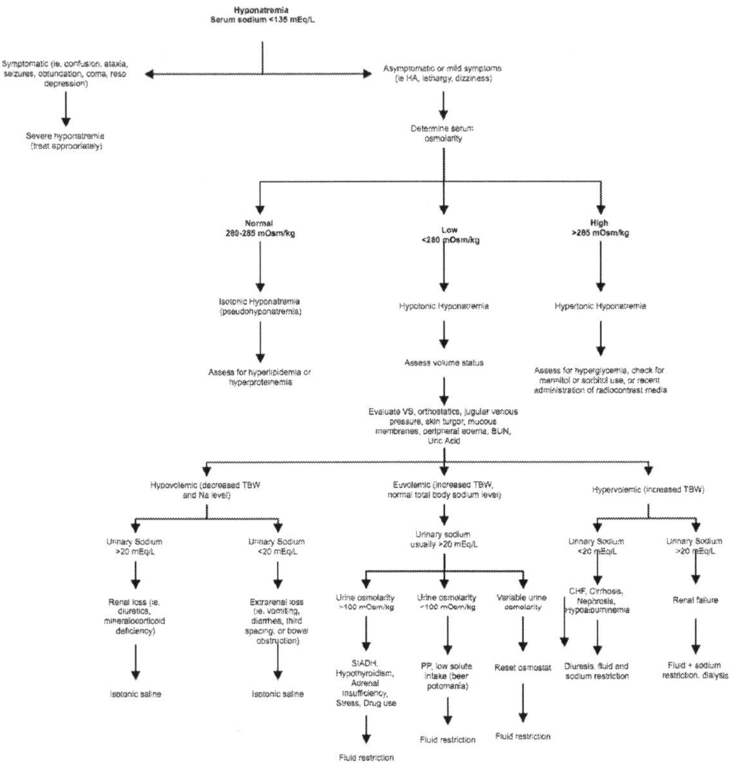

HYPERNATREMIA

- **Definition** - Serum Na is greater than 145 mmol/L.
- **Pathology** - Signs and symptoms are similar to that found in patients with hyponatremia and are due to intracellular dehydration, as high plasma osmolality causes large fluid shifts out of cells.
- **Differential**
    - Impaired water intake: urine osmolality > 700 mOsm/L
        - Neurologic disease (eg, dementia, delirium, coma, stroke)
        - Water unavailable (ie, desert conditions)
        - Osmotic diuresis with impaired water intake
    - Hyperosmolar hyperglycemia
    - Post obstructive diuresis
    - Rare etiologies
        - DI (if associated with decreased water intake)
        - Neurogenic DI (decreased ADH production)
        - Nephrogenic DI (ADH resistance)
        - Long-term lithium ingestion
- **Evaluation**
    - See polyuria work-up on page 514
- **Treatment**
    - Hypovolemic
        - Can give empiric 100cc bolus of 3%Na
        - Free water deficit can be calculated and replaced with either D5W or 0.45NS.

H2O deficit = desired body water – actual body water H2O deficit = (0.5 x IBW kgs) x {(Na actual – Na desired / Na actual) – 1}

- Correction should be no faster than 0.5-1mmol/hour → goal 4-6 mmol/24 hours
    - Calculate fall in serum sodium depending on fluid chosen above
        - D5W = 0 mEq sodium = "0"
        - 0.45NS = 77 mEq = "77"
        - TBW = (0.5 x wt kgs)

("Amount of sodium" – "serum sodium")/(TBW + 1) = # mEq fall per liter of fluid infused

- Take above value and divide by 0.5 to determine over how many hours you should give fluid to prevent too fast of a fall (remember no faster than 0.5 per hour)
- To convert to cc/hr then just divide 1000cc by the above value

1000/ # mEq fall per liter of fluid infused = rate of infusion

- Failsafe: infuse at 1-2cc/kg/hr

- Hypervolemic

- Free water and Lasix. Dialysis may be needed in patients with renal failure

HYPOPARATHYROIDISM

- **Treatment**
  - Vitamin D (calciferol) over 1,25-dihydroxyvitamin D (Calcitrol) as it is less expensive
  - Dosages vary from 25,000 to 100,000 → aim for higher dosage in ↓PTH patients
  - Goal Ca = 8.5 – 9
  - Monitor for hypercalciuria → treat with thiazide diuretic

SUBCLINICAL HYPOTHYROIDISM

- **Definition**[165]
  - ↑TSH and normal T4
  - Commonly precedes overt hypothyroidism within years at a rate of 5-20% yearly → if they have +antibodies
  - Recommend treatment be initiated due to cardiovascular risk → consider starting at 25-50mcg/d and check after 6-8 weeks on therapy
- **Labs**
  - At least one repeat measurement of thyrotropin and free T is indicated, together with a test for antibodies to thyroid peroxidase, after a 2-to-3-month interval.
- **Treatment**
  - Levothyroxine treatment is unlikely to reduce symptoms in persons with modest elevations in thyrotropin levels and with minimal symptoms at baseline
  - Treatment may have benefit in symptomatic patients, particularly in those:
    - Who have a serum thyrotropin level above 10 to 12 mIU per liter.
    - For persons 70 years of age or younger who have thyrotropin levels of 10 mIU per liter or higher, although long-term benefits have not been shown and the risks of such treatment are unknown.
      - For persons older than 70 years of age **or** for persons who have a thyrotropin level of less than 10 mIU per liter, treatment decisions should be guided by individual patient factors, including the extent of thyrotropin elevation and whether the patient has symptoms of hypothyroidism, antibodies to thyroid peroxidase, goiter, or evidence of atherosclerotic cardiovascular disease, heart failure, or associated risk factors.
  - If treatment is started because of symptoms of hypothyroidism, the treatment should be discontinued if no alleviation of the symptoms is observed **after 3 to 6 months** or if adverse effects occur.
  - If no treatment is started, the thyrotropin level should be monitored every 6 to 12 months, and treatment should be initiated if the level increases to 10 mIU per liter or more in persons younger than 70 years of age or if other indications for treatment become apparent.
  - Cutoff values for the levels of thyrotropin and free T for the diagnosis and treatment of subclinical hypothyroidism in pregnant women differ from those in nonpregnant women.
- **Long Term Prognosis**
  - Risk of progression of subclinical hypothyroidism to overt hypothyroidism is approximately 2 to 6% per year
  - Higher risk of progression: women, higher thyrotropin levels, higher levels of antibodies to thyroid peroxidase, low-normal free T levels.
  - Risk of cardiovascular disease.

- Thyrotropin levels of more than 7 mIU per liter → ↑ risks of CHF and fatal stroke

Figure. Thyroid work up based on TSH level

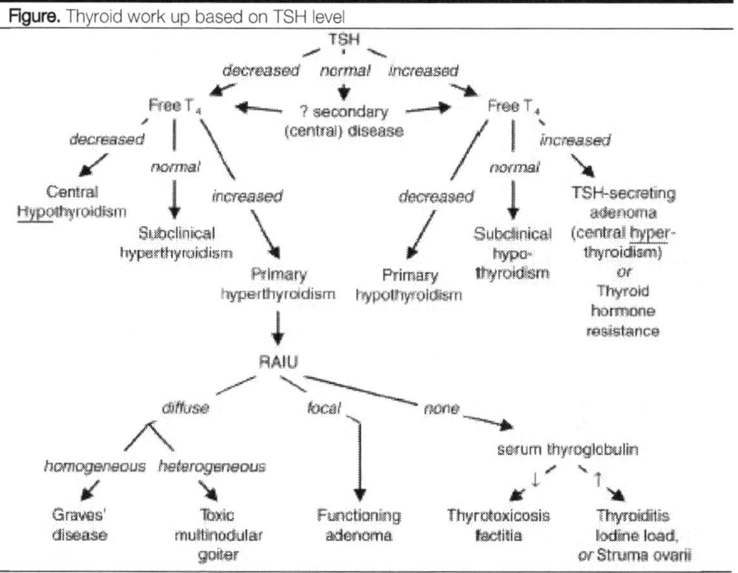

Thyroid Hormone Profiles

Hormone Profile	Associated Condition
↑TSH ↓T4	Hypothyroidism
↑TSH normal T4	Treated hypothyroidism or subclinical hypothyroidism
↑TSH ↑T4	TSH secreting tumor or thyroid hormone resistance
↑TSH ↑T4 and ↓T3	Slow conversion of T4→T3 or thyroid hormone AB artifact
↓TSH ↑T4/↑T3	Hyperthyroidism
↓TSH normal T4/T3	Subclinical hyperthyroidism
↑TSH ↓T4	Central hypothyroidism (r/o pituitary source)
↓TSH ↓T4 and ↓T3	Sick euthyroidism or pituitary disease

HYPERTHYROIDISM

- **Etiology**[166]
  - Graves' disease (60-80%)
  - ABs: +TSI or TBII, anti-TPO, antithyroglobulin, ANA
  - Thyroiditis (either the thyrotoxic phase of subacute thyroiditis or painless)
  - Painful thyroid to palpation
  - +TPO Ab
  - Toxic adenoma (single or multinodular)
  - Rx: amiodarone
- **History**
  - Ask about h/o cancer, radiation exposure, pregnancy and family history of thyroid d/o.

- **Clinical Presentation**
    - Restlessness, sweating, tremor, ↑HR, ↓weight, moist skin, diarrhea, ↑reflexes
    - Consider storm in patients with delirium, ↑Temp, ↑HR, ↑BP with wide gap, GI sx
    - Goiter
    - Ophthalmopathy (seen in only 50%)
    - Pretibial myxedema

Causes of Hyperthyroidism

Disease	FT4	FT3	Uptake Scan (RAIU)	Others
Graves	↑	↑ (T3>T4)	Increased + homogenous	High TSI or thyrotropin receptor Ab
Silent Thyroiditis	↑	↑	Low uptake	Thyroid peroxidase Ab +
Painful subacute thyroiditis	↑	↑	Low uptake	Thyroid-related Ab usually negative
Exogenous Ingestion	↑	↑	Low uptake	Serum thyroglobulin very low or absent
Toxic multinodular goiter	Low/normal/high	↑	Increased/patchy	Thyroid-related Ab usually -
Solitary nodule	Low/normal/high	↑	Increased focal uptake, suppression within surrounding gland	Thyroid-related Ab usually -

- **Thyroid Storm**
    - <u>Precipitants</u>
        - MI
        - Infection
        - Surgery
        - DKA
    - <u>Symptoms/Diagnosis</u>
        - Use SAALE point system
            - Storm likely with >45 points
            - Impending storm if point total 25-44
            - Unlikely storm if <25 points
    - <u>Treatment</u>
        - *Medications*
            - Propranolol @ 240mg or higher (vs. atenolol due to ↑ reduction of T4→T3 conversion)
            - PTU>MMI (↑ reduction of T4→T3 conversion)
            - +/- steroids (suspected concurrent adrenal insufficiency)
            - +/- iodine (SSKI, Lugol) to inhibit further hormone release

        - Acetaminophen
    - *Endocrinology consult*
- **Labs**
    - ↓TSH ↑FT4 and ↑FT3
        - Normal TSH often excludes hyperthyroidism
        - ↑ FT4 or FT3 confirms thyrotoxicosis. If FT4 elevated no need to check FT3, diagnosis is already confirmed.
        - if ↓ or normal FT4 and ↓ TSH, measure FT3; use T3 if FT3 assay not available
        - Normal FT4 and FT3 suggests subclinical hyperthyroidism, lab error, hypothalamic or pituitary disease, nonthyroidal illness, or medication effects.
    - ↑calciuria
    - ↑Ca
    - Anemia
    - Consider measuring thyroid antibodies and serum thyroglobulin if the etiology is still unclear after a thyroid scan
- **Imaging**
    - US
        - Useful in distinguishing cystic from solid nodules (benign vs. malignant)
        - If a solitary or dominant nodule, do FNA to r/o cancer
    - Scintigraphy

      Scanning should not be performed in a woman who is pregnant (with the exception of a molar pregnancy) or breastfeeding. Perform scanning if patients do not have classic Graves (exophthalmos or symmetrically enlarged thyroid)
        - Iodine-123 (123 I) or technetium-99m (99m Tc) can be used for thyroid scanning.
        - Normally, the isotope distributes homogeneously throughout both lobes of the thyroid gland.
        - In patients with hyperthyroidism, the pattern of uptake (eg, diffuse vs nodular) varies with the underlying disorder.
            - Normal: 2-26% (@ 24 hours 8-25%)
            - Increased (40-100%) and homogenous/diffuse: diffuse toxic goiter (Graves)
            - Single/Multiple Foci of Increased Uptake: toxic thyroid adenoma or toxic multinodular goiter
            - Decreased (<2%): thyrotoxic phase of subacute thyroiditis or a nonthyroidal source of thyroid hormone

          Less Common Forms
            - Decreased (<25%): iodide-induced thyrotoxicosis, metastatic thyroid carcinoma or struma ovarii

Medications for treatment of Hyperthyroidism		
Drug	Dosing	Comment
Propylthiouracil	500-1000 mg load, then 250 mg every 4 hours	Blocks new hormone synthesis
		Blocks T4 → T3 conversion
Methimazole	60-80 mg/day	Blocks new hormone synthesis
Propranolol	60-80 mg every 4 hours	Consider invasive monitoring in congestive heart failure patients
		Blocks T4 → T3 conversion in high doses
		Alternate drug: esmolol infusion
Iodine (saturated solution of potassium iodide)	5 drops (0.25 mL or 250 mg) orally every 6 hours	Do not start until 1 hour after antithyroid drugs
		Blocks new hormone synthesis
		Blocks thyroid hormone release
Hydrocortisone	300 mg intravenous load, then 100 mg every 8 hours	May block T4 → T3 conversion
		Prophylaxis against relative adrenal insufficiency
		Alternative drug: dexamethasone

- **Treatment**
  - Pregnancy Specific Goals
  - Thyroid function testing q4w
    - Goals:
      - Maintain mild hyperthyroid state with TSH 0.1-0.3, FT4 just above trimester specific ranges, and TT3/TT4 1.5x nonpregnant range
  - Treatment includes symptom relief, antithyroid pharmacotherapy, radioactive iodine-131 (131I) therapy (the preferred treatment of hyperthyroidism among US thyroid specialists), or thyroidectomy.
  - Antithyroid medications are **not effective** in thyrotoxicosis in which scintigraphy shows **low uptake** of iodine-123 (123I), as in patients with subacute thyroiditis, because these cases result from release of **preformed** thyroid hormone.
  - Patients should be given written or documented verbal instruction to the effect that if they develop high fever (>100.5°F) or a severe sore throat, they should stop the medication and seek medical attention.
  - Many of the neurologic and cardiovascular symptoms are relieved with propranolol.
  - Anti-Thyroid Medications
    - Drug dose should be titrated every 4 weeks until thyroid functions normalize.
    - Best in patients with Graves' disease (or can use radioactive iodine)
    - Some patients with Graves' disease go into a remission after treatment for 12-18 months, and the drug can be discontinued.
      - 1/2 of the patients who go into remission experience a recurrence of hyperthyroidism within the following year.
      - Nodular forms of hyperthyroidism (ie, toxic multinodular goiter and toxic adenoma) are permanent conditions and will not go into remission.
    - Methimazole
      - *Dosing*: 10-20mg PO once daily (in divided q8h dosing) or dose by symptoms severity:
        - mild, 15 mg/day
        - moderate, 30-40 mg/day
        - severe, 60 mg/day

  - *Pregnancy*: use lowest dose to keep free T4 at or slightly above ULN for nonpregnant women; assess monthly and adjust dose as required.
  - *Duration* - taper or discontinue if TSH levels are normal after 12-18 months if for tx of Grave disease
  - *S/E*: risk for agranulocytosis; check LFTs, WBC, TSH
- Propylthiouracil
  - *Dosing* – 50-150 mg PO TID; may ↑ to 400 mg/day for severe hyperthyroidism, very large goiters, or both.
  - *Duration*: as above
  - *Pregnancy*: used in thyrotoxicosis due to Graves' disease in the first trimester only (otherwise switch to MMU for 2nd and 3rd. Use lowest dose to keep mother's total thyroxine (T4) and triiodothyronine (T3) levels slightly above normal range for pregnancy, keep TSH suppressed.
  - *S/E*: risk for hepatocellular necrosis; best in pregnancy; check LFTs, WBC, and TSH

HYPOTHYROIDISM

- **Etiology**
  - Hashimoto's, iodine deficiency, drugs (lithium, iodide, propylthiouracil, sulfonamides, amiodarone), infiltrative disease (*e.g.* sarcoid), genetic enzyme defects, after therapy for other thyroid disease, and secondary to hypopituitarism.
- **Classic Symptoms**: fatigue, sluggishness, hoarse voice, constipation, delayed distal tendon reflexes, and skin changes
- **Screening**
  Done with TSH only
  - Women reaching age 50 YO
  - Those at risk given hx of neck radiation, family history, hx of autoimmune disease, patients with goiter
  - Use third generation TSH assays starting at 35 q5y or more frequent/early if high risk conditions such as pregnancy, female>60, T1DM, h/o neck radiation
- **Diagnosis**
  - Screening: TSH, often elevated above 10, then get FT4 which should be low in hypothyroidism
    - If patient has elevated TSH (often <10) but normal FT4, this is termed **subclinical hypothyroidism** and data is mixed in whether to treat these patients. All pregnant patients with SCH should be treated
      - If FT4 is normal can get anti-TPO antibody to determine risk of progressing to clinical hypothyroidism
    - Thyroglobulin AB (Tg Ab) is often also found in patients with Hashimoto's hypothyroidism (along with anti-TPO AB)
    - Other labs: ↑cholesterol, ↑AST/ALT
  - Hospital - Should not be done due to high likelihood of SES (see next topic)
  - Pregnant patients: FT4, Total T4, TSH (> 2.5 milliunits/L in the first trimester, > 3 milliunits/L in the second trimester, or > 3-3.5 milliunits/L in the third trimester)
- **Types**
  - Primary – 95% of cases; ↑TSH ↓FT4
  - Secondary – due to insufficient stimulation of TSH (due to ↓TRH) caused by either pituitary or hypothalamic issue. Consider this diagnosis in patients with known mass lesion in the pituitary or multiple hormonal deficiencies are also present
- **Causes**
  - Hashimoto's

        - Most common cause in adequate iodine intake countries (whereas iodine deficiency is the most common cause in those countries where deficiency remains)
        - Form of autoimmune thyroid disease
        - +thyroid peroxidase ab
- **Treatment**
    - Levothyroxine: start *low* and go *slow* (↓ risk of AF or MI). Consider starting with 50mcg/d (1.5-1.7 mcg/kg of IBW which is about 100-125mcg/d in healthy adults or 1.0mcg/kg if elderly) taken ½ to 1 hour **before breakfast** with at least 3-4 hours between taking any other medications. Patients with known cardiac disease should be started at lower dose of 12.5-25 mcg/d
        - **Always take on an empty stomach**
        - Full replacement dose can be started initially (no titrating up required) in healthy and young patients (ATA does not define 'young')
            - If elderly or h/o ischemic heart disease, start at ¼ - ½ the level and increase every 6 weeks
            - Mild to moderate can often be treated with solely 50-75mcg
        - First labs obtained after starting therapy should be done after **at least** 2 months!
        - Goal TSH is 2-3 mIU/L → after reaching goal, check every 6 months then every 12 months
        - Often takes 4-6 weeks for TSH levels to reflect effects of therapy.
        - Sole treatment with L-T4 remains first line therapy as T4 is converted peripherally to T3 if sufficient T4 is given
    - <u>Myxedema coma</u>: levothyroxine 5-8 mcg/kg IV load, then daily 50-100 mcg IV, consider adrenal insufficiency, treat underlying precipitant
    - <u>Hypertension</u> – classically patients will have ↑diastolic pressure and ↓pulse pressure.
    - Suggestion of whether the true ULN of TSH is inadequate, and patients should be treated to TSH of 1.0-1.5 mU/l
    - **Thyroidectomy**
        - Risks include voice loss or change in voice
        - TSH is the only pre-surgery lab value required
- **Monitoring**
    - TSH is best to use as a monitoring lab; T4 only checked if concerned of central hypothyroidism
        - Normal TSH considered 0.3-3.0 mIU/mL but up to 5.0 in older adults
    - If checking labs, make sure patient did not take their replacement therapy yet
    - Patients will often have ↑diuresis and weight loss with successful changes in therapy
- **Maintenance Changes**
    - Most common reason for changes is **noncompliance**
    - 12.5-25mcg changes at any time
    - May take 6-8 weeks to note change.
        - Consider obtaining T3 and T4 to look for immediate changes while waiting for TSH to eventually respond
        - TSH can then be used once the T4 and T3 return to normal range
    - Catch-up doses can be taken at the end of the week to maintain a weekly level
- **Adding T3 therapy (aka combination therapy)**
    - Long held belief that those that have normal T4 levels should theoretically have normal T3 levels due to the physiologic conversion from T4□T3 to maintain homeostasis
    - Animal models have shown those with primary hypothyroidism on L-T4 monotherapy is not sufficient to normalize systemic thyroid levels

- Debate ongoing between ATA and AACE due to s/e reported (↑ risk of AF, angina, MI)
- ATA previously advised against combination therapy, but more recently changed their stance to "insufficient evidence to support"
- Numerous studies have addressed potential benefits of combined therapy of triiodothyronine with LT4. Results of these studies have failed to support a potential benefit of combined therapy
- Suggestion of benefit was raised from question if LT4 alone is sufficient to treat hypothyroidism
- Presence of genetic polymorphism may suggest which patients on treatment may benefit from treatment with T3 as well.
  - Symptoms suggestive of the presence of this include patients with high free T4/free T3 ratio
  - Most physicians consider this route when patients on LT4 remain symptomatic
- Levothyroxine remains first-line therapy (effective in 80-90% of patients)

Figure. Evaluation of hypothyroidism

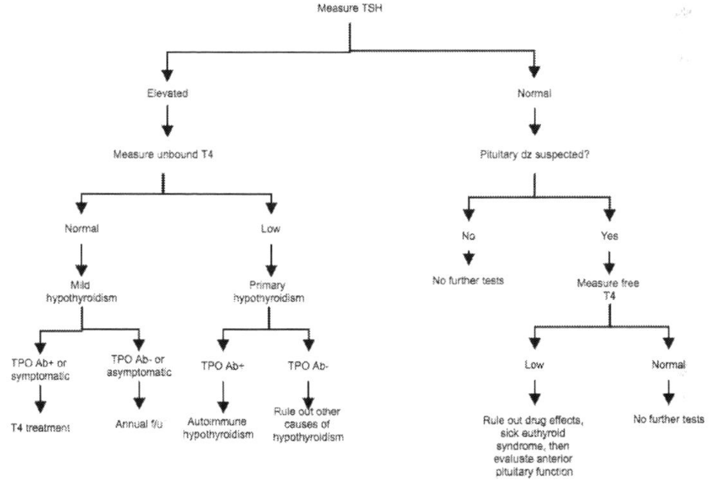

PITUITARY INCIDENTALOMA

- **Overview**[167]
  - Occur in up to 10% of patients undergoing MRI
  - All patients, no matter the size, should undergo clinical and laboratory workup for function
  - All patients with visual complaints (normally bitemporal hemianopsia) undergo formal visual field (VF) testing
- **Labs**
  - Hypersecretion:
    - Prolactin (PLCT)
    - GH/IGF-1

  - ACTH (if clinically indicated, routine measurement is not necessarily recommended)
- Hyposecretion
  - Prolactin
  - TSH
  - Free T4
  - AM Cortisol
  - Testosterone
  - LH
  - FSH
  - IGF-1

Figure. Evaluation and treatment of pituitary incidentalomas

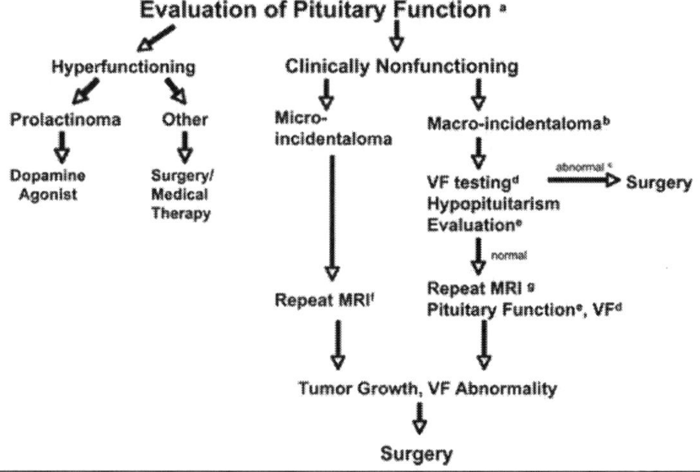

- **Management**
  - <10mm (*microadenoma)*: if 2-4mm and no function (nml PLCT), then no further testing. If 5-9mm, then repeat MRI in 12 months (then 2 years if unchanged, then q3y, etc.)
  - >10mm (*macroadenoma)*: check for pituitary hyper/hypo function with visual field testing. If positive, do surgery. If not positive, follow and do surgery if increasing in size over time and repeat imaging in 6 months (then 1 year if unchanged, then q2y, etc.)
  - Surgery
    - VF deficit
    - Compression on the optic nerve (or close to the chiasm if planning on pregnancy)
    - Unremitting headaches
    - Pituitary apoplexy
    - Hypersecreting adenomas
    - Clinically significant growth

SICK EUTHYROID SYNDROME

- **Physiology**
  - Thought to be due to underlying cytokines released during illness
- **Diagnosis/Labs**
  - Most common pattern seen is ↓T3 with normal T4 and TSH
  - The amount of decrease in T3 can be used to determine the severity of underlying illness. Very poor prognosis is seen when T4 also decreases
  - Ultimate diagnosis is based off hx of normal thyroid labs prior to hospitalization and resolution of labs after discharge
- **Treatment**
  - Not indicated

STEROIDS

Steroid formulations				
Agent	Dose (mg)	Potency	Mineralcort. potency	Half life
Cortisone	25	0.8	0.8	8-12
Hydrocortisone	20	1	1	8-12
Prednisone	5	4	0.8	18-36
Prednisolone	5	4	0.8	18-36
Methylprednisolone	5	5	0.5	18-36
Dexamethasone	0.75	25	0	35-54

- **Emergency Steroids**
  - Immediate high-dose IV hydrocortisone 100 mg bolus followed by infusion of 100-200 mg over the next 24 hours or intermittent IV dosing at 100 mg q6-8 hours.
  - "Stress dose steroids" typically means at least 200-300 mg of hydrocortisone per day.
- **Taper**
  - Physiologic doses of steroids (Hydrocortisone 30 mg (20 mg qAM, 10 mg qPM) OR Cortisone 37.5 mg (25 mg qAM, 12.5 mg qPM) OR prednisone 7.5 mg (5 mg qAM, 2.5 mg qPM)) are around 5-10 mg/day thus any dose of this will not require a taper.[168]
  - When providing therapy of 20 mg for more than 20 days (20/20 rule) a taper is required to ↓ risk for withdrawal
  - If rx is <= 40, cut by half, if greater, then cut by 25%
  - All tapers are different, one example is as such:
    - First Method
      - Decrease dose by 10mg every other week until reaching 20 mg
      - Decrease dose by 5 mg every week until finished
    - Second Method
      - Rx for 40 mgs or above: a reduction of up to 10 mgs every few weeks is acceptable
      - Rx is between 20 and 40mgs: tapering of no more than 5 mgs every few weeks is standard
      - At 20 mgs, taper down in increments of 2.5 mgs every four weeks, and when the dosage gets down to 10 mgs per day, tapering in 1 to 2 mgs every four weeks is best.

TESTOSTERONE

- **Physiology S/E of Exogenous Treatment**[169]
  - Use of AAS results in hypogonadotropic hypogonadism by feedback suppression of the hypothalamic-pituitary-gonadal (HPG) axis via inhibition of pulsatile GnRH release and a subsequent decrease in LH and FSH
  - Younger men may have a more "elastic axis" capable of recovering GnRH pulsation and gonadotropin secretion faster and more completely than older AAS users.
  - It is possible that shorter durations, lower doses, younger ages, and higher T levels at baseline are associated with a quicker recovery of HPG axis function after AAS use.
- **Features Consistent with Testosterone Deficiency**[170]
  - Incomplete sexual development
  - ↓libido and potency
  - ↓early-morning erection
  - Gynecomastia
  - ↓2/2 sexual characteristics (ie. ↓shaving frequency)
  - Small testicles (normal adult: length of 4-7cm and volume 20-25cc)
  - Hot flashes (severe)
  - Low sperm count
  - Osteoporosis
- **Causes/Associated Conditions**
  - Chronic steroid use or other known medication s/e
  - Mod-Sev COPD
  - T2DM
  - Infertility
  - HIV associated weight loss
  - ESRD
- **Initial Labs**
  - Testosterone (total+free) and repeat if initial are low (0800)
  - Secondary Labs
  - Hormones: LH, FSH, SHBG, Prolactin
  - CBC
  - Lipid panel
  - PSA
  - CMP
- **Diagnosis (only if patient has no acute illness)**
  - AM testosterone low per reference lab standards (if no reference, then use 300)
    - Repeat testosterone to confirm
  - FSH/LH low: secondary hypogonadism (pituitary-hypothalamic)
    - Obtain PRL, MRI sella imaging
  - FSH/LH high: primary hypogonadism (testicular)
    - Obtain karyotype imaging to rule out Klinefelter's
- **Side Effects**
  - General: hepatotoxicity, cardiotoxicity, polycythemia, ↑LDL, ↑BP, gynecomastia, testicular atrophy, acne, skin striations, depression, reduced fertility
  - <u>Gel</u>: skin irritation, transfer to partner
  - <u>IM</u>: deep tissue infection, mood fluctuations, ↑↑HCT
- **Contraindications to Therapy**
  - Known history of Breast or Prostate Cancer
  - Prostate nodule palpated
  - PSA>4 ng/ml (or 3 if high risk such as AA)

  - Uncontrolled CHF
  - HCT>50%
  - Severe OSA
- **Threshold for Treatment**
  - US Endocrine Society: T (total) <300 ng/dL or T (free) lower limit of normal
  - Joint Societies: T (total) <230 ng/dL or T (free) <65 pg/mL
  - EAU: T (total) <230 ng/dL or T (free) <60 pg/mL
  - Italian Society of Endocrinology: T (total) <230 ng/dL
- **Management**

  Recommend testosterone therapy for symptomatic men with classical androgen deficiency syndromes aimed at inducing and maintaining secondary sex characteristics and at improving their sexual function, sense of wellbeing, and bone mineral density.

Management Options			
Medication	Dosage	Advantages	Side Effects
1% Gel (ie. Fortesta)	5-10g of gel applied to thighs daily	Corrects symptoms of androgen deficiency, provides flexibility of dosing, ease of application, good skin tolerability	Transfer to female partner, skin irritation
Patch	2-6mg/day (initial: 4mg) applied once a day at night to dry intact skin of back, abdomen or upper thigh	Easy to use; corrects symptoms of deficiency	May remain in the low-normal range; these men may need application of 2 patches daily; skin irritation at the application site occurs frequently in many patients. Cannot use same site for 7 days.
IM (long acting)	Testosterone enanthate 50-100 mg qweek or 100-200mg q2weeks or 250mg q3w	Corrects symptoms of androgen deficiency; relatively inexpensive if self-administered; flexibility of dosing	Requires IM injection; peaks and valleys without consistent levels. Avoid cypionate if soy allergy.
	Testosterone cypionate 50-100mg qweek or 100-200mg q2w		
IM (extra-long acting)	Testosterone undecanoate 1000mg initially f/b 1000mg @ 6	Less frequent dosing among IM preparations	Must monitor patients 30m after dosing; risk for anaphylaxis

	weeks then 1000mg every 10-14 weeks		
Oral	40-80mg; 2 to 3 times/day after meals	Oral	GI s/e; variable clinical and biochemical response

- **Imaging:**
  - DEXA scan qyear
- **Labs (Testosterone, HCT):**
  - Re-evaluate 3-6 months after treatment initiation then annually with repeat testosterone levels
- **Timing Based on Formulation**
  - Oral: 3-5 hrs after ingestion
  - Long-acting IM: midway between injections
  - Extra-long acting IM: before the next dose
  - Dermal: 3-12 hours after application
  - Gel: any time after at least 2 weeks of treatment
- **Goal testosterone is in the mid-normal range of reference lab**
  - If HCT>54% then stop therapy until level <50%
  - Consider monitoring PSA yearly (>1.4 ng/mL in a year or increase in 0.4ng/dL after 6 months)
- **Weaning Off**
  - Medications
    - Weaning testosterone is a lot like weaning glucocorticoids, there is no firm data to guide you.
    - Start by cutting the dose by 25% sequentially over a few weeks. Eg Fortesta 4 pumps x 3 weeks, 3 pumps x 2 weeks, 2 pump x 3 weeks, 1 pump x 3 weeks.
      - The interval of how many weeks will depend on testicular mass and how long they have been on it
        - If they have normal testis and have been on testosterone for under 6mo, they can wean sooner, eg 2 weeks.
        - If longer or with atrophy then longer, in general it can take up 4-6months for the HPG axis to reset.
        - If they are normal at any time after stopping testosterone, you are done.
    - Can consider co-administration of a SERM:
      - Clomiphene citrate 25mg/QOD x 10 weeks then decrease dose to 50% for total of 4 months
        - This is off-label and documentation must note this!
  - Labs
    - After 4 weeks

THYROID NODULE

- **Differential Diagnosis**[171,172]
  - Thyroid cancer (↑ risk if: family hx, excessive radiation exposure, sx such as hoarse voice, dysphagia)
  - Benign adenoma
  - Colloid cyst

- Metastasis

Types of Thyroid Nodules		
Adenomas	Carcinoma	Colloid Nodule
Macrofollicular adenoma (simple colloid) Microfollicular adenoma (fetal) Embryonal adenoma (trabecular) Hurthle cell adenoma (oxyphilic, oncolytic) Atypical adenoma Adenoma with papillae Signet-ring adenoma	Papillary (75%) Follicular (10%) Medullary (5-10%) Anaplastic (5%) Other (ie. Lymphoma 5%)	Dominant nodule in a multinodular goiter
	Cyst	Other
	Simple cyst Cystic/solid tumors (ie. hemorrhagic, necrotic)	Inflammatory thyroid disorders (ie. subacute thyroiditis, chronic l lymphocytic thyroiditis, granulomatous dz) Developmental abnormalities (ie. dermoid, rare unilateral lobe agenesis)

- **Diagnosis**
  - Obtain TSH
  - ↑TSH:
    - Likely cold nodule
    - Obtain US in all thyroid nodules
      - Based on the ATA, obtain FNA if ≥1cm and at least one of the following suspicious signs:
        - **Nodule**: microcalcifications, hypoechogenicity, irregular margins, taller than wider
        - **LN**: microcalcifications, hyperechogenicity, peripheral vascularity, rounded shape, cystic aspect
      - Or if solid isoechoic/hyperechoic ≥1 cm without the above findings or cystic and ≥2cm
        - Often requires 2-4 passes to have diagnostic significance in 80% cases
        - Calcitonin should only be sent for if patient has family hx of medullary thyroid cancer or MEN-2
        - If results confirm cancer, then proceed to RAIU to determine if nodule is functioning.
          - If functioning nodule (↑uptake, hot), can avoid surgery
          - If nonfunctioning nodule (↓uptake, cold) surgery is indicated
    - Monitor with f/u US if <1cm
  - **Normal TSH:**
    - Likely cold nodule
    - See above
  - ↓TSH:
    - Suggests hot nodule (toxic adenoma)
    - RAIU scan to confirm if hot
    - Hot? Treat with I131
    - Cold? Likely malignant, obtain FNA

Figure. Work up of a patient with a thyroid nodule

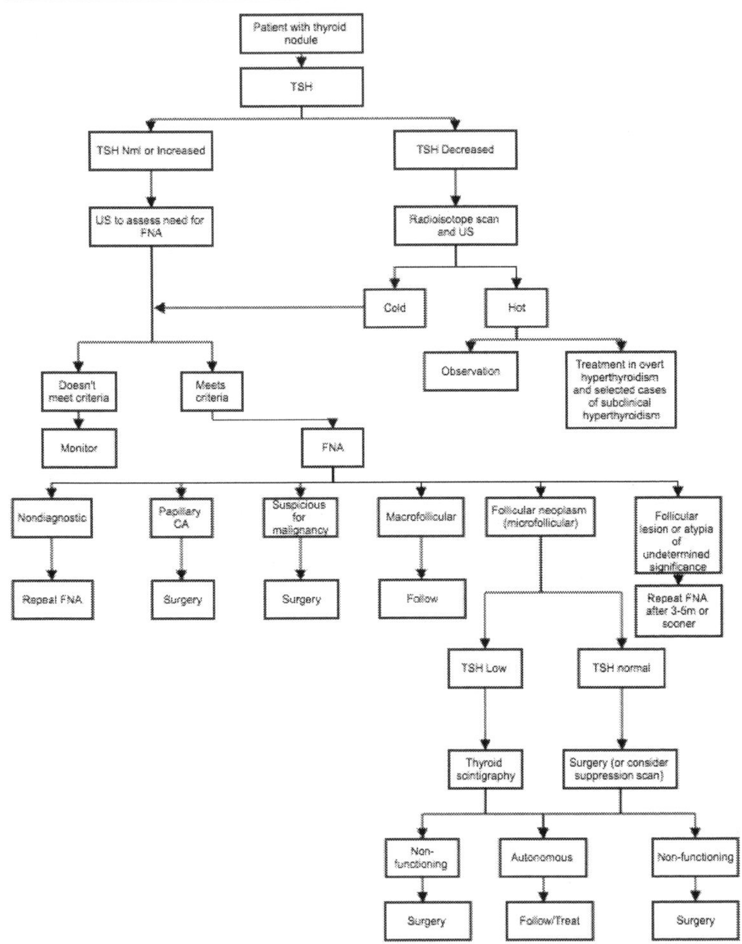

- **Treatment**
  - Functioning nodule, ↑ Ca risk – hemithyroidectomy
  - Benign functioning nodule – radioiodine
  - Nonfunctioning nodules – ethanol injection if solid, therapeutic aspiration if cystic
  - Surgery – indications include: features suggestive of cancer, symptoms 2/2 to nodules presence (hoarse voice, dysphagia); high risk of complications (such as hypoparathyroidism)
  - Levothyroxine – goal is to tx to obtain TSH of 0.3 to ↓ further growth however recent studies have shown better reduction if TSH is at 0.1 however ↑ adverse risks (atrial fibrillation, ↓bone density)
  - Radioiodine – tx of choice for functioning benign nodule; often implemented in cases of functioning nodule (↑uptake on RAIU), c/I in pregnant females, highest

complication is hypothyroidism (test TSH yearly post operatively and continue to monitor for ↑ nodule size)
  - Ethanol injection – indicated in non-functioning nodules, cysts, benign functioning nodules by inducing coagulative necrosis and small-vessel thrombosis; higher efficacy with multiple treatments.

VITAMIN D DEFICIENCY

- **Who should be tested**
  - Evidence of severe deficiency:
    - Low 24 hour urine calcium excretion
    - ↑PTH
    - ↑ALKP
    - ↓Ca or PO4
    - Nontraumatic fractures
    - Osteopenia
- **Risk Factors**
  - Age>65
  - Decreased PO intake (malnutrition)
  - Low sun exposure
  - GI malabsorption (short bowel, celiac, pancreatitis, IBD, amyloidosis)
  - CKD
- **Symptoms**
  - Bone discomfort/pain
  - Generalized pain (may mimic fibromyalgia)
  - Proximal muscle weakness
  - Symmetric low back pain
  - HA
  - N/V
- **Diagnosis**
  - Deficiency: <20 ng/mL
  - Insufficiency: 20-30 ng/mL
- **Testing/Normals**
  - Total 25(OH)D is optimal
  - Normal 25-80 ng/mL
- **Treatment**
  - Contraindications: sarcoidosis, tuberculosis, metastatic bone disease, Williams syndrome
  - Prevention can be done with daily intake of 200-600IU
  - Repletion: Ergocalciferol (D3) 50,000IU orally once/week for 2-3 months or three times a week for 1 month; after finishing you should start daily therapy with cholecalciferol 800-1000IU (max 2000IUj/d)
    - Recheck Vitamin D after 3 months, repeat course if necessary

GERIATRICS

ACTIVITIES OF DAILY LIVING

Daily Living Activities[173] Points (1 or 0)	Independence (1 Point)	Dependence (0 Points)
	NO supervision, direction or personal assistance	WITH supervision, direction, personal assistance or total care
BATHING Points: _________	(1 POINT) Bathes self completely or needs help in bathing only a single part of the body such as the back, genital area or disabled extremity	(0 POINTS) Need help with bathing more than one part of the body, getting in or out of the tub or shower. Requires total bathing
DRESSING Points: _________	(1 POINT) Get clothes from closets and drawers and puts on clothes and outer garments complete with fasteners. May have help tying shoes.	(0 POINTS) Needs help with dressing self or needs to be completely dressed.
TOILETING Points: _________	(1 POINT) Goes to toilet, gets on and off, arranges clothes, cleans genital area without help.	(0 POINTS) Needs help transferring to the toilet, cleaning self or uses bedpan or commode.
TRANSFERRING Points: _________	(1 POINT) Moves in and out of bed or chair unassisted. Mechanical transfer aids are acceptable	(0 POINTS)Needs help in moving from bed to chair or requires a complete transfer.
CONTINENCE Points: _________	(1 POINT) Exercises complete self-control over urination and defecation.	(0 POINTS) Is partially or totally incontinent of bowel or bladder
FEEDING Points: _________	(1 POINT) Gets food from plate into mouth without help. Preparation of food may be done by another person.	(0 POINTS) Needs partial or total help with feeding or requires parenteral feeding.

Score of 6 = High, Patient is independent.
Score of 0 = Low, patient is very dependent

DEMENTIA

- **Overview**[174]
  - Aging —most significant r/f for Alzheimer disease and dementia in general
  - individuals ≥85 yr of age are the most rapidly growing segment of population
  - Pure Lewy body dementia or vascular dementia more common in younger patients
- **Most Comon Types**
  - Alzheimers (AD)
    - *Presentation*: short-term memory loss most common presenting symptom; immediate memory also affected; language variants (eg, logopenic [difficulty repeating or retrieving word]) and visual variants (eg, inability to find objects in visual field) also seen; other symptoms — executive dysfunction; apathy; reactive irritability; most patients with dementia have **delusions** and **disorientation** late in disease. Poor performance on animal fluency suggests medial temporal or temporal lobe disorder (eg, AD).
  - Frontotemporal (FTD)
    - *Presentation*: executive dysfunction and behavioral changes; minimal memory loss; apathy and poor insight; cortical dysfunction, particularly involving language; behavioral disturbances; behavioral and aphasic are the main variants
  - Lewy Body (LBD)
    - *Presentation:* psychosis early in disease suggests LBD. Difficulty with executive functioning and visuospatial skills (ie. clock drawing) more than issues with memory loss (more problems with processing speed). Will perform well on delayed recall. poor performance on animal fluency suggests medial temporal or temporal lobe disorder (eg, AD), Poor performance on letter fluency more suggestive LBD. Insight often intact, so depression common; early visual hallucinations strongly correlated with LB pathology.
  - Prion - sporadic — rapidly progressive; can occur in different sites in brain, so presentation variable; often presents with psychiatric disturbances and painful dysesthesias.
  - Vascular (VD) – stepwise worsening of memory; often in combination with vascular disease; may co-occur with AD, LBD, and other disorders
  - Parkinsons Disease Dementia (PDD)
    - *Presentation:* Difficulty with executive functioning and visuospatial skills (ie. clock drawing). Will perform well on delayed recall. poor performance on animal fluency suggests medial temporal or temporal lobe disorder (eg, AD), Poor performance on letter fluency more suggestive of PD.
- **Step by Step Approach**
  1) Prediagnostic Testing (look for risk factors, medical history of comorbid cardiovascular disease, prior labs such as CBC, glucose, thyroid, B12, RPR, LFTs, UA)
  2) Assess their performance (see screening below)
  3) Asses their daily functioning (determine the level of independence, and degree of disability with ADLs)
  4) Assess behavioral symptoms (NPI-Q, look for drug toxicity, psychiatric diagnoses that may be contributing)
  5) Identify caregiver needs
- **Risk Factors for AD**
  - Female>male
  - Prior head trauma
  - Family history of AD
  - Obesity

- HTN
- DM
- ↑Age
- Smoking

- **History**
  - Warning signs associated with AD
    - Memory loss
    - Difficulty performing familiar tasks
    - Problems with language
    - Disorientation to time and place
    - Poor or decreased judgement
    - Problems with abstract thought
    - Misplacing things
    - Changes in mood/behavior
    - Changes in personality
    - Loss of initiative
- **Screening**[175,176]
  - ACE v2
  - MMSE
  - Mini-COG
  - MOCA

Memory screening and assessment tools				
Tool	Key Features	Time	Cut off Score	Sensitivity/ Specificity
MMSE	Costly Quick and easy Can be used to track progression of decline Insufficient evalution of short term memory (STM)	5-10 minutes	23-24 / 30	79/95
Mini-Cog	Very short (only 3 items) Similar sens/spec to MMSE Poor evaluation of non-AD dementias	3 minutes	Probably normal/ possibly impaired	76/89
MoCA	Best to screen for MCI (look for delayed recall) Free More evaluation of executive fxn and STM Look at pattern rather than score	10 minutes	≤25	100/87

- **Diagnostic Testing**

- Labs
  - Most will be WNL
  - Can consider Vitamin-D (unclear association b/w ↓ levels and ↑ risk for PD)
  - Presenilin-1 and amyloid precursor protein testing in patients with young-onset dementia and strong family history;
  - If dementia strongly suspected, biomarkers may be obtained to strengthen diagnosis of AD (through examination of cerebrospinal fluid [CSF] for β-amyloid [Aβ] and phospho-tau [P-tau], or amyloid imaging)

CSF evaluation/interpretation		
	Aβ-amyloid	phospho-tau [P-tau]
Alzheimer's	↓↓ (<400 pg/mL)	↑↑ (≥60 pg/mL)
Lewy-Body	↓↓	--
Parkinson's Disease	↓↓	--
Fronto-Temporal	--	--
Creutzfeldt-Jakob	--	-- (Tau levels ↑↑)

- Imaging
  - MRI better for identifying vascular disease
    - FTD: often shows more atrophy than expected; look for asymmetry
    - LBD: mild atrophy
    - Prion: cortical ribboning
    - VD: hyperintensities in >25% of white matter; multiple large-vessel infarcts; ≥2 basal ganglia and white matter lacunas
  - Amyloid imaging used to increase diagnostic accuracy (more important for early-onset dementia)
  - FDG-PET:
    - AD: parietal and posterior cingulate hypometabolism
    - FTD: frontal hypometabolism and relatively preserved parietal or posterior cingulate metabolism
    - LBD: hypometabolism in occipital region; scan not highly sensitive.
- Consults
  - Neuropsych testing helpful in early cases or those that are atypical presentations.

- **Dementia with Behavioral Disorders**
  - Evaluation
    - H&P
    - Consider MRI
      - Evaluate for cerebral atrophy, hippocampus involvement
    - Labs to r/o reversible cause
      - B12, folate, CBC, CMP, LFT
      - Optional: syphilis (RPR), HIV, Paraneoplastic ab (r/o autoimmune encephalitis), CSF proteins (tau, P-tau, 14-3-3) to r/o CJD
  - Treatment[177]
    - No clear standard of care
    - Psychosis
      - Most studies conclude that olanzapine and risperidone show the best effects with minimal side effects (↑ risk of stroke) of all atypical antipsychotics
      - Olanzapine 5-10mg
      - Risperidone 1mg (however better to start low at 0.25mg daily)
    - Agitation

      - Quetiapine 25mg qHS titrated to maximum 150mg BID (morning, evening) per "*Quetiapine for agitation or psychosis in patients with dementia and parkinsonism.*"
        - APA recommends that in patients with dementia with agitation or psychosis, if there is no clinically significant response after a **4-week trial** of an adequate dose of an antipsychotic drug, the medication should be tapered and withdrawn.
        - In patients with dementia who show adequate response of behavioral/ psychological symptoms to treatment with an antipsychotic drug, an attempt to taper and withdraw the drug should be made **within 4 months of initiation**, unless the patient experienced a recurrence of symptoms with prior attempts at tapering of antipsychotic medication.
      - Prazosin 1mg daily → increase to 1mg BID (max dose 9mg/d)
    - <u>Depression</u>
      - Seen in up to 30% of patients with AD; often begins before the diagnosis of AD
      - Citalopram was the only antidepressant that showed benefit
    - Other options include Remeron (15mg/22.5mg/30mg)
- **Rapid Onset Dementia**
  - <u>Defined</u> – no specific timeline noted in literature, however considered decline in 1 or more cognitive domains in less than 1 or 2 years however, most occur over weeks to months when they are seen in the medical setting.
  - <u>Differential</u>
    - *CJD* (look for concurrent myoclonus, sleep difficulties, and psychiatric presentation, MRI of the brain will often show a pattern of increased intensity in the DWI of the basal ganglia and cortex)
    - *HIV encephalopathy*
    - *Lyme disease*
    - *Neoplasm*
    - *Frontotemporal dementia*
    - *Dementia with Lewy bodies*
    - *Progressive supranuclear palsy*
    - *Vascular dementia*
    - *Neurosyphilis*
  - <u>Diagnostics</u>
    - Imaging
      - Brain MRI (T1, T2, DWI, FLAIR, with and without contrast)
      - CXR
      - Others to consider: CT head, CT C/A/P, MRA/V, Mammogram, FDG-PET CT, TTE, testicular/pelvic US
    - CSF with
      - 14-3-3 (CJD)
      - Tau (CJD)
      - West Nile Virus
      - Cell count and differential
      - Culture
      - Glucose
      - Protein
      - IgG index
      - Oligoclonal bands (MS)
      - VDRL
      - Neuron specific enolase

    - Cryptococcal antigen
    - Others to consider: Whipple PCR, metagenomic deep sequencing, phosphorylated tau, B2-microglobulin and EBV PCR, amyloid-beta-42
- EEG
    - Periodic sharp wave complexes seen with CJD
- Labs
    - HIV
    - CBC with differential
    - LFTs
    - RPR
    - Rheumatologic screen (ESR, C-RP, ANA)
    - TSH
    - VB12
    - Appropriate medication levels (ie. digoxin, phenytoin, lithium)
    - BMP/CMP
    - UA with culture
    - Urine toxicology
    - Heavy metal screen (urine)
    - Cultures: urine, blood, viral PCR, cytology

Additional Labs to Consider

- SPEP/UPEP
- Blood smear
- INR/PT/PTT
- Homocysteine
- Lyme AB
- Cortisol
- Antithyroglobulin, Anti-TPO
- ANCA, anti-ds-DNA, anti-Smith, SCL-70, SSA/SSB, RF, C3, C4, CH50

Figure. Suggested work up for rapidly progressive dementia

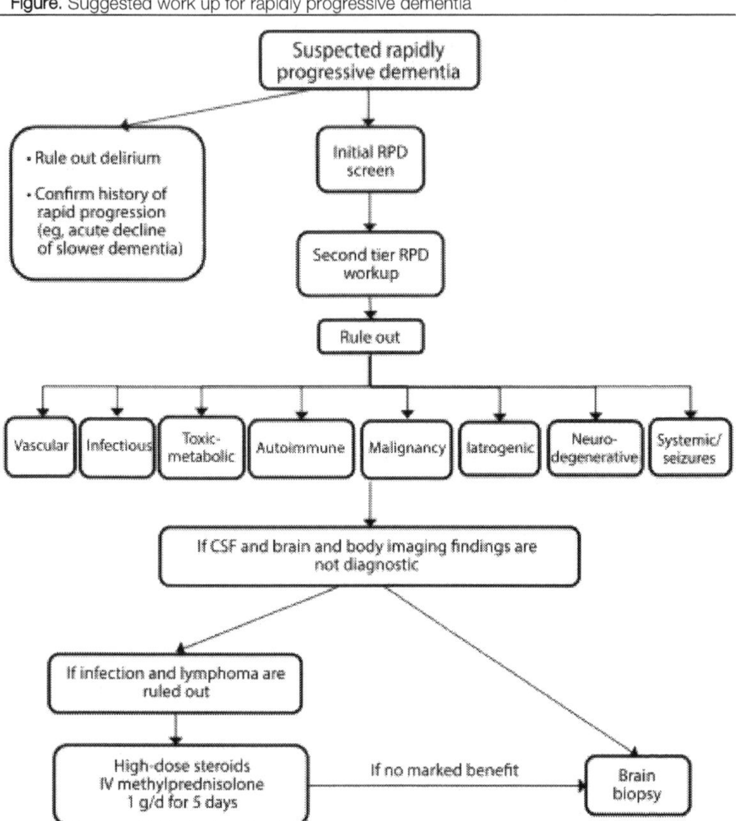

Treatment Options

Cholinesterase inhibitors	Dosing	S/E	Be Aware...	Indications	Combination of NMDA antagonist and cholinesterase inhibitors has been shown to decrease rates of institutionalization
Donepezil (Aricept)	Initially, 5 mg q.d. May increase to 10 mg qd *Take during breakfast*	Nausea vomiting Diarrhea Anorexia Fatigue Vivid dreams **Insomnia**	Substrate of CYPs 2D6, 3A4	Class 1A indication; no meaningful difference between drugs within this class; duration may be from 4-7 years per studies.	
Rivastigmine (Exelon)	PO: Initially, 1.5 mg bid with food. Usual dose is 3-6 mg bid. Transdermal patch: Initially, one 4.6 mg/24 hr patch q.d. May increase to 9.5-13.3 mg qd				
NMDA receptor antagonist					
Memantine (Namenda, Namenda XR)	Immediate-release: Initially, 5 mg q.d. May increase to 10 mg bid. Extended-release: Initially, 7 mg q.d. May increase to 28 mg qd	Headache, dizziness, drowsiness, constipation	Caution with severe hepatic disease. Decrease dose with CrCl<30	Moderate-advanced Alzheimer's disease and vascular dementia	
Atypical antipsychotics					
Olanzapine (Zyprexa, Zyprexa Zydis)	Initially, 2.5 mg qHS. Maximum dose 10 mg qHS	Hyperprolactinemia	Caution with CKD. Substrate of CYPs 1A2, 2D6		
Quetiapine (Seroquel)	Initially, 25 mg qHS. Maximum dose 200 mg qHS	Hypothyroidism, hepatotoxicity	Caution with CKD. Periodic eye exams. Substrate of CYP3A4	First line	
Risperidone (Risperdal)	Initially, 0.25-0.5 mg qHS. Maximum dose 2 mg qHS	Hyperprolactinemia	Decrease dose with CKD. Substrate of CYP2D6		

Other				
Haloperidol (Haldol)	0.25-5 mg total daily dose, dosed q.d.-bid	Drowsiness, dizziness, other CNS side effects, orthostatic hypotension, QT prolongation and TdP, anticholinergic effects, hematologic toxicity, hyperprolactinemia, skin hyperpigmentation, photosensitivity, ocular toxicity, EPS, NMS, TD	Increased mortality in elderly patients with dementia related psychosis. Avoid abrupt withdrawal, extreme temperature, severe hepatic disease. Caution with: pregnancy, seizure disorder, cardiac disease, pulmonary disease. Metabolized by CYPs 2D6 and 3A4	
Agents for sleep disturbances				
Trazodone	Initially, 25 mg qHS. Maximum dose 100 mg qHS	Hypotension, anxiety, blurred vision, priapism	Decrease dose w/elderly, hepatic disease, potent CYP3A4 inhibitors. Caution with cardiac disease, CKD	
Zolpidem (Ambien)	Initially, 5 mg qHS. Maximum dose 10 mg qHS	CNS side effects, anterograde amnesia, sleep-related behaviors (e.g. sleep-talking and sleep-walking	Decrease dose by 1/2 with: hepatic disease, elderly. Caution with: depression, respiratory disorders, history of substance abuse, CYP3A4 inhibitors or inducers. Avoid abrupt withdrawal after >2 weeks use	Second-line

MILD COGNITIVE IMPAIRMENT

- **Overview**[179]
  - For patients for whom the patient or a close contact voices concern about memory or impaired cognition, clinicians should assess for MCI and not assume the concerns are related to normal aging
  - For patients for whom screening or assessing for MCI is appropriate, clinicians should use validated assessment tools to assess for cognitive impairment. For patients who test positive for MCI, clinicians should perform a more formal clinical assessment for diagnosis of MCI
  - For patients with MCI, clinicians should assess for the presence of functional impairment related to cognition before giving a diagnosis of dementia
  - For patients diagnosed with MCI, clinicians should perform serial assessments over time to monitor for changes in cognitive status

Cognitive Impairments	
Normal Aging	• Slight decrease in ability to process new information • Normal functioning of ADLs
MCI	• Mild decline in ≥1 cognitive domain(s) • Normal functioning in ADLs
Dementia	• Significant decline in ≥1 cognitive domain(s) • Irreversible global cognitive impairment • Marked functional impairment • Chronic and progressive, months→years • To r/o Alzheimer's, consider CSF testing for Aβ42 peptide (will be ↓) and ↑ tau protein and p-tau levels.

- **Reversible Causes**
  - Sleep deprivation
  - Depression
  - General medical conditions
  - Medication side effects
- **Treatment Options**
  - Pharmacologic – no promising medications have been shown to be effective in decreasing progression to AD
  - Non-Pharmacologic – treatment with exercise training for 6 months is likely to improve cognitive measures

SLUMS EXAMINATION

- **Overview**[180]
  - SLUMS is a screening tool that was developed to give clinicians a better gauge of early changes in an individual's cognitive levels that could signal the onset of dementia and indicate to physicians when they should pursue further testing to support or rule out a dementia diagnosis.
    - Identifies mild cognitive disorders
    - In contrast, MMSE is often normal in mild cognitive disorders, especially with college education

- Generally, used with the VA geriatric population in a va hospital. Could be used in a skilled nursing facility, inpatient/outpatient rehab clinics. This assessment can be used on individuals that may be experiencing difficulties with orientation, memory, attention, and executive functions. Primarily given to people who are suspected to have dementia or Alzheimer's disease.

Scoring the Exam		
High School Education		Less Than High School Education
27-30	Normal	25-30
21-26	Mild Neurocognitive Impairment	20-24
1-20	Dementia	1-19

END OF LIFE MANAGEMENT

- **Palliative Care**[181]
  - Focuses on providing relief from the symptoms and stress of serious illness
  - Does not seek to make a diagnosis
  - Goal is to improve quality of life for both the patient and family
- **Key Symptoms of Management**
  - Pain
  - Nausea
  - Delirium
  - Fatigue anorexia
  - Anxiety/Depression
- **Advanced Care Planning**
  - Encourage patients to appoint a health care proxy or surrogate decision maker
  - Patients who discuss EOL concerns with a physician earlier are more likely to take a comfort-focused approach to care at the EOL
- **Treatment Options in Primary Care**
  - Pain
    - Morphine 10mg/5ml, 5mg po Q2H prn dyspnea.
    - Morphine 20mg/ml, 5mg SL Q2H prn dyspnea.
    - Morphine 2mg IV Q2H prn dyspnea

HEMATOLOGY/ ONCOLOGY

THE CBC

Lab Analysis[182,183]		
Element	Description	Differential
Left shift	A presence of immature cells with one or two nuclear lobes is called a "shift to the left" as the more lobes that are present, the older the cell is. "Bands" are the immature forms of PMNs (more mature are designated as "segs" and thus have more lobes). A left shift is present in the CBC when > 10-12% bands are seen.	Infection toxemia hemorrhage myeloproliferation
Reticulocyte Count	Indicator of erythropoietic activity. Reticulocytes are juvenile RBCs. The presence of these cells is suggested by basophilia of the RBC cytoplasm on Wright stain (polychromasia). Basophils are commonly seen with CML, s/p splenectomy, PC.	High levels may indicate a bleed, low levels suggest chronic disease, bone marrow suppression, or marrow failure.

Leukocytes	One of the body's chief defenses against infection that become active in sites of infection or inflammation by they crossing the wall of venules and migrating into the tissues. Two major types: granulocytes and agranulocytes. About 70% of circulating leukocytes are mature neutrophils which are the first leukocytes to arrive at sites of infection.	Increased Infection, inflammation (RA, allergies) leukemia, severe stress (physical and emotional), postoperative state (physiologic stress), severe tissue damage (eg, burns), steroids. Decreased BM failure, 2/2 cytotoxic medication, VB12 or folate deficiency.
Eosinophils	Eosinophils make up only about 4% of leukocytes and function in killing parasitic worms, and release chemokines and cytokines with allergies.	Increased Allergies, parasites, skin dz, cancer, asthma. Decreased Steroids, ACTH
Basophils	Make up only 1% at most of leukocytes. Granules contain histamine and have surface receptors for IgE. With rapid degranulation → vasodilation occurs → anaphylaxis → sudden ↓ in BP	Increased Allergies
Monocytes	↑ #'s occur in the early phase of inflammation following tissue injury. Chronic inflammation can lead to excessive tissue damage.	Increased Inflammation, infection

RBC Morphology Differentials

Appearance	Differential
Basophilic Stippling	Lead or heavy-metal poisoning, thalassemia, severe anemia
Spherocytes	Hereditary spherocytosis, immune hemolysis, severe burns, ABO transfusion reaction
Target Cells	Thalassemia, hemoglobinopathies, liver disease, any hypochromic anemia, aftermath of splenectomy
Nucleated RBCs	Severe bone marrow stress (eg, hemorrhage, hemolysis, hypoxia), marrow replacement by tumor, extramedullary hematopoiesis
Schistocytes	DIC, microangiopathic anemia, severe burns, drug effect (ie. tacrolimus)
Polychromasia	Bluish red cell on routine Wright stain suggests reticulocytes
Helmet Cells	Microangiopathic hemolysis (TTP, HUS, HELLP syndrome), hemolytic transfusion reaction, transplant rejection
Howell-Jolly Bodies:	Asplenia
Acanthocytes	Severe liver dz; ↑ levels of bile, fatty acids, or toxins
Heinz Bodies	Drug-induced hemolysis

ANEMIA

Anemia lab analysis					
Disease	Ferritin	TIBC	Iron Sat	Iron	Other
Iron Deficiency Anemia	↓	↑	↓	↓	↑Transferritin
ACD	↑	↓	↓	↓	↑ESR/CRP
Hemochromatosis	↑↑↑	↑	↑		
Sideroblastic Anemia	↑	↓	↑	↑	
Thalassemia	↑	↓	↑	↑	Target cells

- **General Labs**[184,185]
  - MCV, MCHC, RDW
  - Iron panel, B12, Folate, TSH
  - LDH, Haptoglobin, Reticulocyte count, Differential with observation for schistocytes
  - Decreased Production
    - Low MCV
      - Iron Deficiency Anemia
        - Low ferritin
        - High TIBC
        - Low Fe
        - Low Iron Saturation
        - Elevated RDW (newer RBCs are smaller therefore there is a larger spread of cell widths present)
        - Treatment: every other day of PO iron
          - 10cc of iron elixir (ferrous sulfate) mixed in one-fifth of a glass of orange juice and taken 30 minutes prior to breakfast. This will provide 88mg of elemental iron
          - Ferrous sulfate 325mg contains 65mg of elemental iron per tablet
    - Normal MCV
      - Anemia of Chronic Disease, Anemia of Kidney Disease
        RA, COPD, ESRD, Connective tissue diseases
        - High ferritin
        - Low TIBC
        - Low Fe
        - Low iron saturation
    - High MCV
      - B12/folate deficiency (pernicious anemia, malabsorption)
        - B12/folate level, methylmalonic acid, homocysteine level
      - EtOH elevation
      - Thyroid disease
      - Bone marrow disease
  - Increased Destruction
    - High reticulocyte count
    - Obtain haptoglobin, LDH, reticulocyte count, TBILI, peripheral smear
  - Reticulocyte count
    - "Poor man's bone marrow aspirate"
    - Measures RBC production
    - ↑ in acute blood loss, hemorrhage, acute hemolytic anemia

  - ↓ in aplastic anemia, BM infiltration, sepsis (BM failure), disordered RBC maturation (↑B12/folate/iron)

Differential based on reticulcyte count		
Low reticulocyte		Conditions
MCV	Low	Iron deficiency, Thalassemia, ACD, Sideroblastic
	WNL	Acute bleed, hemolysis, ACD, liver dz, sideroblastic, ↓thyroid, MDS, aplastic
	High	B12 deficiency, folate deficiency, drug cause, liver dz, ↓thyroid, MDS
High reticulocyte		Conditions
LDH/BILI	Elevated	AIHA, MAHA, PNH, sickle cell, spur cell, G6PD
	WNL	Subacute bleed, splenic sequestration, liver sequestration

- **Treatment**
  Indications for treatment include symptomatic anemia (weakness, HA, ↓exercise tolerance), pica, and RLS
  - IDA
    - Iron supplementation to target saturation of 20-50% and ferritin of 200-500 ng/dL taken every other day rather than daily.
    - Dosing is dependent on severity of deficiency, age, etc. In general, start Ferrous Sulfate 325mg TID (but given every other day - for example MWF) **not** with food unless the patient has GI s/e in which case can take with food.
    - IV administration is often done in patients who cannot tolerate PO s/e, want quicker repletion (1-2 doses), or have on going blood loss.

PO Iron Replacement Preparations		
Name	Dose	Elemental Iron (mg/dose)
Ferrous sulfate	**325mg TID**	**65**
Ferrous gluconate	300mg TID	36
Ferrous fumarate	100mg TID	33
Iron polysaccharide complex	150mg BID	150
Carbonyl iron	50mg BID-TID	50

IV Iron Replacement Preparations		
Name	Indication	Cumulative Dosing
Iron dextran/LMW ID (INFeD)	IDA where PO administration has failed	Multiple doses of 100mg or single dose of 1000mg (diluted in 250cc NS) given over 1 hour. Always give 25mg prior to the first dose as a test dose over 5 minutes while observing the patient. If no reaction, give the rest of the dose over 1 total hour
Iron sucrose (Venofer)	IDA in non dialysis dependent CKD patients	Goal of 100mg. Administered undiluted as slow IV injection or infusion in diluted solution: Injection: 100 mg over 2-5 min 200 mg over 2-5 min Infusion: 100 mg/100 mL over 15 min 300 mg/250 mL over 1.5 h 400 mg/250 mL over 2.5 h >500 mg/250 mL over 3.5 h
Ferric carboxymaltose (Injectafer)	IDA where PO administration has failed (cannot tolerate or did not respond) and patients with non-dialysis dependent CKD	*1500mg with no test dose required
Ferric gluconate	IDA	Injection: 125 mg over 10 min Infusion: 125 mg/100 mL over 1 h
Ferumoxytol	IDA	510 mg over 20 min; given as 2 doses 7 d apart Observe patient for at least 30 min after administration. Serious hypersensitivity reactions have been observed with rapid IV injection (<1 min).

Consider pre-treatment in patients with h/o asthma, multiple drug allergies, inflammatory arthritis. Options include 125mg methylprednisolone given IV prior to infusion, and possible short course of prednisone for 4 days after if they have arthritis. **Avoid antihistamines in treatment. Consider treating concurrently with **Vitamin C supplementation**

Figure. Anemia workout flow chart

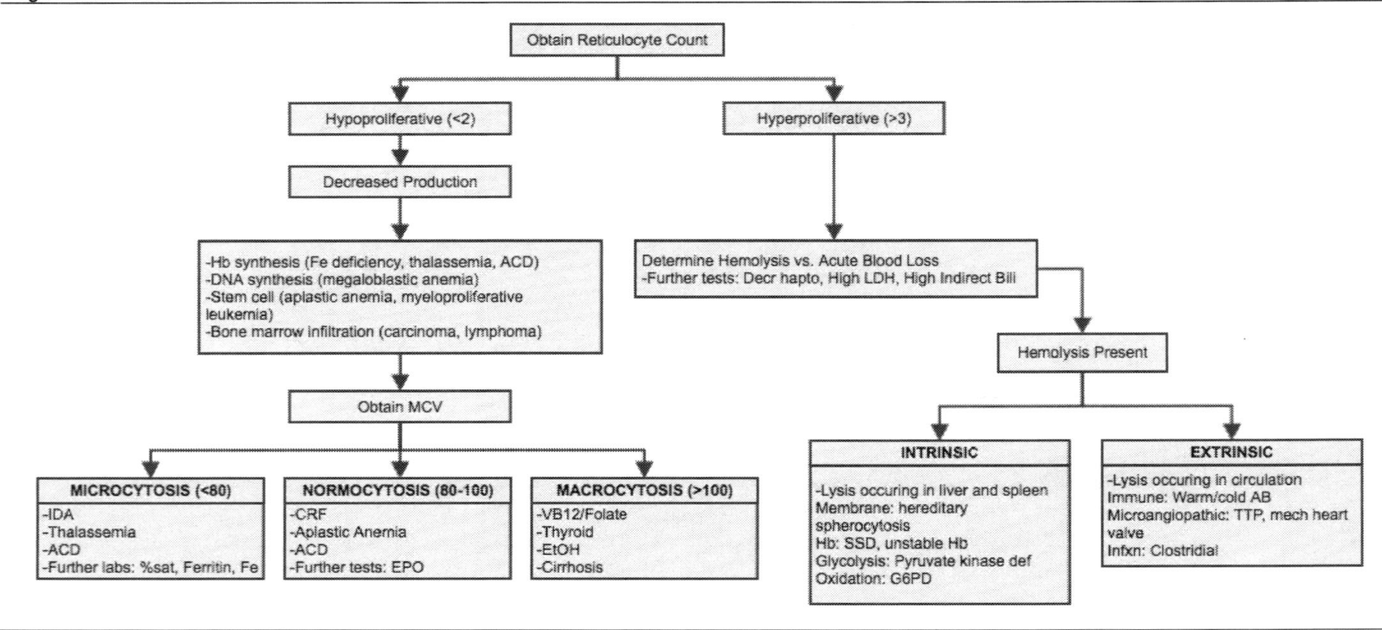

BREAST CANCER SCREENING

Screening with magnetic resonance imaging may be considered in high-risk women, but its impact on breast cancer mortality is uncertain. [186]

Screening Guidelines	
Age	Recommendations
25-40	• For women with an estimated lifetime breast cancer risk of more than 20 percent • Have a BRCA mutation • -or- • Age that is five to 10 years younger than the earliest age that breast cancer was diagnosed in the family
40-49	The risks and benefits of screening should be discussed, and the decision to perform screening should take into consideration the individual patient risk, values, and comfort level of the patient and physician. **The ACS recommends annual screening starting at 45 until 55 then every 2 years thereafter, USPSTF recommends every 2-year starting at 50. ACOG recommends annually starting at 40.**
50-74	There is general agreement that screening should be offered at least biennially to women of this age group
>75	Information is lacking about the effectiveness of screening

****High risk family history includes**
(1) Two first degree relatives with breast cancer, including 1 relative before age 50
(2) Three or more 1st or 2nd degree relatives with breast cancer
(3) 1st or 2nd degree relative with breast & ovarian cancer
(4) 1st degree relative with blateral breast cancer
(5) Breast cancer in male relative

BLOOD TRANSFUSION

PRBCs - 4cc/kg will increase Hb 1gm/dl
Platelets – 1U (6-pack) will increase count by 30,000; 10-60min after transfusion
Fresh Frozen Plasma - 10 ml/kg round up/down to closest unit
Cryoprecipitate - 1 bag / every 5-10kg (Source of fibrinogen and factor VIII)

- **Guidelines**[187,188,189,190]
  - Blood Bank phone: _______ - ___________.
  - Informed consent must be obtained once during each hospital stay using forms present in patient's chart
  - Blood must be infused within 4hrs. It can be split into smaller aliquots.
  - A unit of blood that has been issued and allowed to warm to 10 C but not used cannot be reissued.

- Blood must not be stored in un-monitored refrigerators
- Standard blood filters have a pore size of 170 microns.
- Proper patient identification is essential, mislabeled specimens will not be accepted

Transfusion Guidelines

Component	Threshold/Goal	Indication	Guideline
HGB	Liberal: >10 g/dL Restrictive: >7 g/dL	Hospitalized and Critically Ill, But Hemodynamically Stable **Without** Coronary Artery Disease	AABB 2016, NICE 2014, BCSH 2012, TRICC, FOCUS
	> 8 g/dL	Cardiac or Orthopedic Surgery Patients or Any Patient with Preexisting Cardiovascular Disease	AABB 2016
	> 8 g/dL	Patients with Acute Coronary Syndrome	BCSH 2012 NICE 2014 TRICC FOCUS
	Early resuscitation: >9 g/dL Late resuscitation: >7-9 g/dL	Critically Ill Patients with Sepsis	BCSH 2012
	> 10 g/dL	Symptomatic anemia	AABB 2016
PLT	>20k >50k	CVC placement Lumbar puncture	AABB 2015
	>50k >80k	Major non-neuraxial surgery Neuraxial surgery	AABB 2015
	Insufficient evidence	ICH	AABB 2015
	>100k	Active bleeding	
	>5k	ITP	
	>20k	DIC, hepatic + renal failure, splenomegaly	

- **Components**
  - Whole blood**:** 40% hematocrit; used primarily in hemorrhagic shock.
  - RBC Transfusion
    - *Indications*:
      - Active bleeding and one of the following:
      - Blood loss > 500cc or 15% of blood volume (70 cc/kg body weight)
      - SBP < 100 mmHg or 20% fall in SBP
      - Pulse > 100 bpm

- General anesthesia and Hgb < 9 g/dl
- Chronic, symptomatic anemia (generally Hgb < 9g/dl)
- Chronic transfusions to suppress endogenous Hgb in selected patients with sickle cell disease

- Hgb < 8 g/dl in patients with known coronary artery disease, unstable angina, or acute MI
  - the myocardium is more sensitive to anemia d/t ↑ oxygen requirements
- Hgb < 8 g/dl – undergoing orthopedic surgery, cardiac surgery, and those with pre-existing cardiovascular disease
- Hgb < 7: in hospitalized patients without cardiovascular disease who are hemodynamically stable

- *Dose effect*: 1 unit PRBC (volume = 350 cc) should raise Hgb by about 1 g/dl
- *Complications*
  - Hypocalcemia is most commonly seen in patients with renal or hepatic impairment
  - This is due to their inability to metabolize citrate which is included in the transfusion; the citrate is normally metabolized to lactate
  - The continued presence of citrate binds to calcium causing ↓Ca, however regular calcium testing will be normal, must check **iCa**
  - Prophylactic administration of 10cc of 10% calcium gluconate recommended

Indications for Specialized Transfusions[191]	
Irradiated	Bone marrow transplant recipient Acquired or congenital cellular immunodeficiency Hodgkin's Disease Treatment with purine analogue drugs (fludarabine, cladribine) Blood components donated by 1st or 2nd degree relative Acute leukemias NHL Patients on immunosuppressive medications (**except** HIV, aplastic anemia)
Leukoreduced	Chronically transfused patients CMV seronegative at-risk patients (ie. AIDS, transplant) Acute and chronic leukemia Solid tumor malignancy potentially treated with HRC Thalassemia Potential transplant candidates Previous febrile nonhemolytic transfusion reaction
Washed	IgA deficiency Complement-dependent autoimmune hemolytic anemia Continued allergic reactions (ie. hives) with RBC transfusion despite antihistamines At risk for hyperkalemia (↑K)
Volume reduced	Thalassemia major SSD CHF

Klein et al.[192]

- Platelets
  - One unit of platelets will increase platelet count 30,000/mm^3; usual dose is 1 unit of platelets per 10 kg body weight; single-donor platelets obtained by apheresis are equivalent to 6 platelet concentrate; platelets are stored at room temp; ABO compatibility is not mandatory.
  - A normal platelet count is 150,00-440,000/mm^3.
    - Thrombocytopenia is defined as <150,000/mm^3.
  - Intraoperative bleeding increases with counts of 40,000-70,000/mm^3, and spontaneous bleeding can occur at counts <20,000/mm^3.
    - During surgery platelet transfusions are probably not required unless count is less then 50,000/mm^3.
  - *Indications*
    - Platelet count < 5-10K in ITP or significant purpura
    - Platelet count < 10K in J patients, or patients not predisposed to spontaneous bleeding
      - No change in bleeding events in RCT when compared to < 20K as transfusion threshold
    - Platelet count < 20K and a clinical factor that would be associated with risk of spontaneous bleeding
      - Temperature > 38.5°C
      - Infection
      - Concurrent coagulopathy
      - Disseminated intravascular coagulopathy (DIC)
      - Hepatic or renal failure
      - Marked splenomegaly
    - Platelet count < 50K and surgery or post-op bleeding
    - Platelet count < 50K and invasive procedure (LP, indwelling lines, liver or transbronchial biopsy, epidural puncture)
    - Platelet count < 100K with active bleeding
  - *Premedication*: Tylenol 650 mg p.o. × 1, Benadryl 25-50 mg p.o. OR IV × 1
  - *Post Transfusion*
    - 10-60 minutes after transfusion, recheck platelet level
      - Adequate response → recheck 24 hours later, if count lowers back to original then consider in the differential: sepsis, DIC, medications (vancomycin, heparin, amphotericin)
      - Inadequate response → consider alloimmunization due to presence of antibodies on transfused platelets (HLA-1). Screen patient (HLA) and transfuse HLA-matched platelets
- Fresh frozen plasma (FFP): 250 cc/bag; **contains all coagulation factors** except platelets; 10-15 mL/kg will increase plasma coagulation factors to 30% of normal; fibrinogen levels increase by 1 mg per mL of plasma transfused; acute reversal of warfarin requires 5-8 mL/kg of FFP. ABO compatibility is mandatory.
  - One unit of FFP contains:
    - 200-250 cc volume
    - 400 mg fibrinogen
    - 200 units of other factors (factors V, VII, XI, ATIII, Protein C, Protein S)
  - *Indications*
    - Active bleeding or risk of bleeding if PT and/or PTT> 1.5-1.8× normal.

- Patient with massive bleeding at high risk for clotting factor deficiency while coags pending.
- Common causes of factor deficiency: liver disease, vitamin K deficiency, DIC, hemorrhage, TTP (MAHA+↓PLT; treatment with plasma exchange)
- Reversal of warfarin therapy
  - Minimal evidence that FFP can correct mildly elevated INR (< 1.8).

- *Initial Dosage*
  - 10cc/Kg (round up to nearest 200cc) = #units FFP / 200 cc/unit FFP
- *Common Parameters*

Recommended Coagulation Parameters for Common Procedures		
	Platelet Count*	INR
Lumbar Puncture	≥50,000	≤1.5
Paracentesis	≥30,000	≤2.0
Thoracentesis	≥50,000	≤1.5
Transbronchial Lung Bx	≥50,000	≤1.5
Subclav/IJ Line	≥30,000	≤1.5
Renal Bx	≥50,000	≤1.5
Liver Bx	≥50,000	≤1.5

- Cryoprecipitate**:** 10-20 mL/bag; contains 100 units factor VIII-C, 100 units factor vWF, 60 units factor XIII, and 250 mg fibrinogen;
  - *Indications*
    - hypofibrinogenemia, von Willebrand disease, hemophilia A and preparation of fibrin glue; ABO compatibility not mandatory.
    - Fibrinogen < 100 mg/dl (as in DIC)
    - Preparation of topical fibrin glue for surgical hemostasis
    - Concentrated factor VIII and von Willebrand factor are preferred treatments of Hemophilia A and von Willebrand's disease since cryoprecipitate not virus inactivated, thus carrying a higher risk for virus transmission.
- Albumin**:** 5% and 25% (heat treated at 60 degrees C for 10 hrs).
- 4-Factor Prothrombin Complex Concentrates (50U/kg)[193]: (contains factors 2, 7, 9, 10) for patients who have life-threatening hemorrhage and are within 3–5 half-lives of the last dose of factor Xa inhibitor in intracranial hemorrhage with INR ≥ 1.4 then repeat testing of INR 15-60 m after PCC administration and serially q6-8h for the next 24-48h. Any further corrections required if INR remains >1.4 done with FFP

Blood Products

Component/Product	Composition	Volume	Indications	Expected Change	Formula for transfusion
Whole Blood	RBCs (HCT 40%); plasma; WBCs; platelets	500 ml	Increase both red cell mass and plasma volume (WBCs and Platelets not functional; plasma deficient in labile clotting Factors V and VIII	One unit will increase Hgb 1gm/dl or Hct 3%	
Red Blood Cells (PRBC)	RBCs (HCT 75%); reduced plasma; WBCs; platelets	250 ml	Increase red cell mass in symptomatic anemia (WBCs and platelets not functional)	One unit will increase Hgb 1gm/dl or Hct 3%	Packed cells (mls) = wt (kg) x Hb rise required(g/L) x 0.4
PRBC, Adenine-Saline Added	RBCs (HCT 60%); reduced plasma; WBCs; platelets; 100ml of additive solution	330 ml	Increase red cell mass in symptomatic anemia (WBCs and platelets not functional)	One unit will increase hgb 1gm/dl or Hct 3%	
PRBC, Leukocytes Reduced (prepared by filtration)	>85% original vol. of PRBCs; <5 x 10^6 WBC; few platelets; minimal plasma	225 ml	Increase red cell mass; <5 x 10^6 WBCs to decrease the likelihood of febrile reactions, immunization to leukocytes (HLA antigens) or CMV transmission	One unit will increase hgb 1gm/dl or Hct 3%	
PRBC, Washed	RBCs (HCT 75%); <5 x 10^8 WBC; no plasma	180 ml	Increase red cell mass; reduce the risk of allergic reactions to plasma proteins	One unit will increase hgb .8gm/dl or Hct 2.5%	

PRBC, Frozen & PRBC, Deglycerolized	RBCs (HCT 75%); <5 x 10^8 WBC; no plasma, no platelets	180ml	Increase red cell mass; minimize febrile or allergic transfusion reactions; used for prolonged RBC storage	One unit will increase hgb 1gm/dl or Hct 3%	
Platelets	Platelets(>5.5 x 10^{10}/unit); RBC; WBC; plasma	50 ml	Bleeding due to thrombocytopenia or thrombocytopathy	6-pack will increase platelet count by 30,000	(5 - 10 ml/kg will raise platelet count by 50 - 100x 109 /L)
Platelets, Pheresis	Platelets (>3 x 10^{11}/unit); RBC; WBC; plasma	300 ml	Bleeding due to thrombocytopenia or thrombocytopathy; sometimes HLA matched	One unit will increase platelet count by 30,000-60,000	
Platelets, Leukocyte Reduced	Platelets(>3 x 10^{11}/unit); <5 x 10^6 WBC per final dose of pooled Platelets	300 ml	Bleeding due to thrombocytopenia or thrombocytopathy; <5 x 10^6 WBCs to decrease the likelihood of febrile reactions, immunization to leukocytes (HLA antigens) or CMV transmission	One unit will increase platelet count by 30,000-60,000	
Fresh Frozen Plasma (FFP)	Plasma; all coagulation factors; complement; no platelets	220 ml	Treatment of bleeding due to deficiency in coagulation factors	10-20ml/kg (4-6 units in adults) will increase coagulation factors by 20%	
Cryoprecipitate	Fibrinogen; Factors VIII and XIII; von Willebrand factor	15 ml	Deficiency of fibrinogen and/or Factor VIII; Second choice in treatment of Hemophilia A and von Willebrand's disease	One unit will increase fibrinogen by 5mg/dl	

2. **Orders**:
    - Type, cross match and transfuse __ units with H&H 1 hour after 2nd and 4th units.
        - Do H&H 1 hour after every 2 units of blood given
        - Cross match
            - **Use when transfusion is expected**
                - Blood is set aside for that pt only and is wasted if not used for that patient;
            - ABO-Rh, screen, and crossmatch; 99.95% compatible.
            - Crossmatching confirms ABO-Rh typing, detects antibodies to the other blood group systems, and detects antibodies in low titers.
        - Screen
            - **Use when transfusion is a possibility**
                - Blood is set aside for that pt and is returned to bank if not used; best one to order, unless you know pt will use the blood
            - Hematocrit is determined, if normal, the blood is typed, screened for antibodies, and tested for hepatitis B, hepatitis C, syphilis, HIV-1, HIV-2, and human T-cell lymphotropic viruses I and II. ALT is also measured as a surrogate marker of nonspecific liver infection.
    - Lasix 20 mg IV daily or 20 mg PO prior to each unit of packed RBCs
    - Benadryl 50 mg IV daily-for itch
    - Tylenol 650 mg PO Q 6 hours prn fever greater than 100.4
3. **Reactions**
    - **Hemolytic reactions**
        - Acute hemolytic reactions
            - Occurs when ABO-incompatible blood is transfused resulting in acute intravascular hemolysis; severity of a reaction often depends on how much incompatible blood has been given.
            - Symptoms include fever, chills, chest pain, anxiety, back pain, dyspnea; in anesthetized patients, the reaction is manifested by rise in temperature, unexplained tachycardia, hypotension, hemoglobinuria, and diffuse oozing from surgical site. Free hemoglobin in the plasma or urine is presumptive evidence of a hemolytic reaction.
            - Risk of fatal hemolytic transfusion reaction: 1:600,000 units.
            - Treatment
                - Stop transfusion
                - Vigorous hydration with **NS**
        - Delayed hemolytic reactions
            - Occurs because of incompatibility of minor antigens (e.g., Kidd, Kelly, Duffy, etc) are characterized by extravascular hemolysis.
            - The hemolytic reaction is typically delayed 2-21 days after transfusion, and symptoms are generally mild, consisting of malaise, jaundice, and fever. Treatment is supportive.
    - **Nonhemolytic reactions**
        - Febrile reactions
            - Most common nonhemolytic reaction (0.51.0% of RBC transfusions and up to 30% of platelet transfusions); due to recipient antibodies against donor antigens present on leukocytes and platelets; treatment includes stopping or slowing infusion and antipyretics.
        - Urticarial reactions
            - Characterized by erythema, hives, and itching without fever.
            - Occur in 1% of transfusions and are thought to be due to sensitization of the patient to transfused plasma proteins.
            - Treated with antihistaminic drugs.

- Anaphylactic reactions
  - Anaphylactic reactions are rare; about 1:500,000.
  - Patients with IgA deficiency may be at increased risk of the presence of anti-IgA antibodies that react with transfused IgA.
  - Cause: recipient antibodies react with donor plasma forming immune complexes which activate complement. Reported in patients with congenital IgA deficiency and high titers of anti-IgA IgG.
  - Signs: sudden onset flushing, and hypertension followed by hypotension, edema, respiratory distress, shock.
  - Workup: none (no evidence of RBC incompatibility)
  - **Treatment**
    - *See page 430*
  - Prevention: patients with history of anaphylaxis to blood should receive components depleted of plasma (saline washed RBCs).
- Transfusion related acute lung injury (TRALI)
  - Due to transfusion of antileukocytic or anti-HLA antibodies that interact with and cause the patient's white cells to aggregate in the pulmonary circulation.
  - Risk is 1:6000.
  - Leading cause of transfusion related mortality.
  - Defined as acute lung injury within 6 hours of transfusion.
  - Exam: dyspnea, hypoxia, fever, chills, hypotension with CXR showing b/l pulm infiltrates.
  - Treatment is supportive, mimicking the treatment of ARDS.
- Transfusion Associated Circulatory Overload (TACO)
  - 1-8% of transfusion recipients
  - Risk factors: h/o cardiac disease, kidney disease, h/o reception of multiple transfusions (ie. myelodysplastic patients), rapid administration rate.
  - Defined as respiratory distress within 6 hours with known positive fluid balance, ↑BNP, ↑CVP, CXR with pulmonary edema.
  - Treatment: stop transfusion, diuresis, supportive care.
  - When restarting transfusion, keep rate at 1 mL/kg/hr.
- Graft-vs-host disease
  - Most commonly seen in immunocompromised patients.
  - Cellular blood products contain lymphocytes capable of mounting an immune response against the compromised host.
- Posttransfusion purpura
  - Due to the development of platelet alloantibodies; the platelet count typically drops precipitously 1 week after transfusion.
- Immune suppression
  - Transfusion of leukocyte-containing blood products appears to be immunosuppressive (can improve allograft survival following renal transplants).
  - Blood transfusions may increase the incidence of serious infections following surgery or trauma.
  - Blood transfusions may worsen tumor recurrence and mortality rate following resections of many cancer.

SCREENING TESTS FOR BLEEDING DISORDERS

- **Overview of hemostasis**
  - Platelets normally circulate in inactivated state, when they do become activated (disruption in vascular endothelium (d/t release of VWF, etc.) or due to molecules

(TxA2, ADP) released by other activated platelets) they gain ability to adhere to one another
- This allows for the facilitation of platelet and college adhesion to allow for formation of occlusive plug
- Second set of reactions activate the coagulation cascade leading to thrombin formation
- This allows for stabilization of the thrombus
- Thrombin then converts fibrinogen → fibrin monomers

Expected Lab Changes with Specific Bleeding Disorders			
	Mechanism Tested	Normal	Where Abnormal
PT	Extrinsic and common pathways	<12 sec	Defect in vitamin K-dependent factors, liver diseases, DIC, oral anticoagulants
aPTT	Intrinsic and common pathways	25-40 sec	Hemophilia, von Willebrand's disease, heparin therapy, DIC, deficient XII, XI, IX circulating anticoagulant
Thrombin time	Fibrinogen-fibrin conversion	10-15 sec	Third-stage anticoagulant, fibrin split products, DIC, severe hypofibrinogenemia
Bleeding time	Primary hemostasis platelet function	3-7 min	Platelet dysfunction, von Willebrand's disease, thrombocytopenia

Corresponding factor deficiencies and assay results	
Assay Result	Suspected Deficiencies
↑aPTT; normal PT	XII, XI, IX, VIII, HMWK, PK
↑PT; normal aPTT	VII
↑PT and ↑aPTT	II, V, X, fibrinogen

- **Thrombophilia Work-Up**
  - Activated protein C resistance
  - Factor V Leiden
  - Prothrombin gene mutation
  - Antiphospholipid antibodies194
  - Patients will have prolonged aPTT, ↓PLT
  - Beta-2 glycoprotein I antibody, IgA
  - Cardiolipin antibody, IgA
  - DRVVT
  - Prothrombin Ab
  - Lupus inhibitor
  - Antithrombin deficiency
  - Protein C deficiency
  - Protein S deficiency

Figure. Algorithm for bleeding disorder work-up

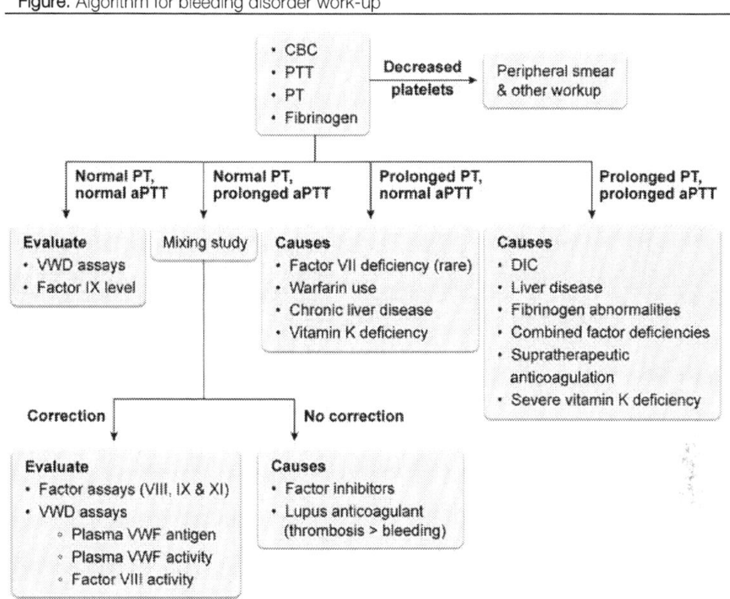

DISSEMINATED INTRAVASCULAR COAGULATION

- **Overview**[195,196]
  - Characterized by the consumption of plasma coagulation factors and platelets after exposure to antigen (ie. infection) due to the over-formation of fibrin with secondary fibrinolysis leading to prethrombotic state and increased bleeding due to consumption of platelets
  - ↑PT, ↑Thrombin Time (TT), and ↑PTT
  - Thrombotic events due to deposition of thrombin in microvasculature
  - Often seen in patients with malignancy, infection (esp GN) and post-surgical
  - Most often affects the liver, kidney (ATN), brain, heart (endocarditis)
- **Diagnosis**
  - Exam
    - Hemorrhage at multiple sites to include mucosal surfaces
    - Petechiae, ecchymosis

Labs in DIC		
Test	Abnormality	Causes Other Than DIC Contributing to Test Result
Platelet count	Decreased	Sepsis, impaired production, major blood loss, hypersplenism
Prothrombin time	Prolonged	Vitamin K deficiency, liver failure, major blood loss
aPTT	Prolonged	Liver failure, heparin treatment, major blood loss
Fibrin degradation products	Elevated	Surgery, trauma, infection, hematoma
Fibrin	Elevated	
D-dimer	Elevated	
Factor VIII	Low	Can help distinguish superimposed DIC in patients with underlying liver failure

- Labs
  - PT, PTT, TT
  - CBC (↓platelets due to thrombin generation)
  - Fibrinogen level (↓due to fibrinolysis; what actually deposits in microvasculature)
  - Blood smear (schistocytes due to trauma experienced by presence of fibrin strands)
  - Fibrinogen degradation products (↑Fibrin D-Dimer assay due to circulating plasmin that degrades fibrin)
  - D-dimer (increased; due to ↑FDP)
- Imaging
  - Consider LE duplex US (to r/o DVT)

- **Treatment**
  - Cryoprecipitate (replaces fibrinogen if <50) → goal ↑100 mg/dl
    or
  - FFP (replaces coagulation proteins/factors, most notably 5 and 8) → may not be necessary with normal liver function
  - Platelets (1-2U per 10kg per day)
  - IV Heparin @ 5000U bolus then 500/h (due to risk of thrombotic events) for first 24 hrs, ↑ to 10U after 24hrs if no improvement in fibrinogen and FDP levels **not supported by experimental data**

ELEVATED INR

Bleeding Patient[197,198]		
	Action	Comment
Any INR	1. Hold warfarin 2. Vitamin K 5-10mg IV 3. Give Factor-4 prothrombin complex concentrate (PCC) 25-50 u/kg 4. Repeat INR in 30min	FFP can be substituted for PCC at 15cc/kg Factor VIIa can be considered in urgent sit.

INR <4.5	1. Lower Warfarin dose or omit dose 2. Monitor more frequently 3. Resume at lower dose when INR therapeutic	
INR 4.5 - 10	1. Hold 1-2 doses of warfarin 2. Monitor INR Frequently 3. Vitamin K not recommended	
INR >10	1. Hold warfarin 2. Give vitamin K 2.5-5mg PO 3. Monitor INR frequently	Vitamin K not routinely recommended if no evidence of bleeding Vitamin K can be used if urgent surgery needed

HEMOLYTIC ANEMIA

- **Types**
  - Intravascular: ↑↑LDH, ↓↓haptoglobin
  - Extravascular: splenomegaly
- **Conditions**
  - G6PD, SSA, HS, PNH, AIHA (warm with IgG vs cold with IgM), MAHA
- **Labs**
  - Bilirubin (↑indirect)
  - Coombs (DAT) → drug induced (consider ABx; -DAT, ↑LDH), autoimmune (+DAT, spherocytes)
  - Smear (spherocytes; schistocytes)
  - ↑LDH
  - ↓Haptoglobin
  - Reticulocyte count (↑ in HA; >2%)
- **Treatment**
  - Steroids

HEPARIN INDUCED THROMBOCYTOPENIA

- **Statistics**
  - Seen in approximately 8% of patients placed on anticoagulation with up to 5% developing thrombotic events
  - UFH associated with 10x higher risk than LMWH
  - Higher incidents in post-surgical and orthopedic patients
- **Defined**
  - Type 1 – 10%; benign; no ↑ risk of thrombosis; unknown pathophysiology; mild transient thrombocytopenia (>100k) seen early in administration and recovers quickly after stopping heparin
  - Type 2 – immune mediated with ↑ risk of thrombosis; occurs 5-14 days after heparin exposure or within 24 hours of re-exposure.
- **Pathophysiology**
  - Immune response (type 2) associated with an antigen in the form of the heparin/PF4 complex (PF4 is a molecule found on platelets). When platelets get activated, PF4

  - gets released and binds to the platelets and heparin then binds to the PF4 (opposite charges, attract).
  - This complex then causes the formation of an IgG AB against the heparin-PF4-plt complex by binding to another region on the platelet. When the AB binds to this Fc region, it causes more activation of platelets and aggregation which ultimately bind to a tissue surface which activates the coagulation system leading to thrombosis
  - Can cause false positives as it is also seen in patients simply exposed to heparin without clinical sx
  - False positives are highest in first 85 days (length of duration for PF4 antibodies to leave circulation)
- **Clinical**
  - Exposure to heparin or LMWH leads to low platelet count (<150,000) or a decrease of 50% or more from baseline with thrombosis resulting in up to 50% of patients
    - Platelets rarely drop <10,000 or cause bleeding
  - Onset is often 5-10 days from initiation of medication (no hx of exposure) or within **hours** if they have been exposed in the past (due to presence of the circulating PF4-heparin ABs
  - 4T's
    - <u>Thrombosis</u>
      - Higher PF4 associated with higher risk
      - Risk is 30x higher and even after discontinuation remains high (seen mostly in orthopedic, surgical, and post cardiac pts)
      - Often occurs after 50% of platelets have decreased
      - Occurs in any vascular territory (arterial or venous) but most often in areas of injury
      - Limb ischemia results in 5-10% of patients
- **Laboratory confirmation**
  - SRA – preferred; detects ^{14}C-Serotonin release from activated platelets: Sn up to 100%, Sp up to 100%
  - PF4 – detects circulating IgG, IgA, and IgM antibodies: Sn 97%, Sp 86%
  - Heparin-induced platelet aggregation
- **How to objectively diagnosis**
  - The resulting clinical probability scores were divided into high (6–8 points), intermediate (4–5 points), and low (<3 points) groups.
    - Low suspicion – no testing
    - Intermediate - SRA
    - High/Intermediate suspicion – PF4-heparin ABs

The 4T's of HIT			
	2 points	1 point	0 point
Thrombocytopenia	PLT count fall >50% and PLT nadir >20	PLT count fall 30-50% or PLT nadir 10-19%	PLT count fall <30% or PLT nadir <10
Timing of PLT count fall	Clear onset between days 5-10 or PLT fall < 1 day (prior heparin exposure within 30 days)	Consistent with days 5-10 fall, but not clear (ie. missing PLT counts); onset after day 10, or fall <1 day (prior heparin exposure 30-100 days ago)	PLT count fall <4 days without recent exposure
Thrombosis or other sequelae	New thrombosis (confirmed); skin necrosis, acute systemic reaction post IV UFH bolus	Progressive or recurrent thrombosis; non-necrotizing (erythematous) skin lesions; suspected thrombosis	None
Other causes for thrombocytopenia	None apparent	Possible	Definite

- **Treatment**
  - Adequate alternatives:
    - Two classes to choose from: direct-thrombin inhibitors or heparinoids. These should be initiated when you **suspect** HIT and then send for above labs to confirm.
      - DTI: lepirudin, argatroban, or bivalirudin
        - Argatroban – significant ↓ risk of death, amputation, and thrombosis.
        - Lepirudin – significant reduction in thrombotic events, no effect on death or amputation, ↑bleeding risk; if hx of use before for HIT, don't use again d/t ↑ risk of AB production
        - Bivalirudin – patient's s/p PCA at high risk of HIT
      - Once you have confirmed the diagnosis (labs have returned), you can switch to a vitamin K antagonist or alternate anticoagulant for 3 months
    - Duration of therapy
      - No hx of thrombosis – until platelet counts recover to stable level or baseline with switch to warfarin for additional 4 weeks
      - Hx of thrombosis – allow platelet counts to recover to 150,000 then transition with bridging to warfarin (5 day bridge) and keep until INR is therapeutic for 48 hours then stop after 3-6 months
  - Not adequate alternatives:
    - Warfarin monotherapy d/t s/e such as venous gangrene and skin necrosis
    - ASA
    - IVC filter
    - LMWH – AB often cross-react
  - Patients often recover in 4-14 days after discontinuation of heparin

NEUTROPENIA

- **Definition**: absolute neutrophil cell count (anc) < 1500
  - Mild – 1000-1500 cells/mm3
  - Moderate – 500-1000 cells/mm3
  - Severe – <500 cells/mm3

ANC = WBC Count x (total % of PMN)
ANC = WBC count × (SEGS/100 + bands/100)

- Risk of serious infection ↑ dramatically when ANC falls below 1000.
- **Management**: when ANC reaches 500 or less, or in patients with impending neutropenia (i.e. patients receiving conditioning chemotherapy with ANC 1000 or less and dropping), institute:
  - Neutropenic precautions (hand washing for all contact with patient; masks, gowns or gloves are not necessary unless the health care worker in contact with the patient is ill, i.e. has a cold or URI)
  - Neutropenic diet (low bacterial, i.e. no fresh fruits or vegetables)
  - Gut sterilizers (pre-printed antibiotic form)
    - Norfloxacin 400 mg p.o. BID
    - Clotrimazole troche 10 mg to dissolve in mouth 4× daily OR nystatin swish and swallow 5 cc 5× daily
    - Nystatin powder to apply to axilla and groin TID
    - Nystatin tablets 1 million units p.o. 4× daily
  - Patients at high risk for febrile neutropenia (AML/MDS, hematopoietic stem cell recipients) should be considered for antibiotic and antifungal prophylaxis with fluoroquinolone and oral triazole in conjunction with ID consultation.

NEUTROPENIC FEVER

- **Definition**[199,200]
  - ANC <=500/mm^3 or an ANC expected to ↓<500 in next 48 hours
    - Remember there are grades with mild defined as <1500
  - 100.4 temp (38.3C) x 2 hours –or- any recorded temp of 101
  - If caused by chemotherapy regimen, consider nadir of ANC to likely occur 12-14 days from day one of therapy
- **Etiology**
  - The majority of documented infections are due to bacterial pathogens derived from the patient's own normal bacterial microflora that colonize the mucosal surfaces of the gastrointestinal tract, the upper and lower respiratory tract, the genitourinary tract, and skin.
  - Damage to these surfaces due to cytotoxic therapy or invasive procedures permits colonizing microorganisms to gain access to deeper tissues.
  - Cytotoxic therapy–induced damage to the patient's cellular defenses allows rapid, unimpeded microbial proliferation
- **Pathogens**
  - GN (E. coli, Pseudomonas, Klebsiella, Enterobacter) and GPC (S. aureus)

Multinational Association for Supportive Care in Cancer Score (MASCC)	
Characteristic	Points
Burden of febrile neutropenia symptoms	
No or mild symptoms	5
Moderate symptoms	3
Severe or morbid symptoms	0
No hypotension (SBP<9)	5

No COPD	4
Solid or hematologic cancer with no previous fungal infxn	4
No dehydration necessitating parenteral fluids	3
Outpatient status on onset of fever	3
Age<60	2

- **Outpatient vs. Inpatient Management**
  A score of 21 or greater identifies low-risk febrile neutropenic patients, who can be managed on an outpatient basis
  - MASCC score < 21 or significant comorbidities with ANC<500 = hospitalization
    - High Risk Features:
      - Age > 70 years
      - Mucositis greater than grade 2
      - Poor performance status (ECOG)
      - Initial ANC < 0.1 × 10^9cells/L
      - Patients with active comorbidities, such as congestive cardiac failure or renal insufficiency
      - Patients with sepsis or septic shock syndrome
      - Documented infection with a defined clinical focus, such as pneumonia (*eg*, community-acquired pneumonia), cellulitis , or intra-abdominal sepsis syndrome
  - MASCC score ≥ 21 or no comorbidities with ↑ANC = outpatient → oral fluoroquinolone + amoxicillin
    - If patient re fevers or continues to fever on tx in 48 hours, should return for hospitalization
- **Workup**
  - Labs
    - CBC
    - HFP
    - Cultures (bacterial, fungal, urine, sputum with viral culture) from any indwelling lines or 2 separate venipuncture sites
    - If Pneumonia:
      - S.pneumo
      - Legionella
      - RSV
      - Influenza
      - Viral Culture
    - UA with culture
    - Lactate (r/o sepsis)
    - Diarrhea
    - C.diff
    - Stool culture
    - Enterovirus RNA
    - Fecal leukocytes
    - CMV (if s/p transplant)
    - C.diff (w/ diarrhea)
  - Imaging/Procedures
    - CXR
    - LP if AMS
- **CLABSI**
  - S. aureus and Pseudomonas
  - Require 14d treatment

        - 4-6 week treatment if complicated by deep tissue infection, endocarditis, thrombosis, or bacteremia x 72 hrs **after** catheter removal
    - Remove catheter
        - Other indications to remove catheter include sepsis without resolution of fever for 72 hours, endocarditis, septic thrombosis.
        - Can remain if documented source is **coagulase negative staph**
- **Prophylaxis**
    - Leukemia
        - ABx: Moxifloxacin 400mg PO daily + Amoxicillin 500mg PO TID (start on day 5)
        - Antifungal: Voriconazole or Posaconazole susp 200mg PO TID or 300mg PO daily
        - Antiviral: Valacyclovir 500mg PO BID or Acyclovir 800m PO BID
    - Lymphoma
        - ABx: Moxifloxacin 400mg PO daily
        - Antifungal: Fluconazole 200mg PO daily
        - Antiviral: Valacyclovir 500mg PO BID or Acyclovir 800m PO BID

Neutropenic Fever Treatment		
Antibiotic regimen		
Monotherapy	Cefepime 2 gm IV q8hrs Meropenem or Imipenem 500 mg IV q6hrs Or if allergic to PCN: Zosyn 3.375g IV q4h	
PLUS		
Any of the following depending on the situation	*Catheter related infection, SSTI*	Vancomycin, linezolid
	Pneumonia:	Fluoroquinolones, Vancomycin
	VRE	Linezolid, daptomycin
	ESBL (E.coli, K.pneumonia) *Severe sepsis* *Hemodynamic Instability*	Carbapenem Vancomycin Vancomycin
Antifungal Treatment *Consider addition of antifungal agent if > 4-7 days of fever on antibacterial agents (50% patients will have resolution of febrile neutropenia s/p initiation of antifungals) and expected neutropenia > 7 days*	Any of the following: Micafungin 100 mg IV q24h if sinus or head CT **not** suggestive of fungal infxn Voriconazole 6 mg/kg q12h for 2 doses, then 4 mg/kg q12h **if** chest CT suggestive of fungal infxn Other Options: Amphotericin B liposomal complex 3 mg/kg q24h Posaconazole 20 mg PO q6h for 7d, then 400 mg PO q12h Itraconazole 200 mg IV q12h for 2d, then 200 mg IV or PO q24h for 7d, then 400 mg PO q24h thereafter Caspofungin 70 mg IV for 1 dose, then 50 mg IV q24hAnidulafungin 200 mg IV for 1 dose, then 100 mg IV q24h	

Complicated case or antibiotic resistance present *(clinically unstable and/or persistent fevers despite appropriate ABx and anti-fungal coverage)*	Vancomycin + Meropenem 1 g IV q8h + Amikacin
Step Down Therapy for discharge	
Ciprofloxacin 750mg PO BID + Augmentin 875mg PO BID -or- Moxifloxacin 400mg PO daily	

- **Duration of therapy**
  - Antibiotics
    - Should be continued until the patient has been afebrile for 4 to 5 days, on the basis of clinical trial definitions of treatment response
      - MASCC → low risk and no documented source → minimum of 7 days duration of therapy
      - MASCC → high risk and no documented source → minimum of 10 days duration of therapy
    - Transition to PO ABx if patient clinically stable

Figure. Fever with neutropenia work-up

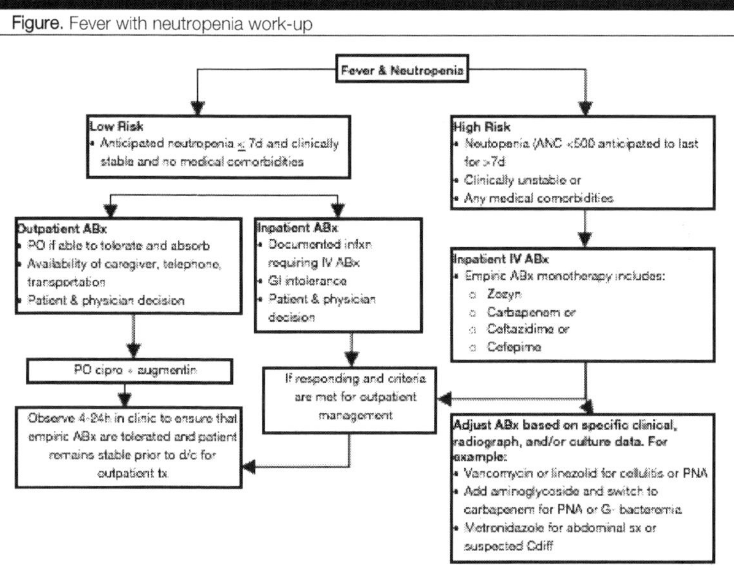

SUPPORTIVE CARE OF CANCER PATIENTS

Treatment Options		
Oral Care and Mucositis [201]	Peridex 15 cc PO swish and spit QAC, QHS	Neutropenic mouth care, antibacterial and antifungal activity Consider IV Narcotics for pain control
	"MMX" Susp, 10 cc PO swish and spit/swallow QAC, QHS, prn (Mylanta/Maalox, Mycelex, Xylocaine)	
	Viscous Lidocaine 2%, 10 cc PO swish and spit/swallow QAC, QHS, prn	
	Hurricane Spray to mouth/throat QAC, QHS, prn	
	Topical Cocaine 2-4% swish or swab Q4hr prn1	
	Stanford Susp 10 cc swish and spit/swallow QAC, QHS, prn	

	Carafate Susp/tab 1 gm swish and swallow/PO QAC, QHS	
Nausea and Vomiting	Compazine 10 mg IV/PO Q6 hr prn (ATC if needed)	Beware of EPS with dopaminergic antagonists
	Droperidol 0.625-1.25 mg IV Q4hr prn2	
	Reglan 10 mg IV/PO QAC, QHS, or Q6hr prn (ATC if needed)	
	Phenergan 25 mg IVPB Q6 hr prn	Consider anti-emetics ATC to prevent sxs.
	Ativan 0.5-2 mg IV/PO/SL Q4hr prn	
	Decadron 4-8 mg IV/PO Q12-24hr prn	
	Marinol 2.5-5 mg PO Q4hr prn	
	Zofran 4 mg IV or 8 mg PO Q4hr prn (ATC if needed)	
Diarrhea	Imodium 2 mg PO after each loose stool, max 8 tabs per day (16 mg)	Anti-motility agents
	Lomotil 2.5 mg PO after each loose stool, max 8 tabs per day	
	Tincture of Opium 0.5-1 cc PO Q4hr prn	
	Metamucil 5 cc PO TID	
	Questran 4 gm PO TID3	
	Lactinex 1 tab/packet PO TID	Probiotic
	Octreotide 100-500 mcg Sub-Q Q8hr	Antisecretory
Constipation	Dulcolax 10 mg PO/PR daily prn	Onset 30-60 minutes
	Glycerin supp PR daily prn	Onset 30-60 minutes
	MOM 30 cc PO Q6hr prn Magnesium Citrate 150-300 cc PO daily prn	Onset 3-6 hrs
	Mineral Oil 30 cc PO prn	Onset 6-8 hrs
	Senokot 2 tabs PO daily prn (up to 4 tabs BID), Cascara 5-10 cc PO QHS prn	Onset 6-10 hrs
	Metamucil 5-10 cc PO daily prn	Onset 12-24 hrs
	Sorbitol 30 cc PO daily prn, Lactulose 30 cc PO daily prn	Onset 24-48 hrs
	Colace 100mg BID	Onset 24-72 hrs
	Polyethylene Glycol 17g daily-BID	
	Psyllium 3.4g up to TID	

VENOUS THROMBOEMBOLISM

- **Those at increased risk (MEDENOX study)**[336,202,203]
  - Current infection
  - Age >50
  - Cancer (kidney, pancreas, lung, colon)
  - History of VTE
  - Immobility
  - Trauma/Surgery
- **Pretest probability of DVT**
  - Well's score for DVT
    - History
    - Ask about family history (inherited thrombosis, Factor V is most common)

        - Recent trauma
        - Prolonged immobilization
        - Cancer
        - Weight loss, loss of appetite, fatigue
- **Differential**
    - Muscle strain, lymphangitis, venous insufficiency, cellulitis
- **Examination**
    - Palpable cord, calf/thigh pain, unilateral edema
    - Look for calf circumference difference or absence of calf swelling **only 2 factors shown to help r/o **
- **Labs**
    - CBC, coagulation panel, UA, ICU panel
    - D-dimer <500 associated with low probability
    - Consider serial D-dimer's in patients experiencing first unprovoked episode q2m starting 1 month after duration of anticoagulation therapy to determine risk of recurrence (PROLONG trial)
        - <500 ng/mL associated with 3.5% yearly risk of recurrence
        - >500 ng/mL associated with 8.9% risk in each of the first 2 years
    - <u>Screening for hypercoagulable state:</u>
      Only should be done in patients with intermediate risk for progression d/t transient risk factors such as small travel, OCP, minor surgery, pregnancy. Should not be done on first episode, provoked VTE.
        - CBC
        - Coagulation panel
        - Protein C and S activity, free protein S
        - Activated protein C → if abnormal then Factor V Leiden gene mutation
        - Prothrombin mutation
        - Antiphospholipid AB (APLAS) with cardiolipin AB (IgG, IgM), DRVVT (lupus anticoagulant), and B2-glycoprotein
            - Presents as a prothrombotic disorder with either (1) vascular thrombosis or (2) pregnancy complications. Bleeding is uncommon and if present, is usually secondary to significant thrombocytopenia, dysfunctional platelets, hypoprothrombinemia, or an underlying disease. Often see ↑PLT and ↑APTT levels.
            - If only one test is positive, repeat in 12 weeks and if it remains positive then diagnosis is confirmed.
        - Antithrombin activity (AT3)
        - Prothrombin gene mutation
            - *Done mostly in those with no risk factors, family history, recurrent disease*
        - +/- SS trait
        - Homocysteine level
- **Imaging**
    - Duplex/compression US → if Wells Score is high and US negative, repeat in 3-4 days d/t chance of false negative
    - 2016 meta-analysis of prospective clinical trials that evaluated use of the Wells rule and D-dimer level to predict PE found that a more appropriate D-dimer threshold should be age adjusted.
        - For patients older than 50 years, the D-dimer threshold is (age × 0.01 μg/mL).
    - Venography only used if noninvasive testing unavailable

- **Inpatient vs. Outpatient**

HESITA criteria
If at least one of the questions is answered with "yes," then the patient should be admitted to hospital.
Hemodynamic instability?
Thrombolytic or embolectomy therapy needed?
Active bleeding or at high risk for bleeding?
Oxygen needed for _24 hours to keep O2 saturation _90%?
PE developed while on anticoagulant therapy?
Intravenous pain medication needed for _24 hours?
Medical or social reason for admission?
Renal impairment (creatinine clearance _30 mL/min)?
Severe liver impairment?
Pregnancy?
H/o HIT?

- **Treatment**

Choosing Therapy		
Indication	Treatment	Misc. Information
Cancer	LMWH	
Once daily therapy requested	Rivaroxaban Edoxaban VKA	
Want to avoid any parental therapy initially	Rivaroxaban Apixaban	VKA, dabigatran, and edoxaban require initial parenteral therapy.
Co-existing liver disease	LMWH	
Pregnancy or risk thereof	LMWH	
Dyspepsia or history of GIB	VKA Apixaban	

  - Bridge required:
    - Warfarin at 5mg/day for a total of 3 months (until INR is 2.0 for at least 24 hours) but may consider starting at 10mg if healthy
    - Dabigatran (Pradaxa) 150mg BID for 6 months (assuming normal SCr; *REMEDY, RESONATE, RE-COVER*). Lovenox bridge required for at least 5 days
    - Edoxaban (Savaysa) 60mg daily for 6 months (30mg if ≤ 60kg in weight; assuming normal SCr; *Hokusai-VTE*). Lovenox bridge required for at least 5 days
    - LMWH, fondaparinux, for **5 days** and until INR 2-3 overlapped with oral anticoagulation for 24 hours
    - Lovenox: 1mg/kg BID (or daily if CrCl <30cc) or 1.5mg/kg SQ q24h
    - UFH: 80U/kg bolus then 18U/kg/hr
      - Alternative dosing is 8k-10k SQ q8h or 15k-20k q12h
      - Adjust dosing for an APTT of 1.5-2.5x control
  - Anticoagulation
    - **Rivaroxaban** 15mg BID for first 3 weeks then 20mg once daily thereafter for 6 months (assuming normal SCr; *EINSTEIN*)
    - **Apixaban** 10mg BID for 7 days followed by 5mg BID for 6 months (*AMPLIFY* trial)[204]
      - Efficacy in patients with PE was similar to that in the patients with deep-vein thrombosis

- Has been shown to be effective for the prevention of recurrent venous thromboembolism in patient's s/p 6 to 12 months of therapy for acute VTE
- Renal dosing is 2.5mg BID if SCr >1.5 or age>80 or weight <60kg

- **Aspirin**
  - In patients with unprovoked VTE or PE, start ASA for further prevention after anticoagulation therapy has finished (*INSPIRE, ASPIRE*)
- Temporary IVC filter indicated if you cannot anticoagulate patient
- OCP → avoid injectable contraceptives. Should aim for progestin-releasing IUD

- **Duration**
  - The risk of VTE recurrence is **greatest in the first year after** the event and remains elevated indefinitely compared with the general population.
  - Lifetime recurrence rates for DVT ranges from 21% to 30%, depending on the population.
  - Reversible VTE Risk Factor (ie. travel, OCP, trauma) – 3 months. ASH does not recommend prolonged therapy. See chart below for full list and calculation of percentage risk.
  - D-Dimer
    - The d-dimer test has been used to stratify risk of recurrent VTE.
    - The d-dimer value is checked **one month after anticoagulation ends**, with an increased level indicating increased risk.
  - Unprovoked (idiopathic) VTE – at least 3 months; if no bleeding issues and tolerated well then consider extended therapy duration. Extended duration of DOAC therapy has been found to be superior to simply using ASA. The study specifically utilized higher dose Rivaroxaban 20mg (*Weitz et al. NEJM 2017 Mar 18*). Men have higher risk than women (1.75 fold) and a positive d-dimer doubles the risk of another event. If extended duration therapy is initiated, it should be re-assessed at least annually to decide if it remains required.
  - Antiphospholipid ABS → extended duration / possibly lifelong
  - Cancer – LMWH for 3-6 months; consider extended treatment until cancer treated
  - Proximal DVT – 3 months (but if no risk factors, asymptomatic may consider serial US w/o tx)
  - Distal (below the knee) DVT – compression stockings

Situation	Management Recommendation
Unprovoked DVT (no cancer)	DOAC (dabigatran, rivaroxaban, etc.) over VKA for at least 3 months. Extended duration of therapy should be considered based on patient risk factors (low (0.8% risk of major bleed)/moderate (1.6% annual risk)/high (>6.5% annual risk) with re-evaluation of extended therapy done at least annually.
Provoked DVT d/t cancer	LMWH for duration of cancer therapy

- **Reversible Risk Factors**
  - Age > 65 years
  - Comorbidity and reduced functional capacity
  - Previous bleeding problems
  - Age > 75 years*
  - Diabetes mellitus
  - Previous stroke
  - Alcohol abuse

- Frequent falls
- Recent surgery
- Anemia
- Liver failure
- Renal failure
- Antiplatelet therapy (NSAID included)
- Metastatic cancer
- Thrombocytopenia
- Cancer
- Poor anticoagulant control

DVT Risk based on RF			
Categorization of Risk	Low Risk (0 Risk Factors)	Moderate Risk (1 Risk Factor)	High Risk (≥ 2 Risk Factors)
Initial risk (0 to 3 months)	1.6	3.2	12.8
Risk beyond 3 months	0.8	1.6	≥ 6.5

- **DVT Prophylaxis**
  Based on *Padua score (medical)* or *Caprini score (if non-ortho surgical patient)*
  - Leg pumps (PCDs) while in bed
  - Elastic compression stockings
  - Lovenox 40 mg SQ daily (unless GFR<30; then use Heparin 5000U SQ TID)
  - Post-operative:
    - *Low Risk (outpatient surg, neurosurg)*
      - PCD
      - Early ambulation
      - UFH until discharge
    - *High Risk (Hx malignancy, ortho surg, hx VTE)*
      - LMWH x 5 weeks
        - Use 30 mg if renal impairment
        - Don't give if bleeding, thrombocytopenic or going to surgery
      - If Creatinine Clearance 30, use Heparin 5000 units SC Q 8 hours (7500 units SC Q 8 hours if obese)
      - For ortho patients, duration of 35 days
- **Recurrent VTE on Anticoagulation Therapy**
  - If patient is on warfarin (assuming therapeutic INR), then switch to treatment-dose LMWH
  - If patient is on LMWH then ↑ dose by 25%
  - If anticoagulation intensity cannot be safely ↑ due to bleeding risk, insert IVC

OPTHALMOLOGY

EYE PAIN

- **History**[205]
  - Ask about vision loss or vision changes → immediate referral (for other referral indictions, see next page)
  - Photophobia or Foreign body sensation → likely corneal process, abrasion, retained foreign body
  - Ask about contact lens use → r/o bacterial and acanthamoeba keratitis
  - HA → r/o AACG, scleritis, cluster HA (usually unilateral), migraines
  - Stabbing pain → scleritis, uveitis, optic neuritis
  - ↓ vision → optic neuritis, scleritis, keratitis, uveitis, AACG, cellulitis
- **Exam**
  - Functional assessment
    - Vision check with snellen chart @ 20'
    - Visual Fields - confrontation testing with wiggle test from boundary of visual field
    - Extraocular movements – have pt keep head stationary and follow fingers
  - Structures
    - Look for eyelid swelling, erythema, lesions, ptosis, rashes, vesicles
  - Differentials
    - Conjunctival injection → conjunctivitis, uveitis, scleritis, keratitis, corneal abrasion
    - Eyelid swelling → hordeolum, orbital cellulitis, preseptal cellulitis
    - Pain w/ extraocular mvmt → optic neuritis, cellulitis, scleritis, AACG
    - +Fluorescein stain → corneal abrasion (linear pattern), keratitis (dendritic pattern), superficial keratitis (punctate pattern)
- **Imaging**
  - MRI with gad in patients with suspected optic neuritis
  - CT orbits if suspecting orbital cellulitis
- **Management**
  - See red flags in next section for indications for urgent referral
  - Corneal abrasion treated with topical NSAID drops, with topical fluoroquinolone (FLQ) or aminoglycoside (AMG) drops in patients who were using contact lenses. See section dedicated to corneal abrasions below.
  - Viral and Bacterial conjunctivitis – see *Conjunctivitis* section below
  - Scleritis – NSAIDs
  - Bacterial keratitis – broad spectrum ABx if not wearing contact lenses, if using, then topical FLQ or AMG
  - Dry eye syndrome – artificial tears QID but refer if persistent

- Orbital cellulitis – optho referral, inpatient admission, IV Vanco + (ceftriaxone, cefotaxime, Augmentin, or Zosyn)

Figure. Work up for the diagnosis of eye pain

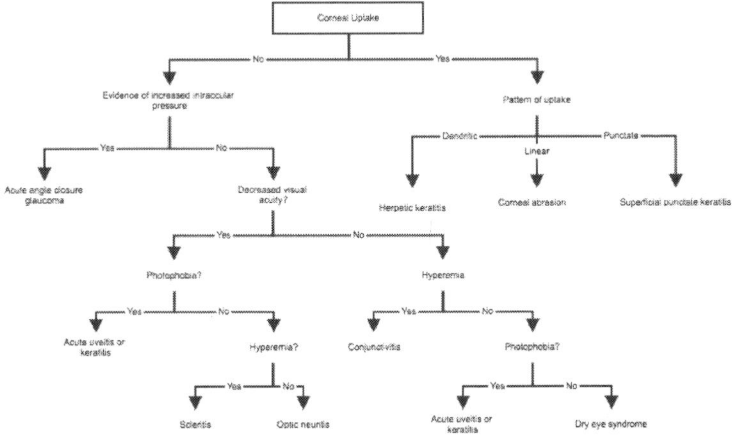

CONJUNCTIVITIS

- **General**[206]
  - The conjunctiva is a thin semitransparent membrane that covers the sclera.
  - Conjunctivitis is an inflammation of the conjunctival tissue due to infection or other irritants.
  - The three most common causes of conjunctivitis are:
    - viral (m/c due to adenovirus)
    - allergic
    - bacterial
- **Historical Features**
  - Patients with viral conjunctivitis present with foreign body sensation, red eyes, itching, light sensitivity, burning, and watery discharge.
    - Usually have a recent history of an upper respiratory tract infection or recent contact with a sick individual.
    - Visual acuity is usually at or near their baseline vision.
    - The conjunctiva is injected (red) and can also be edematous.
  - Patients with bacterial conjunctivitis present with all the above symptoms, **but with mucopurulent discharge and mattering of the eyelids upon waking**.
  - Red Flag Symptoms
    - Visual acuity change (usually one-line change)
    - Copious/muco purulent discharge
    - Photophobia
    - Foreign body sensation
    - Corneal opacity
    - Fixed pupil

        - Trouble keeping eye open
        - Severe HA w/ nausea
        - Pain
        - Constant blurred vision
- **Management**
    - Viral – conservative tx
    - Bacterial – Moxifloxacin, Erythromycin or TMP+polymyxin; alternative is quinolone; azithromycin 1% applied every 2 hours for the first 1-2 days then decrease to QID for the next 5-7 days. If ABx hard to come by, consider povidone-iodine solution 1.25% ophthalmic solution.
    - Allergic – usually lasts <24 hours; can try Olopatadine if recurrent or prolonged course

Diagnosis / Differential of Conjunctivitis			
	Viral	Bacterial	Allergic
Percentage	9-80%	18-57%	90%
Involvement	Unilateral, may progress to bilateral	Unilateral, may progress to bilateral	Bilateral
Stuck shut in morning?	Yes	Yes	Yes
Discharge	Watery; scant; serous	Purulent, green, white, or yellow; thick	Watery; scant
Discharge re-appears after wiping **can help distinguish bacterial from viral**	No	Yes	No
Other	Burning, sandy, gritty sensation, viral prodromal symptoms	Unremitting ocular discharge	Itching
Conjunctiva	Diffuse appearance	Diffuse	Diffuse
Causes	Adenovirus Herpes simplex Herpes zoster Enterovirus	*S. aureus* *H. influenza* *S. pneumonia*	Pollens
Treatment	• May take up to 3 weeks • Cold compress • Artificial tears QID • Antihistamines • Good hand hygiene • *Herpes Zoster* Oral famciclovir 500mg TID x7d or valacyclovir 1g TID x7d • *Herpes Simplex*	• Tobramycin ointment: 3 ×/d for 1 wk • Ciprofloxacin ointment: 3 ×/d for 1 wk Solution: 1-2 drops 4 ×/d for 1 wk • Azithromycin: 2 ×/d for 2 d; then 1 drop daily for 5 d • Trimethoprim/polymyxin B: 1 or 2 drops 4 ×/d for 1 wk • Gentamicin Ointment: 4 ×/d for 1 wk Solution: 1-2 drops 4 ×/d for 1 wk • *2/2 Neisseria Gonorrhea*	• Azelastine 0.05%: 1 drop 2 ×/d A52 • Cromolyn sodium 4%: 1-2 drops every 4-6 h A52 • Ketorolac: 1 drop 4 ×/d B53,54 • Naphazoline/pheniramine: 1-2 drops up to 4 ×/d • Olopatadine 0.1%: 1 drop 2 ×/d

	Topical acyclovir: 1 drop 9 ×/d	Ceftriaxone 1g IM Lavage of eye Azithromycin 250mg PO	

ACUTE MONOCULAR VISION LOSS

- **Definitions/Anatomy**[207]
  - Time Course
    - Transient – vision returned by the time sen by the clinician
    - Acute – instantaneous onset in seconds to minutes
    - Subacute – progression over days to weeks
    - Chronic – insidious over months to years
  - Localization
    - Anterior to optic chiasm results in monocular vision loss
      - Ocular medial (cornea, chamber, lens)
      - Retinal
      - Neurologic (optic nerve, chiasm)
    - Posterior to optic chiasm results in binocular vision loss (ie. pituitary apoplexy)
- **Differential / Questions to Ask**
  - Eye Pain: acute angle-closure glaucoma, optic neuritis (pain worsens with eye mvmt, loss of color vision), keratitis (sharp superficial pain, discharge)
  - Hyperemia: acute angle-closure glaucoma, keratitis, uveitis
  - Headache: GCA, migraine
  - Photophobia: retinal detachment
  - Preceding trauma: keratitis, uveitis, hyphema, lens dislocation

Figure. Relevant anatomy of the eye

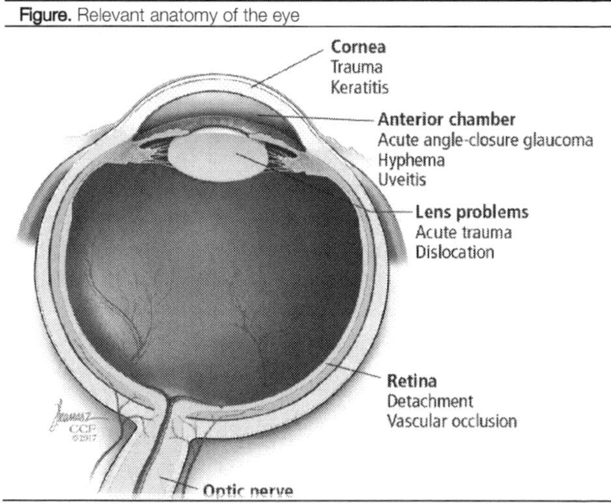

- **Physical Exam**
  - Visual Acuity
  - Visual Field – monocular testing, confrontation testing, central fields using Amsler grid
  - Color Testing
  - Pupillary Examination – size, shape, symmetry
  - Red reflex
  - Direct ophthalmoscopy

- **Diagnostics**
  - Carotid US
  - ECG
  - TTE
  - CT angio/MRA head&neck
  - ESR/CRP

CORNEAL ABRASION

- **General**[208]
  - 3rd leading cause of red-eye behind conjunctivitis and subconjunctival hemorrhage
- **Differential Diagnosis**
  - Acute angle closure glaucoma
  - Conjunctivitis
  - Corneal Ulcer
  - Hyphema (blood in anterior chamber)
  - Dry Eye Syndrome
  - Infective Keratitis (HSV, fungal, bacterial)
  - Uveitis
- **Evaluation**
  - Look for evidence of penetrating trauma, infection, and significant vision loss,
    - Penetrating trauma should be suspected in any patient with extruded ocular contents, or who has a pupil that is dilated, nonreactive, or irregular.
  - In corneal abrasion, the pupil is typically round, and central, and conjunctival injection may be present.
  - The anterior chamber should be inspected for blood (hyphema) or pus (hypopyon).
  - After inspection, visual acuity should be documented.
    - Vision loss of more than 20/40 requires referral.
  - Extraocular movements should be tested and documented
  - Confirm presence of red reflex
- **Urgent Ophthalmology Referral Indications**
  - Penetrating Trauma
  - Corneal opacity
  - Foreign bodies
  - ↓vision >1-2 lines on Snellen
  - Worsening symptoms
- **Management**
  - Topical ABx usually prescribed to prevent superinfection.
  - Topical ABx are used for corneal abrasions caused by contact lens use, foreign bodies, or a history of trauma as there is a higher risk of secondary bacterial keratitis in these cases.
  - Consider providing sunglasses for protection
  - For uncomplicated abrasions, options include erythromycin 0.5% ophthalmic ointment, polymyxin B/trimethoprim (Polytrim) ophthalmic solution, and sulfacetamide 10% ophthalmic ointment or solution
  - Topical antibiotics are generally dosed **four times a day** and **continued until the patient is asymptomatic for 24 hours**.
  - Ointments provide better lubrication than solutions

Figure. Algorithm for management of eye pain possibly due to a foreign body

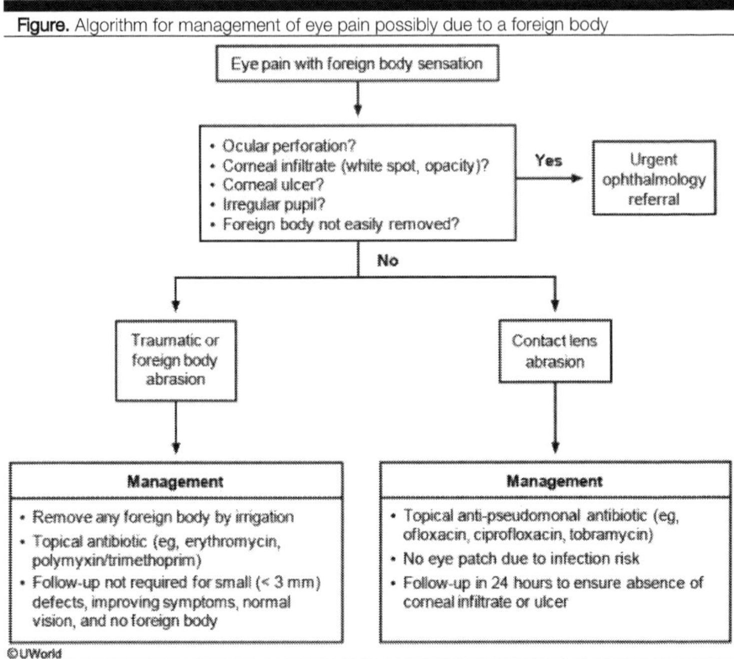

Medication	Dosage
Antibiotics	
Erythromycin 0.5% ointment	0.5-inch ribbon, four times per day for three to five days
Polymyxin B/trimethoprim (Polytrim) solution	1 drop, four times per day for three to five days
Anti-Pseudomonal	
Ciprofloxacin 0.3% (Ciloxan) ointment	0.5-inch ribbon, four times per day for three to five days
Ofloxacin 0.3% (Ocuflox) solution	1 to 2 drops, four times per day for three to five days
NSAIDs	
Diclofenac 0.1% (Voltaren)	1 drop, four times per day for two to three days
Corneal Ulcer	
Ciprofloxacin/Ofloxacin	1 drop every 5 minutes for 3 doses; 1 drop every 15 minutes for 6 hours, then 1 drop every 30 minutes
Scopolamine 0.25% (pain)	1 drop BID
Foreign Body	
Proparacaine 0.5%	1 drop for anesthesia for better evaluation and removal

RADIOLOGY

CXR

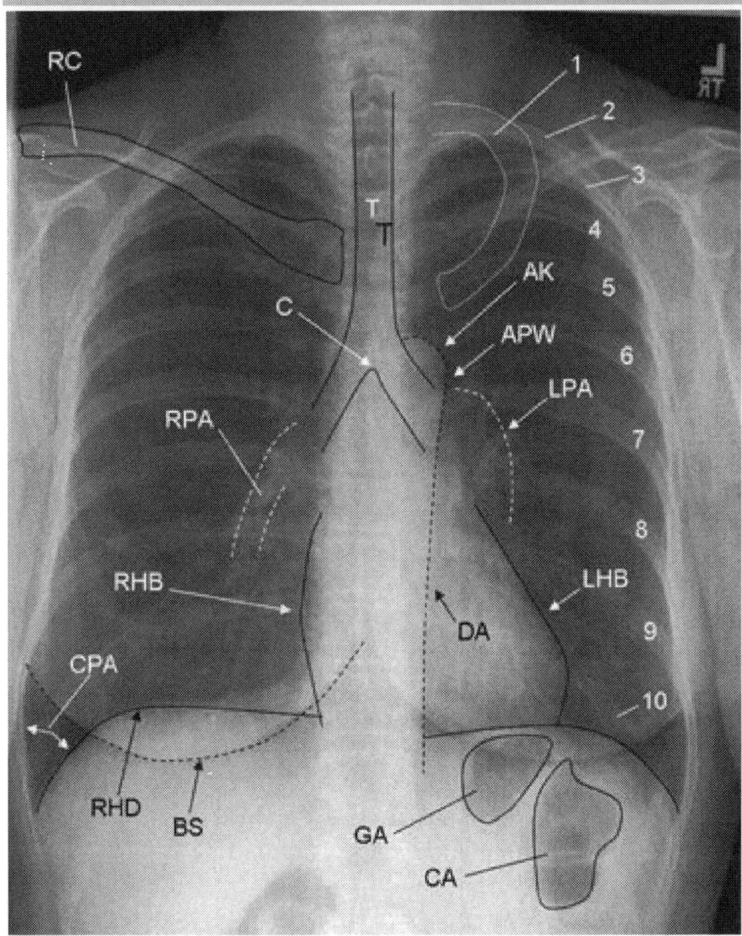

1 = first rib; 2–10 = posterior aspect of ribs 2–10; AK = aortic knob; APW = aortopulmonary window, BS = breast shadow (labeled only on right); C = carina; CA = colonic air; CPA = costophrenic angle, DA = descending aorta; GA = gastric air; LHB = left heart border (*Note:* Most of the left heart border represents the left ventricle; the superior aspect of the left heart border represents the left atrial appendage.); LPA = left pulmonary artery; RC = right clavicle (left clavicle not labeled); RHB = right heart border (*Note:* The right heart border represents the right atrium.); RHD = right hemidiaphragm (left hemidiaphragm not labeled); RPA = right pulmonary artery; T = tracheal air column.

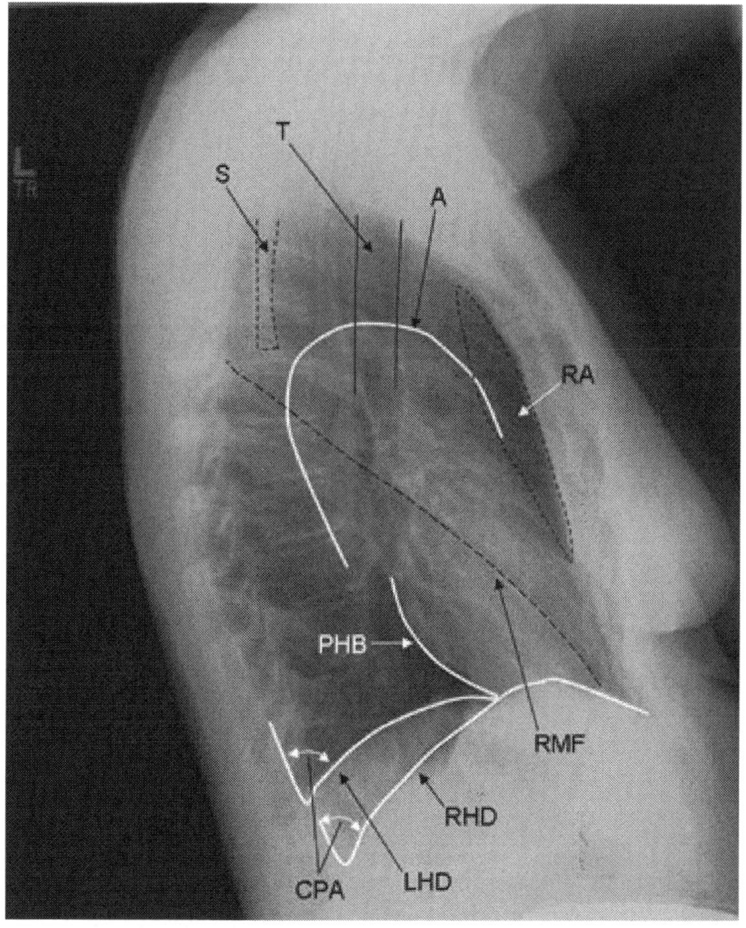
L
T
S
A
RA
PHB
RMF
RHD
CPA
LHD

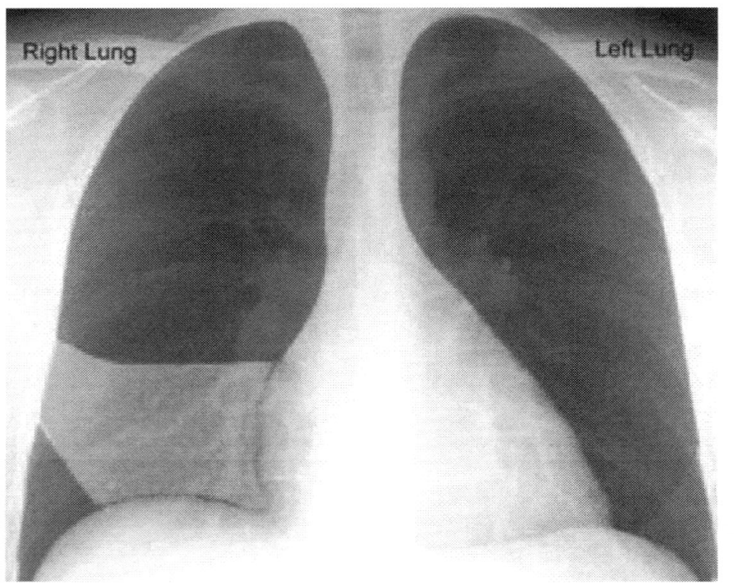

Right and Left Upper Lobes
Right Middle Lobe
Right and Left Lower Lobes

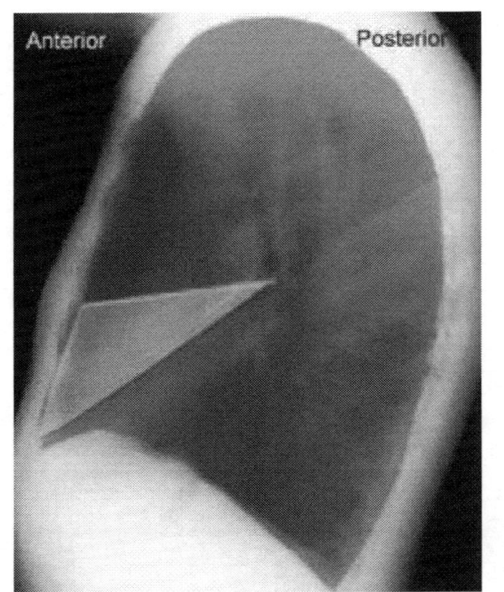

Left Upper Lobe
Major Fissure
Left Lower Lobe

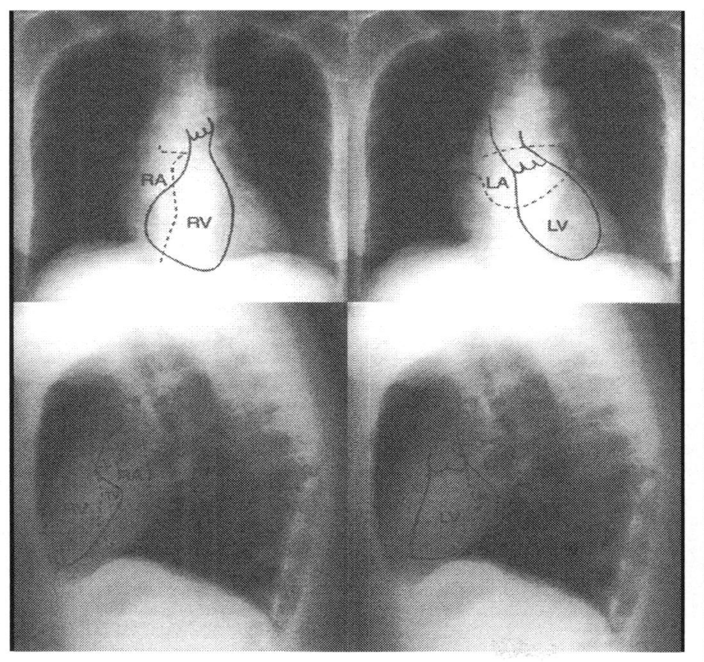
RA
RV
LA
LV

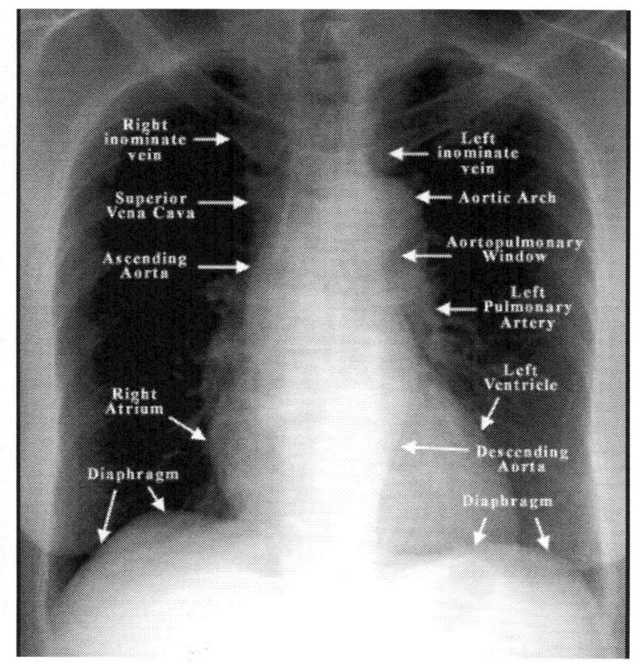
Right inominate vein
Superior Vena Cava
Ascending Aorta
Right Atrium
Diaphragm
Left inominate vein
Aortic Arch
Aortopulmonary Window
Left Pulmonary Artery
Left Ventricle
Descending Aorta
Diaphragm

- **How to Read**[209]
  - Determine the Adequacy of the Film
    - Inspiration: Diaphragm below ribs 8–10 posteriorly and 5–6 anteriorly
    - Rotation: Clavicles are equidistant from the spinous processes
    - Penetration: Disc spaces are seen but bony details of spine cannot be seen
  - PA Film
    - Remember, the film is on the patient's chest and the x-rays are passing from back (posterior) to front (anterior).
    - *Soft Tissues*: Check for symmetry, swelling, loss of tissue planes, and subcutaneous air.
    - *Skeletal Structures*: Examine the clavicles, scapulas, vertebrae, sternum, and ribs. Look for symmetry. In a good x-ray, the clavicles are symmetrical. Check for osteolytic or osteoblastic lesions, fractures, or arthritic changes. Look for rib-notching.
    - *Diaphragm*: Sides should be equal and slightly rounded, although the left may be slightly lower. Costophrenic angles should be clear and sharp. Blunting suggests scarring or fluid. It takes about 100–200 mL of pleural fluid to cause blunting. Check below the diaphragm for the gas pattern and free air. A unilateral high diaphragm suggests paralysis (either from nerve damage, trauma, or an abscess), eventration or loss of lung volume on that side because of atelectasis or pneumothorax.
    - *Mediastinum and Heart*: The aortic knob should be visible and distinct. Widening of the mediastinum is seen with traumatic disruption of the thoracic aorta. In children, do not mistake the normally prominent thymus for widening. Mediastinal masses can be associated with Hodgkin's disease and other lymphomas. The trachea should be in a straight line with a sharp carina. Tracheal deviation suggests a mass (tumor), goiter, unilateral loss of lung volume (collapse), or tension pneumothorax. The heart should be less than one-half the width of the chest wall on a PA film. If greater than one-half, think of CHF or pericardial fluid.
      - **Differential Diagnosis of Mediastinal Mass**[210]
        - Anterior
          1. Thymoma
          2. Teratoma
          3. Terrible Lymphoma
          4. Thyroid mass
          5. Tumor
        - Middle
          1. Bronchogenic cyst or tumor
          2. Lymphoma
        - Posterior
          1. Aneurysm
          2. Esophageal diverticula, tumor
          3. Neurogenic tumor
    - *Hilum*: The left hilum should be up to 2–3 cm higher than the right. Vessels are seen here. Look for any masses, nodes, or calcifications.
    - *Lung Fields*: Note the presence of any shadows from CVP lines, NG tubes, pulmonary artery catheters, etc. The fields should be clear with normal lung markings all the way to the periphery.
      - The vessels should taper to become almost invisible at the periphery.
      - Vessels in the lower lung should be larger than those in the upper lung. A reversal of this difference (called cephalization) suggests pulmonary venous hypertension and heart failure.

- **Kerley's B lines**, small linear densities found usually at the lateral base of the lung, are associated with CHF. Check the margins carefully; look for pleural thickening, masses, or pneumothorax.
- If the lungs appear hyperlucent with a relatively small heart and flattening of the diaphragms, COPD is likely.
- Thin *plate-like* linear densities are associated with atelectasis. To locate a lesion, do not forget to check a lateral film and remember the "silhouette sign." Obliteration of all or part of a heart border means the lesion is anterior in the chest and lies in the right middle lobe, lingula, or anterior segment of the upper lobe. A radiopacity that overlaps the heart but does not obliterate the heart border is posterior and lies in the lower lobes.
- Examine carefully for the following:
  - Coin lesions: Causes are granulomas (50% which are usually calcified), (histoplasmosis 25%, TB 20%, coccidioidomycosis 20%, varies with locale); primary carcinoma (25%), hamartoma (<10%), and metastatic disease (<5%).
  - Cavitary lesions: Causes are abscess, cancer, TB, coccidioidomycosis, Wegener's granulomatosis.
  - Infiltrates: Two major types
    1. *Interstitial pattern*. "Reticular." Causes are granulomatous infections, miliary TB, coccidioidomycosis, pneumoconiosis, sarcoidosis, CHF. "Honeycombing" represents end-stage fibrosis caused by sarcoid, RA, and pneumoconiosis.
    2. *Alveolar pattern*. Diffuse, quick progression and regression. Can see either "butterfly" pattern or air bronchograms. Causes are PE, pneumonia, hemorrhage or PE associated with CHF.
- **Regions That Commonly Hide Pathology**
  - Apical
  - Paratracheal
  - Perihilar
  - CPA
  - Retrocardiac

- *Lines/Devices* –
  - ETT - If the patient is intubated, check the position of the endotracheal tube (ETT; should be a minimum of 2 cm above the carina with 3 to 5 cm being ideal). Good rule of thumb is it should be near the medial ends of the clavicles.
  - Central venous catheters - should follow expected venous courses and should generally terminate in the superior vena cava (SVC), near the level of the **carina** (cavo-atrial junction) along the right aspect of the mediastinum. The end of the catheter should travel along the long axis of the superior vena cava (vertically).
  - Nasogastric (NG) and enteric feeding tubes may be partially visualized. Ensure they do not coil in the esophagus or extend outward into the lung due to endobronchial placement.
  - Chest tubes –
    - More common in the ICU environment
    - Should lie between the visceral and parietal pleura with its position on the CXR determining its intent: anterosuperior for drainage of PTX while posteroinferior for pleural effusions.
    - Verify function by ensuring all fenestrations in the tube are within the thoracic cavity. The last side-hole in a thoracostomy tube is indicated by a

gap in the radiopaque line. If this interruption in the radiopaque line is not within the thoracic cavity or there is evidence of subcutaneous air, then the tube may not have been completely inserted.

- Pacemakers –
  - *Single chamber* – look for the electrode tip in the right atrial (RA) appendage (if it is atrial paced) or the right ventricular (RV) apex (for ventricular paced).
  - *Dual chamber* – the electrode tips will be both in the RA and RV
  - *Biventricular* – electrode tips will be in the RA, RV, and coronary sinus (to stimulate the LV)
  - *ICD* – electrode tips in the apex of the RV

ABDOMINAL FILM

- **How to Read**[211]
  - Bones – start with the spine, then ribs then finish with the pelvis and upper femurs. Common pathology includes arthritis, fx, and osteolytic/osteoblastic lesions.
  - Lines/Tubes – NG/OG and other enteric tubes. These should terminate in the LUQ with appearance of the proximal port past the GE junction. Enteric tubes should farther, moving past the GE junction into the right abdomen then **crossing midline** to the left to terminate in the jejunum.
  - Soft Tissue – look for masses (fibroids in the uterus) , calcifications (GB, pancreas, phleboliths), and free air under the diaphragm.
  - GI Structures
    - *Gastric bubble* (larger size may be suggestive of an obstruction)
    - *Bowel gas pattern* – common to see a small amount of air in the colon but is commonly absent in the SI. Large fecal burden in the colon may be seen in the elderly. If the colon is obstructed, it may distend. If there is loss of the haustral markings (do not completely cross the lumen), this is concerning (r/o toxic megacolon).
      - >6cm in colon is pathologic
      - >3cm in small intestine is pathologic
    - *Air fluid levels* - nonspecific

ECHOCARDIOGRAPHY

- **3 basic views**[212]

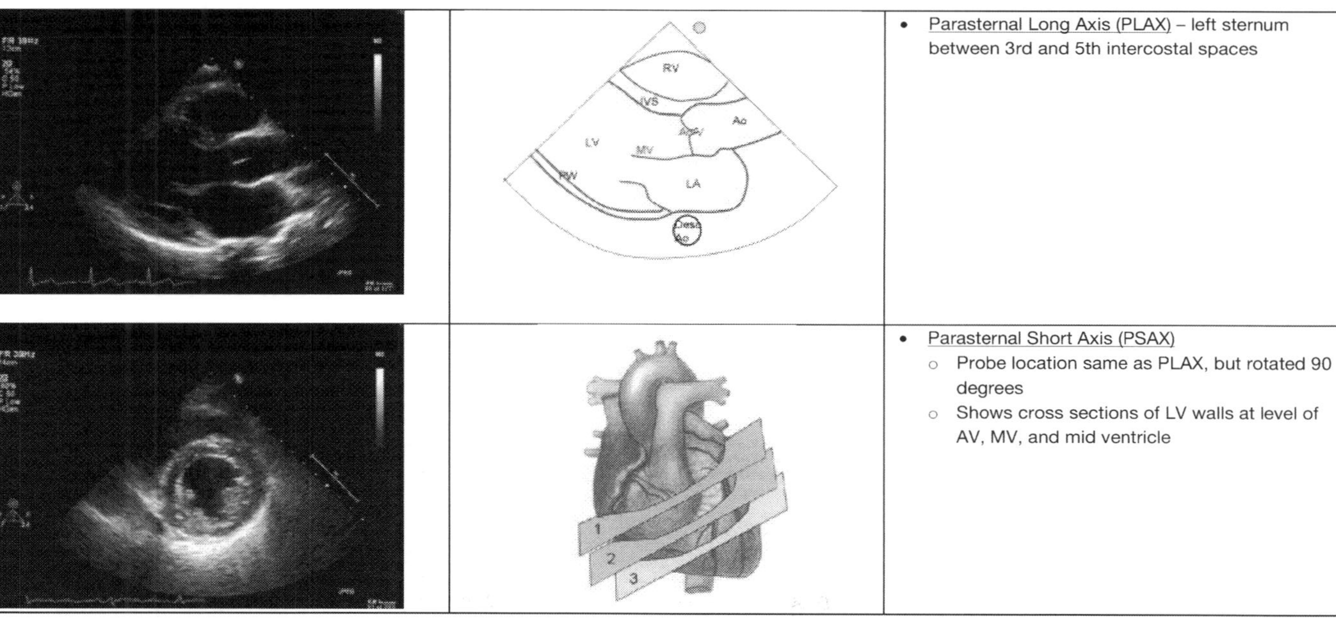

		• <u>Parasternal Long Axis (PLAX)</u> – left sternum between 3rd and 5th intercostal spaces
		• <u>Parasternal Short Axis (PSAX)</u> ○ Probe location same as PLAX, but rotated 90 degrees ○ Shows cross sections of LV walls at level of AV, MV, and mid ventricle

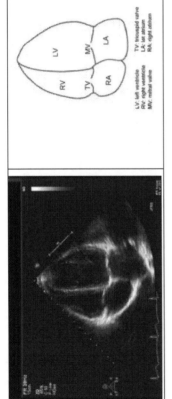

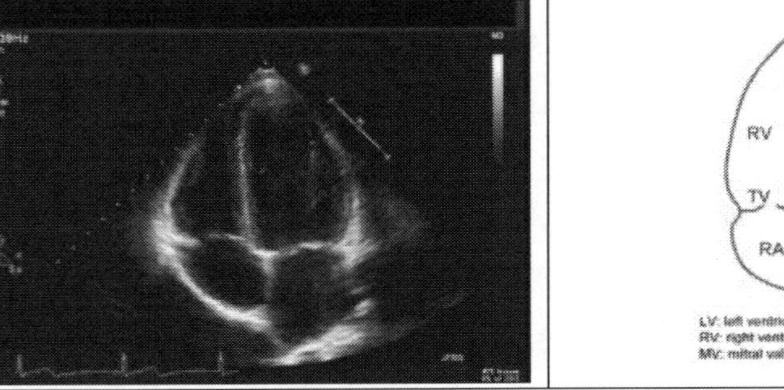	RV LV TV MV RA LA LV: left ventricle RV: right ventricle MV: mitral valve TV: tricuspid valve LA: left atrium RA: right atrium	• Apical 4 Chamber ○ Probe at LV apex max impulse

US

- **General Instructions**[213]
  - Determine the image orientation.
    - Taken in one of two planes: longitudinal (long) and transverse (trans).
    - In long images, the left side of the sonogram shows structures toward the patient's head. The right side shows structures toward the feet.
    - In trans images, the left side of the sonogram shows structures on the patient's right side and vice versa. The top of the image is the skin, where the transducer, or camera, is resting.
  - Measurement orientation.
    - Three measurements are taken of structures: length, height, and width.
      - Length is measured on the long image from left to right.
      - Height is the depth, from the top of the image towards the bottom.
      - Width is taken in the trans image from left to right.
  - Differentiate between cystic and solid.
    - Cysts are fluid-filled sacs. A cyst with no debris is black on the sonogram because no signal is returned to the ultrasound system.
      - Ultrasound waves get stronger when they pass through fluid and will demonstrate increased, or enhanced, through-transmission.
      - This is evident by brighter, and sometimes clearer, structures behind the cyst.
    - Solids are bright and white. Variations of gray are the result of varying fluid contents of structures.
  - Evaluate the fat or air content.
    - Ultrasound does not travel well through fat and air, so images may be of poor quality and structures difficult to see when more fat or bowel is present.
      - This is sometimes an indication of a pathology.
  - Asses blood flow.
    - Doppler is used to determine the presence, direction and velocity of blood flow.
    - Continuous Doppler demonstrates red and blue signals.
      - Generally, red represents blood moving toward the camera, and blue represents blood moving away from the camera.
      - Pulsed Doppler can be used to determine the resistance of blood flow. High peaks represent high resistance, and low peaks represent low resistance.
- **Gallbladder**
  - Look for shadowing:
    - Stones
    - Sludge
  - Look at anterior wall for thickening
  - Echogenicity should be ↑ in comparison to the liver
  - Check cystic duct for patency (normal 6-7mm)
- **Kidney**
  - Cortex decreases with ↑ pathology
  - Compare size of both kidneys
  - Kidney cysts do NOT create shadows
- **Testicular**
  - Calcifications
  - Extra vs. Intraparenchymal
  - Should be homogenous

MRI

- **When to Use MRI**
  In general, MRI imaging is at least equal to CT imaging. MRI is superior to CT for imaging of brain, spinal cord, musculoskeletal soft tissues, adrenal and renal masses, and areas of high CT bony artifact. However, spiral CT may now have overcome some of these disadvantages.
- **Advantages**
  - No ionizing radiation
  - Display of vascular anatomy without contrast
  - Visualization of linear structures: Spine and spinal cord, aorta, and cava
  - Visualization of posterior fossa and other hard to see CT areas
  - High-contrast soft tissue images
- **Disadvantages**
  - Claustrophobia due to confining magnet (Newer open MRI scanners may obviate this problem.)
  - Longer scanning time resulting in motion artifacts
  - Unable to scan critically ill patients requiring life support equipment
  - Metallic foreign bodies: Pacemakers, shrapnel, CNS vascular clips, metallic eye fragments, and cochlear implants are contraindications
  - MRI Contrast: Gadolinium (gadopentetic dimeglumine) is an ionic contrast agent
- **How to Read**
  - SE T1-Weighted Images
    - Provide good anatomic planes due to the wide variances of T1 values among normal tissues.
      - Brightest (high signal intensity): Fat
      - Dark or black: Pathological tissues, tumor or inflammation, fluid collections
      - Black (low signal intensity): Respiratory tract, GI tract, calcified bone and tissues, blood vessels, heart chambers, and pericardial effusions
  - SE T2-Weighted Images
    - Pathology prolongs T2 measurements, and normal tissues have a very small range of T2 values. T2-weighted images provide the best detection of pathology and a decreased visualization of normal tissue anatomy. Tumor surrounded by fat may be lost on T2 imaging.
      - Brightest: Fat and fluid collections
      - Bright: Pheochromocytomas
  - FLAIR
    - Highlights pathology

CT

- **Head**
  - Technique - With Our Without Contrast
- **Mnemonic**[214]
  - Blood Can Be Very Bad
    - Blood—Acute hemorrhage appears hyperdense (bright white) on CT.
      - This is due to the fact that the globin molecule is relatively dense and hence effectively absorbs x-ray beams.
      - As the blood becomes older and the globin breaks down, it loses this hyperdense appearance, beginning at the periphery. The precise localization of the blood is as important as identifying its presence.
  - Cisterns—Cerebrospinal fluid collections jacketing the brain; the following four key cisterns must be examined for blood, asymmetry, and effacement (representing increased intracranial pressure):

- Circummesencephalic—Cerebrospinal fluid ring around the midbrain; first to be effaced with increased intracranial pressure
- Suprasellar (star-shaped)—Location of the circle of Willis; frequent site of aneurysmal subarachnoid hemorrhage
- Quadrigeminal—W-shaped cistern at top of midbrain; effaced early by rostrocaudal herniation
- Sylvian—Between temporal and frontal lobes; site of traumatic and distal mid-cerebral aneurysm and subarachnoid hemorrhage

- Brain—Examine for:
  - Symmetry—Sulcal pattern (gyri) well differentiated in adults and symmetric side-to-side.
  - Gray-white differentiation—Earliest sign of cerebrovascular aneurysm is loss of gray-white differentiation; metastatic lesions often found at gray-white border
  - Shift—Falx should be midline, with ventricles evenly spaced to the sides; can also have rostrocaudal shift, evidenced by loss of cisternal space; unilateral effacement of sulci signals increased pressure in one compartment; bilateral effacement signals global increased pressure
  - Hyper/hypodensity—Increased density with blood, calcification, intravenous contrast media; decreased density with air/gas (pneumocephalus), fat, ischemia (cerebrovascular aneurysm), tumor
- Ventricles—Pathologic processes cause dilation (hydrocephalus) or compression/shift; hydrocephalus usually first evident in dilation of the temporal horns (normally small and slit-like); examiner must take in the "whole picture" to determine if the ventricles are enlarged due to lack of brain tissue or to increased cerebrospinal fluid pressure
- Bone—Highest density on CT scan; diagnosis of skull fracture can be confusing due to the presence of sutures in the skull; compare other side of skull for symmetry (suture) versus asymmetry (fracture); basilar skull fractures commonly found in petrous ridge (look for blood in mastoid air cells)

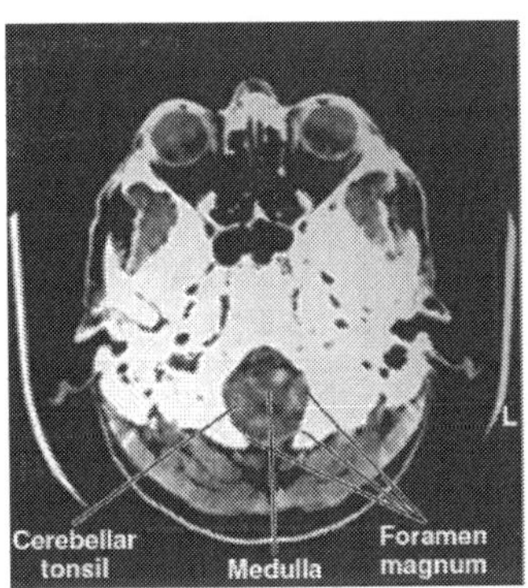

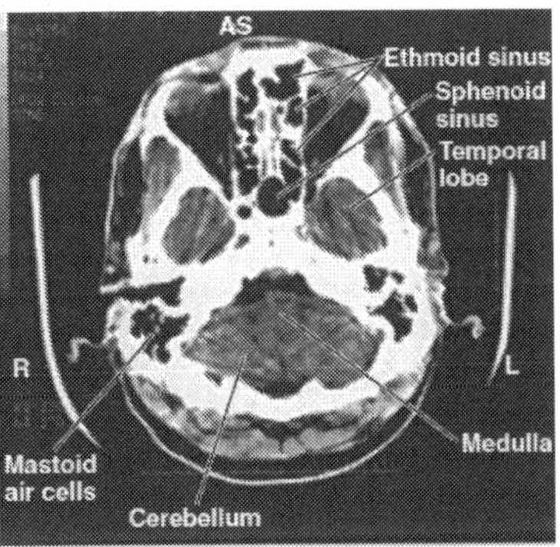

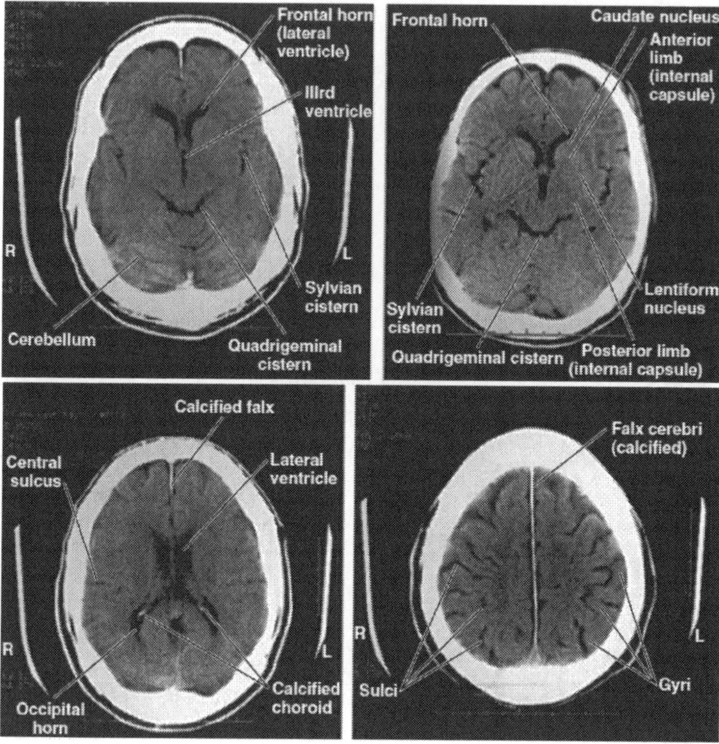
Frontal horn (lateral ventricle)
IIIrd ventricle
R
L
Sylvian cistern
Cerebellum
Quadrigeminal cistern
Frontal horn
Caudate nucleus
Anterior limb (internal capsule)
Lentiform nucleus
Sylvian cistern
Quadrigeminal cistern
Posterior limb (internal capsule)
Calcified falx
Central sulcus
Lateral ventricle
R
L
Calcified choroid
Occipital horn
Falx cerebri (calcified)
R
L
Sulci
Gyri

Abdomen

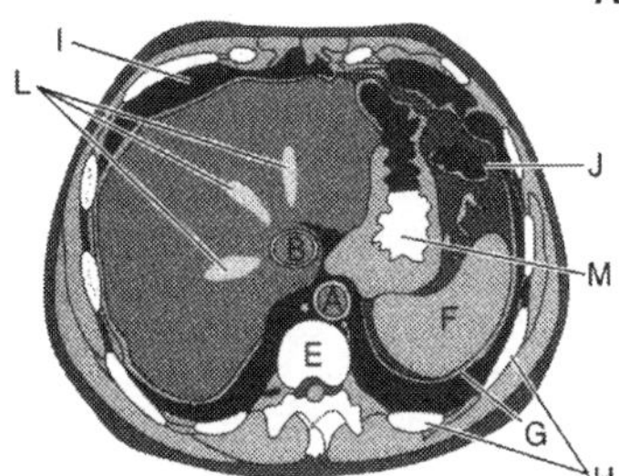

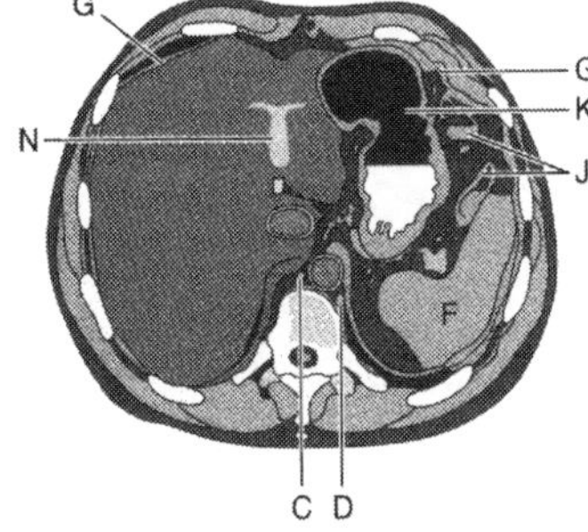

A = Aorta
B = IVC
C = Azygos vein
D = Hemiazygos vein
E = Vertebral body
F = Spleen
G = Diaphragm
H = Rib
I = Lung
J = Splenic flexure
K = Stomach
L = Hepatic veins
M = Gastric fundus
N = Left portal vein
O = Falciform ligament
P = Left adrenal gland
Q = Left kidney
R = Pancreatic tail
S = Small bowel
T = Right portal vein
U = Right adrenal gland
V = Celiac axis
W = Splenic vein
X = Pancreatic body
Y = Gastric antrum
Z = Common bile duct
AA = Main portal vein
BB = Right kidney
CC = SMA
DD = Collecting system
EE = Transverse colon
FF = Duodenal bulb
GG = Head of the pancreas
HH = Gallbladder
II = Left renal vein
JJ = Descending colon
KK = Superior mesenteric vein (SMV)
LL = Uncinate process of the pancreas
MM = Crus of the diaphragm
NN = Right renal artery
OO = Third portion of the duodenum

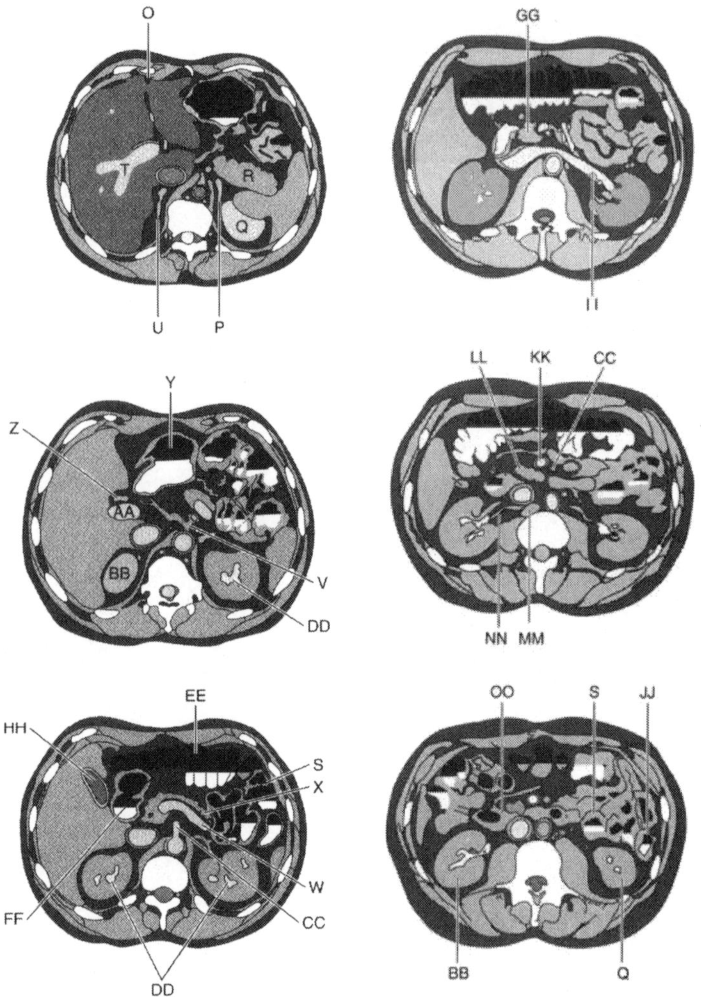
O
T
R
Q
U
P
GG
II
Y
Z
AA
BB
V
DD
LL
KK
CC
NN
MM
EE
HH
S
X
W
CC
FF
DD
OO
S
JJ
BB
Q

LUNG NODULES

Recommendations for Follow-up and Management of Nodules Smaller than 8mm Detected Incidentally at Non screening AT in Patients >35YO		
Nodule Size (mm)	Low-Risk Patient	High-Risk Patient
≤4	No follow-up needed	Follow-up AT at 12mo; If unchanged, no further follow-up
>4-6	Follow-up AT @ 12mo; if unchanged, no further follow-up	Initial follow-up AT at 6-12mo then at 18-24mo if no change
>6-8	Initial follow-up AT @ 6-12mo then at 18-24mo if no change	Initial follow-up AT @ 3-6mo then @ 9-12mo and 24mo if no change
>8	Follow-up AT @ around 3,9, and 24mo, dynamic aontrast-enhanaed AT, PET, and/or biopsy	Same as for low-risk patient

Low risk – minimal or absent history of smoking and other known risk factors
High risk – History of smoking or other known risk factors

- **General**
  - Diameter of ≥8 mm, ground-glass density, irregular borders, and doubling time between one month and one year are suggestive of malignancy.
- **Differential Diagnosis**
  - Nonspecific granuloma
  - Hamartoma
  - Infectious granuloma (ie. aspergillosis, cocci, crypto, histo)
  - Malignancy (ie. adeno, small cell, mets, squamous)

Radiologic features suggestive of benign vs. malignant nodule		
Feature	Benign	Malignant
Size	<5mm	>10mm
Border	Smooth	Irregular or spiculated
Density	Dense, solid	Nonsolid or "ground-glass"
Calcification	Typically, a benign feature, especially in "concentric," "central," "popcorn-like," or "homogeneous" patterns	noncalcified, or "eccentric" calcification
Doubling time	<1mo; more than 1 year	1mo-1year

- **Risk Factors**
  - Older patients, those with a history of extrathoracic cancer, and those with recent smoking histories are at highest risk of malignancy, whereas younger patients with no history of smoking are at lowest risk.
- **Screening**
  - For asymptomatic smokers and former smokers ages 55 to 77 years who have smoked 30 pack-years or more **and** either continue to smoke or have quit **within** the past 15 years, annual screening with low-dose CT should be offered. Furthermore, if none of the previous are met but if still considered high risk of having/developing lung cancer based on clinical risk prediction calculators then still do CT

- Individuals who have accumulated fewer than 30 pack-years of smoking or who are younger than age 55 years or older than age 77 years, or who have quit smoking more than 15 years ago, and do not have a high risk of having/developing lung cancer based on clinical risk prediction calculators.
- individuals with comorbidities that adversely influence their ability to tolerate the evaluation of screen-detected findings, or tolerate treatment of an early stage screen-detected lung cancer, or that substantially limit their life expectancy

V/Q SCAN

- **Mechanism** – micro albumin particles embolize into the pulmonary artery occluding the vasculature
- **Analysis**[215]
  - 2 series are obtained: perfusion and ventilation
  - Look for **mis**match defects were you see defect on perfusion that is not seen on the ventilation scan → this represents pathology
    - It is considered a *V/Q Mismatch.*
  - Matched defects are likely due to infection vs. effusion
- **Size**
  - Determining the size of a defect can be difficult.
  - A knowledge of segmental anatomy is essential, and use of a schematic chart (right) is encouraged to increase reading reproducibility and inter observer agreement
  - In general, the actual size of a perfusion defect is UNDER estimated by exam interpreters
    - Small defect (*small subsegmental*): Less than 25% of a segment.
    - Moderate defect (*moderate subsegmental*): > 25%, but < 75% of a segment.
    - Large defect (*segmental*): Greater than 75% of a segment.
- **Interpretation**
  - High Probability (80-100% likelihood for PE:
    - Greater than or equal to 2 large mismatched segmental perfusion defects or the arithmetic equivalent in moderate or large and moderate defects.
    - A high probability lung scan confirms a very high likelihood for pulmonary embolism and **justifies treatment with anticoagulation (unless contraindicated).**
    - *Caveat* - It has been suggested that 2.5 mismatched large segmental defects (or the arithmetic equivalent) is a better threshold for calling a scan high probability, as it associated with a 100% probability of PE in the PIOPED population.
  - Intermediate Probability (20-80% likelihood for PE
    - One moderate to 2 large mismatched perfusion defects or the arithmetic equivalent in moderate or large and moderate defects.
    - Single matched ventilation-perfusion defect with a clear chest radiograph.
    - *Caveat* - Single ventilation-perfusion matches are borderline for "low probability" and thus should be categorized as "intermediate" in most circumstances by most readers, although individual readers may correctly interpret individual scintigram with this pattern as "low probability".
    - Difficult to categorize as low or high, or not described as low or high.
  - Low Probability (0-19% likelihood for PE
    - Perfusion defects matched by ventilation abnormality provided that there are: (a) clear chest radiograph and (b) some areas of normal perfusion in the lungs. Extensive matched V/Q abnormalities are appropriate for low probability, provided that the CXR is clear.
    - Any perfusion defect with a substantially larger chest radiographic abnormality.

        - Any number of small perfusion defects with a normal chest radiograph.
        - Non segmental perfusion defects (e.g., cardiomegaly, enlarged aorta, enlarged hila, elevated diaphragm).
        - Multiple matched V/Q abnormalities, even when relatively extensive, are low probability for PE. The prevalence of PE in patients with extensive matched V/Q defects and no CXR abnormality was 14% (low probability).
    - Normal Study: No perfusion defects or perfusion exactly outlines the shape of the lungs seen on the chest radiograph (note that hila and aortic impressions may be seen, and the chest radiograph and/or ventilation study may be abnormal).

Clinical Science Probability				
Scan Probability	80 - 100%	20 - 79%	0 - 19%	All Probabilities
High	96%	88%	56%	87%
Intermediate	66%	28%	16%	30%
Low	40%	16%	4%	14%
Near normal/ normal	0%	6%	2%	4%
Total	68%	30%	9%	28%

CERVICAL SPINE SERIES

- **Presentation**
    - Adequacy - An adequate film should include all 7 vertebrae and c7-t1 junction. It should also have correct density and show the soft tissue and bony structures well.
    - Alignment
        - Assess four parallel lines. These are:
        - Anterior vertebral line (anterior margin of vertebral bodies)
        - Posterior vertebral line (posterior margin of vertebral bodies)
        - Spinolaminar line (posterior margin of spinal canal)
        - Posterior spinous line (tips of the spinous processes)
    - Bone - Check anterior portions for Schmorl nodes or anterior lipping, commonly seen with OA
    - Cartilage - The predental space (distance from dens to c1 body) should not measure more than 2-3 mm in adults and 5mm in children. If the space is increased, a fracture of the odontoid process or disruption of the transverse ligament is likely.
    - Joints
        - Check uncovertebral joints for adequate space
        - Check uncinate processes
    - Disc
    - Soft tissue
        - Nasopharyngeal space (c1) - 10 mm (adult)
        - Retropharyngeal space (c2-c4) - 5-7 mm
        - Retrotracheal space (c5-c7) - 14 mm (children), 22 mm (adults).

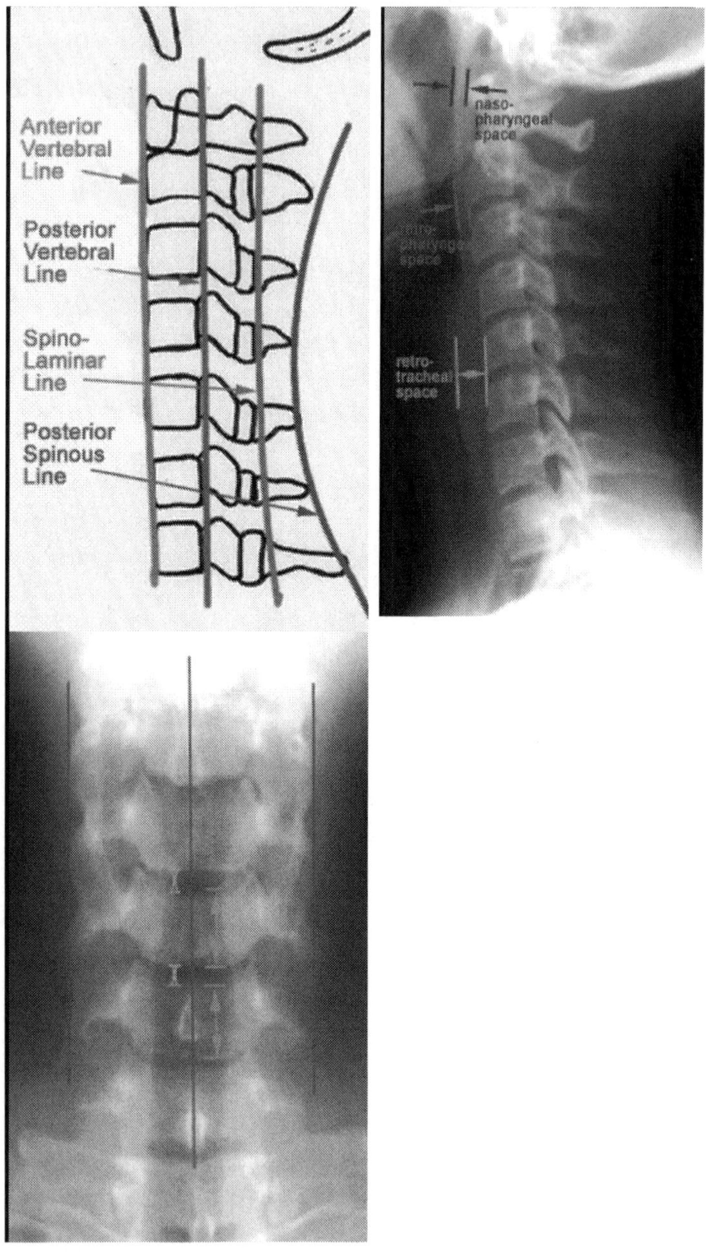
Anterior Vertebral Line
Posterior Vertebral Line
Spino-Laminar Line
Posterior Spinous Line
naso-pharyngeal space
retro-tracheal space

RADIOGRAPHIC IMAGING OPTIONS

Contrast vs. Noncontrast Imaging

Non-Contrast	Contrast
o Expiratory Chest: ▪ Visualization of small pneumothorax o Lateral Decubitus Chest: ▪ Allows small amounts of pleural effusion or subpulmonic effusion to layer out; as little as 175 mL of pleural fluid can be detected o Lordotic Chest: ▪ Evaluation of apices and lesions of the right and left upper lobes, TB, sarcoidosis o Portable Chest and AP Films: ▪ Imaging of critically ill patients who cannot stand for a routine PA CXR; diagnosis of pneumothorax, pneumonia, and edema; verification of vascular line or tube placement. Not accurate in evaluation of heart or mediastinal size because the standard x-ray is PA (beam from behind), and the AP technique magnifies these structures o Rib Details: ▪ Delineation of rib abnormalities when plain CXR or bone scan findings suggest fracture or other metastatic lesions o Abdominal ▪ Abdominal Decubitus: ▫ Obtain instead of upright abdominal film for imaging of debilitated patients. Patient's left side is down to show free air outlining the liver and right lateral gutter.	• Angiography o A rapid series of films obtained after a bolus contrast injection through a percutaneous catheter. Imaging of aorta, major arteries and branches, tumors, and venous drainage with late "run-off" films. Helical CT scans also generate angiographic images. ▪ **Cardiac angiography**. Definitive for diagnosis and assessment of severity of CAD. Significant (> 70% occlusion) stenotic lesions can be seen: 30% involve single vessels, 30% involve two, and 40% involve three vessels. ▪ **Cerebral angiography**. Evaluation of intra- and extracranial vascular disease, atherosclerosis, aneurysms, and A-V malformations. Not used for detection of cerebral structural lesions (use MRI or CT instead) ▪ **Pulmonary angiography**. Visualization of emboli, intrinsic or extrinsic vascular abnormalities, A-V malformations, and bleeding due to tumors. Most accurate diagnostic procedure for PE but only used if findings on helical CT or lung V/Q scan are not diagnostic • Barium Enema (BE) o Examination of colon and rectum. Indications include diarrhea, crampy abdominal pain, heme-positive stools, change in bowel habits, and unexplained weight loss o **Air-contrast BE**. Done with the double-contrast technique (air and barium) to better delineate the mucosa. More likely to show polyps than standard BE

- Acute Abdominal Series ("Obstruction Series"):
  - Includes flat and upright abdominal films (KUB) and CXR. Initial evaluation of acute abdomen
- Cross-Table Lateral Abdominal:
  - Identification of free air in debilitated patients.
- KUB, Supine and Erect:
  - Short for "kidneys, ureter, and bladder"; also known as flat and upright abdominal, scout film, and flat plate. Useful when the patient complains of abdominal pain or distention, and for initial evaluation of the urinary tract (80% of kidney stones and 20% of gallstones are visualized on KUBs). Look for calcifications, foreign bodies, the gas pattern, psoas shadows, renal and liver shadows, flank stripes, the vertebral bodies, and the pelvic bones. On the upright, look for air-fluid levels of adynamic ileus and mechanical obstruction and for free air under the diaphragm, which suggests a perforated viscus or recent surgery; however, an upright CXR (especially the lateral view) is often best for spotting pneumoperitoneum.

  - **Gastrografin enema**. Similar to barium enema, but water-soluble contrast agent is used (clears colon more quickly than barium). If Gastrografin leaks from the GI tract, it is less irritating to the peritoneum (does not cause barium peritonitis). Therapeutic in evaluation of obstipation and colonic volvulus; depicts postop anastomotic leak
- Barium Swallow (Esophagogram)
  - Evaluation of swallowing mechanism, esophageal lesions, and abnormal peristalsis
- Cystogram
  - Bladder is filled and emptied with a catheter in place; used to evaluate bladder filling defects (tumors, diverticula) and bladder perforation. Can also be done with CT (CT cystogram is more sensitive for perforation with trauma)
- Enteroclysis
  - Intubation of the proximal jejunum and rapid infusion of contrast material. Better than an SBFT in evaluation of polyps and obstruction (eg, adhesions, internal hernia); used to evaluate small-bowel sources of chronic bleeding after negative upper and lower endoscopy
- Endoscopic Retrograde Cholangiopancreatography (ERCP)
  - Contrast material is endoscopically injected into the ampulla of Vater to visualize the common bile and pancreatic ducts for obstruction, stones, and ductal pattern
- Intravenous Pyelography (IVP):
  - Contrast study of the kidneys and ureters; limited usefulness for evaluating bladder. Indications include flank pain, kidney stones, hematuria, UTI, trauma, and malignancy. Bowel prep helpful but not essential. Creatinine must be < 1.8 mg/dL. Largely replaced by CT urography. Nephrotomogram

are images of kidney sections for further definition of the three-dimensional location or nature of renal lesions and stones.

- <u>Retrograde Pyelography (RPG):</u>
    - Contrast material injected into the ureters through a cystoscope. Imaging of patients allergic to IV contrast medium or with elevated creatinine, if kidney or ureter cannot be visualized with other imaging techniques, and in the presence of renal mass, ureteral obstruction, or filling defects in the collecting system
- <u>Small Bowel Follow-Through (SBFT):</u>
    - Usually done after a UGI series. Delayed films show jejunum and ileum. Evaluation of diarrhea, abdominal cramps, malabsorption, and UGI bleeding
- <u>Upper GI (UGI) Series:</u>
    - Includes esophagography and imaging of stomach and duodenum. Visualization of ulcers, masses, hiatal hernia and to evaluate heme-positive stools and upper abdominal pain
- <u>Voiding Cystourethrography (VCUG):</u>
    - Bladder is filled with contrast material through a catheter, then catheter is removed, and the patient voids. Diagnosis of vesicoureteral reflux, examination of urethral valves, and evaluation of UTI

MUSCULOSKELETAL

BACK EXAMINATION

- **Duration**[216]
  - Acute (6-12 weeks) vs. Chronic (>12 weeks
- **Types**
  - Nonspecific
  - With radiculopathy
  - 2/2 cause
- **Differential**
  - MSK
    - Herniation (Leg pain>back pain; anterior radiation is likely L1-3, past knee is L4-S1 → positive straight leg raise)
    - Strain (worse with movement, better with rest)
    - Spondylolisthesis (leg pain>back pain but better with flexion of spine; if better with extension consider spondylolysis)
  - Infection
  - Malignancy
  - Fracture
  - Osteoporosis
  - Inflammatory

Figure. Relevant anatomy of the lumbar spine

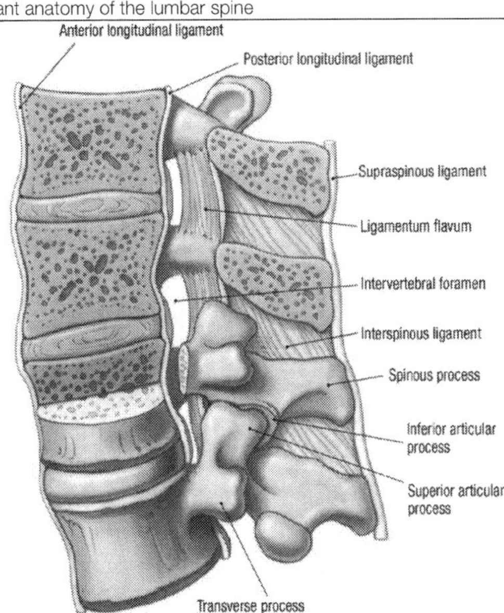

Condition	History	Exam
Axial Pain		
SI Joint	Gluteal Pain Off-midline pain below L5 Worse with rising from sitted position	Compression - Compression of the iliac crest in the lateral position Distraction - Downward pressure on the anterior superior iliac crest FABER - Flexion abduction external rotation of the thigh and hip Gaenslen - Hyperextension of the leg on the affected side Thigh trust - Adduction of the flexed hip on the affected side Fortin finger - Pain localized 1 fingerbreadth of the posterior iliac crest Gillet - Flexion of the leg toward the chest while standing
Facet Joint	Age>65 Pain worse with standing (load) Pain improves with sitting Paraspinal distribution	
Intervertebral Disk	Age<45	

	Worse with sitting Midline pain	
Spinal Stenosis	Age>65 Neurogenic claudication Improved with flexion Pain in buttocks/legs	+Romberg Wide-based gait No pain with spinal flexion Thigh pain with >30sec of back extension
Muscle/Ligament	Delayed onset Decreased mobility	Spasms palpable
Radicular Pain		
Herniated Disk	Known traumatic event Onset 1-2 days after event Sharp/Burning sensation with clear dermatome Improved with sit/laying	Straight leg raising - Patient supine and hip flexed with knee extended Cross straight leg raising - Pain with passive extension of the contralateral Muscle weakness - During ankle dorsiflexion or extension of the great toe Impaired reflexes - Achilles tendon (S1 radiculopathy) Forward flexion - Pain with bending forward in the standing position

- **Examination**
  - Sciatica symptoms
    - Yes
      - Urinary retention, saddle anesthesia, motor weakness, b/l neuro findings
        - Yes → MRI
        - No → ↓activity, NSAIDS, f/u as outpatient
    - No
      - Red Flag Symptoms
        - Age>50
        - Hx of cancer
        - Wt loss
        - Pain >1 month
        - Pain @ HS
        - Not responsive to initial therapy
        - Neurological symptoms
        - Hx of IVDA
        - Recent UTI
      - Yes → Back XR + ESR and if abnormal then MRI
      - No → ↓ activity, NSAIDS, routine f/u and if not improved then do XR with ESR
- **Neurologic Exam**

Disk Herniation						
Nerve Root	Motor deficiency	Sensory deficiency	Reflex	Central	Paracententral	Lateral
L1	None	Inguinal	Cremasteric			
L2	Hip flexion Hip adduction	Proximal anterior/medial thigh	Cremastic			

L3	Hip flexion	Anterior/medial thigh	Patella	Above L2-L3	L2-L3	L3-L4
L4	Knee extension	Anterior leg/medial foot	Patella	Above L3-L4	L3-L4	L4-L5
L5	Dorsiflexion\great toe	Lateral leg/dorsal foot	Medial hamstring	Above L4-L5	L4-L5	L5-S1
S1	Plantar flexion	Posterior leg/lateral foot	Achilles tendon	Above L5-S1	L5-S1	

- **Treatment**
  - Non-Pharmacologic
    - Exercise
    - Pilates
    - Yoga
    - Heat therapy in conjunction with education or NSAIDs is more effective than education or NSAIDs alone at 14 days.
    - PT: McKenzie method and spine stabilization
    - TENS has not been shown in evidenced based literature to be effective for chronic LBP.
  - Pharmacologic
    - Nonsteroidal anti-inflammatory drugs, acetaminophen, and muscle relaxants are effective treatments for nonspecific acute low back pain.
      - Add the muscle relaxer or opiate for short term based on severity of pain
        - Moderate-quality evidence shows that non-benzodiazepine muscle relaxants (e.g., cyclobenzaprine [Flexeril], tizanidine [Zanaflex], metaxalone [Skelaxin]) are beneficial in the treatment of acute low back pain.
          - Skelaxin is non-sedating, 800mg TID
        - There is moderate-quality evidence that muscle relaxants combined with NSAIDs may have additive benefit for reducing pain.
        - Most pain reduction from these medications occurs in the first 7 to 14 days, but the benefit may continue for up to four weeks.
      - Change NSAID type if repeat visits

KNEE EXAMINATION

- **History**[218]
  - Location
    - Anterior
    - Medial
    - Lateral
    - Posterior
  - Characterization of pain
    - Dull
    - Sharp
    - Achy
  - Mechanism of injury
    - Onset
    - Rapid
    - Insidious
  - Associated sounds heard during injury (ie. popping associated with ligamentous injury)
  - Swelling immediately after injury
  - Recent infections
- **Historical Data**

- Injury → suspect ligamentous or meniscal tear
- Popping sensation → consider ACL tear
- Swelling → within hours with ACL tear but if it occurs overnight then consider meniscal
- Locking → meniscal tear
- Buckling → quad weakness, trapped meniscus, ligamentous instability, patellar dislocation
- Pain with climbing/descending stairs → PFPS
- Squatting ↑ pain → meniscus tear
- Jumping pain → patellar tendonitis

- **PMHx**
  - Gout (monosodium urate)
  - Pseudogout (calcium pyrophosphate)
  - Surgeries
  - RA
  - DJD
- **Differential**
  - By Anatomy
    - <u>Patellar Tendon</u>
      - *Cause:* Commonly injured when patient has foot firmly planted in ground and flexes quadriceps
      - *Symptoms:* swelling and tenderness in the anterior portion of the knee; cannot bear weight
      - *Examination*: Unable to actively extend knee (d/t quadriceps requirement)
      - *Treatment*: orthopedic referral due to risk of quadriceps atrophy with ↓ROM of knee
    - <u>Pes Anserine Bursitis[219]</u>
      - *Risk*: m/c in long distance runners, DM
      - *Anatomy:* At point where sartorius, gracilis, and semitendinous tendons meet
      - *Cause*: trauma
      - *Diagnosis: Purely clinical with on imaging required*
        - Pain at medial joint line anterior aspect, approximately 5cm distal to the medial joint line
        - Pain when going up stairs or downstairs
        - Sensitivity to palpation
        - Sometimes local swelling
      - *Treatment*: rest, cryotherapy, NSAIDS
    - <u>ACL</u>
      - *Cause:* direct trauma to anterior portion of knee
      - *Symptoms:* popping sensation, inability to ambulate directly after, ↑pain and laxity upon performance of the anterior drawer test or Lachman maneuver
      - *Examination:* Anterior drawer test with ≥1cm laxity in comparison to other knee
    - <u>PCL</u>
      - *Cause:* posterior directed force on flexed knee (dashboard being struck; hyperextension)
      - *Symptoms*: not associated with much pain or effect on ROM
      - *Examination*: posterior drawer test is positive
    - <u>MCL/LCL</u>
      - *Cause:* dramatic varus or valgus stress; uncommon
      - *Symptoms*: local tenderness

        - *Examination:* local tenderness over joint lines, abnormal valgus and varus stress testing
    - Meniscus
        - *Cause:* sudden twisting movement of knee when knee is firmly planted in ground
        - *Symptoms:* locking sensation to knee
        - *Examination:* McMurray's test (place one hand over the anterior aspect of the knee, with fingers and thumb on the medial and lateral joint lines. Grasp the patient's heel with the other hand and externally rotate the tibia, using the first hand to apply valgus force at the knee during passive flexion and extension. The maneuver is repeated when applying internal rotation and varus stress to test the lateral meniscus) shows popping sensation with audible click/pop during extension
        - *Treatment*: Active rehabilitation is as effective as arthroscopy for improving pain and function in patients with nontraumatic medial meniscal tears and is as good as meniscectomy for improving physical function in patients with meniscal tears and osteoarthritis.
    - Prepatellar Bursitis
        - Inflammation of the bursa sac d/t direct pressure to the patella
        - Trauma directly to knee or a fall or continuous kneeling
    - Patellofemoral Syndrome
        - M/c in W>M age <45
        - Sx: worsened with climbing stairs, extended sitting
        - Dx: patellofemoral compression test (medial and lateral pressure onto the patella with knee in extension → pain)
    - Osteoarthritis[220]
        - *Treatment*
            - PT and exercise are the foundation of therapy
            - If locking or catching sensation → likely meniscal tear requiring ortho referral
            - If BMI> 25 then lose weight through monitored exercise program
            - Otherwise, treat with Tylenol (1300mg TID) +/- NSAIDs with addition of Tramadol/Injections/Brace if ineffective. If continued pain, can consider opiates or ortho referral.
- By Mechanism Of Injury
    - Varus stress → LCL damage
    - Valgus stress → MCL damage
    - Deceleration with twisting/pivoting motion → ACL
    - Twisting while pivoting on knee → Meniscal tear

- **Exam**
    - Duck walk – to perform successfully, must have intact ligament system, no meniscal damage, no OA
    - Standing – look for resting deformities
- **Imaging (to r/o fracture)**

  Ottawa Knee Rules

  1) Age>55
  2) Tenderness @ head of fibula
  3) Isolated patellar tenderness
  4) Cannot flex > 90 degrees
  5) Cannot bear weight and/or complete 4 steps

  if suspect osteoarthritis then obtain weight bearing films

Figure. Superficial landmarks on knee examination

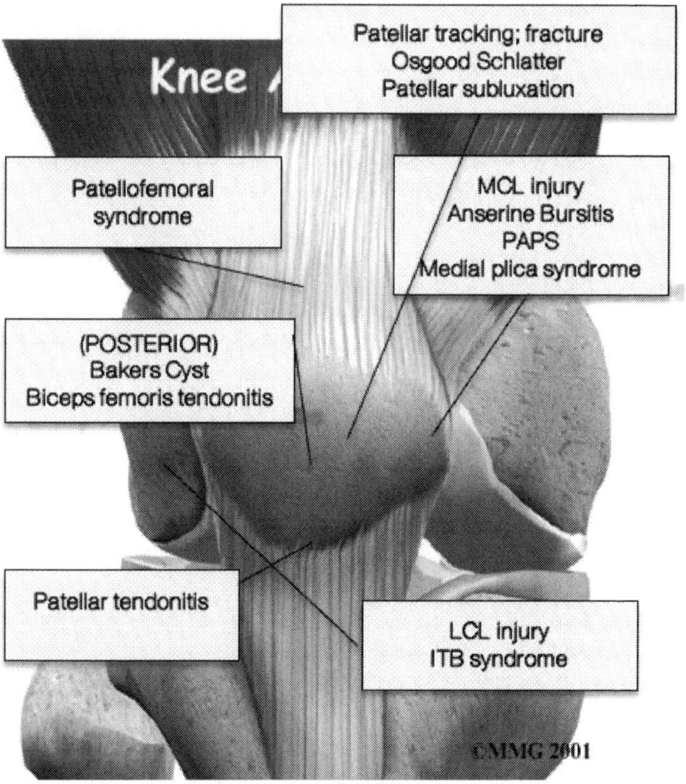

Evaluation of knee pain based on location of pain

Location	Pathology	Mechanism	Symptoms	Evaluation	Treatment
Joint Lines	Meniscal Tear	Sudden twisting or pivoting	"Locking" Slow onset effusion or recurrent Pain with squatting	• Tenderness of the joint line • McMurray's test (place one hand over the anterior aspect of the knee, with fingers and thumb on the medial and lateral joint lines. Grasp the patient's heel with the other hand and externally rotate the tibia, using the first hand to apply valgus force at the knee during passive flexion and extension. The maneuver is repeated when applying internal rotation and varus stress to test the lateral meniscus) shows popping sensation with audible click/pop during extension	• RICE • PT to strengthen the muscular support of the knee • Consider evaluation by Orthopedic Surgery (↑ likelihood in severe twisting injuries, concurrent ACL tear, knee locking, pain w/ McMurray, no improvement with 3-6 weeks of PT)
N/A	Ligament Tear	PAL: dashboard; hyperextension LAL: medial force MAL: lateral force AAL: twisting while planted foot; quick start and stop; hyperextension	"Popping" "Giving way" Immediate swelling <2hrs Cannot walk immed. after	▪ ACL ▫ Anterior drawer test with ≥1cm laxity in comparison to other knee ▫ Lachman's test - The test is performed with the patient in a supine position and the injured knee flexed to 30 degrees. The physician stabilizes the distal femur with one hand, grasps the proximal	• RICE • PT • Surgical evaluation

				tibia in the other hand, and then attempts to sublux the tibia anteriorly ▪ PCL ▫ Posterior drawer test is positive ▪ MCL/LCL ▫ Local tenderness over joint lines, abnormal valgus and varus stress testing	
Anterior	Patellofemoral (PFPS)	Overuse Training Errors Recent alteration in training program History of knee trauma or surgery	Pain with walking up and down stairs Squatting Kneeling "Giving way" Gradual onset anterior knee pain Theatre sign (prolonged knee flexion) Pain under/behind or around patella	Positive Patellar Grind Test - Accomplished by pressing the patella away from the femoral condyles while asking the patient to contrast the quadriceps muscles. A positive test is represented by sudden patellar pain and relaxation of the muscle. The opposite test involves lifting the patella away from the knee joint while passively bending and straightening the knee. If this relieves pain, the patellofemoral joint is likely the source. Other Tests - Pain with squatting, patellar tilt pain Patients often have more pain with rest and complain of giving-way sensation	Often caused by weak quadriceps, hip strengthening, hip flexors, and IT band 3x/week for 8 weeks PT, bracing (limited evidence to support the use of the lateral patellar buttress brace), patellar taping, normal gait biomechanics

Anterior Superior	Patellar Tendonitis (Jumper's Knee)	Jumping Uphill running Squatting Stand from sitting	Anterior knee pain that is tender on exam	Focal pain to the inferior pole of the patella and proximal tendon. Pain with single-leg decline squat is characteristic.	Rest NSAIDs NO STEROIDS! Surgery if not improved after 3 months
Medial	Medial Plica Syndrome	Genetic Overuse	Anterior knee pain Snapping sensation as the plica moves over the femoral condyle	Palpable band parallel to the medial border of the patella	MRI for diagnosis PT
	Pes Anserine Bursitis	Tendinous insertion of the Sartorius, Gracilis, and Semitendinosus get inflamed	Pain on medial knee Increased pain w/ flexion and extension	Tenderness to medial aspect of knee posterior and distal to the joint line No effusion Reproduced pain with valgus move	• Rest • Consider steroid injection
Lateral	IT Band Syndrome	Distance runners Analysts	Pain reproduced after reaching certain milage	Noble compression test - The examiner applies pressure along the palpable iliotibial band approximately 2 cm proximal to the lateral femoral epicondyle while passively flexing the knee from 0 to 60 degrees. A positive result is pain at 30 degrees of flexion. Noble test - With the patient in a supine position, the physician places a thumb over the lateral femoral epicondyle as the patient repeatedly flexes and extends the knee. Pain symptoms are	Rest Decrease distance Changing shoes Stretching+NSAID combo Steroid injections

				usually most prominent with the knee at 30 degrees of flexion.	
	Popliteus Tendinitis	Excessive use of quadriceps	Posterior lateral aspect of the knee Downhill running	Webb test - internally rotate the leg in the supine patient, the knee is flexed at 90 degrees, with the patient then forcing external rotation while the examiner provides resistance. A positive test produces pain with the maneuver.	Test NSAIDs

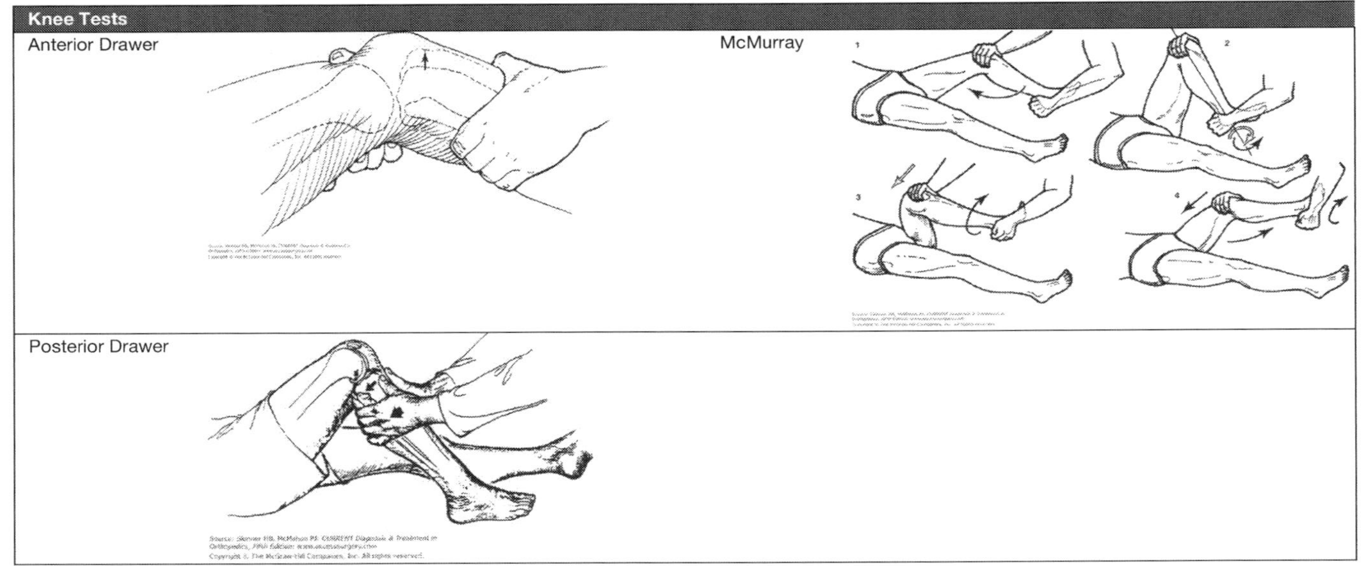
Knee Tests
Anterior Drawer
McMurray
1
2
3
4
Posterior Drawer

APPROACH TO KNEE EFFUSION

- **Etiologies**[221,222]
  - Hemorhagic
    - Traumatic (ligament injury, meniscal injury, articular injury)
    - Anticoagulants
    - Hemophilia
  - Inflammatory
    - RA
    - Gout
    - Septic arthritis
    - Reactive arthritis
  - Infectious
    - Gonorrhea (younger patients)
    - Lyme
    - TB
  - Non-Inflammatory
    - OA
    - Cancer
- **History and Physical**
  - Recent trauma → fracture (look for ecchymosis, deformity, acute swelling)
  - Knee 'gives way', unstable, aut or pivot movement → AAL tear (positive drawer sign, acute swelling <4 hrs after incident)
  - Cannot squat, clicking/locking → Meniscal tear (joint line tenderness, +Apley's, +McMurray, acute swelling <4 hrs after incident)
  - Repetitive causational movement → overuse syndrome
  - Recent sex, no trauma, fevers, chills→ Infectious (look for erythema, swelling, +joint aspiration)
  - Night pain, fevers, weight loss → tumor (+imaging, joint aspiration)
- **Imaging**
  - Most common: AP, lateral, axial patellar. Get lateral @ 15-30 degrees flexion if effusion suspected
  - MRI not necessary to diagnose AAL/PAL tear, simple AP enough with PE
  - Ottawa Rules
    1) Inability to bear weight after incident or in ER (no more than 4 steps)
    2) Age 55+
    3) Isolated tenderness to the patella or head of fibula
    4) Cannot flex more than 90 degrees

Joint Fluid Analysis

Findings	Normal	Noninflammatory	Inflammatory	Septic	Hemorrhagic
Color	Clear	Yellow	Yellow to green	Yellow	Red
Clarity	Transparent	Transparent	Opaque	Opaque	Bloody
Viscosity	High	High	Low	Variable	Variable
WBC per mm^3	< 200	200 to 2,000	2,000 to 50,000	50,000 to 200,000	200-2500
PMNs	< 25%	< 25%	> 50%	> 75%	50-75%
Mucin	Good	Good	Good to	Poor	Unk

clot			poor		
Protein g/dL	N/A	1-3	3-5	3-5	4-6
Glucose mg/dL	N/A	=blood	<blood	<<blood	=blood

Figure. Evaluation of the swollen knee

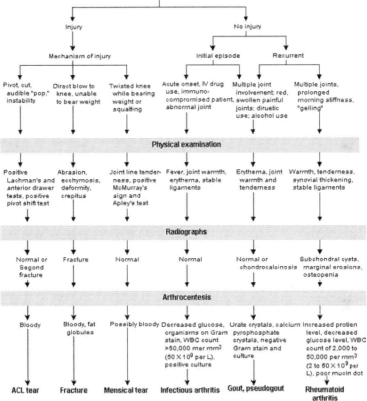

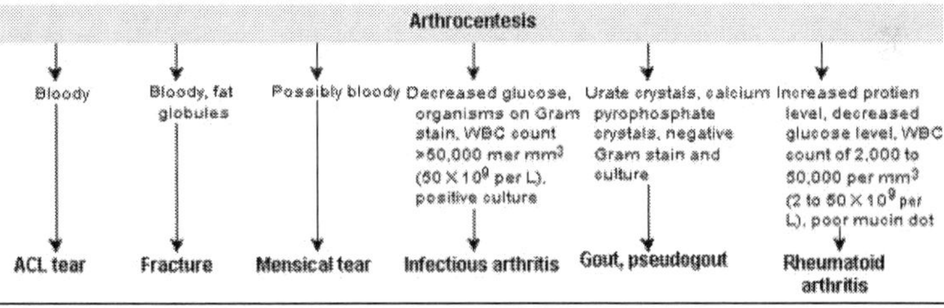

LEG/ANKLE/FOOT PAIN DIFFERENTIAL

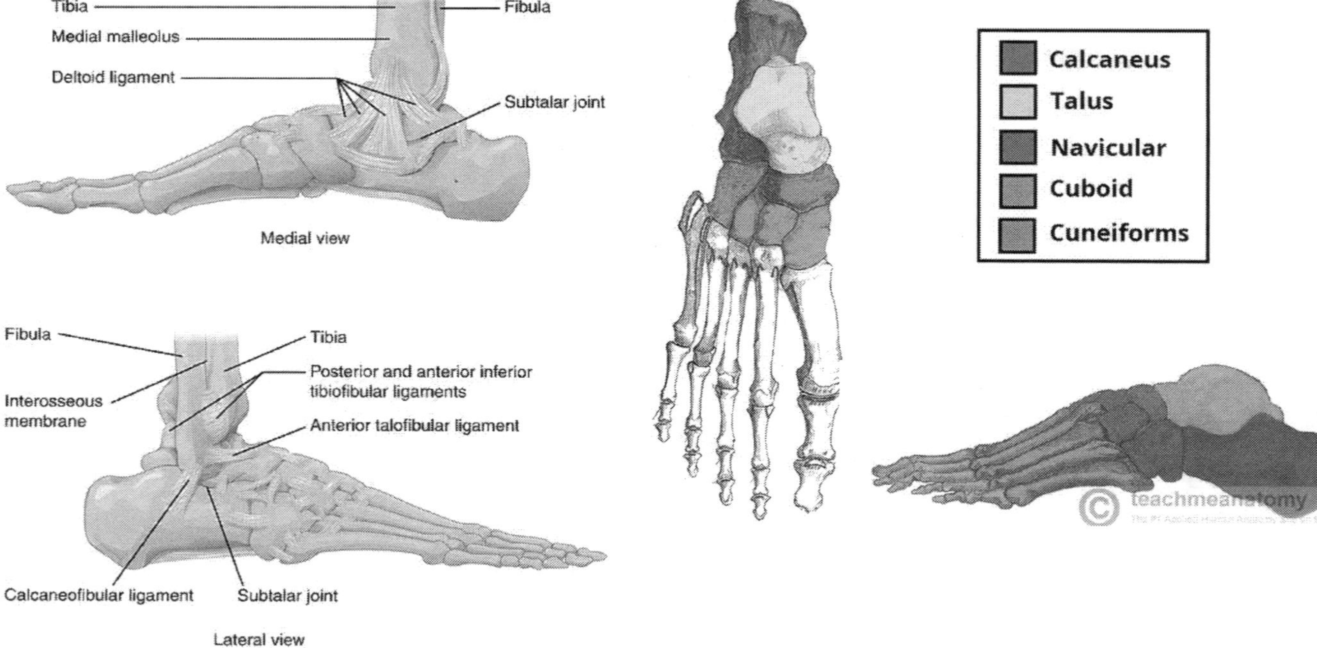
Tibia
Fibula
Medial malleolus
Deltoid ligament
Subtalar joint
Medial view
Fibula
Tibia
Interosseous membrane
Posterior and anterior inferior tibiofibular ligaments
Anterior talofibular ligament
Calcaneofibular ligament
Subtalar joint
Lateral view
Calcaneus
Talus
Navicular
Cuboid
Cuneiforms
teachmeanatomy

Evaluation of ankle/foot pain

Location	Pathology	Mechanism	Symptoms	Evaluation	Treatment
Ankle	Achilles Tendinopathy	Overuse	Posterior heel pain	Pain/swelling/tenderness at 2-6cm above insertion into the calcaneus	Eccentric heel-lowering exercises performed with toes on a step so that the heel can be lowered below the toes Shock wave therapy has limited evidence of benefit, with improvement in patients with insertional tendinopathy but not for those with the more common midportion tendinopathy. Injections and surgical techniques have insufficient evidence of benefit.16,41
Foot	Plantar Fasciopathy (Plantar Fasciitis)		Pain typically located at the medial calcaneal tubercle and is worse with early morning ambulation, and improves with activity	Tenderness over the medial calcaneal tubercle that extends along the plantar fascia, often with crepitus, thickness, or swelling Plantar fascia thickness of more than 4 mm on ultrasonography or plain radiography can support the diagnosis	Passive stretching of the plantar fascia (e.g., pulling back toes with a hand or towel and active strength training (e.g., heel raises) are recommended. A meta-analysis showed that foot orthoses with arch support led to improvement in pain and function after 11 weeks.

				The Windlass test, in which the toes are passively extended, can elicit pain by stretching the fascia	Local steroid injections reduce pain at one month but not afterward.

Leg Pain Differential

Location	Pathology	Mechanism	Symptoms	Evaluation	Treatment
Tibia	Medial Tibial Stress Syndrome (Shin Splints)	Overuse	Presents with pain over the middle or distal one-third of the posteromedial tibial border	The most sensitive physical examination finding is tenderness to palpation over the posteromedial tibial border. XR is useful if a tibial stress fracture is suspected. MRI is more sensitive and specific than bone scans for dx.	Treatment is conservative. Relative rest and calf stretching are recommended because evidence links tightness in the soleus and posterior tibialis to medial tibial stress syndrome.
Tibia	Tibial Stress Fracture	Rapid increases in activity	Present with pain and tenderness on palpation, most commonly in the middle to distal 1/3 of the anterior tibia	Patients with significant pain or difficulty walking should undergo MRI.	Temporary (6 to 8 weeks) vacation from running, with continued weight bearing unless walking is painful. Return to activity should be slow and dependent on pain levels. Surgery may be considered for failure of union.

SHOULDER EXAMINATION

- **History**[223,224]
  - Scapular winging, trauma, recent viral illness → Serratus anterior or trapezius dysfunction
  - Seizure and inability to passively or actively rotate affected arm externally → Posterior shoulder dislocation
  - Supraspinatus/infraspinatus wasting → Rotator cuff tear; suprascapular nerve entrapment
  - Pain radiating below elbow; decreased cervical range of motion → Cervical disc disease
  - Shoulder pain in throwing athletes; anterior glenohumeral joint pain and impingement → Glenohumeral joint instability
  - Duration (acute<6 weeks; subacute 6-12 weeks; chronic >3 months)
  - Pain or "clunking" sound with overhead motion → Labral disorder
  - Nighttime shoulder pain → tear
- **Examination**

Figure. Demonstration of different shoulder range of motion positions

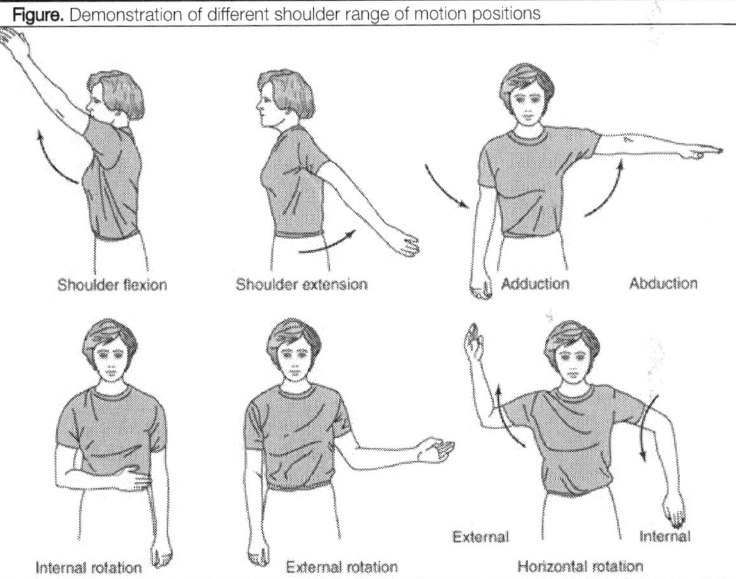

Muscle Specific Testing		
Demonstration	Muscle	Test Name
	Subscapularis	"Bear-hug test" Lift Off
	Infraspinatus Teres Minor	External-rotation test
	Supraspinatus	Empty Can Test

- **Common Diagnoses**
  - Impingement
    Lateral pain, subacute, worse with movement overhead. Neer and Hawkins are best.
    - *Subacromial Bursitis* - Pain occurs during arm elevation **beyond 90°** (impingement position) and is frequently referred down the upper arm (deltoid region) to the mid-humerus.
    - *Supraspinatus/rotator cuff tendonitis* - Pain occurs especially during active or resisted **abduction** and frequently radiates down the upper arm (deltoid region) to the mid-humerus.
  - Biceps tendonitis - Pain during forward flexion and forearm supination is usually felt anteriorly in the region of the bicipital groove.
  - Rotator Cuff Tear – sudden onset, drop arm positive, pain at night, weakness
  - Adhesive Capsulitis / Frozen Shoulder – distant injury with minimal ROM, inability to reach over head
  - GH arthritis
  - AC joint arthritis

- **Diagnosis (see table below and following diagnostic maneuvers)**

Imaging modality	Advantages	Disadvantages
MRI	95% sensitivity and specificity in detecting complete rotator cuff tears, cuff degeneration, chronic tendonitis and partial cuff tears No ionizing radiation	Often identifies an apparent "abnormality" in an asymptomatic patient
Arthrography	Good at identifying complete rotator cuff tear or adhesive capsulitis (frozen shoulder)	Invasive Relatively poor at diagnosing a partial rotator cuff tear
Ultrasonography	Accurately diagnoses complete rotator cuff tears	Less useful in identifying partial cuff tears Operator-dependent interpretation
MRI arthrography	Reliably identifies full-thickness rotator cuff tears and labral tears	Invasive
CT scanning	May be useful in diagnosis of subtle dislocation	Ionizing radiation

- **Treatment**
    - Impingement/RCD – ice/heat, analgesics, HEP, if no improvement after 3 months then referral to orthopedics
    - Tear – consider surgical referral

Systematic evaluation of the shoulder

Order	Test	Description
1	Appearance	Symmetry, bulk, deformities, atrophy above or below the scapular spine. Atrophy in the space below the scapular spine suggests RCD or injury to the suprascapular nerve.
2	Palpation	Sternoclavicular joint, clavicle, acromioclavicular joint, lateral acromion, biceps tendon in the groove between the greater and lesser tubercle of the humerus. Remember: some patients can be tender at many points, but you are trying to recreate the pain that they have been experiencing at home. The anterior joint line can be palpated.
3	ROM	ROM testing identifies limitations in ROM and localizes pain. Start with these basic ROM tests with the patient standing. Test active ROM first and add passive ROM if the patient has pain or limited motion. All maneuvers start from the anatomic position with arms at the side and palms facing forward. • Flexion - 160-180 degrees • Extension - 40-60 degrees • Abduction - raise arm from side to overhead; normal is 180 degrees. - 0-90 is determined by supraspinatus and deltoid. - After 90 degrees, trapezius and serratus anterior - **Painful arc** is 60-120 and is indicative of subacromial impingement - 120-180 is due to AC joint pathology • Adduction - 45 degrees • External Rotation - hold arms in front of body with elbow bent 90 degrees and palms facing in moving away from center. Normal is 55-80 degrees. Pain here localizes to teres minor and infraspinatus. • Internal Rotation - hold arms in front of body with elbow bent 90 degrees and palms facing in and move towards center. Normal ROM is 45 degrees. Pain here localizes to the subscapularis.

4	Impingement/RCD	• <u>Hawkins-Kennedy</u> - Patient holds arm at 90 flexion with elbow at 90 flexion. Place downward pressure on the forearm and passively internally rotate the arm. *Positive test: Tear* *Muscle: supraspinatus/teres minor/infraspinatus* *Movement* – internal rotation • <u>Neer's</u> - The patient internally rotates their hand (thumb toward the ground). Place your hand on the back of the patient's shoulder to stabilize the scapula. Forward flex the patient's straight arm by grasping just below the elbow and lifting. *Muscle: No specific group* *Movement: Flexion* *Positive test: Impingement subacromial structures to humeral head*	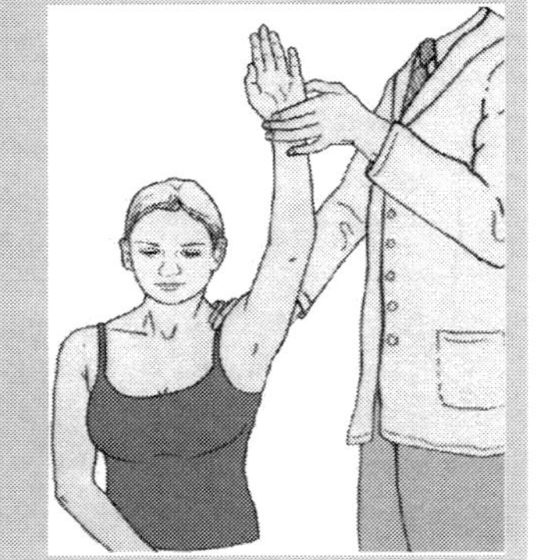

- Empty Can - Patient starts with a straight arm at 90 abduction. The arm is then brought forward 30 toward center on the horizontal plane and the thumb rotated toward the floor. Apply gentle pressure downward above the elbow while patient attempts to resist this pressure. Pain suggests impingement of the **supraspinatus**. Weakness suggests a partial- or full-thickness tear.

  Muscle: Supraspinatus
  Movement: adduction
  Positive test: Tear

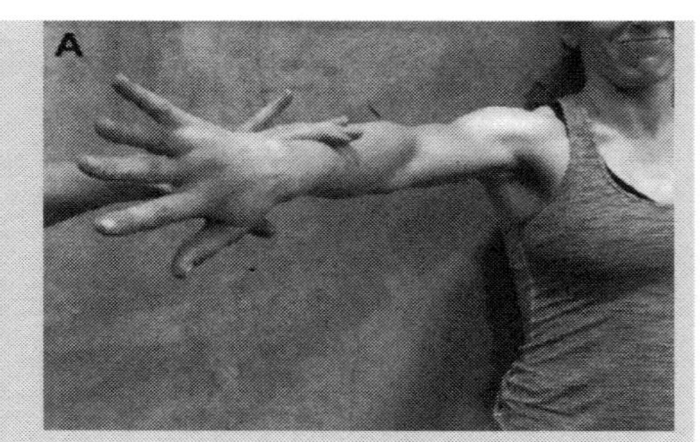

- Lift Off - Patient internally rotates shoulder. Place the back of their hand against the small of the back. Internal rotation against resistance. Examiner resists patient's attempt to force their hand away from their back. Weakness suggests a subscapularis muscle tear or impingement

  Muscle: Subscapularis
  Movement: Internal rotation
  Positive test: Impingement

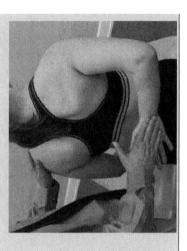

- <u>External Push Off</u> - Placing the patient's arm at the side in neutral rotation and with the elbow flexed. Support the elbow and instruct the patient to maintain this position while you apply moderate to firm pressure at the distal forearm, attempting to internally rotate the arm.

  Positive test: Impingement
  Muscle: Infraspinatus + Teres minor

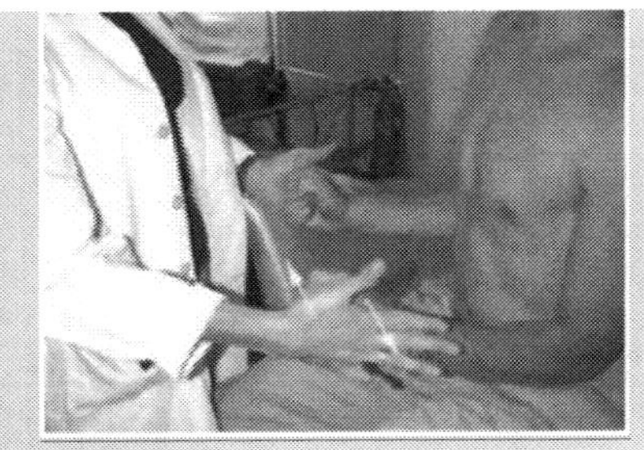

- <u>Belly Press</u> - A positive "belly-press" test is the inability to hold the elbow in front of the trunk while pressing down with the hand on the belly. A positive belly press test indicates subscapularis tendon insufficiency.

  Muscle: Subscapularis
  Movement: Internal rotation
  Positive test: Impingement

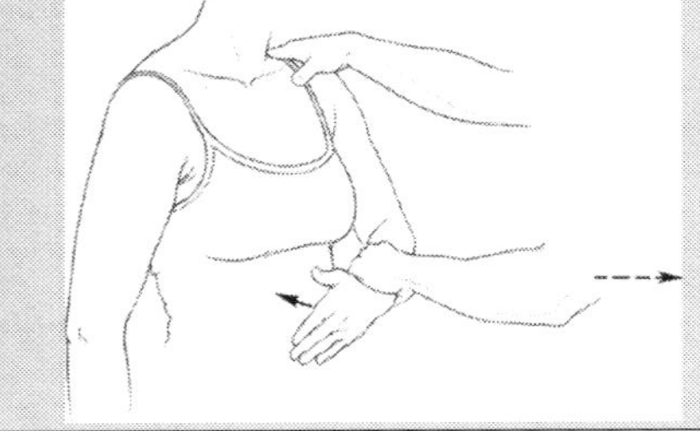

		• <u>Drop Arm</u> - Passively abduct shoulder to 160 degrees. Once at the position, the patient will now attempt to slowly bring arm back to their side by adducting. If the arm suddenly drops, or gives way with a tap, consider rotator cuff tear *Positive test: Tear*	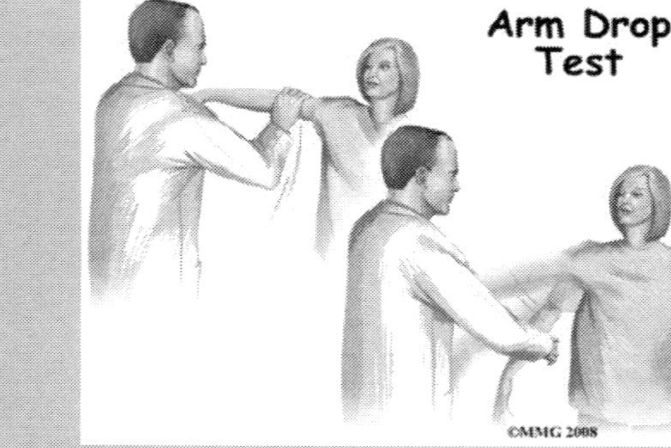
5	Other tests if not suspecting impingement or RCD	*Concern for biceps pathology* • <u>Speed's</u> - Forward flex arm to 50 degrees. Keep palm up. Elbow should be slightly flexed at 15 degrees. Provide resistance against patient trying to keep shoulder up (examiner pushes down). Pain suggestive of biceps tendonitis • <u>Yergason's</u> - The patient flexes their elbow to 90. Provide resistance to supination. A positive test is pain in area of bicipital groove.	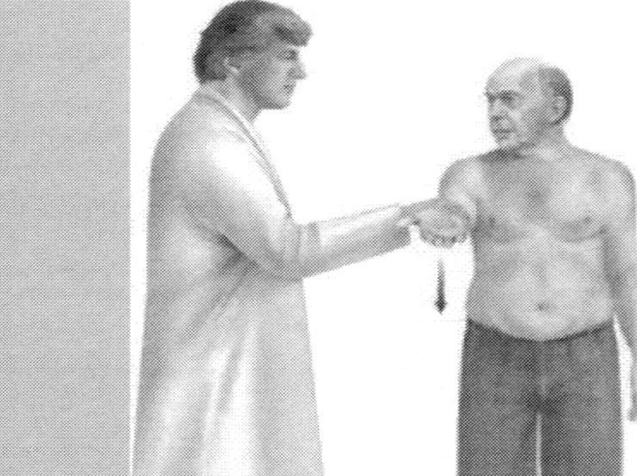

*Concern for **labral** tear (lateral or anterior shoulder pain)*

- O'Brien - Performed to rule out labral cartilage tears that often occur following a shoulder subluxation or dislocation. The test involves flexing the patient's arm to 90 degrees, fully internally rotating the arm so the thumb is facing down (palm down) and adducting the arm to 10 degrees. Once positioned properly, the clinician applies downward force and asks the patient to resist. The test is then repeated in the same position except that the patient has his arm fully supinated (palm up). A positive O'Brien test for labral tear is pain deep in the shoulder with palm down more than the palm up.

  The O'Brien test can also be used to identify AC joint pathology. The patient would typically complain equally of pain directly over the AC joint with the palm down or up.

  - Speed's - examiner places the patient's arm in shoulder flexion, external rotation, full elbow extension, and forearm supination; manual resistance is then applied by the examiner in a downward direction. The test is considered to be positive if pain in the bicipital tendon or bicipital groove is reproduced.
  - Crank - This test is usually performed with the patient in sitting but can also be performed with the patient in supine or standing. The examiner flexes the patients elbow to 90 degrees and elevates the patient's arm to approximately 160 degrees in the scapular plane. In

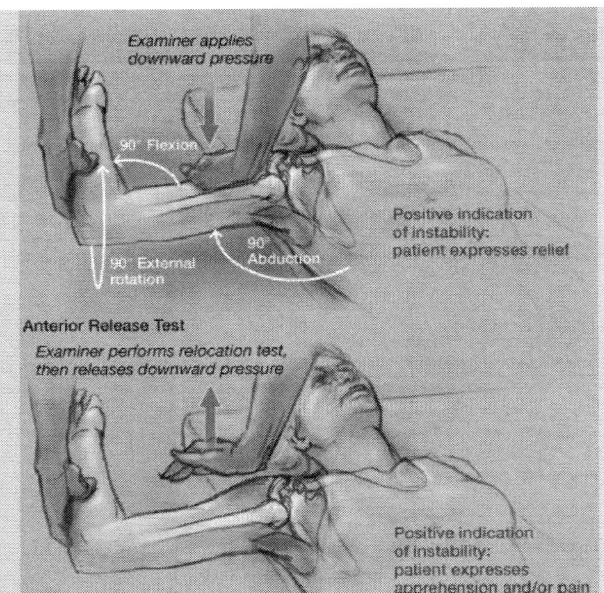
Examiner applies downward pressure
90° Flexion
90° External rotation
90° Abduction
Positive indication of instability: patient expresses relief
Anterior Release Test
Examiner performs relocation test, then releases downward pressure
Positive indication of instability: patient expresses apprehension and/or pain

	this position, the examiner applies a gentle compressive force on the glenohumeral joint along the axis of the humerus while simultaneously moving the humerus into internal and external rotation	

NEUROLOGY

Figure. Eye muscles and associated directions of function

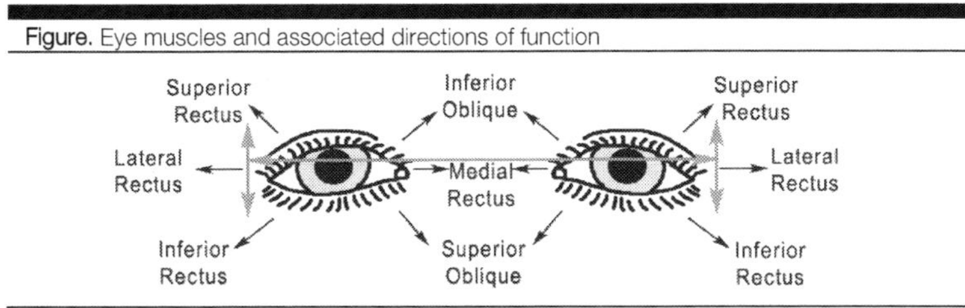

Figure. Anterior dermatomes

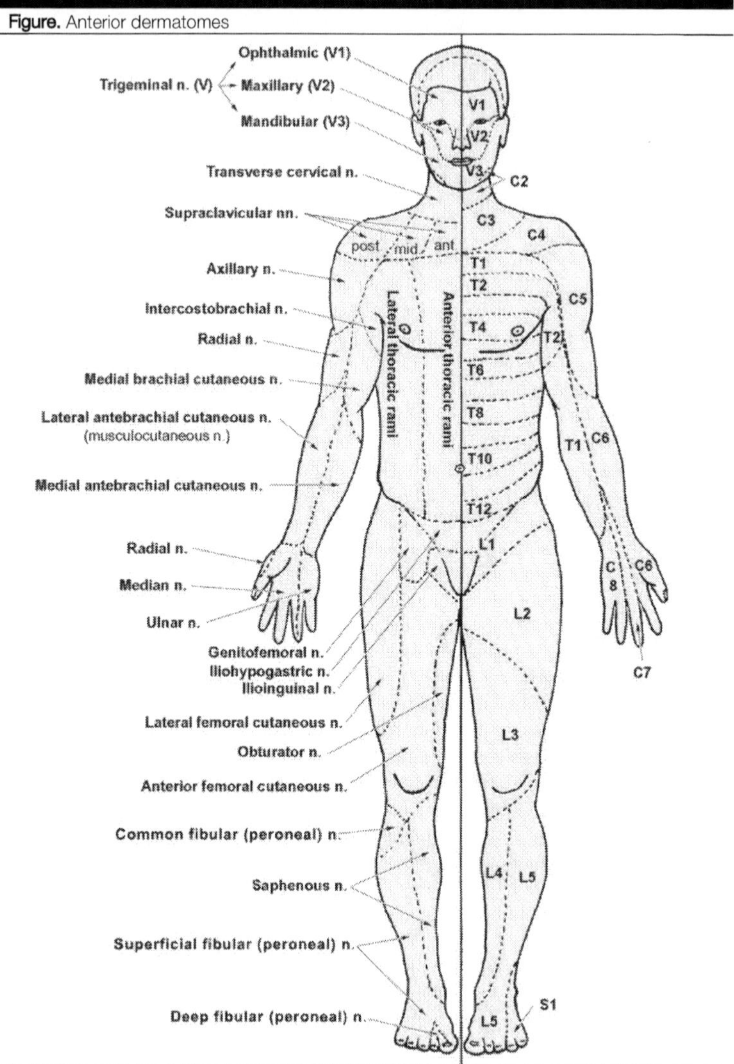

Ophthalmic (V1)
Trigeminal n. (V)
Maxillary (V2)
Mandibular (V3)
Transverse cervical n.
Supraclavicular nn.
post
mid
ant
Axillary n.
Intercostobrachial n.
Radial n.
Medial brachial cutaneous n.
Lateral antebrachial cutaneous n.
(musculocutaneous n.)
Medial antebrachial cutaneous n.
Radial n.
Median n.
Ulnar n.
Genitofemoral n.
Iliohypogastric n.
Ilioinguinal n.
Lateral femoral cutaneous n.
Obturator n.
Anterior femoral cutaneous n.
Common fibular (peroneal) n.
Saphenous n.
Superficial fibular (peroneal) n.
Deep fibular (peroneal) n.
Lateral thoracic rami
Anterior thoracic rami
V1
V2
V3
C2
C3
C4
T1
T2
C5
T4
T2
T6
T8
T1
C6
T10
T12
L1
C8
C6
L2
C7
L3
L4
L5
S1
L5

Figure. Posterior dermatomes

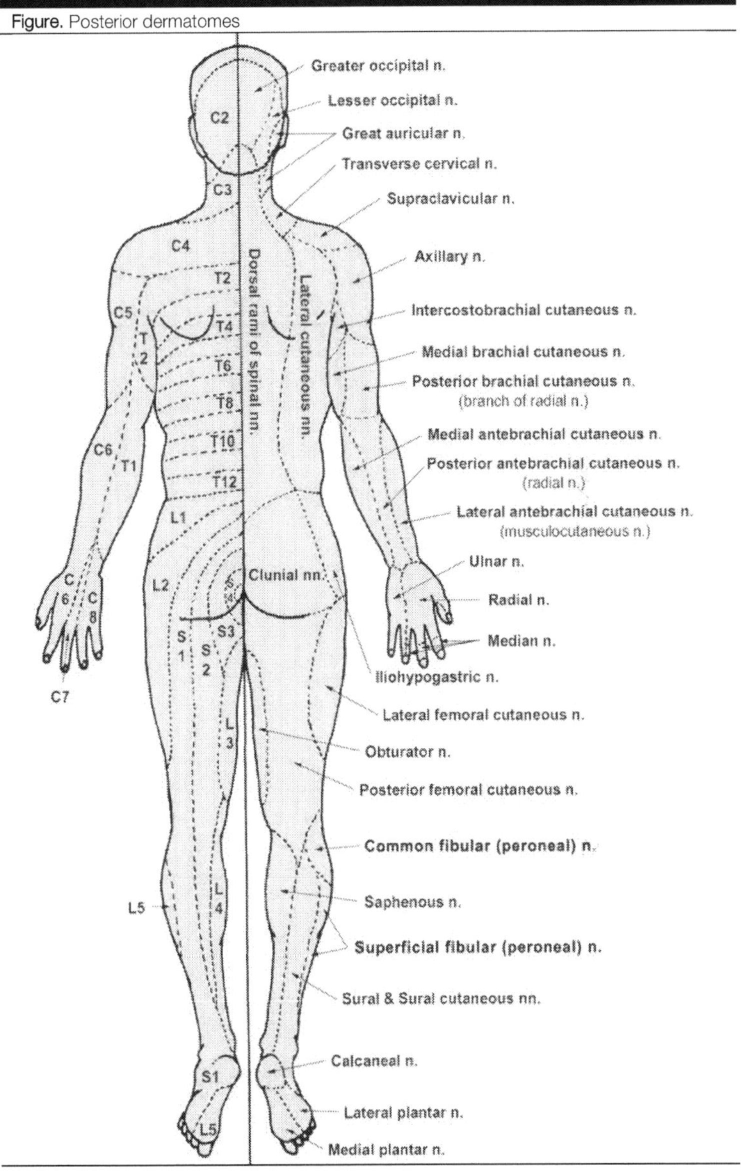

NEUROLOGICAL EXAM

- MS: AA&Ox3, appropriately interactive, normal affect
- Attention: WORLD backwards, MOY backwards, digit span 4 forwards, 3 back

- Speech: fluent w/o paraphasic error, repetition, naming, reading, writing intact
- Memory: x/3 at 5 minutes, x/3 with prompting
- Calculations: 9 quarters = $2.25
- L/R confusion: No L/R confusion
- Praxis: Able to mimic brushing teeth and blowing out match with either hand.
- Cranial Nerves
  - CN: I--not tested
  - II, III--PERRLA, VF by confrontation, optic discs sharp
  - III,IV, VI—EOMI w/o nystagmus, no ptosis
  - V--sensation intact to LT, masseters strong symmetricallyVII--face symmetric without weakness
  - VIII—hearing grossly intact
  - IX,X--voice normal, palate elevates symmetrically, gag intact
  - XI--SCM/trapezii 5/5
  - XII--tongue protrudes midline, no atrophy or fasciculation.
- Motor: normal bulk and tone, no tremor, rigidity or bradykinesia, no pronator drift. No orbital movement.
- Strength
- Coordination: rapid alternating and point-to-point (FNF, HTS, TTF) movements intact.
- Language: receptive and expressive language intact
- Visuospatial: normal clock-drawing
- Motor:
  - Upper extremity
    - Shoulder abduction (c5 – deltoid/supraspinatus) 5/5
    - Shoulder adduction 5/5
    - Elbow flexion (c5/c6 -biceps brachii – musculocutaneous nerve) 5/5
    - Elbow extension (c7 -triceps -radial nerve) 5/5
    - Wrist flexion (c7 – fcr/fcu – median/ulnar) 5/5
    - Wrist extension (c6 – ecr/ecu – radial nerve) 5/5
    - Finger adduction (t1-interossei-ulnar) 5/5
    - Thumb radial abduction (c7 – apl – radial nerve) 5/5
    - Thumb opposition (c8/t1 -opponens pollicis – median nerve) 5/5
  - Lower extremity
    - Hip flexion (l1/l2 – iliopsoas muscle) 5/5
    - Hip extension (l5/s1 – gluteus maximus muscle) 5/5
    - Knee flexion (l5/s1 -hamstrings -sciatica nerve) 5/5
    - Knee extension (l3/l4 -quadriceps femoris muscle -femoral nerve) 5/5
    - Ankle dorsiflexion (l4/l5 -tibialis anterior muscle -deep peroneal nerve) 5/5
    - Ankle plantarflexion (s1 – gastrocnemius muscle -tibial nerve) 5/5
    - Ankle eversion (l5/s1 -peroneus longus/brevis – superficial peroneal nerve) 5/5
    - Ankle inversion (l4/l5 -tibialis posterior muscle – tibial nerve) 5/5
    - Extensor hallucis longus (l4/l5 – ehl/edls – deep peroneal nerve) 5/5
    - Flexor hallucis longus (s1 – fhl, fdls – tibial nerve) 5/5
- Sensory:
  - Lateral spinothalamic – pinprick, temperature nl
  - Dorsal columns – proprioception nl
  - Cortical – graphesthesia nl, proprioception nl

SYNCOPE / LOSS OF CONSCIOUSNESS

- **Definition**[225, 226]

- Transient global cerebral hypoperfusion characterized by rapid onset, short duration, and spontaneous complete recover
- Presyncope refers to the symptoms (nausea, LH, sweating, weakness, visual changes) that occur before syncope without actual LOC

- **Admission**
  - Definitely admit:
    - HPI: chest pain
    - PMH: CAD, CHF, ventricular arrhythmia
    - PE: CHF, valvular disease, focal neurologic deficit or disorder
    - ECG: ischemia, arrhythmia, bundle branch block, prolonged QT
  - Strongly consider admission:
    - HPI: age > 70, exertional syncope, frequent syncope, cardiac disease suspected
    - PE: tachycardia, moderate to severe orthostasis, injury
- **Initial Assessment**
  - EKG
    - Rule out arrhythmias such as Brugada, VT, AF
  - Postural BPs
  - Optional
    - TTE
    - CT (if head trauma)

Figure. Differential diagnosis to consider for transient loss of consciousness

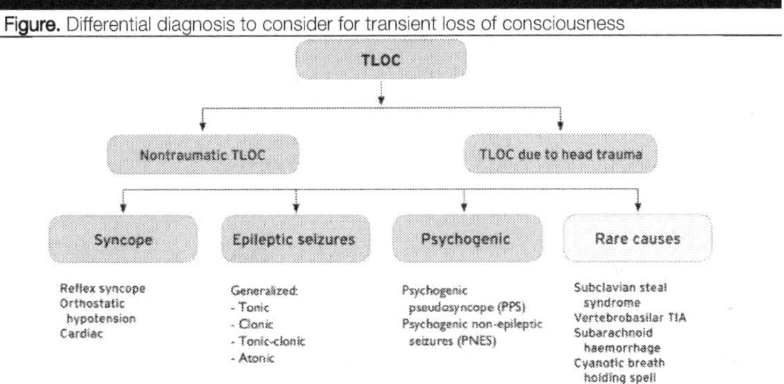

- **Major Causes/Classification**[227]
  - Reflex
    - Posture
    - Provoking event (ie. micturition, GI stimulation, cough, laughing)
    - Prodromal symptoms
  - Orthostatic Hypotension
    - Medications (vasodilators, anti-depressants)
    - Hemorrhage, diarrhea, vomiting
    - Autonomic failure 2/2 nervous system dysfunction - POTS, postural orthostatic hypotension, vasovagal syncope. Secondary failure from DM, amyloidosis, etc.
  - Cardiac
    - Bradycardia (sinus node dysfunction, AV conduction dz)
    - Tachycardia (SVT, VT)
    - Structural (AS, ACS, HCM, tamponade, PE, dissection)
- **Mimics of syncope**
  - Metabolic: hypoxia, hypoglycemia, hyperventilation

- Subclavian Steal
- Intoxication
- Epilepsy
- Carotid TIA

Differential Diagnosis	
Reflex	
Vasovagal	Emotional distress
Situational	Cough, sneeze GI stimulated (swallow, defecation) Micturition Post-exercise Post-prandial
Atypical	
Orthostatic Hypotension (Consider tilt table testing)	
Primary Autonomic Failure	MSA, Parkinson's disease, Lewy Body Dementia
Secondary Autonomic Failure	DM, amyloidosis, uremia, spinal cord injuries
Drug-induced	EtOH, vasodilators, diuretics, anti-depressants
↓Volume	Hemorrhage, diarrea, vomiting
Postprandial Hypotension	Defined as drop in SBP by 20 or more points within 2 hours of eating; important to ask patient when the events occur (around meal time); symptoms include dizziness, near syncope, syncope, weakness, angina. Mechanism is not fully understood. Patients at higher risk include those on BP medications, diuretics, low salt diet. Treatment includes avoiding sitting for long periods after eating, liberal salt intake if possible with adequate fluids, avoid EtOH.
Cardiac	
Arrythmia	• Bradyarrhythmia o Sinus node dysfunction o AV conduction disease / Heart block • Tachyarrhythmia o Supraventricular arrhythmia o Ventricular arrhythmia (MOST important one to exclude risk of sudden cardiac death in patients with history of cardiac disease) • Other o QT prolongation o Brugada
Structural	Valvular disease (aortic stenosis, mitral stenosis, pulmonary stenosis), global ischemia, aortic dissection, obstructive cardiomyopathy, left atrial myxoma, prosthetic valve dysfunction, pulmonary embolus, pulmonary hypertension (careful cardiac auscultation and obtain ECHO)

- **Evaluation**
  - Exam: Supine and standing BP, BP (look for unexplained ↓SBP below 90 mmHg), GIB on rectal exam, HR<40 bpm, new SEM
    - Orthostatics: abnormal ↓ in SBP by ≥20mmHg or DBP ≥10mmHg or overall ↓ in SBP to <90mmHg
    - Consider tilt table testing if orthostatic hypotension suspected
  - Diagonstics: ECG, TTE if previous known heart dz present or concern for structural heart dz

        - *ECG findings*: look for bifascicular block, complete heart block or second degree type 2 block, ↑QRS duration, inappropriate sinus bradycardia (or slow afib), ↑ST segment, LVH, Type 1 Brugada, sVT or nsVT, dysfunction in implanted pacemaker, QTc>460ms
        - *Carotid sinus massage*: ventricular pause >3s or a ↓ in SBP of >50mmHg concerning for carotid hypersensitivity (often seen with tight collars, shaving, rotating head history leading to syncope)
    - Labs: CBC, TROP, d-dimer, ABG
- **Management**
    - Answer the following questions to determine management:
        - Is there a serious underlying cause that can be identified? Often r/o with above diagnostics and history/exam
        - What is the risk of a serious outcome?

High and Low risk symptoms in evaluation of syncope
High-risk (should be admitted)
Major
• New onset chest pain, SOB, DOE, abdominal pain, or HA
• Syncope during exercise or when supine
• Sudden onset palpitations leading to syncope
Minor (only considered high risk if below findings found with structural heart dz or ECG findings)
• No prodromal symptoms or short (<10 seconds) prodrome
• Family history of SCD at young age
• Syncope while sitting
Low-risk (typically can be sent home)
• Typical reflex syncope suspected based on hx (LH, warmth, sweating, n/v)
• Unpleasant sound, smell, pain leading to syncope
• Syncope after prolonged standing or in crowded place
• Syncope after meal
• Syncope after cough, defecation or micturition
• Syncope after rotating head or shaving

        - Should the patient be admitted to hospital?
            - *High risk* → admit and monitor for at least 24 hours in the hospital
            - *Mix of High and Low Risk* → admit and monitor for at least 24 hours in the hospital
            - *Low Risk* → can be d/c home
- **Treatment**
    - Reflex → lifestyle education, ↑fluids, ↑salt intake, ↓BP medications, pharmacologic meds (ie. fludrocortisone 0.1-0.3mg/d), pacemaker (if asystole was noted),
    - HOCM/ARVD/BBB/↑QTc/Sinus Node Disease → refer to Cardiology. Consider holter or prolonged ECG if necessary.
    - Seizure → refer to Neurology

ALTERED MENTAL STATUS

- **General**
    - Stabilize first, then diagnose
- **Differential**

  - HE IS OUT OF IT
    - **H**emorrhage/Hepatic Encephalopathy → LFTs, NH3, CT head
    - **E**tOH (intoxication or withdrawal)/Electrolytes → EtOH, CIWA, CMP
    - **I**schemia (MI, CVA, bowel, etc.) → Cardiac enzymes, CT head/abd
    - **S**ugar (low/high) → accucheck
    - **O**verdose → drug levels, UDS, antidoes
    - **U**remia → CMP
    - **T**hyroid (low or high) → TSH/FT4
    - **O**xygen (hypoxia) → Pulse ox, ABG
    - **F**its (seziures) → EEG
    - **I**nfection/Iatrogenic → FFWU, delirum precautions
    - **T**rauma/Temperature/Toxins → Vital signs, osmolar gap
- **Exam**
  - Vitals
  - Temp
    - Hypothermia: sepsis, hypothyroidism
    - Hyperthermia: infection, thyroid storm, adrenal crises
  - Neurological exam
- **Diagnostics**
  - Imaging
    - CT head
    - EKG
    - CXR
    - Consider LP
  - Labs
    - Bedside glucose measurement (give 1 amp D50 if suspected hypoglycemia)
    - TSH
    - CBC → look for anemia, new or ↑WBC
    - CHEM7 → electrolyte abnormalities, uremia
    - LFTs → look for acute liver failure
    - TSH
    - ABG → hypo or hypercapnic resp failure
    - UDS
    - NH3 → encephalopathy however understand NH3 is not req'd for diagnosis
- **Treatment**
  - Give 1 amp D50 if suspected hypoglycemia
  - Narcan 0.4-2mg IV or IM if suspect narcotic overdose (if patient does not respond to initial dose, consider fentanyl as source which may require multiple doses)
  - Thiamine 100mg in alcoholics (give before glucose)
  - Oxygen

CONCUSSION

- **Defined**: no standard universal definition of concussion or mTBI, diagnosis is based primarily on characteristics of immediate sequelae after the event. Generic definition is a condition in which there is a traumatically induced alteration in mental status, **with or without** an associated loss of consciousness (LOC). No single test score can be the basis of a concussion diagnosis.
- **Epidemiology**[228,229,230]
  - Highest risk sports include hockey, rugby, football, and soccer
  - Military highest risks with blast injuries
- **Symptoms**

- Exercise intolerance
- Headache
- Increased emotions
- Nausea
- Tinnitus
- Irritability
- Drowsiness
- Poor balance
- Slowed verbal output
- Noise/Light sensitivity
- Difficulty remembering
- Sleep disturbances
- Difficulty concentrating

- **Signs**
  - LOC
  - Altered heart rate (HR) and BP response to submaximal exercise
  - Post traumatic amnesia
  - Eye movement abnormalities
  - Seizure
  - If symptoms are worsening over time, alternative explanations for the patient's symptoms should be considered.
- **Examination**
  - Vitals
    - Autonomic dysregulation - abnormal blood pressure (BP) control, temperature regulation, and disruption of endocrine, analgesic, and circadian functions may occur after head injury.
    - Orthostatic Hypotension – 20mmHg or greater reduction in SBP or 10mmHg drop in DBP with or without symptoms after standing
      - Obtaining: lay down for 2 minutes, obtain VS, then stand, wait for 1 minute, and re-do VS. Wait 2 minutes, and obtain a second set of VS
      - Lack of HR change is more concerning for underlying neurologic injury, whereas a change is c/w likely concurrent hypovolemia
      - In POTS there will be tachycardia without a change in BP
      - Seated position is not recommended to do
  - Mental Status Exam
    - SCAT, SAC
    - Orientation
    - Immediate and delayed recall
    - Concentration, mood, affect, insight, judgement
  - Neurologic Exam
    - CN 2-12 with CN 2, 3, and 7 being ost often injured
    - DTRs
  - MSK Exam
    - Head and neck
    - Neck isometrics
    - Cervical proprioception with ROM
    - Jaw
    - Thoracic Spine
    - Spurling Test
  - Balance
    - Static and/or dynamic balance assessment
    - In athletes, have them keep their eyes closed and do tandem gait with feet-together

- Vestibulo-occular
  - Screening ocular examination
  - Pupillary reactivity
  - Visual acuity
  - Nystagmus (vertical may lead to difficulty with jumping; horizontal may lead to difficulty tolerating car rides due to motion sickness)
  - Convergence (difficulty with near vision work)
  - Saccades
  - Smooth pursuits (difficulty may mean patient has issues reading or using electronic devices)
- **Diagnosis** - clinical diagnosis when more severe conditions (ie. ICH) have been ruled out. Based solely on subjective symptoms. The GFAP blood test may be utilized in specific scenarios to assist in diagnosis.
- **Diagnostic Testing**
  - Labs: The Banyan Brain Trauma Indicator measures the serum proteins UCH-L1 and GFAP within 12 hours of head injury. Levels of these proteins can help indicate whether a patient has a low probability of intracranial lesions and thus can eliminate the need for unnecessary CT imaging. Test results can take 3 to 4 hours.
  - The purpose of neuroimaging is to assess for other etiologies or injuries, such as hemorrhage or contusion, that may cause similar symptoms but require different management.
  - Guidelines
    - *Canadian CT Head Rule* – CT imaging is required in the following situations:
      - The patient fails to reach a Glasgow Coma Scale score of 15—on a scale of 3 (worst) to 15 (best)—within 2 hours
      - There is a suspected open skull fracture
      - There is any sign of basal skull fracture
      - The patient has 2 or more episodes of vomiting
      - The patient is 65 or older
      - The patient has retrograde amnesia (ie, cannot remember events that occurred before the injury) for 30 minutes or more
      - The mechanism of injury was dangerous (eg, a pedestrian was struck by a motor vehicle, or the patient fell from > 3 feet or > 5 stairs).
    - *The New Orleans Criteria*- CT imaging is required in the following situations:
      - Severe headache
      - Vomiting
      - Age over 60
      - Drug or alcohol intoxication
      - Deficit in short-term memory
      - Physical evidence of trauma above the clavicles
      - Seizure.
  - Post-TBI dysfunction
    - LH
    - FSH
    - Testosterone (men), estradiol (women)
    - IGF
    - Free thyroxine, TSH
    - 0800 cortisol
- **Treatment**
  - Data suggests that most adults will recover in 2-4 weeks, if patients have symptoms that persist beyond **2 weeks** it may be indicative of a more servere injury.
  - Rest (physical and cognitive)

        - Initial therapy involves several days of cognitive and physical rest, followed by a gradual return to physical and cognitive activities.
            - The optimal period of rest suggested by recent studies is 3 to 5 days after injury, followed by a gradual resumption of both physical and cognitive activities as tolerated, remaining below the level at which symptoms are exacerbated.

- **Returning to Activity** – physiologic recovery is delayed behind symptomatic recovery, thus, if patients are feeling better, their body may not be completely healed. This is the basis behind "return to play" protocols.

  All Adults
    - After the rest period, patients may gradually resume cognitive and physical activities while avoiding those that result in severe symptom exacerbation.
        - Recommended modifications include reduced workload, shortened workdays, and frequent breaks to allow provocable symptoms to improve and cognitive stamina to recover.
        - For those whose symptoms persist **beyond 1 month**, there is evidence that noncontact aerobic activity is helpful in promoting recovery.
    - Light physical activity (typically walking or stationary bicycling), followed by more vigorous aerobic activity, followed by some resistance activities.
    - Mild aerobic exercise (to below the threshold of symptoms) may speed recovery from refractive postconcussion syndrome, even in those who did not exercise before the injury.

  Athletes
    - Once aerobic reconditioning produces no symptoms, then noncontact, sport-specific activities are begun, followed by contact activities.
    - Have patients return to the clinic once they are symptom-free for repeat evaluation before clearing them for high-risk activities (eg, skiing, bicycling) or contact sports (eg, basketball, soccer, football, ice hockey).
- **Pharmacologic Treatments**
    - <u>Post-Traumatic Headache</u>
        - Most common type is migraine, followed by tension
            - *PRN*: Analgesics (NSAIDs) are often used initially by patients to treat posttraumatic headache.
            - *Prophylactic*:
                - In adults, nortriptyline 20 mg or gabapentin 300 mg at night as an initial prophylactic headache medication, increasing as tolerated or until pain is controlled, though there are no high-quality data to guide this decision.
                - The ideal prophylactic medication depends on headache type, patient tolerance, comorbidities, allergies, and medication sensitivities. Gabapentin, amitriptyline, and nortriptyline can produce sedation, which can help those suffering from sleep disturbance.
    - <u>Dizziness</u>
        - Patients should be encouraged to begin movement—gradually and safely—to help the vestibular system accommodate, which it will do with gradual stimulation. It usually resolves spontaneously.
        - Referral for a comprehensive balance assessment or to vestibular therapy should be considered if there is no recovery from dizziness **4 to 6 weeks after the concussion**.
    - <u>Sleep Disturbances</u>
        - Sleep hygiene education – minimize screen time, keep consistent sleep schedule, avoid naps, minimize use of nicotine, caffeine, and alcohol
        - Consider use of **melatonin** which can help in patients with TBI

        - Use of medications above for HA may also cause sedation s/e which can help with sleep
        - Order of treatment: sleep hygiene → melatonin → amitriptyline / nortriptyline → trazodone
    - Mental Fogginess
        - Amantadine may be helpful in recovery phase
    - Anxiety/Depression
        - Consider referral to BH
        - SSRI, SNRI and TCAs may improve depression after concussion
- **Referring Out**
    - Approximately 10% of athletes have persistent signs and symptoms of concussion beyond 2 weeks. If concussion is not sport-related, most patients recover completely within the first 3 months, but up to 33% may have symptoms beyond that.
    - If their recovery is prolonged (ie, longer than 6 weeks), they likely need to be referred to a concussion specialist.
    - High risk for persistent symptoms:
        - High-force mechanism of injury
        - History of multiple concussions
        - Underlying neurologic condition
            - Intractable pain and emotional lability after initial injury

HEADACHES

- **Diagnosis**[231]
    - Migraine – two of four pain features (unilateral, pulsatile, moderate-severe intensity, associated with routine activity) AND at least one of the following (nausea, photophobia/phonophobia). Often occur 1-5x/month lasting 4-72 hours at a time. F>M with + family history
    - Cluster – most often in males; 15min-3 hrs duration, associated with rhinorrhea, tearing, often occurs multiple times throughout the day, periorbital.
- **Types**
    - Primary
        - Tension
        - Migraine w/ or w/o aura
        - Cluster
        - Pseudotumor cerebrae
        - Trigeminal autonomic cephalgia
    - Secondary
        - Temporal arteritis
        - Mass lesion
        - SAH
        - SDH
        - Stroke
        - Vascular malformation
        - Acute glaucoma
- **Red Flags**
    - First HA in patients >55
    - Sudden onset with maximum intensity reached within 5 minutes
    - Pain worse with valsalva type maneuvers (ie. cough)
    - Recent head injury in the last 3 months
    - Associated with fever

- PMHx of HIV or immunosuppression
- Focal neurologic signs
- Pain associated with local tenderness, e.g., region of temporal artery
- Vomiting that precedes headache
- Associated conjunctivitis
- Papilledema on exam

- **Treatment**
  - GCA – prednisone 1mg/kg (up to 60mg) and ASA 81mg; labs include ESR, CRP, CBC, temporal artery biopsy within 7 days of steroid initiation
  - Cluster – 100% O2 at 6-12L/min using nonrebreather for 15min; can also give SQ sumatriptan or zolmitriptan nasal spray; prophylactic tx with verapamil/lithium/topiramate for prevention

Headache types and characteristics

Symptom	Migraine with or without aura	Tension-type headache	Cluster headache	Medication-overuse headache
Aura	Yes	No	No	No
Headache duration	4-72 hrs	30m-7d	15-180m	Some or all of the day
Frequency	Episodic, variable	1-15 days per month, variable	1 on alternate days to 8 per day, often for 7 days to 1 year when episodic	Daily >15d/month, for more than 3 months
Laterality	Unilateral	Bilateral	Unilateral	Unilateral/Bilateral
Character of pain	Pulsating	Pressing/tightening	Knife-like, severe, excruciating	Pressing/ tightening/pulsating
Severity of pain	Moderate/ severe	Mild/moderate	Severe/ Very severe	Mild/moderate/ Severe
Aggravated by movement	Yes	No	No	No
Eased by movement	No	No	Yes; restless	No
Nausea +/- movement	Yes	No	No	No
Photophobia/ phonophobia	Yes	No	No	No
Red/watery eye	No	No	Yes	No
Watery or blocked nose	No	No	Yes	No

- **Generic Treatment Options**
  - Tylenol 650 mg PO Q 4-6 hour prn HA
    - 15 mg/kg Q 6 hours
  - Naprosyn 500 mg PO bid prn HA
  - Diclofenac
  - Fioricet 2 tabs q4h **avoid in pts with hx of addiction
- **Headache Cocktail (EM)**
  - Combination of:
    - Toradol 30mg IV or 60mg IM
    - Benadryl (optional but encouraged)
    - Reglan 10mg IVP
      vs
      Prochlorperazine 10mg IVP
    - IV NS (1L)
    - Optional: Decadron 4mg IV

      No relief in 15 minutes...

  - **C/I if risk for SAH
    - Phenergan 12.5mg IVP or Demerol 25mg
    - Toradol 30mg IV

MIGRAINE HEADACHES

- **Define**[232,233,234]
  - Two of four pain features (unilateral, pulsatile, moderate-severe intensity, symptoms impact daily activity) AND at least one of the following (nausea, photophobia/phonophobia). Often occur 1-5x/month lasting 4-72 hours at a time. F>M with + family history.
  - Often occur 1-5x/month lasting 4-72 hours at a time.
  - F>M with + family history.
- **Duration**
  - Episodic – fewer than 15 headache days per month
  - Chronic – at least 15 headache days per month
- **Types**
  - Migraine without aura (4-72 hours)
  - Migraine with aura (4-72 hours; visual changes last 15-20 minutes prior to HA)
    - Aura only occurs in 30% of patients
    - Typically characterized by any neurological event that can be a combination of visual, hemisensory, or language abnormalities, with each symptom developing over at least 5 minutes and lasting a maximum of 60 minutes.
  - Status migrainosus (>72 hours)
  - Migraine with Brainstem Aura (MBA)
    - Patients often present with basilar symptoms such as vertigo, dysarthria, tinnitus, diplopia, b/l visual sx, hypacusis, ataxic gait, impaired consciousness.
  - Transformed
    - Initially episodic in duration but becomes more frequent and classified as chronic.
  - Retinal Migraines - spreading cortical depression that occurs in the retina. Fairly rare.
  - Abdominal Migraines - characterized by abdominal pain or vomiting as part of the headache syndrome. Symptoms predominate over the HA. Seen primarily in children

  - and adolescents, although can manifest as cyclic abdominal pain and vomiting in adults.
  - Hemiplegic Migraines - must have exam-confirmed motor weakness, as well as other aura (including dysphasia). Triptans are avoided in the management
- **Differential Diagnosis**
  - Tension – does not have associated nausea and disability; not associated with activity, usually non pulsatile, bilateral and lasts from 30 minutes to 7 days. It is better described as vise-like that wraps around the head.
  - Aneurysm
  - GCA/PMR
  - SAH
  - Meningitis
  - Glaucoma
  - IIH
  - TIA
  - Intracranial neoplasia
- **Known Precipitants**
  - Stress
  - Foods
  - Weather changes
  - Smoke
  - Hunger
  - Fatigue
  - Bright light sensitivity
  - Menstruation - thought to be related to the sudden drop in estrogen levels
  - Hormones
- **Evaluation/Work-up**
  - Clinical diagnosis; physical exam is done to rule out secondary causes
    - Focal neurologic abnormality (consider mass)
    - Fever (consider inflammation, infection)
    - DBP>120 mmHg (consider malignant HTN)
    - Papilledema (consider pseudotumor; mass; meningitis)
    - Tender temporary arteries
    - Nuchal rigidity
  - Imaging
    - In general imaging is only obtained if abnormal unexplained findings found on exam, or atypical features such as worsening with Valsalva, awaken from sleep due to HA, HA onset after age 50, aura lasting more than 1 hour, or progressively worsening.
    - CT imaging if HA are typical and have not changed in quality or quantity
    - Other imaging other than CT and MRI to consider include lumbar puncture, IOP, CT sinuses, MR angiogram
  - Symptoms Suggestive of Secondary Headache
    - New onset headache in >50 YO
    - Headache lasting >72 hours
    - Visual/sensory/language sx lasting >1 hr
    - Sudden onset with neurological symptoms
    - Abnormal neuro exam
    - Fever, systemic sx
  - Concerning Symptoms
    - Change in quality of HA or frequency
    - Daily or continuous

  - Changes in mental status or personality
  - Associated jaw pain (especially in older patient; consider GCA)
  - New onset after 50 years old (consider neoplasm)
- **Consultation** - Referral is indicated if the headache is atypical, remains difficult to classify, or fails to respond to recommended management strategies
- **Pregnancy** – must rule out pre-eclampsia and pregnancy-induced HTN. Best preferred therapies are MgOH and rest. Sumatriptan (nasal delivery system or nasal spray) for <9 days/month okay during pregnancy. For short term therapy, Tylenol and NSAIDs are best. Do not advise use of NSAIDs past 32 weeks. Preventive therapy has at least Category C rating. Best for now is beta blockers but should be tapered off the last few weeks of pregnancy.
  - During Lactation – sumatriptan and eletriptan are considered safe in the lowest effective dose.
- **Overuse Headache** – common in patients using OTC NSAIDs for 15 of the 30 days in a month with headaches occurring >10 days of the month. Consider use of Tylenol or Naproxen, these are less likely to cause overuse HA. In the acute setting, if needing to stop medication(s) immediately, steroid tapers have been used as well as gabapentin and hydroxyzine.
- **Treatment**
  - See table on next page
  - Menstruation related[235]
    - Remember women with aura cannot be on combined hormonal contraceptives (CHC) due to ↑ risk for stroke.
    - Common treatments include antihypertensives, anticonvulsants, and hormonal prophylaxis (ie. transdermal estradiol gel 1.5mg applied 7 days starting on day 10 after ovulation and continued through the 2nd day of menstruation bleeding. Another option includes CHC throughout (skipping placebo period), ensuring at least **30** mcg of EE is prescribed. Overall goal is to prevent EE level from ↓ below 10mcg.

Hormonal treatment options for Menstrual Migraines		
Medication	Dose	Pearl
Continuous Formulation *NuvaRing* *Lybrel (Ashlyna)*	 Vaginal Ring 20mcg EE+ 0.09 mg levonorgestrel once daily x 365d	Women on the ring may notice ↑ sensitivity on week 4 and may require changing out the ring every 3 weeks as a result
Extended Formulation *LoSeasonique* *Any 20-mcg EE CHC used in an extended manner* *Any 30-mcg EE CHC used in an extended manner*	 20 mcg EE and 0.1 mg levonorgestrel for 84 d, followed by 7 d of 10 mcg EE 20 mcg EE used >2 mo without placebo 30 mcg EE used >2 mo without placebo	 Add conjugated equine estrogens, 0.9 mg daily to achieve 30 mcg of EE
Monthly Formulation *Lo Loestrin Fe 1/10* *Natazia*	 10 mcg EE and 1 mg norethindrone for 24d, f/b 10 mcg EE for 2d and then placebo for 2d Gradually ↓ estradiol valerate dose from 3 to 2 to 1 mg ↑ dienogest dose from 2 to 3 mg	 Ultralow doses may be a/w ↑ breakthrough bleeding, which may improve with time

Acute and chronic reatments for migraines in either inpatient our outpatient settings

Acute/Abortive

Contraindications of DHE and Triptans:

- Uncontrolled HTN, CAD, CVA, prego, coronary spasm
  - Causes vasoconstriction
- Avoid concurrent use with SSRI (serotonin syndrome)

Clinic Setting / Inpatient	Home/Outpatient
• Abortive ER Cocktail: o Promethazine 25mg IM (caution with IV administration) (or Reglan 10 mg IV or Chlorpromazine 0.1 mg/kg IV (to 25mg IV or IM) over 20 minutes, may repeat after 15 minutes to max of 37.5mg, o Pretreating with 5ml.kg of NS may prevent hypotensive effects) o +/-Dexamethasone 4mg o Toradol 15mg o Benadryl 50mg • Dihydroergotamine 0.5-1mg (start with 0.33 if first time) IM/SC/IV x1 & may be repeated in 1 hour. OR • Prochlorperazine 10mg IV or 25mg rectal • Promethazine 12.5-25mg IV (or 25mg rectal) • Ketorolac 60mg IM is very effective in severe cases[236] • <u>Triptans</u> o Sumatriptan 4 or 6mg SC (may repeat 6 mg SC in 1 hr if not effective max 12mg/d). Other form is Sumatriptan PO 100mg at first visit (50mg if s/e noted)	• <u>Mild (limit to <14d/month):</u> o ASA 600-900 mg PO Q 4 hours x2 o Ibuprofen 400-800 mg PO Q 6 hours x2 o Excedrin Migraine 2 tabs q3h (max 4 tabs/d) o Prodrin 1 tab q2-3h (max 3 doses) o Diclofenac 50mg dissolved q2-4h (max 150mg/d) o Ibuprofen 800mg q3h (max 2.4g) o Magnesium 400-500mg/d • <u>Moderate:</u> o Consider DHE nasal spray as alternative. o Doxepin 10→25/50mg/d o Duloxetine 30-60mg/d or Venlafaxine 75-200mg/d • <u>Severe:</u> o Triptans *Instruct patients to take up to 3x/week and alternate with NSAID; works within 2 hrs*

○ Rizatriptan 5-10mg (5mg if taking propranolol concurrently; 10mg if no beta blocker on board) ○ Zolmitriptan 5mg nasal (first line tx for cluster) ○ Zolmitriptan 5mg PO (2.5mg if s/e)	▪ Sumatriptan 50-100 mg PO **q3h prn** (max 200mg) or nasal spray 40mg/d PLUS Aleve 440-500mg ▪ Rizatriptan 10mg PO q4h prn (max 3 doses) ▪ Zomig 2.5/5mg q3-4h prn (max 10mg/d) → nasal better for severe symptoms such as nausea/vomiting

Preventative

- Indicated if freq >2x/week or 4+ days/month or acute tx unsuccessful, prolonged auras >1hr, disabling nature of HA, interfere with daily routine. Consider tapering off therapy after 6-12 months of stability.
- Habits - Counsel patients on getting consistent, quality sleep and stress management with yoga or meditation.
- Dietary – missed or delayed meals are common trigger. Other triggers include caffeine, artificial sweeteners, additives (ie. MSG)
- A common measure of success for migraine prevention is at least a 50% reduction in migraine attack frequency or days, which is the clinical trial end point recommended by the Clinical Trials Subcommittee of the International Headache Society
- Avoid OCP in patients with migraine with aura if possible.

Name	Great For	Side Effects
Depakote 250-500mg BID or Depakote ER 500-1000mg daily	Concurrent anxiety or mood stabilization	Nausea, fatigue, tremor, weight gain. Contraindicated in pregnancy!
Frovatriptan 2.5mg BID	Best for **menstrual** related migraines. Best to start therapy 2 days before expected period and continue for total duration of 6 days	Best for **menstrual** related migraines
Propranolol LA 80mg/d to max dose of 160-240mg/d Metoprolol succinate 100mg/d increased q1-2w to max of 200mg/d	Anxiety, palpitations, **HTN**	fatigue, reduced exercise tolerance, nausea, dizziness, insomnia, ED, and depression

Timolol 5-30mg/d		
Amitriptyline 10mg QHS ↑ by 10mg q1-2w to target dose of 20-40mg qhs	Parasthesias, depression **Insomnia**, Anorexia, IBS, fibromyalgia	drowsiness, weight gain, and dry mouth
Fluoxetine 40mg/d		
Gabapentin 300mg/d ↑ by 300mg q3-5d to target 1200-1500mg/d divided TID		
Tizanidine 8mg TID		
Topiramate 25mg QHS ↑ by 25mg/d per week to target 100mg/daily divided BID or daily in ER formulations	Refractory migraine, aura, **overweight**, bipolar, depression, **may ↓ effectiveness of OCP at doses ↑200mg**	Parasthesias, fatigue, anorexia, nausea, ↓concentration
Magnesium Oxide 400-500mg/d		Diarrhea
Botox injections	**>15 episodes/month** (8 must be migrainous) lasting 3 months duration with each HA ≥ 4 hrs/d Avoid s/e of other medications	
Fremanezumab (single high dose of 675mg SQ quarterly or 3 monthly doses of 225mg SQ)	Patients on multiple medications (few drug drug interactions noted) May work quicker than other preventive meds	Cardiovascular abnormalities (↑ risk if known history) No reversal strategy
Venlafaxine 37.5/d for 1 week then increase weekly by 37.5mg to target 150mg/d	Concurrent anxiety or depression	Beware in pts with HTN, h/o seizure disorder, and MAOI use within 14 days.
Open Label		
Pregabalin 150mg BID Zonisamide 100-400mg Atenolol 50mg/d Olanzapine 2.5-35mg/d Controversial: Butterbur Coenzyme-Q10 Riboflavin		

PARKINSON'S DISEASE

- **Clinical Features**[237]
  - Tremor – resting tremor; worse when ask patient to do mental calculations; gets worse with progression of disease
  - Bradykinesia – generalized slowness of movement; patient may state "I want to move, I just can't get my legs to move"; also seen as the 'shuffling gait'

Gait Type	Description
Parkinsonian	• Patient will take small steps without raising feet • When stopping, patient appears to "freeze"
Senile Gait	• "Walking on Ice" • Feet wide apart, knees and hips flexed • Walk as if they are expecting to fall
Spastic Paraparesis	• Dragging of each leg with steps • No flexion of the knees • Due to circular leg movements (scissor gait)
Distal LMN disease	• Steppage gait • Foot drop • Excessive elevation of legs during walking (toes touch floor before heals)

USMLEWorld

  - Masked Facies
  - Cogwheel Rigidity – resistance of passive movement throughout a joint
  - Postural instability - ↑ tendency to fall; tested by standing behind patient and pulling their shoulders back – normal response is for pt to only have to take one step backward to get balanced whereas in PD patients may fall
  - Others
    - ↓eye blinking
    - blurred vision
    - dysphagia
    - kyphosis
    - fatigue
- **Differential Diagnosis**
  - Tremors

Differentiating Essential Termor from Parkinson's Disease		
	Essential Tremor (ET)	Parkinson Disease (PD)
Onset of disease	Bilateral arm involvement	Unilateral tremor, associated with stooped posture, shuffling gait, memory loss
Body affected by tremor	Arms most commonly then head, legs, larynx, trunk	Stooped posture, shuffling gait
Tremor characteristics	Associated with purposeful movement	Tremor in arms at side
Latency period	Immediate	Longer (several seconds)
Source: DeLong MR, Luncos JL. Parkinson's disease and other movement disorders. In: Kasper DL, Fauci AS, Longo DL, et al, eds. Harrison's Principles of Internal Medicine. Vol 2. 16th ed. New York: McGraw-Hill. 2005:2406-2418.		

- **Labs/Diagnostic**
  - Clinical impression
    - Bradykinesia + tremor or rigidity must be present
  - Response to DA
- **Dementia**
  - Memory difficulty, altered personality, difficulty multi-tasking
  - Lewy Body type is associated with visual hallucinations and altered cognition
- **Treatment**
  - Based on impairment

Pharmacologic Management of Parkinsons Disease				
Generic name	Trade name	Starting dose	Maintenance dose	Mechanism
Trihexyphenidyl	Artane	1 mg BID	2 mg BID-TID	Anticholinergic
Benztropine	Cogentin	0.5 mg BID	1 to 2 mg BID-TID	Anticholinergic
Amantadine	Symmetrel	100 mg BID	100 mg BID-TID	?
Selegiline	Eldepryl	5 mg	5 mg qam	MAO B inhibitor
Carbidopa/ levodopa	Sinemet	25/100 mg TID	25/250 mg TID-QID	Dopamine precursor
Carbidopa/ levodopa	Sinemet CR	25/100 mg TID	50/200 mg TID	Dopamine precursor
Apomorphine	Apokyn	2 mg SC test dose	2 to 10 mg SC TID	Dopamine agonist
Bromocriptine	Parlodel	2.5 mg daily	5 to 10 mg QID	Dopamine agonist
Pramipexole	Mirapex	0.125 mg TID	1.5 mg TID	Dopamine agonist
Ropinirole	Requip	0.25 mg TID	1.0 mg TID	Dopamine agonist
Entacapone	Comtan	200 mg with L-dopa	600 to 800 mg a day	COMT inhibitor
Tolcapone	Tasmar	100 mg TID	100 to 200 mg TID	COMT inhibitor

SENSORY/MOTOR DEFICITS

- **Localization**
  - Supratentorial (cerebral cortex and subcortical regions, including the basal ganglia, hypothalamus, and thalamus)
  - Posterior fossa (cerebellum, brainstem, and cranial nerves)
  - Spinal cord (including extramedullary, intramedullary, cauda equina, and conus medullaris lesions)
  - Peripheral
    - Peripheral are localized further from proximal to distal: radiculopathy, plexopathy, peripheral neuropathy, neuromuscular junction, and muscle.
- **Diagnostic Testing**
  - CT is a good starting point for TIA/Stroke for acute hemorrhage
    - In hyperacute stages, MRI is far superior

CT preferred	MRI preferred
Suspected acute hemorrhage Skull Fractures Meningiomas	Subacute and chronic hemorrhage Ischemic stroke Posterior fossa and brainstem tumors and lesions Dx of MS Evaluation of the spinal cord

- **UMN vs. LMN**
  - UMN damage occurs above the red nucleus resulting in a dicorticate posture (with arms flexed and hands fisted)
  - LMN damage occurs below the red nucleus and above the vestibulospinal and reticulospinal tracts resulting in a decerebrate posture

Differentiating UMN vs. LMN disease		
	UMN	LMN
Tone	↑	↓
Fasciculations	None	Present
Muscle	No atrophy	Atrophied
Babinski	Present	Negative
Reflexes	Increased/Clonus	Decreased
Pattern of weakness	Pyramidal/regional	Distal/segmental
Hoffman	+	-
Spasticity	+	-

SEIZURE

- **Defined**
  - Epileptic seizure – transient occurrence of signs and/or symptoms due to abnormal excessive or synchronous neuronal activity in the brain
  - Epilepsy – at least 2 unprovoked seizures on separate days, generally 24/h apart
  - Status epilepticus – single seizure episode lasting 5+ minutes or 2 or more sequential seizures without full recovery of consciousness
- **Questions to ask**
  - Curent or new medications (ie. Wellbutrin, tramadol)
  - History of childhood/febrile seizures or even seizures as an adult
  - Family history?
  - History of head trauma (fx; TBI does not necessarily ↑ risk)
  - Does the patient recall any part of the event
  - Any warning signs prior to event
  - Any witnesses
  - Incontinence, lateral tongue/cheek biting?
- **Admission Criteria**[238,239]
  - First unprovoked seizure evaluation:
    - Clinically significant abnormality on neuroimaging or labs which require admission
    - Abnormality on neurologic exam/failure to return to baseline status

- Patient does not have a responsible adult to stay with for 24hrs following discharge
- Patient has not been given written instructions regarding driving and duty restrictions
- Second (or more) unprovoked seizure not on medication:
  - MRI Brain and/or EEG has not been performed
  - Abnormality on neuroimaging or labs which require admission
  - Abnormality on neurologic exam/failure to return to baseline status
  - Patient does not have a responsible adult to stay with for 24hrs following discharge
  - Patient has not been given written instructions regarding driving and duty restrictions
  - AED therapy can be started in the ER (initiation of therapy alone does not require admission)
  - If admitted neurology will consult in the inpatient setting

- **Etiology**
  - Primary
    - Idiopathic (accounts for 2/3 of new seizures in the general population)
    - Head trauma (m/c in 5-35 YO; ICH or SAH)
    - CVA (m/c after age 50)
    - Post-syncopal (often accompanied by tonic or myoclonical activity)q
    - Mass lesion (glioblastoma, astrocytoma, and meningiomas)
    - Genetic (often d/t mutations in genes affecting sodium, calcium, and potassium channels)
    - CNS infection (encephalitis, meningitis 2/2 to HSV, H.influenza, TB, cysticercosis)
  - Systemic Disorders
    - ↓glucose (<30), ↓sodium (<120), ↓calcium
    - Uremia
    - Hepatic encephalopathy
    - Drug toxicity (TCAs, anti-psychotics, insulin, isoniazid) or withdrawal (EtOH)
    - ↑HTN (emergency)
    - Pseudoseizure (usually psychiatric history present to suggest conversion disorder, normal EEG)
  - Provoked – occurring within 7 days of acute brain insult secondary to:
    - Structural – head injury, NS intervention, stroke, CNS infxn, malignancy
    - Metabolic/toxic – EtOH w/d, liver or kidney failure

Figure. Seizure classifications

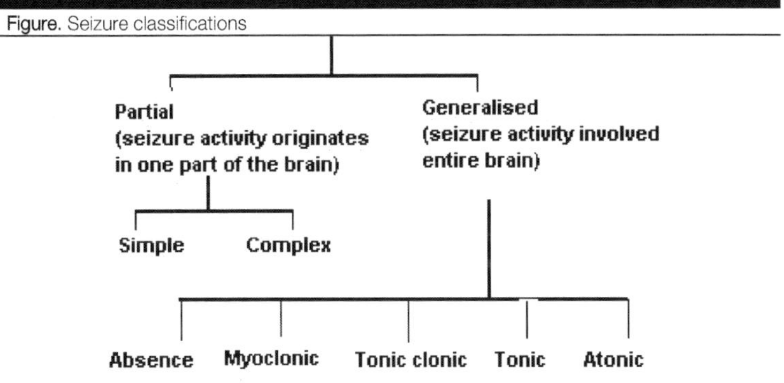

- **Types**
  - Acute
  - Symptomatic – occur in the setting of EtoH w/d, hypoglycemia, head trauma
  - Unprovoked – absence of provoking factors
- **Classification Scheme**

  Epileptic seizures are classified by whether or not the seizure is localized to 1 area of a lobe (focal) or is widespread, involving both cerebral hemispheres (generalized)
  - Focal (originates in a single focus; can become generalized; most commonly affecting the temporal lobe)
    - *Simple* – no loss of consciousness; motor/sensory/ or autonomic phenomena are in the beginning; affect only single cortex region (face, limb), sweating, vomiting. May end in Todd's Paralysis which may be an indiction of an underlying brain mass.
    - *Complex* – partial seizures with impaired consciousness; also begin with an aura which then leads to loss of consciousness; characterized by coordinated involuntary muscle movements (automatism)
    - *Partial seizures with secondary generalization*
  - Generalized
    - *Tonic clonic* – loss of consciousness without warning aura; patients will have stiffening and bilateral tonic-clonic activity is observed.
    - *Absence* – m/c in childhood with rare occupance in adolescence; brief LOC with eye blinking, rare loss of motor tone, immobile
      - Typical
      - Atypical
      - Absence with special features (myoclonic, eyelid myoclonia)
    - *Myoclonic* – single or repetitive jerks are observed; usually bilateral and involving face, trunk, UE, very brief lasting <1s with no post-ictal confusion
  - Focal – may or may not have impairment of consciousness or awareness; may have todd's paralysis after event
  - Unknown
  - Status Epilepticus
    - Seizures prolonging for $\geq$ 30 minutes without spontaneous cease
- **Phases**
  - Tonic phase – contraction of limbs flexion then extension of the back and neck, tongue biting occurs with contraction of mastication muscles; may become cyanotic
  - Clonic phase – alternative contraction and relaxation for additional 30-60s ending with flaccid muscles, urinary incontinence can occur d/t effects on detrusor muscle
- **Diagnosis/Workup**
  - EEG
    - The EEG (routine) should be considered as part of the neuro diagnostic evaluation of the adult with an apparent unprovoked first seizure because it has a substantial yield (Level B)
    - Only 1/3 will be abnormal
    - Can help not only classify the type of seizure but also beneficial for surgical localization
  - Neuroimaging
    - Brain imaging using CT or MRI should be considered as part of the neurodiagnostic evaluation of adults presenting with an apparent unprovoked first seizure (Level B).
  - Labs
    - Blood glucose, CBC, and electrolyte panels (particularly sodium, mg, Ca), toxicology screening, LFTs

- Prolactin is nonspecific!
- Lumbar Puncture
  - Helpful in patients who are febrile, but there are insufficient data to support or refute recommending routine lumbar puncture (Level U).

- **Treatment/Prophylaxis (see table on next page)**
  - Treatment Physiology
    - Benzodiazepines enhance neurotransmission of GABA at the GABAA receptor, increasing the frequency of chloride ion channel opening in response to GABA.
    - Valproate prolongs sodium channel inactivation, attenuates calcium mediated transient currents and augments GABA.
  - Treatment aimed at seizure freedom with no side effects
  - In women of child-bearing age, add folic acid 1mg/d (do not use pre-natal vitamin only)
    - If using contraception, avoid enzyme inducer medications such as Phenobarbitol, phenytoin, carbamezapine, and primidone as they ↓ efficacy of OCP
    - Combined OCPs can ↓ lamotrigine levels by up to 50%
  - Anti-epileptic drug therapy (AED) often for those with ≥ 2 unprovoked seizures or a single seizure with high risk occupation or (ie. bus driver) high risk for recurrence (abnormal EEG, abnormal MRI, nocturnal occurrence) or known strutural abnormality (CT or MRI).
    - After first unprovoked seizure however, consider pros and cons of starting AED
- **Status Epilepticus**
  - *Defined* – continuous convulsve seizure ≥5 minutes or > 2 seizures w/o resolution of postictal encephalopathy
  - *Orders*
    - Bedside glucose, serum glucose, ABG, U&E, Ca, FBC, EKG
    - Consider anticonvulsant levels, tox screen, LP, BCx, UCx, EEG, CT head, CO level
    - Pulse ox and continuous cardiac monitoring

Pharmacologic Management of Epilepsy

Drug	Doses	Loading / Initial Dose[1]	Maint. Dose[1]	Therapeutic Serum Levels	Pearl
Phenytoin(Dilantin) *S/E include gum hyperplasia, SJS, cerebellar atrophy* Fosphenytoin is form for IM or IV use	100 mg; 30, 50 mg also available	Oral loading: 1,000 mg in two to four divided doses over 12-24 hours Intravenous loading: 1,000-1,500 mg (15-18 mg/kg) not exceeding 50 mg/min	300-400 mg/day in a single dose or divided doses	10-20 g/mL	Narrow spectrum (used for focal onset seizure)
Carbamazepine (Tegretol) *S/E include aplastic anemia, ↓WBC, rash (SJS), ↑LFT, ↑PR interval, ↓Na*	200, 300 mg; XR: 100, 200, 400 mg	100 mg twice a day; increase by 200 mg/day to maintenance dose	400-1,600 mg/day in three or four doses, or in two doses if XR form	4-12 g/mL	Narrow spectrum (used for focal onset seizure); good for concurrent migraine d/o, ↓Na,
Oxcarbazepine(Trileptal) *S/E include ↓Na, rash, ↑LFT*	150, 300, 600 mg	300 mg twice a day	600-2,400 mg/day in two doses	12-30g/mL*	Narrow spectrum (used for focal onset seizure)
Phenobarbital(Luminal) *S/E include rash, SJS*	15, 30, 60, 100 mg	180 mg twice a day for 3 days or same as maintenance dose	90-180 mg/day in a single dose	20-40 g/mL	Broad spectrum
Valproic acid(Depakote, Depakene) *S/E include ↑LFTs, ↑NH3, ↑wt, ↓hair, SJS, osteoporosis, tremor*	250 mg	Same as maintenance dose	750-3,000 mg/day in two or three doses	50-150g/mL	Broad spectrum; good for concurrent mood and HA d/o; do DEXA scan if on for 3-5 years. **Avoid in pregnancy**
Lamotrigine(Lamictal) *S/E include **SJS esp in Asian pop.**, not good to use with OCP*	50, 100, 200 mg	25 mg twice a day then slowly increase[2]	200-500 mg/day in two doses[2]	5-15 g/mL*	Broad spectrum; good for concurrent mood d/o

Levetiracetam(Keppra) *S/E include GI upset*	250, 500, 750 mg	250-500 mg twice a day	1,000-3,000 mg/day in two doses	10-40g/mL*	Broad spectrum; Good for women of child bearing age

Status epilepticus treatment

Time		Treatment
STABILIZATION PHASE	0-5min	Stabilize patient via monitoring of O2 sat, EKG, establishing IV access Labs: CBC, CHEM7, AED, UDS, ABG, TOX screen 50cc D50W if finger glucose < 60mg/dl f/b Thiamine 200mg IV, Consider naloxone 0.4-2mg IV added to D5 if history suggests
CONSIDER INTUBATION, EEG, AND ICU TRANSFER		
INITIAL THERAPY PHASE	5-20min	• Consider intubation • Give thiamine 200mg IV and D50W 50cc • Fosphenytoin: Load 15-20 mg/kg PE IV at max 150 mg/min. Keep on cardiac monitoring (goal therapeutic level: 22-25 μg/mL) • Levels should be checked >2 h after an IV load or >4 h after an IM load. • May give an additional 500 PE IV if no response. • Valproate 1 g over 15-20 min (20-40 mg/kg) can be given **if patient is allergic to phenytoin**. Therapeutic level is 70-140. May give an additional 500 mg after 20 min. • Dilantin 1,000 mg IV at <50 mg/min. May give an additional 500 mg IV if no response after 20 min. (Note: Do not give w/ glucose or dextrose due to precipitation.) • Levetiracetam 1000-4000mg over 5-15min (additional dose 1500-3000mg)

IV Access Available	No IV Access Available
Drip Lorazepam 0.1mg/kg (@ 2mg/min; max 4mg) may repeat once Diazepam 0.15-0.2 mg/kg (max 10mg/dose) may repeat once IV phenobarbital 15mg/kg/dose x1	Midazolam 10mg IN Diazepam 0.2-0.5mg/kg PR (max 20mg) over 5 minutes x1 Versed 5 mg IM if no IV access

Phase	Time	Therapy
		Non-Drip Lorazepam 2mg IV over 2min *max 0.1-1.5mg/kg*
SECOND THERAPY PHASE	20-40min	• IV fosphenytoin 20mg PE/kg IV max 1500mg PE/dose x 1 • IV valproate: 40 mg/kg over ~10 min max 3000mg/dose x1 • IV levetiracetam 60mg/kg max 4500mg/dose x 1 • IV phenobarbital: 15 mg/kg x1 *Other Options* • IV propofol: Load 1-2 mg/kg; repeat 1-2 mg/kg boluses every 3-5 min until seizures stop, up to a maximum total loading dose of 10 mg/kg. Initial IV rate: 2 mg/kg/h. IV dose range: 1-15 mg/kg/h. If still having seizures, switch to midazolam, valproate, or pentobarbital.
THIRD THERAPY PHASE	40-60min	• IV pentobarbital: Load 5 mg/kg at up to 50 mg/min; repeat 5 mg/kg boluses until seizures stop. Initial IV rate: 1 mg/kg/h. IV dose range: 0.5-10 mg/kg/h; traditionally titrated to burst suppression on EEG but titrating to seizure suppression is reasonable as well. Therapeutic level: 30-45 mcg/mL. • Pt will need to be admitted to an intensive care unit. Begin EEG monitoring as soon as possible if patient does not rapidly awaken or if any continuous IV Rx is used. • Consider CT brain or MRI brain. Evaluate for & correct underlying causes.

- When patient has stopped...
  - Phenytoin or Fosphenytoin (preferred) 20 mg/kg IV in 3 doses @ 50 mg/min (25 mg/min in cardiac pt) over 2 hours (any shorter you ↑ risk for cardiac rhythm disturbances). Again, can use valproic acid if allergies exist to above.
  - Ensure glucose and thiamine were already given
  - Consider EEG
  - Consider MRI, brain
  - Must give while on cardiac monitor (may prolong QRS)
    - If either Phenytoin or Fosphenytoin ineffective then try Phenobarbital
  - Phenobarbital 20 mg/kg @ 100 mg/min
    - May repeat up to 30 mg/kg
    - May cause hypotension and depressed respirations

UNRESPONSIVE PATIENT

- **Common Causes**
  - Hypoglycemia
  - CVA/subdural hematoma
  - Postictal state
  - Cardiovascular (hypotension, arrhythmia)
  - Drug (narcotic, sedative, EtOH)
  - Metabolic/respiratory encephalopathy
  - CNS tumor/meningitis
- **Questions to Ask**
  - Any recent narcotics, sedatives, falls? Hx of DM? *Think D50, narcan*
  - History of alcoholism? *Think thiamine*
  - Any trauma? *Think CT head, c-spine precautions*
  - History of depression? *Think overdose*
- **Exam**
  - Vital signs
    - Clear the airway, stabilize c-spine if necessary
    - If inadequate ventilation with O2, use NRB
    - ↑RR → obstructed airway, aspiration, PNA, DKA
    - ↓RR → poisoning, ↑ICP
    - ↓HR → hypoxia, CHB, ↑ICP, digoxin
    - ↑HR → airway obstruction, pain, ↓volume, SVT, VT, AF
    - Rectal temp (coma common in T<86F
  - Physical Exam
    - Neuro Exam
      - Measure GCS score
      - Limb strength, muscle tone and reflexes, neck stiffness (except in neck injury).
      - Lateralizing signs - facial or limb weakness, may be caused by a stroke, intracranial bleeding or preexisting problems
      - Ocular nerve palsy or divergent squint with coma s/o Wernicke's encephalopathy
      - Look for signs of seizure activity which may indicate non-convulsive status epilepticus.
- **Interventions**
  - Make sure there is IV access.
- **Treatment**

  (airway →breathing →circulation)
  - Diagnostics
    - Consider EKG, CXR
    - CT head to r/o SAH, CVA, injury

- Labs
  - Get a stat fingerstick, Chem 7, ABG, UDS
- Medications
  - Coma cocktail:
    - Dextrose 1 amp
    - O2
    - Naloxone 2mg IV
      - Remember that narcan may need to be repeated multiple times in patients with fentanyl overdose.
        - Dosing:
          - IV/SQ: Narcan 0.4mg (can do 0.2mg initially if patient is opiate naïve) repeated q3-5 minutes
          - Intranasal: 4.0mg intranasal repeated q3-5 minutes until effect.
          - Drip: often done in patients on methadone; use 2/3 of total effective dose of naloxone per hour (typically 0.25-6.25mg/hr) and provide ½ of that bolus dose about 15 minutes after starting the drip to prevent a drop in naloxone levels
    - Thiamine 100mg IV
    - Magnesium 1-2g IV in alcoholics
    - Ceftriaxone IV if meningitis suspected

ACUTE STROKE/CVA

- **Evaluation**[240,241,242,243,244,245,246,247]
  - If any of these signs are present, the probability of a stroke is 72%[248]
    - Facial droop: Ask patient to smile; sign is present if one side does not move as well as the other
    - Arm drift: Ask patient to close eyes and hold arms out for 10 s; sign is present if one arm does not move or drifts downward
    - Abnormal speech: Sign is present if the patient slurs speech or uses wrong words
  - Obtain vitals including oxygen saturation. Keep patient on a continuous cardiac monitor and obtain frequent vital sign measurements and neurologic checks every 1-2 hours.
  - Blood glucose check: Keep BS <200 avoiding dextrose-containing solutions for the first 24 hours.
  - In young women presenting with stroke like symptoms and predominant headache consider cerebral venous thrombosis.
- **Types**
  - Ischemic (80-87%) – large vessel (ICA, basal ganglia, cerebellar), small vessel (ie. lacunar), embolic, unknown
    - Lacunar
      - Pure motor or pure sensory
      - Face-arm or arm-leg syndromes
    - TACI
      - Dysphasia, visual-spatial disorder, or dyscalculia (subtract 7's)
      - Visual field defect
      - Ipsilateral motor/sensory defect in 2 areas (face, arm, or leg)
    - PACI
      - 2 of 3 in TACI
    - PCI
      - Ipsilateral CN defect with ctl motor/sensory
      - **Bilateral** motor/sensory defect

        - Cerebellar dysfunction
        - Visual defect
  - Hemorrhagic (13-20%)
    - Risk factors on admission (3/4 = 99% spec for hemorr):
      - Vomiting
      - Headache
      - Elevated WBC
      - Decline in neurological status within 3 hrs of admission
      - Decreased LOC
  - CVT[249]
    - Risk factors associated with thrombogenic states (pregnancy, hypercoagulable d/o, trauma, stasis, OCP)
    - Symptoms
      - HA (diffuse, progresses in severity over weeks)
      - Papilledema (d/t ↑ICP; consider in patients who present with sx c/w PTC/IIH)
      - Neurological signs: hemiparesis, aphasia

- **Workup**
  - History and Physical: focus on when symptoms began (i.e. when patient was last known to be symptom/deficit free as this will determine possible eligibility for thrombolytics), look for focal neurologic findings
    - Supinator
    - Spinatus (tests by external rotation)
    - Wrist flexors
    - Fingers
    - Psoas
    - Dorsiflexion (tests by heel walk)
  - Mimic: look for Bell's Palsy which presents with facial paralysis (upper **and** lower) along with often a change in taste perception and hearing. Treatment with steroids recommended.
- **Determing severity of stroke in acute setting**

  The NIHSS was developed to help physicians objectively determine the severity of an ischemic stroke. The higher the score, the larger the stroke likely to be found on imaging. Must be performed within 48 hours of presentation.
  - Minor: NIHSS score $\leq$ 3
  - Moderate: NIHSS score 15-24
  - Severe: NIHSS score $\geq$ 25
  - Severity: NIH stroke scale recommended & document vitals and time

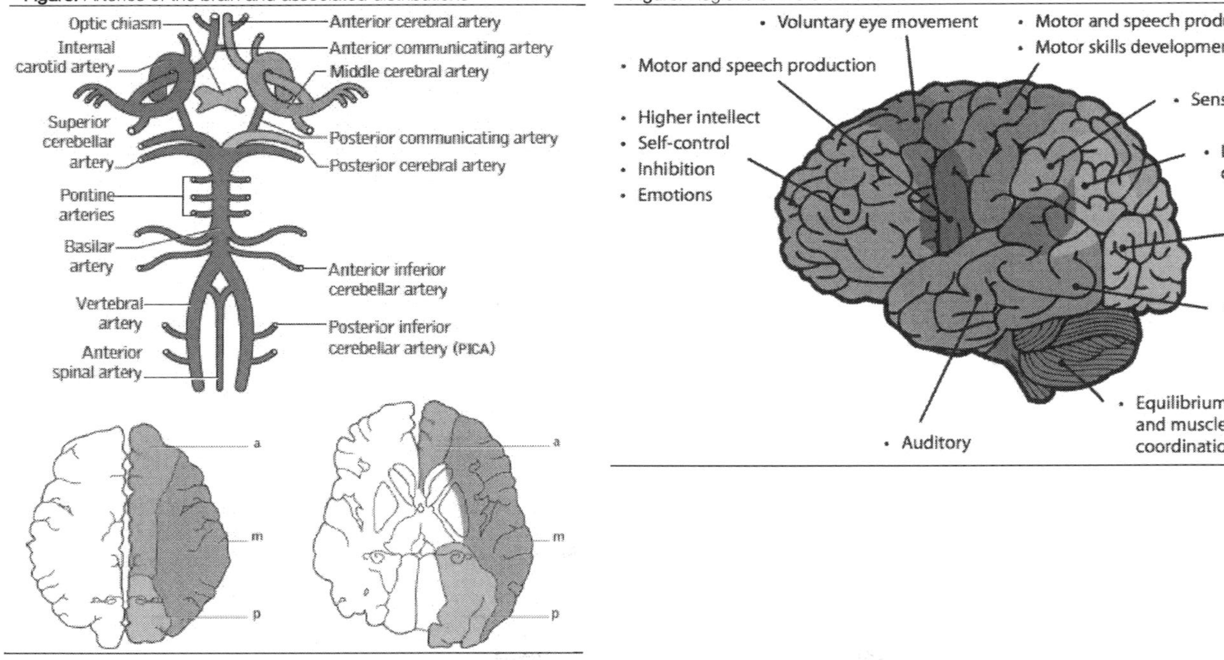

Figure. Arteries of the brain and associated distributions

Figure. Regions of the brain and associated functions

Clinical symptoms based on arterial involvement in stroke

Artery	Findings
Anterior Cerebral	Legs weaker than arms, frontal lobe signs (agitation, lack of motivation)
Middle Cerebral	Aphasia (if dominant side ie. R sided weakness, then expect aphasia), Arms weaker than legs Contralateral hemiplegia and hemianopia Unilateral neglect (if R MCA affected)
Posterior Cerebral	Visual hemianopia
Basilar	Cortical blindness (blind with preserved pupillary reflexes) Same side (L or R) should be affected on each eye's field of vision
Vertebral	The most common clinical features included • vertigo (57%) • unilateral facial paresthesia (46%) • cerebellar signs (33%) • lateral medullary signs (26%) • visual field defects (15%).
Brain Stem	Quadriplegia Hemiparesis Double vision Impaired swallowing → often require intubation Sensory loss across entire half of body

- **Location**
    - Large vessel vs. small vessel (lacunes)
    - Large Vessel: arm/face>leg or leg>arm/face with sensory **and** motor
        - 2/2 thrombosis of intracranial vessels or embolus from aortic arch, carotids
    - Small Vessel: arm/leg/face equal with sensory **or** motor
        - 2/2 lipohyalinosis, HTN, DM2
        - Modify stroke RF's: LDL, BP, diabetes, smoking
- **History**
    - Sx c/w hemorrhagic include HA, meningismus, vomiting, coma
    - HA should make you consider hemorrhagic vs hemiplegic migraine if hx of migraine w/aura
    - Trauma → r/o SAH
    - Young patient → always consider CVT
- **Disposition location**
    - Ward/Tele – no risk for cerebellar involvement, no hemorrhage
    - PCU – concern for cerebellar involvement (and thus herniation)
- **Management**
    - <u>Labs</u>
        - ICU Panel → glucose level required prior to any TPA
        - Lipid panel
        - ECG
        - TROP
        - A1c
        - CBC
        - ESR/CRP if considering CVT
        - Hypercoagulable w/u if considering CVT
        - Coagulation panel
        - Oxygen saturation
        - <u>Selected patients</u>
            - Toxicology screen
            - Blood alcohol level
            - Pregnancy test
            - Arterial blood gas tests (if hypoxia is suspected)
    - <u>Imaging</u>
        - **NCCT scan within 20 minutes of arrival**
        - **CTA should be obtained in patients presenting within 6-24 hours of symptoms with evidence of large vessel occlusion in the anterior circulation**
        - CT (with contrast) or CTA recommended in hemorrhagic stroke to evaluate for hematoma expansion
        - TTE
            - Aortic atherosclerotic plaque
            - Left atrial enlargement
            - Left ventricular hypertrophy
            - ASD/PFO
        - Carotid US *(NACET)*
            - Patients with carotid artery stenosis should be tx with ASA, high-dose statin and referred to vascular surgery for endarterectomy if high grade lesion (70-99%) in the 1-2 weeks following hospitalization.
                - Patients that are candidates include those with TIA or ischemic stroke within the distribution of the affected vessel.
        - EKG, CXR

- Stat head CT without contrast to rule out bleed → obtain within 20 minutes of presentation
- Stat MRI/DWI of brain and MRA of brain and neck
- Consider CT angiogram to r/o aneurysmal source if hemorrhagic stroke noted

- Orders
  - Telemetry
  - NPO
  - Maintain oxygen ≥ 94%
  - Walk with assist
- Consults
  - Swallow evaluation - to reduce risk of aspiration and pneumonia, ALL patients with stroke should have swallowing evaluated
  - PT/OT

Criteria For Determining Thrombolytic Use (TPA) In Ischemic Strokes	
Inclusion criteria	Exclusion criteria
1. Age >18 years 2. Clinical diagnosis of ischemic stroke with a defined onset of symptoms <3 hours from time TPA is to be started 3. CT scan shows no evidence of intracranial hemorrhage	1. INR>1.7 2. PLT<100 3. Seizure at onset or low glucose 4. Recent surgery or hemorrhage 5. ICH present 6. Recent stroke or head trauma (in past 3 months) 7. Recent heparin use in past 48 hours 8. SBP>185, DBP>110 9. Hypoglycemic (<50) 10. Recent surgery in past 3 months 11. Some consider avoiding if NIHSS score of >22 due to ↑ risk for hemorrhagic conversion

BP in Ischemic Stroke[250]	
No-TPA	TPA
First 48 hours goal: Systolic BP <220 mm Hg; diastolic BP <120 mm Hg **If blood pressure drops below 120/80; intravenous crystalloids should be given (assuming no evidence of CHF present) **Further Management:** All patients get ASA 325mg/d within 48 hours Systolic BP >220 mm Hg or diastolic BP 121-140 mm Hg 1. Labetalol 10-20 mg IV over 1-2 min. May repeat or double every 10 min to a maximum dose of 300 mg	**Indications:** *0-3 hours: IV-TPA* *3-6 hours: IV-TPA ** controversial* *3-8 hours: mechanical embolectomy* *>8 hours: anticoagulation/antiplatelet* **Pretreatment:** SBP <185 or diastolic <110 Labetalol 10-20mg IV over 1-2min may repeat once Nicardipine 5mg/h IV; titrate up by 2.5mg/h every 5-15min; max 15mg/h Clevidipine 1-2mg/h IV; titrate by doubling dose q2-5min (max 21mg/h)

2. Nicardipine 5 mg/h IV infusion as initial dose; titrate to desired effect by increasing by 2.5 mg/h every 5 min to maximum of 15 mg/h (target 10%–15% reduction **in first 24 hours**)
3. Nitroprusside 0.5 microm/kg/min IV; titrate to goal

Diastolic BP >140 mm Hg

- Sodium nitroprusside 0.5 microm/kg per min IV with continuous BP monitoring (target 10%–15% reduction)

During and After TPA:

Goal <185/110 for first 24 hrs

Measure BP every 15 minutes for 2 hours → then every 30 minutes for 6 hours → then hourly for 16 hours

Further Management:

SBP 180-230 or DBP 105-120

- IV 10 mg labetalol over 1-2 min; may repeat or double labetalol q10min to a maximum dose of 300 mg or can start with the initial bolus dose of labetalol and then follow-up with a continuous labetalol infusion administered at a rate of 2-8 mg/min

SBP >230 or DBP 121-140

- IV 10 mg labetalol over 1-2 min; may repeat or double labetalol q10min to a maximum dose of 300 mg or can start with the initial bolus dose of labetalol and then follow-up with a continuous labetalol infusion administered at a rate of 2-8 mg/min
- Nicardipine 5 mg/h IV infusion as initial dose, titrate by increasing 2.5 mg/h q 5 min to maximum of 15 mg/h.
- If the blood pressure is not controlled with above two, consider starting an infusion of sodium nitroprusside

DBP >140

- Nitroprusside 0.5 microm/kg/min IV infusion; titrate as desired

- **Treatment**
  - Ischemic
    - Blood pressure – *see above*
    - *Glucose* – consider insulin if BG>140-180 mg/dL; replace K if also giving insulin!
    - Embolus
      - *Thrombolytics*
        - Dose: TPA (alteplase) 0.9 mg/kg (max 90mg; consider lower dose of 0.6 mg/kg in Asian population per *ENCHANTED* study) IV as 10% over 1 min, then 90% over 1 hr
        - Indications: ischemic stroke (CT neg for hemorrhage) with neurological deficits with pt presentation **within 3-4.5 hrs** of sx onset and pt BP <185/110
          - Exclusions: possible SAH, surgery in past 14d, head trauma or MI in past 3mo, GI bleed in past 21d, ANY hx of ICH, any active bleeding, INR>1.7, thrombocytopenia, hypoglycemic (<50)
          - Considered: >80YO, any use of oral anticoagulant, NIH>25
        - Monitoring
          - Patient should be monitored carefully for signs of symptomatic ICH, which include changes in level of alertness, headaches, nausea, vomiting, and worsening neurologic examination findings.
          - The blood pressure should be maintained below **180/105 mm Hg** after thrombolysis to prevent this complication
          - Frequent vital sign checks and neurologic examinations are recommended for the first 24 hours.
      - *Endovascular mechanical embolus removal*
        - MERCI reasonable option to extract intra-arterial thrombi
    - *Antiplatelet* – Start combination ASA 325mg on presentation then 81/d (after 24-48 hrs of presentation if TPA administered) *Class I* along with Plavix (300-600mg load then) 75mg/d and continued together for 10-21 days, then ASA 81mg/d alone thereafter indefinitely. *(FASTER, CHANCE, POINT)*
      - Only do combination therapy for minor stroke or high-risk TIA
      - *Contraindications: ASA allergy, GIB, TPA*
        - *If allergy, consider Plavix alone*
      - Continue for 2 weeks then consider prolonged anticoagulation options
    - *HDL* – continue statin if already on one, poor indication to start if not on already (Level B) with goal LDL of ≤ 100
    - *Oxygen* – maintain >94%, only supplement if needed
    - *Fever* – Tylenol as needed
    - *Statin* – high dose; no specified target LDL level *(SPARCL Trial)*
    - *Anticoagulation* – use SCDs or prophylactic dose (Grade 1A)
      - Chemical prophylaxis is often okay by HD#4 if imaging shows stability
    - *Breathing* - IS use is encouraged due to ↑ risk for PNA
    - *Hemodynamics* - Consider PRN fluid for SBP<120
    - *Edema* - Decompressive surgery within 48 hrs reduces mortality; restrict free water; correct hypoxemia, hypercarbia and hyperthermia. Elevated HOB>30degrees and avoid anti HTN agents that increase vasodilation
    - *Increased ICP* –
      - STAT mannitol
        - 100 g IV bolus, followed by 0.5-1 g/kg
        - Contraindications: low BP, anuria secondary to renal disease, serum osm > 340. Hold dose for Na > 160, serum osm > 340, or osm gap > 10.
      - Hypertonic saline:

        - Goal sodium 145-155
        - 3% saline, 40-50 cc/h can go through peripheral IV for up to 12 h, then needs a central line.
        - Contraindications: Na > 160.
    - Hyperventilation: For goal pCO_2 30
- <u>Hemorrhagic strokes (ICH):</u>

Physical symptoms based on site of ICH	
Site	Findings
Basal Ganglia	Hemiplegia Homonymous hemianopsia Gaze palsy Stupor, Coma
Cerebellum	Neck stiffness Facial weakness **No** hemiparesis Stupor / Coma
Thalamus	Hemiparesis Hemi-sensory loss Upgaze palsy Nonreactive miotic pupils Eyes deviate **toward** the hemiparesis
Cerebral Lobe	Associated with seizures Occipital lobe causes CTL homonymous hemi. Eyes deviate away from hemiparesis
Pons	**Pinpoint** reactive pupils Deep coma Paralysis

USMLEWorld

    - Consult neurology and neurosurgery
    - Early intense SBP reduction best (*INTENSE*-2), keep SBP <140 with IV nicardipine, labetalol (any rapidly titratable medication)[252]
        - The lower the better, however few studies have shown adverse effects with very low SBP (this was rare).
    - On Anticoagulation
        - Warfarin: rapid correction with FFP, 3 Factor PCC (20-40cc; contains Factors II, IX, and X)), rFVII (Factor VII not part of 3-F-PCC but if you do 4-F-PCC it is included) and/or IV Vitamin K (5-10mg) recommended
        - DOAC: consider specific reversal agent
        - ASA not indicated until 2-4 weeks after stroke onset if hematoma has resolved
    - DVT prophylaxis
        - LMWH can be restarted assuming 48 hour CT imaging shows no active bleeding
    - Glucose
        - Should be monitored, manage hyper and hypoglycemia as needed with goal of (80-110 for FBG)
    - ↑ICP:
        - Ventricular drainage for hydrocephalus reasonable if ↓LOC (esp GCS 8)
        - STAT mannitol
            - 100 g IV bolus, followed by 0.5-1 g/kg

        - Contraindications: low BP, anuria secondary to renal disease, serum osm > 340. Hold dose for Na > 160, serum osm > 340, or osm gap > 10.
      - Hypertonic saline:
        - Goal sodium 145-155
        - 3% saline, 40-50 cc/h can go through peripheral IV for up to 12 h, then needs a central line.
        - Contraindications: Na > 160.
      - Hyperventilation: For goal pCO2 30
      - Avoid corticosteroids
    - In general:
      - Activate the STROKE TEAM (call page operator)
      - Q2-4 hour neuro checks.
      - For DVT prophylaxis, use intermittent pneumatic compression together with elastic stockings (can consider elevation to LMWH or UFH if patient non ambulatory after 4 days and no bleeding noted on CT)
      - PT, OT, speech therapy.
      - Passive full ROM exercises of paralyzed limbs should be started during the first 24 hours.
      - NPO if patient is at risk of aspiration.
- **Subarachnoid Hemorrhage**[253]
  - 50% of patients die within the first 6 months
  - Etiology
    - M/c causes include rupture of aneurysm or AVM
    - Atypical: mycotic aneurysm
  - Symptoms
    - Headache → LOC
    - Seizure activity (given risk, prophylactic anticonvulsants are often given)
  - Examination
    - Fundoscopic exam reveals hemorrhage, dilated pupil
    - EKG → look for T wave inversions d/t release of catecholamines 2/2 myocardial ischemia
  - Classification
    - *Hunt-Hess Grades*
      - Grade I: Mild headache with or without meningeal irritation
      - Grade II: Severe headache and a non-focal examination, with or without mydriasis
      - Grade III: Mild alteration in neurologic examination, including mental status
      - Grade IV: Obviously depressed level of consciousness or focal deficit
      - Grade V: Patient either posturing or comatose
  - Imaging
    - On CT-head, look for blood around the COW
      - Intraparenchymal – MCA, PCA
      - Interhemispheric/Intravascular – ACA
    - To identify location, CT angiograms are often ordered
  - LP – if CT negative with high suspicion, look for xanthochromia
  - Intubation
    - Often in HH Grades III-V
    - Target PaCO2 30-35, any lower and ↑ risk of vasospasm
  - Treatment
    - **Triple H Therapy**

        - *Hypertension*: goal CPP>70 or SBP 160-180 if clipped; 140-160 if unclipped; If vasospasm exists then goal is >130
            - ↓BP = labetalol
            - ↑BP = NE, phenylephrine
        - *Hemodilution*: goal HCT of 30-33% using albumin 5% 250cc q6h
        - *Hypervolemia*: goal CVP of 5-7 using NS @ 150cc/hr or 1/2NS if ↑Na
        - Mannitol (osmotic agent, ↓ICP by 50%, lasts 4 hours)
        - Consider prophylactic anticonvulsant
    - Statin therapy if LDL>100[254]
    - CCB
        - Nimodipine 60mg PO/NG q4h for 21 days
- Monitoring
    - Neuro checks q1h
    - Pulse oximetry
    - EtCO2
    - UOP
    - Serum Na
- Complications
    - Rebleed (peaks within 24 hours of event)
    - Hydrocephalus (peaks within 24 hours of event)
    - Hyponatremia (SIADH, cerebral salt wasting, within first week of event)
    - Vasospasm (worst is day 7-10; ↑risk with higher HH grade; prevention with nimodipine, tx with HHH)
        - HHH
            - Hemodilution (HCT 30-35%)
            - Hypertension (vasopressors phenylephrine, NE)
            - Hypervolemia (CVP>12)

- **Prevention of medical complications as an inpatient[255]**
    - IS use due to ↑ risk for PNA
    - VTE prophylaxis → as above; LMWH can be started if 48 hour imaging shows no active bleed
    - Speech pathology c/s for risk of dysphagia
    - Hyperglycemia management with SSI
    - Titrate NC to >92% due to risk for hypoxia
    - Ambulation/bed turns for bed sores
    - Telemetry due to cardiac abnormalities (arrest, CHF, arrhythmias)
    - PPI prophylaxis
    - Evaluation for depression
- **Secondary Prevention of Strokes (All Types)**
    - Most important factors (based on INTERSTROKE case study) to control in the patient are:
        - Lifestyle (↑exercise, ↓smoking, ↓alcohol, ↓weight)
        - BP management (ACEi+thiazide) for optimal reduction of 10/5mmHg rather than ACE alone (PROGERSS trial)
            - PRoFESS did not show ARB>placebo
        - Cholesterol reduction (Simvastatin (40mg/day based on Heart Protection Study) or Atorvistatin 80mg (SPARCL) recommended if LDL>=100 **with goal of reducing to 70** (or overall reduction by 50%)
            - May be contraindicated if patient has hx of intracerebral hemorrhage
            - No utility in treating ↓HDL
        - Lifestyle factors
            - Consider screening for OSA

- Recommend regular exercise
- Weight control (Screen for obesity and consider dietary consultation as outpatient)

- PFO do not require treatment unless history of DVT (CLOSURE 1 study)
- Antiplatelet therapy (unless anticoagulation indicated)[256]:
  - **Non cardioembolic, minor stroke, high risk TIA, lacunar, or cryptogenic:**
    - Clopidogrel 75mg daily combined with ASA 81mg/d
      - Only done in high risk TIA (see below) or minor stroke
        - Start therapy **within** 24 hours of stroke and continue together for 21 days then stop Plavix and continue ASA indefinitely.
      - Plavix failures may be due to CYP450 genetic abnormalities as liver modification is required to create active metabolite
      - More beneficial than ASA alone and lower bleeding risk *Level 2; MATCH, CHANCE (sub-analysis) trial*
      - Plavix>ASA if hx of PAD *(Clopidogrel versus Aspirin in Patients at Risk of Ischemic Events (CAPRIE) study)*
      - *POINT* and *CHANCE* trials suggested possible benefit of initial dual therapy with Plavix+ASA for 90 days or 21 days respectively and then continuation of Plavix indefinitely in patients with TIA and high ABCD2 score.
    - ASA 25mg+dipyridamole 200mg BID
      - More beneficial than ASA alone
      - Higher hemorrhage risk
    - ASA 75-100mg once daily
  - **Cardioembolic (atrial fibrillation):**
    - Edoxaban (*ENGAGE AF-TIMI 48*) 60mg/d (consider 50% dose reduction if GFR<50)
    - Dabigatran 150mg BID (unless CrCl <30 cc/min) (Grade 2B)
    - Warfarin

    If patient does not desire anticoagulant then...
    - ASA + Plavix (Grade 1B)
- **Carotid Stenosis** - best to treat with endarterectomy over stenting when occlusion >70% (NASCET trial)

TIA

- **Definition**[257,258]
  - Brief episode of neurological dysfunction lasting <1 hour without evidence of acute infarction (no residual sx)
  - Importance lies in the fact that patients may be at early risk for future stroke and other vascular events
- **Indications for Hospitalization/Risk Determination:**
  - Obtain ABCD2 score to determine **risk** of re-stroke in 7 days → score **≥3 warrants** admission if symptoms occurred within the past 72 hours
    - Age>60 (1pt)
    - BP>140/90 (1 pt)
    - Clinical features
    - **Unilateral** Weakness (2pt)
    - **Abnormal speech**: Sign is present if the patient slurs speech or uses wrong words (1pt)
    - Duration: 10-59m (1pt), >60m (2pt)

        - DM2 (1pt)

    Risk of CVA in 7 days: 6-7 (11.7%), 4-5 (5.9%), 0-3 (1.2%)
    >>high is considered scores of 6-7

    - If concurrent risk factors (AF, multiple TIAs, hypercoagulable state, symptoms > 1 hour, sx carotid artery disease >50%) or high ABCD2 score (>6)
- **Labs**
    - CBC
    - CMP
    - Lipid panel in AM
    - HgA1c
- **Imaging**
    - TTE (r/o ASD therefore consider bubble study)
    - MRI TIA protocol
    - Consider carotid duplex US
    - Telemetry monitoring with EKG qAM
- **Consults**
    - PT/OT evaluation
    - Speech pathology
    - Neurology
- **Treatment**
    - Non-Cardioembolic TIA
        - First event: ASA 325mg (alternative is Plavix if ASA allergy) then 81mg/d with Plavix 75mg/d combination (if high risk TIA: defined as ABCD2 score of 6+) for 21 days then 81mg/d alone thereafter indefinitely.
            - If already on ASA
                - Considered failure
                - Start Plavix 75mg or Aggrenox
    - Cardioembolic TIA
      Concerning for underlying AF as the source
        - Long term oral anticoagulation with target INR of 2-3
        - If cannot tolerate above and nonvalvular AF (rheumatic disease, hemodynamically significant MS):
            - ASA 325mg
            - Plavix 75mg
    - Concurrent STEMI/USA
        - Start ASA 325mg and Plavix 75mg
- **Prevention**
    - LDL goal < 100; all patients will benefit from statin regardless of LDL
    - BP goal <140/90
    - Fasting glucose goal of <126
    - All smokers should be counseled to quit
    - Lifestyle changes if BMI>25
    - Physical activity for 3-4x/week lasting at least 10 minutes
    - ↓Salt intake

VERTIGO

Evaluation of Vertigo		
	Peripheral Vertigo	Central Vertigo
Pathophysiology	Disorder of vestibular nerve (cn viii)	Disorder of brain stem or cerebellum
Severity	Intense	Less intense
Onset	Sudden	Slow
Pattern	Intermittent	Constant
Nausea and vomiting	Usually present	Usually absent
Exacerbated by position	Yes	No
Hearing abnormalities	Yes	No
Focal neurologic deficits	No	Yes
Fatigability of symptoms	Yes	No
Nystagmus	Horizontal	Vertical
DDx	FB Cerumen impaction Acute otitis media BPPV Meniere's dz Vestibular neuronitis Trauma Motion sickness Neuroma Ototoxic Medications	Infection (ie. encephalitis, meningitis) Vertebrobasilar Migraine Brainstem hemorrhage Infarction Migraine Tumor MS Temp. lobe epilepsy

SOURCE: USMLEASY

- **Differential Diagnosis**
  - BPPV (dx with Dix-Hallpike Maneuver, episodic positionally induced vertigo)
  - Vestibular neuritis (not induced with movement like BPPV)
  - Labyrinthitis (may be associated with unilateral hearing loss, single acute event like VN)
  - Migraine
  - Severe VB12 deficiency
  - Cerebellar stroke (associated sx include headache, instability, diplopia, wide based gait, ataxia, vomiting, nystagmus)
  - Multiple Sclerosis (d/t plaques at CN 8, vision changes (optic neuritis), look for hx suggestive of relapse/remittance, dx with MRI)
  - Medication toxicity (ie. phenytoin)

Vertigo Treatment Based on Situation		
Scenario	Class	Treatment
Vestibular nausea/motion sickness	Histamine ACh	Meclizine 25mg q6h Scopolamine 1ptch q3d Benadryl 25mg q6h
Migraine-associated *(consider Migraine with Brainstem Aura diagnosis)*	Dopamine	Metoclopramide 10mg q4h Promethazine 25mg q6h
Gastroenteritis	Dopamine Serotonin	Promethazine 25mg q6h Zofran 2mg PO

Pregnancy	Unknown	Ginger 250mg q6h Pyridoxine 25mg x 1 Zofran 2mg PO Methylprednisolone 40mg IV

- Check Orthostatic BP
  - Defined as a ↓ in SBP of ≥20 mmHg and DBP ≥10 mmHg within 5 minutes of standing.
  - Meclizine 25 PO tid (1/2-1-tab PO tid)

SEDATION SCALES

Motor Activity Assessment Scale (MAAS)		
Score	Description	Definition
0	Unresponsive	Does not move with noxious stimulus*
1	Responsive only to noxious stimuli	Opens eyes OR raises eyebrows OR turns head toward stimulus OR moves limbs with noxious stimulus*
2	Responsive to touch or name	Opens eyes OR raises eyebrows OR turns head toward stimulus OR moves limbs with when touched or name is loudly spoken
3	Calm and cooperative	No external stimulus is required to elicit movement AND patient is adjusting sheets or clothes purposefully and follows commands
4	Restless and cooperative	No external stimulus is required to elicit movement AND patient is picking at sheets or tubes OR uncovering self and follows commands
5	Agitated	No external stimulus is required to elicit movement AND attempting to sit up OR moves limbs out of bed AND does not consistently follow commands
6	Dangerously agitated, uncooperative	No external stimulus is required to elicit movement AND patient is pulling at tubes or catheters OR thrashing side to side OR striking at staff OR trying to climb out of bed AND does not calm down when asked
* Noxious stimulus, suctioning OR five seconds of vigorous orbital, sternal, or nail bed pressure		

Richmond Agitation-Sedation Scale (RASS)		
Score	Term	Description
+ 4	Combative	Overtly combative or violent; immediate danger to staff
+ 3	Very agitated	Pulls on or removes tube(s) or catheter(s) or has aggressive behavior toward staff
+ 2	Agitated	Frequent non purposeful movement or patient-ventilator dyssynchrony
+ 1	Restless	Anxious or apprehensive but movements not aggressive or vigorous
0	Alert and calm	
- 1	Drowsy	Not fully alert, but has sustained (> 10 seconds) awakening, with eye contact, to voice

- 2	Light sedation	Briefly (< 10 seconds) awakens with eye contact to voice
- 3	Moderate sedation	Any movement (but no eye contact) to voice
- 4	Deep sedation	No response to voice, but any movement to physical stimulation
- 5	Unarousable	No response to voice or physical stimulation

PULMONOLOGY/ CRITICAL CARE

ANAPHYLAXIS

- **General**[259,260]
    - Most cases are immunoglobulin E (IgE)–mediated.
    - Antibodies exposed to a particular allergen attach to mast cells and basophils, resulting in their activation and degranulation.
    - A variety of chemical mediators are released including histamine, heparin, tryptase, kallikrein, platelet-activating factor, bradykinin, tumor necrosis factor, nitrous oxide, and several types of interleukins.[5]
- **Presentation**
    - Signs and symptoms usually develop within five to 30 minutes of exposure to the offending allergen but may not develop for several hours.

- A biphasic reaction is a second acute anaphylactic reaction occurring hours after the first response and without further exposure to the allergen.

- **Labs**
  - Diagnosis if clinical
  - Plasma histamine within 1 hour of symptoms
  - Tryptase levels do not increase until 30 min after onset of symptoms and peak 1-2 hours after
- **Treatment**
  - Supine with legs elevated
  - Pepcid: 20mg IVPB or Zantac 50 mg IV over 5 min
  - Benadryl 50mg IV
  - 100% O2 NRB
  - Albuterol 2.5 mg nebulized
  - Fluid bolus of 1-2L 0.9NS to maintain urine output and BP (often ↓BP).
  - What is pt allergic to? Discontinue medication if found to be the cause
  - Epinephrine 1:1000 0.01 ml/kg to max 0.5 ml IM (normotensive)
    - **Usual initial dose is 0.3-0.5 ml IM/SC**; Repeat every 5-15 minutes as necessary.
    - Give 0.1-0.2 ml of total dose at site of antigenic exposure
    - 1 cc of 1:1000 epinephrine is 1 mg
    - Epinephrine 1 mg IM may be repeated every 3-5 minutes up to a maximum of 3 mg.
  - Epinephrine IV if hypotensive or respiratory failure
    - 0.3 mg & if no improvement→ continuous drip at 1-4 mcg/min of 1:10,000 dilution
  - Diphenhydramine 50 mg IV/IM/PO may be given every 2 hours prn up to a maximum of 400 mg.
  - Racemic Epinephrine neb 0.5 cc in 2.5 ml NS to temporize airway management
  - Solu-Medrol 125-250 mg IV q6h or repeat w/ 50mg/d vs 1-2mg/kg/d x 48 hours
    - Or Prednisone 60 mg PO
  - If 2/2 taking beta blocker → Glucagon 3.5-5mg IV x1 and 0.5 mg peds with prn infusion 1-5 mg/hr
    - Useful in refractory cases, especially in pts on β-Blockers

COUGH

- **Definitions**[261,262]
  - Acute – likely viral upper respiratory illness; on average lasts 18 days
  - Chronic - cough persisting for longer than 8 weeks
- **Causes**
  - Acute – likely viral
  - Chronic – smoking (COPD), medication side effect (ie. ACE inhibitors), upper airway cough syndrome (UACS; post nasal drip), airway bronchospasm (asthma), GERD
    - **UACS** – most often caused by allergic rhinitis, non-allergic rhinitis/vasomotor, rhinitis medicamentosa, infection (chronic bacterial sinusitis), allergic fungal sinusitis, deviated septum.
    - **Asthma** – routine testing using PFTs with methacholine challenge; can mimic non-asthmatic eosinophilic bronchitis except the PFTs are normal but bronchoscopy and lavage will reveal elevated eosinophil counts.
    - **Cough hypersensitivity syndrome** - symptoms suggestive of pharyngeal and laryngeal hypersensitivity, such as throat tickling, irritation or blockage, and dysphonia. It's a cough that is often triggered by low levels of thermal, mechanical, or chemical exposure. Patients with cough hypersensitivity

syndrome develop cough in response to stimuli and their concentrations, which would not otherwise elicit cough.

- **GERD** - Reflux triggers cough due to the effect of acid on the proximal part of the esophagus. Look for other symptoms of acid reflux (ie. Heartburn) but understand that they may be absent (silent reflux) in as many as 75% of cases of a reflux-induced cough. PH esophageal monitoring may confirm the presence of silent reflux, although anti-reflux therapy does not always resolve a cough.
- **Neurogenic** – unexplained cough in excess of 8 weeks with normal diagnostic testing (ie. CXR, pH monitor).

- **Diagnosis**[263,264]
  - Predominance of cough
    - Lasts 1 to 3 weeks
    - With or without sputum
  - Can be accompanied by other respiratory and constitutional symptoms
  - Physical exam suggesting pneumonia:
    - Heart rate >100 beats per minute
    - Respiratory rate >24 breaths per minute
    - Temperature >100.4F (38C)
    - Lung findings suggest a consolidation process
- **Diagnostic Testing**
  - CXR
    - Dyspnea or blood/rust colored sputum
    - Pulse>100
    - RR>14
    - T>100F
    - Focal consolidation on lung exam
  - CT Chest if patient is smoker or suspecting chronic lung disease
  - CT Sinus if suspecting UACS
  - PFTs
  - pH monitor
  - Sputum (for eosinophil count) if suspecting asthma or NAEB
- **Treatment**
  - At least 90% of acute bronchitis episodes are viral → antibiotics not routinely recommended (per AAFP, evidence rating A)
  - Over-the-counter medications are recommended as first-line treatment for acute cough
    - Consider using dextromethorphan, guaifenesin, or honey to manage acute bronchitis symptoms (per AAFP, evidence rating B)
      - Three placebo-controlled trials show that dextromethorphan, 30 mg, decreased the cough count by 19% to 36% compared with placebo
      - One study comparing benzonatate, guaifenesin, and placebo showed significant improvement with the combination of benzonatate and guaifenesin, but not with either agent alone.
    - RCT showed that in comparison to placebo, no benefit from NSAID in decreasing severity or duration of cough in patients with acute bronchitis.
    - First generation anti-histamine (Benadryl) + decongestant or as alternative: second generation antihistamine (Claritin) + nasal corticosteroids. If no response to this, then trial asthma treatment with inhaled corticosteroids. If still no response, then high-dose PPI (ie. 40mg daily or BID).
      - UACS – first generation anti-H1; intranasal steroids, ipratropium
      - Asthma – PFTs
      - GERD – PPI

- Neurogenic - May have paradoxical vocal cord movements. Consider treatment with voice rehabilitation or speech pathology. Can consider pharmacologic therapy with Gabapentin, Pregabalin, or Amitriptyline however data regarding their efficacy is sparse. High dose tramadol (50mg TID) has been used by laryngologists (start at 25mg QHS then increase to BID; after coughing has stopped, wean off).
- Viral Bronchitis/Supportive
  - Robitussin AC 10/100/5ml 1 tsp (5ml) PO Q 4-6 hours prn cough
  - Benzonatate (Tessalon Pearls) 100 mg PO Q 8 hours prn cough
  - Dextromethorphan 15-30 mg PO 4 times daily
  - Most effective: Codeine Phosphate 10-30 mg Q 4-6 hours
  - Diphenhydramine HCl 25 mg Q 4-6 hours
- In patients with evidence of bronchial hyper responsiveness, consider treatment with
  - Albuterol for 1 to 2 weeks (per AAFP, evidence rating B)
  - Robitussin in those with cough for 2 to 3 weeks
  - Tylenol prn
  - Smoking cessation
  - Education: cough likely to last 3 weeks or more

HEMODYNAMIC MONITORING IN THE ICU

Hemodynamic variables			
Item	Acronym	Normals	Interpretation
Volume Status			
Stroke volume variation	SVV	<10%-15%	For ventilated patients, SVV is highly sensitive and specific for **preload responsiveness**. More variation may be indicative of **low volume** status and remember **the correlation between SVV and Frank-Starling Curve.**
Stroke volume index	SVI	35-45	Similar as above
Central Venous Pressure	CVP	8-12	A measurement of **cardiac preload** by looking at the pressure within the thoracic veins. It may be low in low volume states and elevated in either high volume states or RV dysfunction.
Passive Leg-Raising Test			Lift the legs at a 45 degree angle with the patient supine which can result in appx 150cc of blood return to predict responsiveness to cardiac output by providing an endogenous **fluid challenge** by monitoring CO after 60-90s
Cardiac Function			
Cardiac Index	CI	2.5-4.5	Assessment of cardiac output based on the patients BMI.

			Basically, this will tell you how well the heart is pumping. Dobutamine and other inotropes will help increase CI.
Cardiac Output	CO	3-7 L/m	Affected by arrhythmias and ↑HR
Pulmonary Capillary Wedge Pressure	PCWP	2-12 mmHg	An indirect measurement of R atrial pressure and thus, when elevated, can point towards ventricular dysfunction
Other			
Central Venous Oxygen	ScvO2	≥70	Used as a marker of balance between systemic oxygen supply and demand obtained through a VBG from a central line. May require vasopressors +/- transfusions to improve.
Mean Arterial Pressure	MAP	≥65	
Systemic Vascular Resistance	SVR	900-1200 dyn/s/cm^2	

ARDS

- **Clinical**[265]
  - Dyspnea, cyanosis, and diffuse crackles not explained by cardiac process often in 6-72 hrs of event
  - Respiratory distress further shown by tachypnea, tachycardia, and diaphoresis
  - Causes
    - Direct Insult to Lung: PNA, aspiration, pulmonary contusion, vasculitis, drowning
    - Indirect Insult to Lung: sepsis, acute pancreatitis, massive blood transfusions (TRALI), trauma, drug overdose, severe burns
- **Berlin Definition**

Criteria	
Item	Defined
Timing	Within 1 week of a known clinical insult or new or worsening respiratory symptoms
ALI	• Mild: 200 mm Hg < PaO2/FIO2 ≤ 300 mm Hg with PEEP or CPAP ≥5 cm H2O • Moderate: 100 mm Hg < PaO2/FIO2 ≤ 200 mm Hg • Severe: PaO2/FIO2 ≤ 100 mm Hg
Oxygenation	• Mild: PEEP or CPAP ≥5 cm H2O • Moderate-severe: PEEP ≥5 cm H2O
Chest Imaging	Bilateral opacities–not fully explained by effusions, lobar or lung collapse, or nodules
PAWP	Respiratory failure not fully explained by cardiac failure or fluid Overload (nml TTE, pro-BNP<300)

- **Severity Calculator**

  - Based off the CESAR study, patients with severe ARDS should be referred to an ECMO center. The severity can be determined by the Murray calculator found <http://cesar.lshtm.ac.uk/murrayscorecalculator.htm>
  - Variables include:
    - Ratio of arterial oxygen tension to the fraction of inspired oxygen (PaO2/FiO2)
    - Positive end-expiratory pressure (PEEP)
    - Lung compliance (TV/(PIP-PEEP))
    - Chest radiograph quadrants with infiltrates (normal = 0; 1 per quadrant)
- **Treatment**
  - Cornerstone of therapy is mechanical ventilation to reduce ventilation induced lung injury → this can increase the systemic inflammatory response leading to the development of MOSF (multi-organ system failure). This is done through the **lung protective strategy of ventilation** by aiming for low tidal volumes (TV) and low inspiratory pressures.
    - Target TV should be at 0.6cc/kg (up to 0.8cc/kg) of ideal body weight with a maximum plateau pressure (P_{PL}) of 30[266]
    - Consider higher PEEP in moderate and severe ARDS
- **Adjunctive Therapies**
  - Reduced tidal volume - to protect the lungs may lead to hypercapnia and respiratory acidosis. Extracorporeal CO2 removal has not been found to be helpful.
  - Prone ventilation - should be initiated. It encourages homogenous lung ventilation to help distribute the mechanical forces in the lung. Benefits were seen in those with PaO2/FiO2 ratio ≤ 150 mmHg when performed for at least 16 hours/d.
  - Nitric Oxide - did not show mortality benefit
  - Nutritional support: improved survival and oxygenation when using low carb high fat enteral formulas
  - Corticosteroids: not helpful
  - ECMO: not promising (*CESAR)*
  - Neuromuscular blockade: controversial but promising; may ↓ barotrauma.
  - Fluid-conservative: When giving Lasix for diuresis, if total protein <6, consider co-administration of albumin[267] Does not improve survival.
- **Complications to Expect**
  - Barotrauma – due to PEEP on damaged lung tissue; prevented by keeping **plateau pressure** < 30
    - Plateau Pressure: marker of alveolar trauma; pressure maintained during inspiratory hold maneuver. Static pressure that give an estimate of lung compliance. Ideally maintained ≤ 30 cm H20. Differential: **PTX, Pulm Edema, PNA, Atelectasis, R mainstem intubation**
    - Peak Pressure: marker of upper airway pressures (trachea/bronchi); equals the sum of the resistive pressure (flow x resistance) and the plateau pressure. Dynamic pressures that *measure the resistance to flow of air*. Ideally maintained ≤ 35 cm H20. Differential: **bronchospasm, mucus plug, biting ET tube**.
  - Delirium – often treated with sedation and NM blockade
  - Infection – often VAP
  - DVT (lack of mobility)
  - GI bleed (stress ulcers)

Initial ventilator settings								
Calculate predicted body weight (PBW)								
Male =	50 + 2.3 [height (inches) - 60] **OR**							
	50 + 0.91 [height (cm) - 152.4]							
Female =	45.5 + 2.3 [height (inches) - 60] **OR**							
	45.5 + 0.91 [height (cm) - 152.4]							
Set mode to volume assist-control								
Set initial tidal volume to 8 mL/kg PBW								
Reduce tidal volume to 7 and then to 6 mL/kg over 1 to 3 hours								
Set initial ventilator rate ≤35 breaths/min to match baseline minute ventilation								
Subsequent tidal volume adjustment								
Plateau pressure (Pplat) goal ≤30 cm H_2O								
Check inspiratory plateau pressure with 0.5 second inspiratory pause at least every four hours and after each change in PEEP or tidal volume.								
If Pplat >30 cm H_2O, decrease tidal volume in 1 mL/kg PBW steps to 5 or if necessary, to 4 mL/kg PBW.								
If Pplat <25 cm H_2O and tidal volume <6 mL/kg, increase tidal volume by 1 mL/kg PBW until Pplat >25 cm H_2O or tidal volume = 6 mL/kg.								
If breath stacking (auto PEEP) or severe dyspnea occurs, tidal volume may be increased to 7 or 8 mL/kg PBW if Pplat remains ≤30 cm H_2O.								
Arterial oxygenation and PEEP								
Oxygenation goal PaO_2 55 to 80 mmHg or SpO_2 88 to 95 percent								
Use these FiO_2/PEEP combinations to achieve oxygenation goal:								
FiO_2	0.3	0.4	0.5	0.6	0.7	0.8	0.9	1.0
PEEP	5	5 to 8	8 to 10	10	10 to 14	14	14 to 18	18 to 24
PEEP should be applied starting with the minimum value for a given FiO_2.								

High PEEP arm of the ALVEOLI trial

High PEEP group							
FiO2	0.3	0.4	0.5	0.5-0.8	0.8	0.9	1.0
PEEP	12-14	14-16	16-18	20	22	22	22-24

SOLITARY PULMONARY NODULE

Defined

- <3cm
- Round opacity
- Surrounded by pulmonary parenchyma
- Without regional LN

Pearls

- Solid nodules <6mm in low risk patients do not require further w/u
- Solid nodules between 6-8mm should have repeat CT imaging
- Solid nodules >8mm should have f/u CT imaging (+PET) sooner (3 months)

Assessment[148]

SPN Evaluation			
	Low cancer risk	Intermediate Cancer risk	High cancer risk
Diameter of nodule (cm)	<0.8	0.8-2.0	≥2.0
Age (years)	<40	40-60	>60
Smoking	Never	Current (<20/d)	Current (>20/d)
Cessation?	Quit > 15 years ago	Quit 5-15 years ago	<5
Nodule characteristics	Smooth	Scalloped	Spiculated Corona radiata
Cancer risk	<5%	5-65%	>65%

Figure. Recommended work up flow for a solitary pulmonary nodule

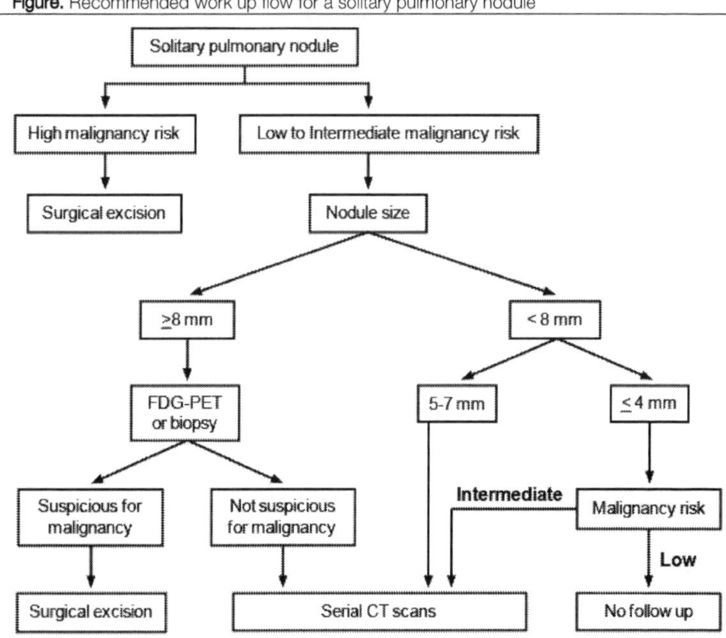

Intervention

- High Risk - Surgical excision
- Intermediate Risk
  - <1cm nodule
    - Serial CT scans
  - >1cm nodule
    - FDG-PET scan
      - Hot – excise
      - Cold- serial CT scans
- Low Risk
  - <6mm, solid, noncalcified, age<35 → serial CT scans (see Fleischner Report Criteria) **not required** unless patient is high risk. If high risk, CT remains optional. CT should be considered though in patients with spiculated margins on the nodule, and/or a nodule in the upper lobe.
  - For patients with solid SPNs that have been stable on serial CT over a two year period, or with subsolid SPNs that have been stable over a five year period, no further diagnostic testing req' d.

COPD

- **Pathophysiology**[268,269,270,271]
  - Hallmark is sudden and marked imbalance between respiratory load and capacity.
  - The inciting event is a flare up in inflammation in the airways that leads to increased airway edema, bronchospasm, and increased sputum production.

- All these lead to an increase in the elastic and resistive loads and worsening of airflow resistance, with consequent increase in the labor of breathing.
- Patients respond with rapid, shallow, ineffective breaths
- There is increased dead space breathing, leading to further deterioration in alveolar ventilation.
- Severe airflow resistance leads to dynamic hyperinflation, which results in a flattening of the diaphragm that further increases the work of breathing.

- **Symptoms**
  - SOB
  - Chest tightness
  - Cough
  - Confusion
  - ↑HR
  - ↑RR
  - Wheezing
  - Fatigue
  - Fever
  - Malaise
- **Diagnosis**
  - Clinical symptoms suggestive of SOB/DOE + Risk Factors + PFTs (decreased FEV1/FVC below LLN or 70%) + Imaging + Negative A1AT screen

Winnipeg Criteria Staging of COPD	
Type 1	All three of the following symptoms: • increase in sputum volume • increase in sputum purulence • increase in shortness of breath
Type 2	Any two of the following symptoms: • increase in sputum volume • increase in sputum purulence • increase in shortness of breath
Type 3	Any one of the following symptoms: • increase in sputum volume, • increase in sputum purulence, • increase in shortness of breath, *plus at least one of the following:* • upper respiratory tract infection lasting 5 d • fever • increase in wheezes • increase in cough • increase in heart rate ⩾ 20%

- **Etiology**
  - Medication noncompliance
  - Exposure (tobacco, allergies, air pollution)
  - CHF
  - Infection
  - PE

  - PTX
- **Labs**
  - CBC
  - Blood eosinophil count can be used to monitor risk for exacerbations and higher levels may mean that patients are more likely to have a beneficial response with the addition of ICS (COPENHAGEN GENERAL POPULATION STUDY).
  - BMP, Mg, Phosphorus
  - All patients should be screened for alpha-1-antitrypsin deficiency once after initial diagnosis is confirmed of COPD
  - 12 lead EKG
  - BNP (r/o CHF)
  - Troponin
  - ABG (O2, CO2)
    - ↓O2 = CPAP
    - ↑CO2 = BiPAP
    - Mechanical ventilation for pH<7.36, CO2>45mm
    - Repeat 30-60min after providing O2
    - BNP (to rule out underlying HF)
- **Inhaler Technique**
  - MDI (Metered Dose Inhaler)
    - Instructions
      1. Must shake before use for about 5 seconds with the cap on, drug is in a suspension
      2. Take the cap off and hold upright
      3. Breath out completely
      4. While pressing the inhaler, slowly breath in and as deep as possible
      5. Hold breath for about 10 seconds
    - Can use spacer if patient has problems with coordinating breaths or has arthritis
  - DPI (Dry Powder Inhaler)
    - Medication is in a loose powder form
    - Easier to use
    - Activated by the breath, no timing required like with MDIs
  - Soft Mist Liquid Inhaler
    - Think of this as a combination between an MDI and a nebulizer
    - Less of the medication gets stuck in the upper airway and no propellant is present
  - Nebulizer
    - Allows for a large dose of medication without any required coordination
    - Problem is they are not portable and take a while to set up
- **Treatment**
  - In mild COPD it is reasonable to start with one bronchodilator (LABA or SABA)
  - In moderate/severe COPD dual bronchodilator therapy with LABA+LAMA combinations are helpful
  - *ICS are rarely used but when necessary are added to single bronchodilator therapy (moderate disease) before going to dual bronchodilators **or** if patients are not responding to LABA+LAMA combinations then add ICS **or** patients have ↑serum eosinophils **or** have asthma like symptoms.*

GOLD Criteria

Grade/Symptoms	Class	Risk	PFTs	Treatment
I (mild)	A	Low (<1 exacerbation & no hospitalizations/year)	FEV1/FVC <70% FEV1 ≥ 80% predicted	SABA prn or Anti-cholinergic
II (moderate)	B		FEV1/FVC <70% FEV1 50-80%	SABA + LAMA or LABA (LAMA preferred per *UPLIFT*)
				If further exacerbations... Combine LAMA+LABA ***Or*** *Try the other long acting bronchodilator alone*
III (severe)	C	High (≥ 2 exacerbations or ≥1 hospitalization/year)	FEV1/FVC <70% FEV1 30-50%	SABA + LAMA
				If further exacerbations... LAMA+LABA (indacaterol/glycopyrronium) -or- LABA+ICS if above is not effective (*TORCH*)
IV (very severe)	D		FEV1/FVC <70% FEV1 ≤ 30% or FEV1 <50% + chronic resp failure	SABA + LAMA+LABA or LABA+ICS (*FLAME*) *(LABA+ICS preferred in patients with asthma component or ↑blood eosinophils)*

				If further exacerbations… • Add ICS (triple therapy; *IMPACT*) • Long term O2 if hypoxemic (PaO2 ≤ 55% or SpO2 ≤ 88%) • Consider lung reduction surgery • Consider roflumilast if FEV1 <50%+chronic bronchitis • Consider stopping ICS if no improvement while on it (patient with low eosinophil count and rare exacerbation history) • Consider macrolide (in former smokers)

- Short acting bronchodilators scheduled
  - Include beta-agonists and anticholinergic bronchodilators via neb or MDI
  - Patients with severe dyspnea may benefit from nebulizer due to poor inhalation technique and can later be transitioned to MDI
- LABA/LAMA combinations (moderate/severe disease) (*FLAME*)
  - These combinations improve lung function compared to placebo and have a greater impact on patient reported outcomes compared to monotherapies.
  - LABA/LAMA improves symptoms and health status in COPD patients, is more effective than long-acting bronchodilator monotherapy for preventing exacerbations and decreases exacerbations to a greater extent than ICS/LABA combination.
  - **Options**
    - **Indacaterol+glycopyrronium** 27.5/15.6 & 110/50 *(FLAME, LANTERN)*
    - Formoterol+aclidinium 12/400
    - Formoterol+glycopyrronium 9.6/14.4
    - Vilanterol+umeclidinium 25/62.5
- Triple Therapy (LAMA+LABA/ICS) shows improved lung function but evidence is scarce *(IMPACT)*
- +/- Antibiotics (↑sputum production, frequency)
  - Goal is to improve airflow and decrease hyperinflation of lungs
  - Provided in the acute setting
  - May benefit patients with mild exacerbations and **purulent** sputum
  - Levofloxacin 500mg PO daily x 3-10 days vs. 750mg PO daily for 7 days
  - Doxycycline 100mg PO BID x 3-10 days
  - Azithromycin (250 mg·day−1 or 500 mg three times per week) or erythromycin (500 mg two times per day) for 1 year reduces the risk of exacerbations in patients prone to exacerbations.
  - Amoxicillin-clavulanate 875 mg, Tab, PO, q12h
  - Chronic Use:
    - Azithromycin use showed a reduced exacerbation rate in former smokers only and was associated with an increased incidence of bacterial resistance and impaired hearing tests. Long-term azithromycin therapy may be considered in patients who have frequent exacerbations despite optimal maintenance inhaler therapy.
    - Pulse moxifloxacin therapy in patients with chronic bronchitis and frequent exacerbations does not reduce exacerbation rate.
- Beta Agonists
  - Duoneb 2ml Q 6 hours with Q 4 hours prn SOB/Wheezing
  - Xopenex (Levalbuterol) 1.25/3ml neb Q 4-6 hour prn SOB/wheezing (hold for tachycardia)
  - Neb: Albuterol 2.5 mg & Atrovent 0.5 mg in 3 cc NS q 4 hours
    or
  - MDI: 4-8 puffs (90 mcg per puff) with a spacer q1-4 hour as needed
- Anticholinergics (*UPLIFT*)
  - Nebulizer
  - Ipratropium (Atrovent) 0.5mg (500mcg) by neb q4h daily (or PRN SOB wheezing), or desaturation
    vs
    Ipratropium/Albuterol (Duoneb) by neb every 4 hours PRN SOB, wheezing
  - MDI
  - Spiriva (Tiotropium) 18mcg 2 puffs by MDI q4h PRN
- Systemic Glucocorticoids

        - Associated with greater FEV1, ↓hospitalization relapse, and improved oxygenation
        - No associated mortality benefit
        - Caution in patients with concurrent DM
        - No efficacy difference in PO vs. IV
            - PO: prednisone 30-60mg daily for 7-14 days
            - IV: Methylprednisolone 60-125mg IV Q6H
    - Oxygen
        - Target PaO2 60-70; SaO2 of 88-92%
            - NC→Simple Mask→VM
            - BiPAP is best if hypoxia and hypercapnia above baseline; IPAP 8-12; EPAP 3-5 with changes to IPAP to alleviate dyspnea
    - Inhaled Steroids
      NOT recommended in the acute setting; here for reference
        - Used per GOLD for categories C + D (higher risk patients)
        - Work best in patients with ↑ serum eosinophils, not responding to LABA+LAMA or have asthma like symptoms. If patients have a low eos count (<100), you may actually ↑ exacerbations if you use ICS.
        - ICS ↑ risk for pneumonia
        - Understand risks of w/d if stopping this medication class
        - Advair (Fluticasone/salmeterol) 250/50 daily vs. BID
        - Flovent (Fluticasone) 110mcg 2 puffs BID
        - If patient is already on and want to switch to LABA/LAMA, no increased risk of exacerbations seen with w/d of medication (*WISDOM*)
    - Roflumilast
        - Improved lung function and reduced exacerbations in participants with frequent exacerbations and hospitalization history
        - **Best to be added in patients on fixed-dose LABA+ICS**
        - Cannot be used concurrently with theophylline
        - Not to be used in acute setting
        - Often added in patients with severe (group D) disease
- **Management/Tracking Progression**
    - COPD Assessment Test (CAT) score
    - Modified Medical Research Council (MMRC) score
- **Preventive/Secondary Management**
    - Smoking cessation is key
    - Influenza and pneumococcal vaccinations are important in ↓ risk for lower respiratory tract infections
    - Long term oxygen improves survival in patients with low resting oxygenation level
    - **Air Travel**[272]
        - When planes travel >8000ft, normal oxygenation drops to 89-94% in healthy passengers
        - Patients with severe COPD may not be able to compensate and may develop LH, chest pain, neurological sequela in the extremities, palpitations, and dyspnea
        - The following patients should be tested:

Air travel oxygen management in COPD	
Resting Pulse Ox	Management
>95%	No testing required
92-95%	Testing if RF such as previous dyspnea during air travel, cannot walk to 50m w/o respiratory distress, mod/severe pulm HTN, FEV<50% are present → hypoxia altitude simulation test
<92%	Supplement with oxygen without testing
On home O2	Increase flow to 1-2L/min from baseline

Figure. Determining o2 requirements during air travel in patients with COPD

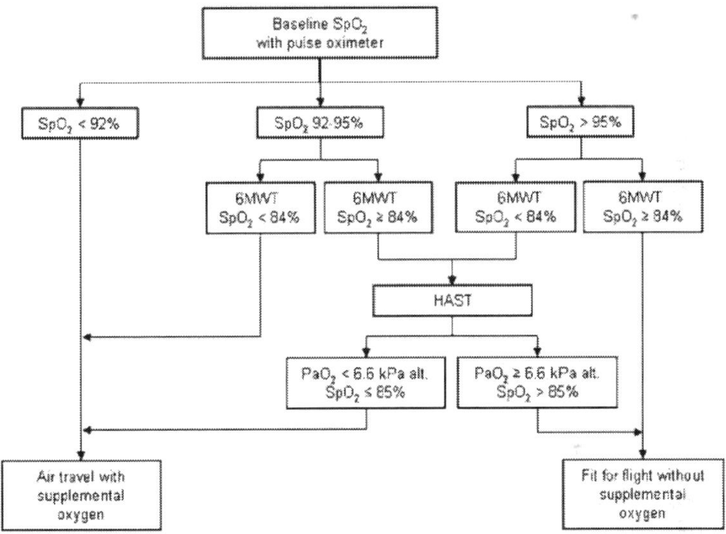

- **COPD Exacerbation**
  - Defined - AECOPD is an event characterized by an acute or subacute change in a patient's baseline dyspnea (particularly with exertion), cough, and/or sputum production (volume [more phlegm or unexpectedly less], purulence) over 2 to 3 days, enough to warrant concern and a call for advice and help with a change in treatment and management
  - General Facts
    - Treat for 10-14 days duration
    - Precipitated by m/c respiratory tract infections, aspiration, pollution, allergies, PE, poor adherence.
    - SABA+/-SAMA, are recommended as the initial bronchodilators to treat an acute exacerbation.
    - Maintenance therapy with LABA or LAMA should be initiated as soon as possible before hospital discharge.
    - Systemic corticosteroids improve lung function (FEV1), oxygenation and shorten recovery time and hospitalization duration.
      - 5-day course is just as good as 14-day course (*REDUCE*)

- ABx, when indicated, shorten recovery time, and reduce the risk of early relapse or treatment failure, and hospitalization duration.
  - It is important to target Streptococcus pneumoniae, Haemophilus influenzae, and Moraxella catarrhalis during AECOPDs.
  - Remember the possibility for Pseudomonas species to cause AECOPDs in more severely affected patients and when patients do not experience clinical improvement after 2 days of treatment.
    - Non-invasive mechanical ventilation should be the first mode of ventilation used to treat acute respiratory failure.
    - Exacerbations associated with an increase in sputum or blood eosinophils may be more responsive to systemic steroids
    - Symptoms usually last between 7 to 10 days during an exacerbation,
- Acid-Base

Acid-base correction			
Condition	∆In PCO2	∆In HCO3	pH
Acute	Every ↑10	↑1	↓.1
Chronic	Every ↑10	↑4	↓.015
Acute on Chronic	Every ↑10	↑1	↓.1

- Oxygen to target saturation of 90 to 92% and PaO2 of 60-65 mmHg with gradual increases in FiO2 by 4-7% (from 24-28%).
  - Venturi masks are preferred means of O2 delivery because they permit a precise delivered fraction of inspired oxygen (FiO2) such as 24, 28, 31, 35, 40, or 60 percent.
  - Nasal cannulae can provide flow rates up to 6 L per minute with an associated FiO2 of approximately 40 percent
- Imaging – CXR to r/o PNA, PTX, or aspiration
- Diagnostics – EKG to r/o cardiac source, ABG
- Labs – CBC, BNP, BMP
- Treatment
  - **Beta Agonists**
    - Goal is to use combination SABA and SAAC
      - Albuterol 5mg via neb q4h prn→ transition to MDI 4-8puffs q1-4h prn
      - Ipratropium (AC) 500 micrograms via nebulizer q6h prn → transition to 2 puffs via MDI q4h prn
      - Others
        - Xopenex (SABA) 1.25/3ml neb Q 6-hour prn SOB/wheezing
        - DuoNeb 2ml Q 4 hours with Q 2 hours prn SOB/Wheezing
  - **Oxygen Therapy**: if SaO2 <88% or PaO2 <7 kPa with goal 88-92%
  - **Solu Medrol** 125 mg-200mg IV now (admit) then 80 mg IV Q 6-8 hours OR Solu Medrol **40mg** IV Q 24 hours
    - Duration of Prednisone 40mg/d = 5 days (no benefit to prolonged 7-14 day course)
  - **Antibiotics**
    - Levofloxacin (750 mg IV) for 6-7 days
    - Amoxicillin 500mg q8h PO
  - **Physiotherapy**: aids in sputum expulsion
  - **Non-Invasive PPV** - Consider if patient does not improve with above interventions or if ↑RR, ↓pH or ↑PaCO2 suggestive of impending failure
  - **Intubation**: Consider if not improving to NIPPV or pH <7.26 and PaCO2 ↑

EXERCISE-INDUCED BRONCHOSPASM

- **Pathophysiology**[273]
  - Strenuous exercise is known to create a hyperosmolar environment by introducing dry air in the airway with compensatory water loss, leading to transient osmotic change on the airway surface. The hyperosmolar environment leads to mast cell degranulation with release of mediators, predominately leukotrienes, but also including histamine, tryptase, and prostaglandins. In addition, eosinophils can also be activated, producing further mediators, including leukotrienes. In turn, this might lead to bronchoconstriction and inflammation of the airway
- **Symptoms**
  - Interestingly, patients will have worse symptoms 5-30 minutes after cessation of activity rather than during
  - EIB: Symptoms: wheeze, stridor, throat tightness, chest pain/tightness, dyspnea
  - VCD Symptoms: throat tightness, inspiratory stridor, voice change
- **Diagnosis**
  - EIB
    - Diagnosis of EIB relies on performing a standardized bronchoprovocation challenge in a subject who has been shown to have normal to near-normal PFT results both before and after bronchodilator
    - Expect reversible lower airway obstruction (12% bronchodilator response)
    - PFT will show 10% reduction in FEV1
    - In a subject who has no history of current clinical asthma, normal PFT results, and no response to bronchodilator, an exercise challenge with a treadmill or cycle or in the sport venue or a surrogate challenge, such as EVH, can be indicated.
    - With exercise challenge, the patient should achieve a heart rate at least 85% of maximum value (95% in children) for 6 minutes after 2 to 4 minutes of ramping up.
  - VCD
    - PFT - flattening of the inspiratory loop; FIF ratio of >1.5; symptoms immediately stop after stopping activity whereas with EIB the symptoms persist for appx 30 minutes after stopping. Gold standard diagnosis requires direct fiberoptic laryngoscopy
- **Evaluation**
  - If baseline pulmonary function test results are normal to near normal (before and after bronchodilator) in a person with suspected EIB, then further testing should be performed by using a standardized exercise challenge or eucapnic voluntary hyperpnea (EVH). Consider CPEX in those with continued symptoms without clear diagnosis, especially if concurrent chest pain is present.
- **Differential Diagnosis**
  - Exercise Induced Laryngospasm – likely inspiratory stridor, whereas you would expect expiratory stridor in asthma or EIB, also symptoms improve immediately after stopping exercise.
  - Exercise Induced Anaphylaxis – patient will have rash, pruritus, urticaria and low blood pressure
- **Treatment**
  - Short-acting β2- agonists to provide bronchodilation and broncho protection.
    - Best to be used if patient does have decreased FEV1 on PFTs

- Avoid using these for a long period of time as it can lead to tolerance, safer to use LTRA's
  - Better to be used intermittently, <4x/week before exercise
- Inhaled steroids – can decrease frequency and severity but not fully eliminate; do not use this daily with concurrent LABA (like you would in asthma or COPD) as it can lead to tolerance
- Leukotriene receptor antagonists (LTRAs) – better to use these daily (does not lead to tolerance) however they only help in 50% of patients (ie. Montelukast)
- Cromolyn Compounds
- Pre-exercise warm-up, nasal breathing, wearing a mask in cold weather
- Dietary supplementation with fish-oil (omega-3-fatty acid)
- Combination therapy (with inhaled corticosteroids and long-acting β2-agonists [LABAs]), are recommended for inflammation.
- Combination therapy that includes a LABA should not be used in persons with normal or near-normal baseline lung function (ie, FEV1 >80% of predicted value) because regular use of short-acting β2-agonists and LABAs can cause tolerance, limiting their ability to provide bronchoprotection and bronchodilation.

- **Consults**
  - Cardiologist or pulmonologist - to perform cardiopulmonary testing when breathlessness with exercise, with or without chest pain, might be caused by heart disease or other conditions in the absence of EIB.
  - Psychological evaluation - when the symptoms (eg, hyperventilation and anxiety disorders) are in the differential diagnosis of EIB.

HYPOXIA

- **Physiology**
  - The arterial pH is the main respiratory drive as it is affected by CO2 and is monitored by <u>peripheral</u> (carotid body; PNS/CNS effects) and <u>central</u> (brainstem; monitor H+ levels) chemoreceptors
  - Linear relationship exists between MV (TVxRR) and CO2; this is why with intubated patients these are the variables you monitor to alter CO2 levels
    - ↑CO2 leads to ↓consciousness, ↑CBF (aka ICP, which is why you hyperventilate pts with suspected ↑ICP), decreased myocardial contractility
  - MV is not as closely correlated with PaO2 when PaO2 levels drop below 60. This is the theory behind COPD patients and their ultimate respiratory drive as their PaO2 is often low due to a chronic elevated PaCO2 therefore their senses are 'blunted' to any abnormal levels due to chronically being in this state, as a result they rely on hypoxia instead to drive respirations.
- **Classifications**
  - <u>Mild</u> - PaO2/FIO2 > 200 mmHg
  - <u>Moderate</u> - PaO2/FIO2 100-200 mmHg
  - <u>Severe</u> – PaO2/FIO2 < 100 mmHg
- **A-a gradient**
  - PAO – PaO (Alveolar oxygen – capillary oxygen)
  - PAO is calculated and PaO is obtained from blood gas
  - PAO = 150 – (1.25 x PACO)
  - Normal gradient 5-20, anything > 20 is abnormal
  - Only causes below that ↑A-a gradient are diffusion defect, V/Q, hypoventilation, Low FiO2, and true shunt
    - Shunt will not improve with supplemental oxygen, require PEEP
    - V/Q mismatch WILL improve with oxygen

- **Five major causes include:**
  - ↓RR / Low alveolar PO2 – low oxygen delivered from lungs into HGB therefore low O2 available to tissues; caused by depressed RAS, respiratory muscle injury, spinal cord injury, NMJ disease (MG), kyphoscoliosis.
  - Diffusion impairment - seen in conditions such as pulmonary fibrosis, interstitial/alveolar edema
  - V/Q mismatch – large areas of lung that are under perfused
    - Major cause of hypercapnia in COPD patients due to emphysema which makes it more difficult to remove CO2 from the lungs due to ↑dead space
    - COPD patients compensate for the ↑ dead space by ↑MV (RR primarily) to try and blow off CO2
  - Shunt – R→L shunt seen with atelectasis, PNA, ARDS, CHF
  - ↓FIO2 – high altitudes

Causes of Hypoxia

Classification	PA_{O2}	Pa_{O2}	Ca_{O2}	P_{O2}	C_{O2}	Increased FI_{O2} Helpful?
↓RR	Low	Low	Low	Low	Low	Yes
Diffusion impairment	N	Low	Low	Low	Low	Yes
Right-to-left shunts	N	Low	Low	Low	Low	No
V/Q mismatch	N	Low	Low	Low	Low	Yes

- **Treatment**
  - Patients with moderate to severe ARDS respond best to prone positioning and NMBD
- **Outcome**
  - Calculate the oxygenation index (see Formulas below)

INTERPRETATION OF PFT'S

Contributor: Eric Crawley, M.D. [274,275,276]

Figure. Lung volumes to consider when interpreting PFTs

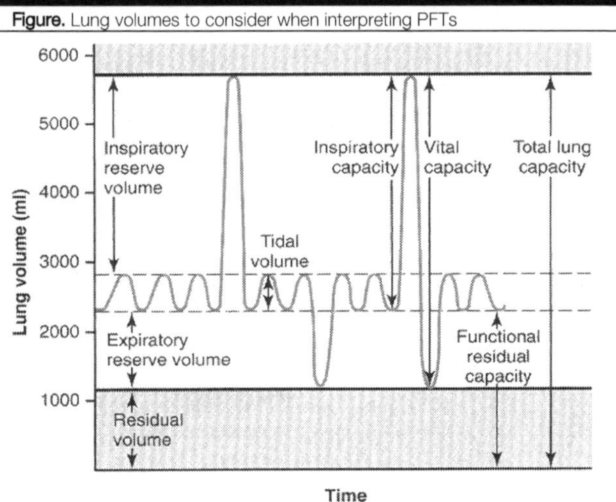

- **Background**
  - Tool used to diagnose and manage respiratory, or suspected respiratory, problems
  - Gold standard for diagnosis of obstructive lung disease (NLHEP, NHLBI, WHO)
  - Used for the diagnosis of lung disease (detect presence thereof)
  - Helps to quantify the extent of disease if present and can be utilized to measure the benefit of therapy administered
- **Types**
  - Spirometry – includes measurement of exhaled or inhaled air during forced maneuvers
  - Diffusion capacity – measures diffusion of CO, can help evaluate parenchyma
  - Lung volumes – obtains total lung volumes to include TLC, RV, etc.
- **Definitions**
  - FVC—Forced vital capacity; the total volume of air that can be exhaled during a maximal forced expiration effort. Will be displayed graphically as to the right. It's important to ensure that a full 6 seconds is seen of effort with an obvious plateau with no early termination/cut-off. Healthy people can exhale the FVC in 4-6 seconds, with COPD patients, you will see this extended to 15+ seconds.
    - Ideally the FVC value is within 150cc of the VC
    - Often in healthy patients this will be quite close to the VC if not equal
    - In obstructive and restrictive disease, we will see this value decreased (mucus plug, bronchial narrowing, CF, asthma, PF, MG, GBS)
  - FEV1—Forced expiratory volume in one second; the volume of air exhaled in the first second under force after a maximal inhalation. Represented on the graph to the bottom right.
  - FEV1/ FVC ratio—The percentage of the FVC expired in one second.
  - FEF25-75%—Forced expiratory flow over the middle one half of the FVC; the average flow from the point at which 25 percent of the FVC has been exhaled to the

point at which 75 percent of the FVC has been exhaled. This is rarely used but used if the FEV1/FVC was questionable, you can use this to confirm evidence of obstructive disease if it is also low.
  - MVV—Maximal voluntary ventilation; measure of how rapidly and deeply someone breaths in and out; decreased in patients with poor test performance or NM disease
  - Flow volume loop - provides important clues about the quality, acceptability, and reproducibility of the maneuver, which is determined by national standards and controlled by each individual laboratory.
- **Lung volumes**
  - ERV—Expiratory reserve volume; the maximal volume of air exhaled from end expiration.
  - IRV—Inspiratory reserve volume; the maximal volume of air inhaled from end inspiration.
  - RV—Residual volume; the volume of air remaining in the lungs after a maximal exhalation.
  - VT—Tidal volume; the volume of air inhaled or exhaled during each respiratory cycle.
  - Lung capacities
  - FRC—Functional residual capacity; the volume of air in the lungs at resting end expiration.
  - IC—Inspiratory capacity; the maximal volume of air that can be inhaled from the resting expiratory level.
  - TLC—Total lung capacity; the volume of air in the lungs at maximal inflation (TLC=IC+FRC)
  - VC—Vital capacity; the largest volume measured on complete exhalation after full inspiration (but not forced)
    - Conditions associated with decreased VC:
- **Lung cancer, pulm edema, PNA, surgical tissue resection, OLD, PTX, pregnancy (limited movement of diaphragm), tumors, scleroderma and kyphoscoliosis due to limited chest wall movement)**
- **Normal Values**
  - Pulmonary Normal value (95 percent function test confidence interval)
  - FEV1 80% to 120%
  - FVC 80% to 120%
  - Absolute FEV1 / FVC Within 5% of the predicted ratio
  - TLC 80% to 120%
  - FRC 75% to 120%
  - RV 75% to 120%
  - DLCO > 60% to < 120%
- **Others Not Commonly Used**
  - Peak Expiratory Flow (aka Peak Flow) – in liters with normal being 100-850 cc/min, used often with asthmatics, and patients with MG. it's the maximum flow obtained during a FVC and measures the large airway function. You can give a patient their own peak flow meter and use it to help them monitor their own asthma function. The patient should know what their "normal" is along with their personal best.
    - For asthmatics specifically, you can use this to determine likelihood of having an exacerbation by the % reduction in PEF from their personal best (<80% is worrisome)
  - Reports will have the following information:
    - Actual – what the patient performed
    - Predicted – what the patient should be able to perform based on epidemiology
    - % Predicted – actual/predicted
    - FVC – flow volume loop, exhibited below:

Figure. Flow volume loops for common pulmonary conditions

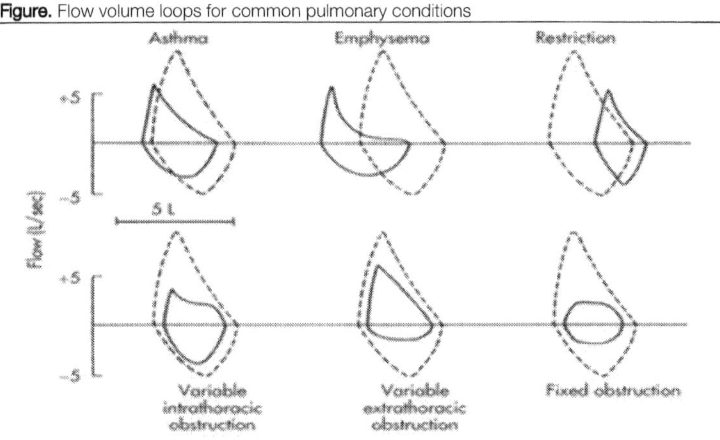

- **Interpretation**
  - Ensure the following are present:
    - Volume/time curve reaches a plateau lasting at least 6 seconds
    - Results are 'reproducible' which means that on at least two attempts, the values were within 0.2L of one another
    - FVL show no evidence of abnormalities

Figure. Interpretation of pulmonary function tests in flow-chart format

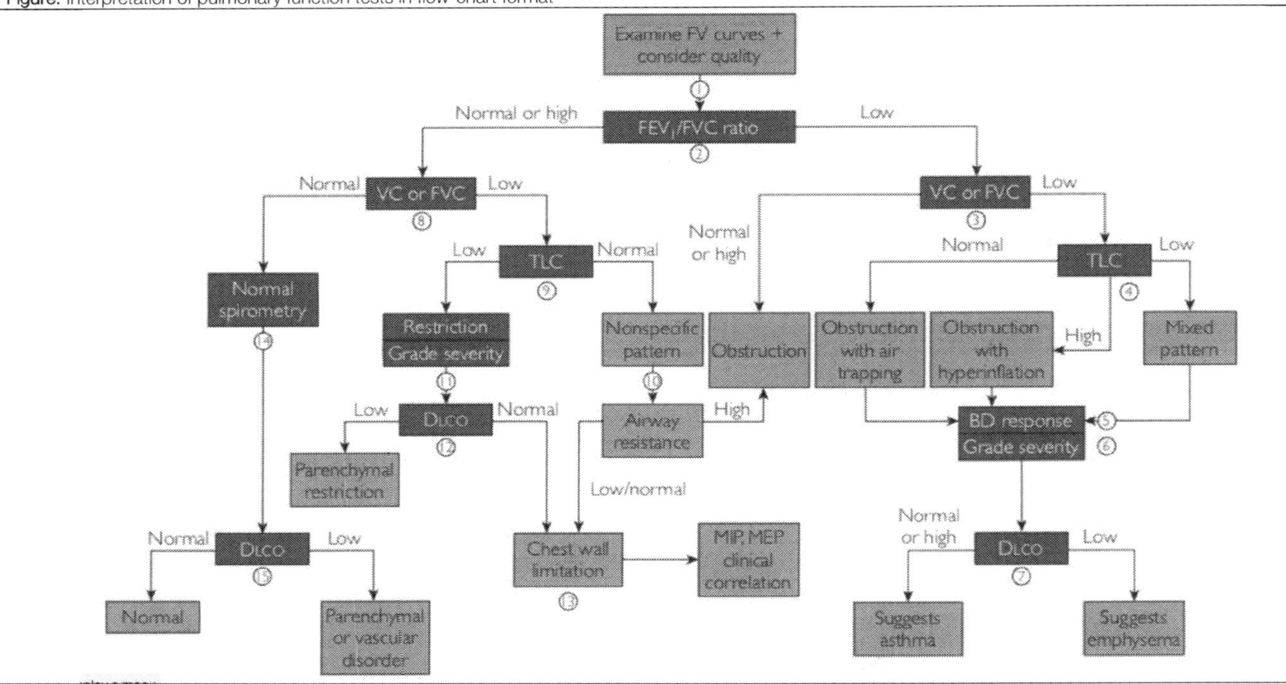

<table>
<tr><th colspan="2">Step by Step Evaluation of PFT</th></tr>
<tr><th>Step</th><th>Evaluation</th></tr>
<tr><td><u>STEP 1</u></td><td>Look at the flow volume loop:
• Look for scooped or scalloped appearance c/w COPD
• Narrow loops are c/w restrictive disease
• Inspiratory flows are disproportionately reduced from lesions in the upper/extrathoracic airway
• Expiratory flows are disproportionately reduced from lesions in the lower/intrathoracic airway (trachea, main stem)
• Restrictions in both inspiratory and expiratory suggest a fixed lesion</td></tr>
<tr><td><u>STEP 2</u></td><td>Look at FEV1:FVC ratio:
This will tell us if there is an obvious obstructive or restrictive defect present
<table><tr><th>Obstructive</th><th>Restrictive</th><th>Mixed</th></tr><tr><td>FEV1/FVC < 70%
FVC nml or ↑</td><td>FEV1/FVC nml
FVC ↑</td><td>FEV1/FVC <70%
FVC↓</td></tr></table>• GOLD: <70% ← the expert consensus criteria to use for patients >65 years
• ATS: Less than the LLN ← the expert consensus criteria to use for patients <65 years
• Anything less than the predicted lower limit of normal (<70%)→obstructive pattern</td></tr>
<tr><td><u>STEP 3</u></td><td>Look at FVC
• If it is reduced in the presence of a reduced FEV1/FVC then mixed pattern present, this is because most patients with a restrictive defect have a low FVC
• If reduced in the presence of a normal FEV1/FVC then restrictive pattern present
• Officially use the LLN to determine if FVC is reduced, but the below can help categorize the severity:
Look at FEV1
• Officially use the LLN to determine if FVC is reduced, but the below can help categorize the severity:
• Only of benefit if there was an obstructive process going on in step 1
• If FEV1 is disproportionally reduced relative to FVC, then a mixed picture may be present (obstruction and restriction)</td></tr>
<tr><td><u>STEP 4</u></td><td>Confirm Restrictive Pattern→Defect
• If pattern above is consistent with restrictive pattern, then obtain full volumes along with DLCO (↓DLCo, ↓TLC compared to LLN, ↓RV compared to LLN)</td></tr>
<tr><td><u>STEP 5</u></td><td>Assess Severity
• Determine severity based on the percentage of FEV1
  o FEV1>70% predicted: mild.
  o FEV1 60-69% predicted: moderate obstruction.
  o FEV1 50-59% predicted: moderate severe obstruction.</td></tr>
</table>

	o FEV1 35-49% predicted: severe obstruction. o FEV1 <35% predicted: very severe obstruction.
STEP 6	Reversibility? • Ensure patients have not taken their medication at least 4 hours prior to testing in lab • If obstructive defect, determine reversibility based on the increase in FEV1 and/or FVC after bronchodilator challenge o 12% **and** 200cc in either FEV1 or FVC • If mixed pattern was present, then if the patient has full reversibility to the LLN of the FVC then this is suggestive of pure obstructive defect but if it doesn't, it confirms restrictive disease
STEP 7	Bronchoprovocation • If PFT is normal (FEV1>70%) but you still suspect disease (ie. EIB, allergen-induced) then perform testing with methacholine challenge, exercise testing, or mannitol inhalation. o Methacholine: 20% reduction in FEV1 is diagnostic o Exercise: 10% or more reduction in FEV1 or FVC is diagnostic if it occurs over two time points (ie. 1/3/5/10/15/20/30/45 min) • If FEV1/FVC was normal but FEV1<70% go ahead and give them albuterol as trial

- Lung volumes:
  - Obstructive pattern:
    - ↑TLC (hyperinflation)
    - ↑RV (gas trapping)
    - If you suspect a defect but don't see it on initial testing (ie. asthma, EIB, allergen-induced), consider bronchoprovocation testing with methacholine challenge
  - Restrictive pattern:
    - ↓FVC
    - ↓TLC
    - Severity:
      - Mild : TLC or FVC 65 - 80% predicted
      - Moderate : TLC or FVC 50 -65% predicted
      - Severe : TLC or FVC < 50% predicted
    - ↓RV
    - Diffusion Capacity (DLCO2) (Parenchymal Process)
      - ↓DLCO2 + normal spirometry: early ILD, pHTN, pulmonary vascular disease, anemia, early emphysema.
      - ↓DLCO2 + obstruction: emphysema, bronchiolitis obliterans, cystic fibrosis, bronchiectasis
      - ↓DLCO2 + restriction: ILD, hypersensitivity pneumonitis, drug toxicity, CHF.
      - ↑DLCO2: polycythemia, pulmonary hemorrhage, asthma, intracardiac shunt
  - Mixed pattern:
    - ↓FEV1/FVC and ↓FVC and the severity is monitored by the FEV1 specifically
    - These are more difficult to interpret:
      - With the reduced ratio and reduced FVC specifically, if the bronchodilator leads to improvement (remember 12% and 200cc) then its suggestive of a pure obstructive defect → COPD. If there is no response to

bronchodilator, then get full pulmonary testing to evaluate for evidence of restrictive defect (ie. TLC, RV reduced)

- **Differential**
  - Obstructive
    - α1-antitrypsin deficiency
    - Asthma
    - Bronchiectasis
    - Bronchiolitis obliterans
    - Chronic obstructive pulmonary disease
    - Cystic fibrosis
    - Silicosis (early)
  - Restrictive
    - Chest wall
      - Ankylosing spondylitis
      - Kyphosis
      - Morbid obesity
      - Scoliosis
      - Drugs (adverse reaction)
        - Amiodarone
        - Methotrexate
        - Nitrofurantoin (Furadantin)
    - Interstitial lung disease
      - Asbestosis
      - Berylliosis
      - Eosinophilic pneumonia
      - Hypersensitivity pneumonitis
      - Idiopathic pulmonary fibrosis
      - Sarcoidosis
      - Silicosis (late)
    - Neuromuscular disorders
      - Amyotrophic lateral sclerosis
      - Guillain-Barré syndrome
      - Muscular dystrophy
      - Myasthenia gravis
- **Summary**
  - FEV1, FVC, TLC and DLCO are pretty much the major variables to know
  - An obstructive defect is indicted by a low FEV1/FVC ratio which overall is defined as < 70%
  - Reversible obstruction (ie. asthma) is evaluated by post bronchodilator response (12% or 200cc improvement)
  - Suspect a restrictive lung disease in patients with a normal FEV1/FVC ratio but the FVC itself is <80%. DLCO is best to obtain at this point to r/o IPF or other diffusion defects

INTUBATION

- **Indications for intubation**[4]
  - Respiratory rate > 35-40 for extended period of time (minutes can count in a severely debilitated patient.
  - pCO2 > 60 in patient who does not chronically retain CO2
  - pO2 < 50-55 despite therapy and high FiO2 in patient without chronically low values

- Gross respiratory distress, especially if it is apparent that patient is tiring or too weak to continue arduous respiration for much longer
- Signs/symptoms of acute respiratory failure:
  - Resp rate > 35
  - Tachycardia
  - PaCO2 > 55 (acute)
- Cyanosis
- Change in mental status
- PaCO2 < 70 on supplemental O2

Be sure that patient is not a DO NOT INTUBATE before initiating process. Call anesthesia to place the tube and consult pulmonary for ventilator management.

NOTE: Most people get into trouble by thinking about intubation too late, rather than too early. Don't intubate without calling your resident -- unless it's too late to wait!

- **Intubate if:**
  - Response to tx is inadequate.
  - Airway obstructed or unstable.
  - Work of breathing becomes overwhelming w/ other organ system failure.
  - Inability to protect airway (decreased LOC with no gag/cough).
  - Severe metabolic acidosis with respiratory distress

Sedation / Induction medications used in the intubation of a patient

Drug	MOA	Dose	Onset	Duration	Elimination	Positive Considerations	Negative Considerations
Etomidate		0.3 mg/kg (usual dose ~20 mg IV)	10-15 seconds	4-10 minutes		• **First line sedative for rapid sequence intubation (RSI).** • Rapid onset • Short duration • No hypotension, lowers ICP	• tendency to induce vomiting (use with paralytic) • C/I in adrenal insufficiency
Midazolam (Versed)	GABAergic	1-15 mg/hr	2-5 min	2-4h	Liver	• Good when used in combination with fentanyl • CV stability (no bradycardia, little hypotension) • Low cost • Anti-convulsant properties	• Risk of ICU delirium (benzos) • Accumulation • Active metabolite • Use lower dose in elderly • High risk for respiratory depression • Daily awakenings and scheduled dose taper can minimize accumulation
Lorazepam (Ativan)	GABAergic	1-15 mg/hr	5-20 min	4-6h	Liver		• Accumulation (long T1/2) • Consider only using boluses • Propylene glycol toxicity at high doses

Propofol (Diprivan)	GABAergic	15-50 mcg/kg/m RSI dose is 0.5 mg/kg, sedative dose is 1 mg/kg	30-90s	3-10m	Liver	• Effective sedation • No risk of accumulation • Easily titratable with no need to bolus • Fast recovery, so good for patients in whom neuro exam must be checked frequently (can turn off and check neuro exam in ~10 minutes) • Some data to suggest use in benzo-refractory delirium tremens	• ↓BP • ↑TRIG due to lipid emulsion • Check TRIG 48 hrs after use • Propofol related infusion syndrome (PRIS) rare but associated with ST elevation, acidosis, electrolyte imbalance, rhabdo, CV collapse • Expensive, • Depresses myocardial contractility
Dexmedetomidine (Precedex)	Alpha-2 agonist	0.4-1.5 mcg/kg/m	15-30m	20-30m	Liver	• Unique sedative profile (can remain arousable) • ↓ICU delirium • Opioid sparing • No respiratory suppression	• Most common adverse events include bradycardia and hypotension • Avoid if patient on paralytic/NMBA • Avoid in hemodynamic shock • High cost
Thiopental	Barbiturate	3-5 mg/kg SE: 15-20 mg/kg IV loading dose over 10-15m	<30 seconds	5-10m	Mostly liver	• Great for RSI in neuro patients (high ICP, CVA, **status epilepticus**). • Rapid onset, ultra-short acting.	• <u>Disadvantages</u>: **not routinely used**, causes hypotension–reduce dose or use alternative sedative. Monitor K levels.

							• Contraindications: severe hypotension.
Ketamine		1.5 mg/kg IV	45-60s	10-20m		• Good option for patients with reactive airway disease or who are hypovolemic, hemorrhaging, or in shock	• ↑HR and ↑BP • ↑Intraocular pressure • Not recommended in hypertensive patients • Use in caution in those with CVD

Pain medications used in the intubation of a patient								
Drug	MOA	Dose	Equianalgesic Dose	Onset	Duration	Elimination	Positive Considerations	Negative Considerations
Fentanyl (DOC for continuous analgesia)	Opioid	25-300 mcg/h	100mcg	1-2m	1-2h	Liver	• Short DOA • Eliminated 1-2h after infusion is D/C • Low risk of accumulation	• Very potent • Dosing error risk • Respiratory suppression • Constipation/ileus • Fentanyl induced Rigidity (rare, a/w large bolus doses)

								Contraindications: increased ICP, end stage liver disease, severe respiratory depression (not yet intubated)
Morphine	Opioid	2-30 mg/h	10mg	2-8m	2-6h	Liver	• Most clinicians are familiar with dosing • Longer duration of action allows for bolus dosing without continuous infusion	• Histamine release • Flushing • ↓BP • Constipation/ileus
Hydromorphone (Dilaudid)	Opioid	0.5-10 mg/h	3.5mg	2-8m	2-4h	Liver	• Longer DOA allows bolus dosing without continuous infusion • Can be used in renal dysfunction • No or less histamine release	• Less histamine release • Constipation/ileus

Rapid Sequence Intubation Step by Step

	Class	Medication	Time to Effect	Miscellaneous Information

1	Preparation	• Monitors, laryngoscope, fiberoptic, crico kit, ETT/stylet/syringe, all medications, suction, IV, rescue devices, fluids hanging, pressors if possible, place CXR order
		• LEMON for difficult airway
		  o Look, Evaluate (3-3-2 rule), Mallampati, Obstruction evidence, Neck mobility
		  o Risk
		    ▪ Mallampati Score (1→4; easy→hard)
		    ▪ Thyromental distance (more = better)
		    ▪ ROM
		    ▪ Size of neck
		    ▪ Size of open mouth
		    ▪ Neck instability (RA, Down's, OA)
		  o Sniff
		    ▪ Put pillow rolls under shoulder
		• Preoxygenation with 100% O2
		  o 100% O2 for 5 minutes OR 2-6 Full Vital Capacity breaths of 100% O2
		  o Denitrogenizes alveoli to allow much longer time before desaturation occurs		

2	Pain medication	Fentanyl 2-10mcg/kg		
3	Premedication	Atropine 0.01-0.02 mg/kg	1-2min	Antisialagogue Inhibits bradycardic response to hypoxia
		Glycopyrrolate 0.005-0.01 mg/kg	1-2min	Antisialagogue Inhibits bradycardic response to hypoxia
4	Induction/Sedative	Etomidate 0.3mg/kg Versed 0.3mg/kg Propofol 1-2mg/kg	15-45 sec 30-60 sec 15-45 sec	Good for ↓BP patients; ↓cortisol (avoid in sepsis) Can ↓BP, good for status epilepticus patients

		Ketamine 1-2mg/kg	30 sec	Good for patients with bronchospasm, can ↓BP, no analgesic properties
		Fentanyl 2-5mcg/kg	1-3min	Arrythmia, increases secretions; elev BP, elev HR
				May lower BP, minimal histamine release
5	Paralytic	Succinylcholine 1-1.5 mg/kg	30s-1min	↑K, ↓HR, GBS, ↑muscle fasciculations, ↑IOP, avoid in burn/crush pts or severe infxn
		Rocuronium 0.6-1.2 mg/kg	45s-1min	Nondepolarizing, rapid onset, used with succinylcholine c/I
		Vecuronium 0.1-0.2 mg/kg	2-3m	Higher doses mean quicker onset and longer duration
6	Confirmation	Check placement with end-tidal CO2, t/c NGT, OGT, CXR (ETT should be just below head of clavicles)		

Intubation/Medications		
	RSI	**Maintenance**
Induction		
Etomidate	30mg	N/A
Ketamine	150mg	50mg/hr
Paralytic		
Succinylcholine	100mg	N/A
Rocuronium	150mg	N/A
Pain		
Fentanyl	50mcg	50mcg/hr

Vent Settings

- Mode: AC
- Rate = 12
- VT = 500cc (6cc/kg; ARDSNet Protocol)
- I:E ratio: 1:2 or 1:3
- FiO2 = 1.0 (wean down rapidly to < 60% to avoid oxygen toxicity).
- PS (pressure support) = 5-10 (5cm H20 needed to overcome resistance of endotracheal tube).
- IFR: 80cc
- PEEP (positive end-expiratory pressure) = 0-15 (start low; cautious use in asthmatics and COPD patients as "auto PEEP" occurs often).

Neuromuscular Blockade Agents[277278]

	Agent	Onset of Action	Duration of Action	Recommended Bolus Dose	Infusion Rate
Short-Acting	Mivacurium	2min	17min	150 mcg/kg	1-15 mcg/kg/min
	Rocuronium	0.7-1min	30-60min	0.6-1.2 mg/kg	10-40 mcg/kg/min
	Succinylcholine	0.5-1min	5-10min	1-2 mg/kg	2.5 mg/min
Intermediate-Acting	Atracurium	2	30 min	0.5 mg/kg	5 mcg/kg/min
	Cisatracurium	2	30 min	100-200 mcg/kg	1-5 mcg/kg/min
	Pancuronium	2-3	60-90min	0.05-0.1 mg/kg	0.05-1 mg/kg q2 prn
	Vecuronium	1.5	30-60min	0.08-0.1 mg/kg	0.1-0.2 mg/kg q2 prn
Long-Acting	Doxacurium	6	80 min	50 mcg/kg	N/A
	Pipecuronium	3-5	70-120 min	50-100 mcg/kg	N/A

Figure. View of different support modes on ventilator[279]

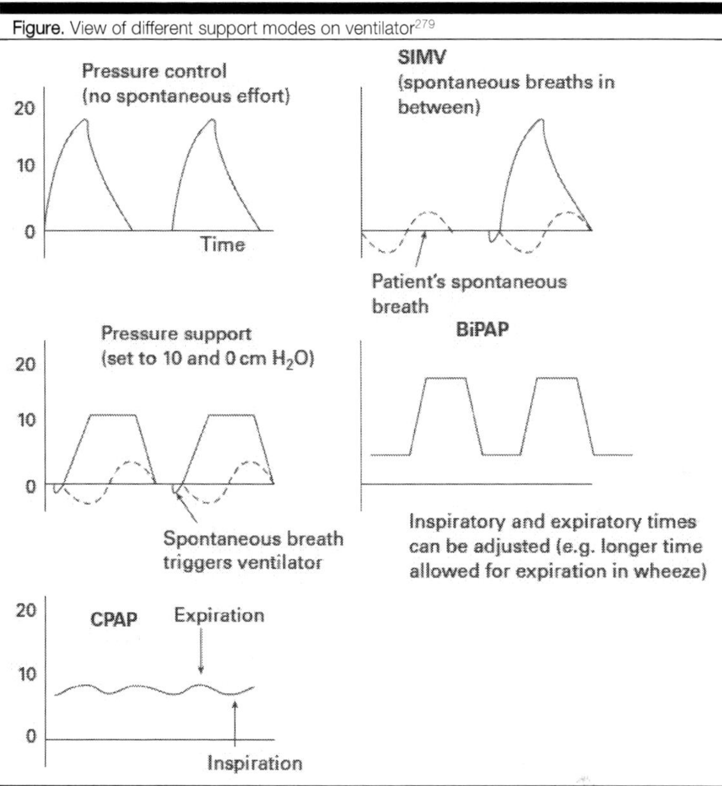

Figure. Example timeline for RSI

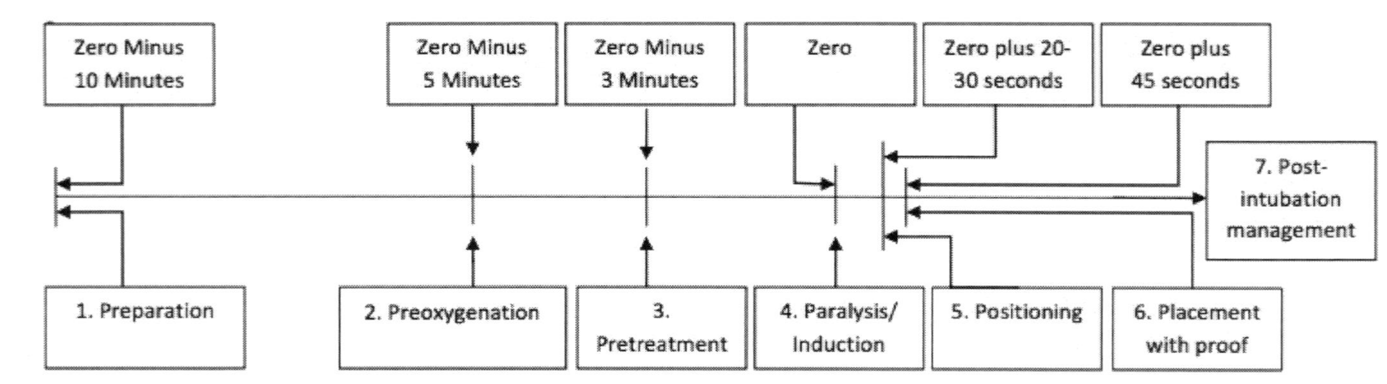

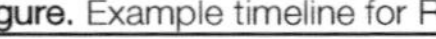

Step 1: Preparation	Step 2: Preoxygenation	Step 3: Pretreatment	Step 4: Paralysis with induction
Assemble all necessary equipment, medications, etc.	Replace the nitrogen in the patient's functional reserve with oxygen – "nitrogen wash out; oxygen wash in"	Ancillary medications are administered to mitigate the adverse physiologic consequences of intubation • Lidocaine 100mg can be given in patients with head injury, TBI, ↑ICP to help protect the patient from ↑ in ICP that occur with intubation	See prior tables

		• Fentanyl 2-3mcg/kg; given to help decrease catecholamine discharge 2/2 to intubation and thus ↓ risk from ↑BP in patients with CVD, aortic dissection, etc.
Step 5: Positioning	**Step 6: Placement with proof**	**Step 7: Post-intubation management**
Position patient for optimal laryngoscopy	Assess mandible for flaccidity, perform intubation, confirm placement	Long-term sedation /analgesia/paralysis as indicated

- **Rapid Sequence Intubation**
  - Used in anyone at risk for aspiration. Major difference is that there is no bag-mask ventilation following induction, as this could introduce air into the GI track causing vomiting.
    1) Be prepared to perform surgical airway in event airway control is lost
    2) Ensure suction is on and you are able to delivery PP ventilation
    3) Equipment:
       - Laryngoscope
       - Blade
       - NPA/OPA
       - Suction
       - Bougie
       - Glideslope
       - Fiberoptic
       - LMA
    4) Preoxygenate to 100% O2 for 5 minutes
    5) The application of pressure to the cricoid cartilage (to close esophagus and ↓ aspiration) is no longer recommended for use in the ER setting. It has not been tested for appropriateness in pre-hospital care.
    6) **Administer induction drug** (etomidate 0.3 mg/kg or 20mg)
       Depresses adrenal function
    7) **Administer pain drug** (fentanyl 0.3mcg/kg)
    8) **Administer paralyzing drug**: 1-2mg/kg succinylcholine IV (or 100mg)
       Avoid if ↑K, crush injuries, burns, CRF, neuromuscular disease
    9) After relaxation, start intubation
    10) Inflate cuff and confirm placement
        - Auscultation
        - B/L chest rise
        - CO2
        - O2 waves on monitor
        - Release cricoid pressure
    11) Ventilate
    12) CXR
        ETT should be 3-7cm from the carina (Remember 357 magnum) often just below the clavicles
        Insertion depth of ETT from corner of mouth of 21cm for women, 23cm for men

VENTILATOR REVIEW

- **Overview**
  - Vocabulary:
    - **Presentation: MODE/TV/RATE/PEEP/FIO2 WITH PEAK **, PLATEAU ***, PULLING TV OF ******
    - *Pressure support* – pressure that augments a spontaneous breath
      - "10 over 5" or "10/5" – (pressure support) above (PEEP). The assigned pressure support, which is above and beyond the continuous PEEP, for spontaneous breaths.
    - *PEEP* – positive end expiratory pressure. Pressure that is maintained at the end of expiration to prevent alveolar collapse. This in effect increases compliance, and thus oxygenation.
    - *I:E ratio* – the inspiratory time to expiratory time ratio. Normal is 3:1.

- Pressures
  - *Peak* – PIP - measure of airway resistence - common causes include coughing, mucous, bronchospasm, ETT occlusion, RMS intubation, PTX, ↑TV
    - Management – disconnect patient from ventilator and bag with 100% O2, if patient is difficult to bag consider suctioning ETT (if not, then likely d/t bronchospasm or asynchrony and can re-connect to vent), look for tracheal obstruction, PTX, RMS intubation, bronchospasm. Treat with bronchodilators, steroids, and pull back ETT.
  - *Plateau* – Pplat - a measure of how compliant the lung is
  - Static = (Peak – Plateau). A measure of resistance in the circuit.
  - Minute Ventilation (total volume ventilated in 1 minute)
- Modes of ventilation
  - **Volume-based ventilation:**
    - Assist-Control.
      - "assist" – refers to assisting a spontaneous breath
      - "control" –refers to a fully controlled breath without spontaneous effort
      - Delivers set volume of air upon patient initiated breath
      - Controls breath at predetermined frequency and tidal volume (TV) if patient breath not initiated
      - On AC rate 12 with TV 700, patient will receive 12 ventilator delivered breaths/minute, each with a volume of 700 cc. If the patient initiates a breath on his/her own, the vent will also deliver volume of 700 cc. Tachypnea in this mode may cause respiratory alkalosis.
    - SIMV – intermittent mandatory ventilation
      - "mandatory" – refers to assigned rate of full mandatory breaths
      - All other breaths are spontaneous or assisted with pressure support
      - "synchronized" – refers to synchronization of mandatory breaths with pt's diaphragm
      - Intermittently supplies mandatory frequency of breaths at predetermined volume or pressure that is synchronized with patient breathing efforts
      - Commonly used in conjunction with PSV during weaning process
      - On SIMV rate 12 with TV 700, patient will receive at least 12 breaths/min, each with volume of 700cc. If patient initiates > 12 breaths/min, the vent provides no support during those breaths unless pressure support is added. This mode prevents over-ventilation in patients with rapid respiratory rates; however, SIMV requires more respiratory muscle work than AC.
  - **Pressure-based ventilation:**
    - Pressure Control
      - Set the PEEP and initial rate. Then adjust inspiratory pressure to obtain desired tidal volume.
        - Watch for patient agitation (sedate), tachypnea (sedate), and auto-PEEP (reduce set respiratory rate, ↓inspiratory time, ↑expiratory time, use bronchodilators+inhalted steroids; see Figure below).
      - Volumes will vary.
      - Flow rate will vary.

Figure. Appearance of flow volume in normal patient vs. patient with auto-PEEP

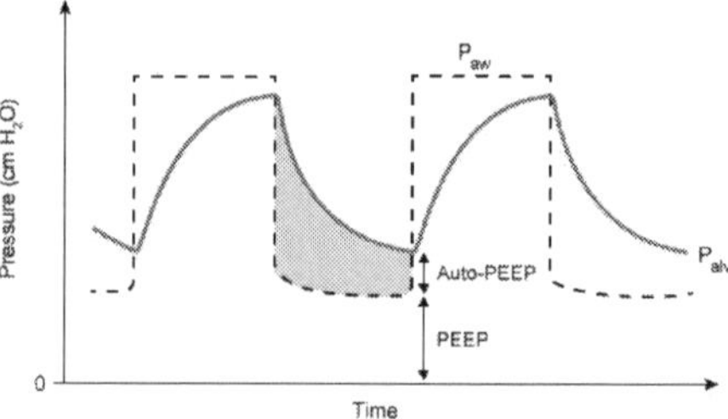

- Pressure Support
  - Augments spontaneous breathing. Helps overcome tubing.
  - Supports patient breathing by delivering air at **predetermined pressure**
  - Adjunctive positive end-expiratory pressure (PEEP): **constant pressure** applied to maintain functional residual capacity & aid gas exchange
  - PRVC – pressure regulated volume control
  - Adjusts I:E time and other factors to accomplish a rate with volume minimums and pressure maximums.
- Bi-Level[280]
  - Concept of alternating between two different pressures of CPAP
  - Pressure controlled, not respiratory rate dependent, allows for spontaneous breathing
  - Variables: Phigh, Plow, Thigh, Tlow
  - **Good if low PaO2 and maxed on FiO2 and PEEP, allows for higher PaO2/FiO2 ratio**
  - Indications: ARDS, CHF
  - Contraindications: COPD, barotrauma
  - Settings:
    - Start with the "respiratory rate": 60/RR gives you your cycle time. Example RR 15 gives cycle time of 4 seconds
    - Set T1 and T2: Example I:E ratio 4:1 results in T1 of 3.2 seconds and T2 of 0.8 seconds
    - Set P1 and P2: Set P2 at the PEEP set on previous mode of ventilation. Set P1 to appropriate TV
  - Pearls
    - ↑O2 - ↑P1 or ↑T1
    - ↓CO2 - ↑T2 or ↓P2

- **Noninvasive ventilation:**
  - CPAP – continuous positive airway pressure
    - Vent maintains constant positive pressure during entire respiratory cycle. This is equivalent to setting PEEP to the desired CPAP level and setting pressure support to zero.
    - Tight fitting mask, only temporary, can't eat
    - Stents open alveoli with continuous pressure. No rate, no volume.
    - Indications: OSA, COPD, **hypoxemia** but not hypercapnia
  - BiPAP – bidirectional positive airway pressure

- Tight fitting mask, only temporary, can't eat
- IPAP – inspiratory positive airway pressure (ventilation)
- EPAP – expiratory positive airway pressure (oxygenation)
- Can set rate (not that helpful)
    - In BiPAP "10/5", the IPAP is 10, the EPAP is 5. In SIMV "10/5", the IPAP is 15, the EPAP is 5.
- Best for COPD or CHF with CO2 retention (**hypercapnia**)

Characteristics of non-invasive ventilation

	CPAP[281,282]	BiPAP
Set Variables	CPAP, FiO2	IPAP, EPAP, RR_{set}, FiO2
Dep. Variables	TV, RR	TV
End-Trigger Trigger	N/A	Patient determines
Notes	= to EPAP (on BiPAP) and cont. PEEP	IPAP=inspiratory positive airway pressure (i.e. PS; effects CO2); EPAP=expiratory positive airway pressure (i.e. PEEP; effects O2) Caution if pressure >=15 → can lead to ↓BP
Initial Settings	CPAP = 5-15 cmH2O	IPAP = 8-10; EPAP = 3-4 Mode: spontaneous ↑EPAP 1-2cm with IPAP constant for ratio 1:2.5
Populations	COPD (acute exacerbation) Acute Cardiogenic PE	Acute Cardiogenic PE (CHF)
Indications	Hypoxemia but not exhausted Weaning off ventilator	Hypercapnia (retained CO2)
Modifications		Continued hypercapnia = ↑IPAP in 1-3cm interv.
Contraindications	• Cardiac/Resp arrest • Acidosis (pH<7.10) • ARDS • Organ failure • Cannot protect airway • Cannot clear secretions • Recent facial surgery • Upper airway obstruction	

- **Generic Initial vent settings**
    - Mode: AC or SIMV.
    - Rate = 12 (lower rate in COPD/asthma).
    - VT = 6cc/kg (ARDSNet Protocol)
    - I:E ratio: no less than 1:2; up to 1:4.
    - FiO2 = 1.0 (wean down rapidly to < 60% to avoid oxygen toxicity).
    - PS (pressure support) = 5-10 (5cm H20 needed to overcome resistance of endotracheal tube).
    - PEEP (positive end-expiratory pressure) = 0-15 (start low; cautious use in asthmatics and COPD patients as "auto PEEP" occurs often).
        - **Auto-PEEP**
            - Check w/ expiratory pause
            - ↓MV (↓TV, ↓RR)
            - Provide long expiratory phase (I:E ratio)

  - ↓air flow resistance with use of bronchodilators and steroids
  - Providing external PEEP may be beneficial

- **Tweaking the Vent**
  - ↑/↓ vent rate → ↑/↓ CO2 and ↑/↓ pH.
  - ↑/↓ FIO2 → ↑/↓ PaO2 (adjust FiO2 in increments of 10-20%).
  - Adding PEEP can increase PaO2 (then you can FiO2).
  - **Low pO2**: ↑FiO2, ↑PEEP (to recruit more alveoli).
  - **High pCO2** : ↑TV or ↑RR (suction, bronchodilators), check for auto-PEEP

  Recheck ABG 30 min after change

Figure. Titrating the vent based on ABG

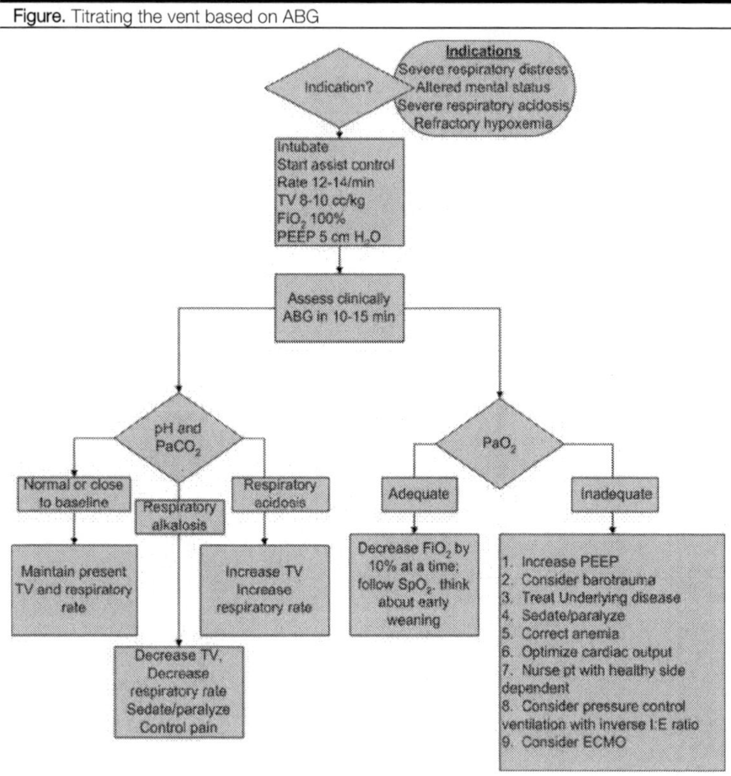

Common Vent Settings by Condition

Condition	Mode	RR	TV (ml/kg)	FIO2	PEEP	Add'tl vent issues	Pearls
Airway protection	AC SIMV PS	10-14	8-10	Wean to sats 92%	5	Peak flow 60 L/min	Maintain on MV until upper airway issues resolved. Patients with hepatic encephalopathy are prone to develop a respiratory alkalosis, so TV may need to be reduced
Asthma exacerbation	AC	8-12 (low)	6-8		0-5	High peak flows Allow adeq. Exp time	Permissive hypercarbia Higher peak airway press. Monitor for auto-PEEP Do **not** attempt to get normal ABG
COPD exacerbation	AC	8-12 (low)	6-8		0-5	High peak flows Allow adeq. Exp time	Monitor auto-PEEP Avoid posthypercapnic alkalosis Permissive hypercarbia Extubate to NIPPV
Hypoxemic respiratory failure with pneumonia or pulmonary edema	AC	High rates (16-24) due to high V_E requirements	6-8		5-10	High V_E requirements	Manage secretions
ARDS	AC PS APRV	High often up to 30	6		5-15	I:E of 1:1 or 1.5:1, allow permissive hypercarbia to pH of 7.20	Consider neb nitrous oxide Monitor for barotrauma Often require heavy sedation Avoid neuromuscular blockade
Postoperative respiratory failure	AC	10-16	8-10		5	Verify placement of all lines and tubes	Wait out the clearance of sedatives and paralytics Prone to hypoventilate after extubation Watch for atelectasis

Weaning parameters[283]	
Method of Assessment	Value
Vital capacity	10 mL/kg
Tidal volume	> 4 mL/kg
Minute ventilation	<15L
Respiratory rate	< 30 breath/min
Dynamic compliance	> 22 mL/cm H2O
Static compliance	> 33 mL/cm H2O
PaO2/FiO2 ratio	> 0.35
Negative inspiratory force (NIF)	20-30 cm H2O
Dead space to tidal volume ratio	0.6
Rapid shallow breathing index (RSBI)	< 105 breaths/min/L
Crop index	> 13 mL/breath/min
Pressors	Not present

- **When to attempt weaning (PS mode)**
  - PaO2/FiO2 ratio > 150
  - Patient can take spontaneous breaths if vent resp-rate reduced
- **Weaning Modes**
  - Preferred method: spontaneous breathing trial (30-120 minutes), T-piece or CPAP x 1-2 hours, check Tobin Index.
  - Decrease SIMV rate (2-4 breaths/min Q12h) ® decrease PS ® T-piece trials.
  - PS wean by decreasing PS until patient on CPAP (i.e., IPAP=PEEP)
  - During weaning, follow ABG, RR, HR and BP to determine when extubation is appropriate.
- **Failure to Wean**
  - F Fluid overload - diurese if indicated.
  - An Airway resistance - check endotracheal tube; is it obstructed or too small?
  - I Infection - treat as indicated.
  - L Lying down, bad V/Q mismatch - elevate head of bed.
  - T Thyroid, toxicity of drugs - check TFT's, check med list.
  - O Oxygen - increase FiO2 as patient is taken off ventilator.
  - W Wheezing - treat with nebs.
  - E Electrolytes, eating - correct K/Mg/PO4/Ca; provide adequate nutrition.
  - An Anti-inflammatory needed? Consider steroids in asthma/COPD.
  - N Neuromuscular disease, neuro status compromised - think of myasthenia gravis, ALS, steroid/paralytic
    neuropathy, etc; assure that patient is in fact awake and alert.

EXTUBATION CRITERIA

Required Criteria

1. The cause of the respiratory failure has improved.
2. Tidal volume > 5cc/kg
3. Respirations spontaneous and >8/min
4. NIF of -10 to -15
5. Patient showing purposeful movement
6. Temperature of 35 C or greater
7. Hemodynamic stability
8. PaO2 ≥ 60 on FiO2 40, Pco2 ≤ 55 mmHg

- **Weaning Predictors**

  - Rapid shallow breathing index – the ratio of respiratory frequency to tidal volume (f/VT). It is the most extensively studied and commonly used weaning predictor. Aim for RSBI <100 breaths/min/L
  - Minute ventilation: aim for 5-6L/min
- **Good Parameters for Successful Extubation**
  - $FiO_2 < 0.5$ *with* PEEP ≤ 5 cmH_2O
  - $PaO_2 > 70$ mmHg ** lower values may be appropriate in $SpO_2 > 90\%$ chronically hypoxemic patients
  - RR < 30 *with* PS ≤ 5cmH_2O
  - pH > 7.2
  - No respiratory distress
  - Patient able to obey commands
  - Patient able to protect airway and cough
  - Patient able to cope with amount of secretions
  - Reason for intubation resolved
- **Bedside Equipment**
  - Oxygen source
  - Suction
  - Oral/Nasal airways
  - Face masks
  - Endotracheal tubes
  - LMA
  - Pulse ox
  - Cardiac Monitors
  - CO_2 detectors
  - Ambu bags
- **Risk Factors**
  - ICU patient
  - Age > 70 or < 24 months
  - Hemoglobin <10 mg/dL
  - Longer duration of mechanical ventilation
  - Medical or surgical airway condition
  - Frequent pulmonary toilet
  - Loss of airway protective reflexes
- **Post Extubation**
  - NIPPV for 24 hours

PLEURAL EFFUSION

- **Causes**[284,285]
  - HF
  - Bacterial pneumonia
  - PE
  - Malignancy
  - Viral infection
  - Cardiac surgery
  - Pancreatitis
- **Thoracentesis**
  - Diagnostic and therapeutic
  - Emergently indicated in patients with respiratory distress or cardiac decompensation
  - Indications:

    - Effusion on decubitus chest XR is >10mm (with or without loculations, thickened pleura or encompassing more than ½ of the hemithorax)
    - Chest tube should be considered if + gram stain, pH<7.2, or glucose <60
  - Can help diagnose: malignancy, empyema (pus and + gram stain), TB, fungal infections, hemothorax, etc.
- **Characterization**
  Done via the Light's Criteria Rule through comparison of serum and pleural protein and LDH

Lights Criteria
- If at least one of the three is present the fluid is considered an exudate:
  - Pleural:Serum Protein ratio is > 0.5
  - Pleural:Serum LDH ratio is > 0.6
  - Pleural LDH value in total is > 2/3 upper limit of normal LDH for the lab's normal LDH

Transudative vs Exudative Pleural Effusion

Variable	Transudative	Exudative
Concept	Physiologically due to an imbalance of oncotic pressures in the chest (↓albumin) resulting in the shift of fluid from peritoneal/retroperitoneal/etc. spaces	Physiologic basis is behind concept that inflammation of the lung and pleura leads to increased capillary and pleural membrane permeability allowing for increased movement of fluid.
Labs	pH 7.4-7.55 + normal glucose + few WBCs (<1000)	pH < 7.3 + low glucose ▫ pH of 7.3 or below itself is an indication for thoracostomy
Differential	▫ CHF ▫ Cirrhosis ▫ Nephrotic syndrome ▫ Peritoneal dialysis (within 48hrs of starting dialysis) ▫ Urinothorax (in presence of obstructive uropathy)	▫ Infection (PNA, abscesses, hepatitis, TB) ▫ Malignancy ▫ Inflammation (pancreatitis, uremia, ARDS) ▫ PE (can be either) ▫ Sarcoidosis ▫ Esophageal perforation (↑amylase)

- **Stages/Classification**
  - Stage 1 - not infected but exudative, generally echo-free on pleural ultrasound, free flowing, and with minimal to no enhancement on CT scan.
  - Stage 2 - generally fibropurulent; likely infected; usually loculated with echogenic fluid, debris, and septations; and associated with pleural enhancement.
  - Stage 3 - organized empyemas with significantly thickened, scarred pleural membranes. The effusion described in this scenario is infected and consistent with an empyema.
- **Fluid Analysis**

Pleural Fluid Analysis: Appearance	
Color	Suspected Diagnosis
Yellow	Transudates
Blood	Malignancy/Trauma/PE
White	Chylothorax, cholesterol effusion, empyema → centrifuge and see below
Brown	Long standing bloody effusion
Black	Aspergillosis
Green	Biliothorax

Pleural Fluid Analysis: Consistency	
Type	Suspected Diagnosis
Clear supernatant above white cells	Empyema (if malodorous, consider anaerobic source)
Viscous	Mesothelioma
Debris	Rheumatoid pleurisy
Turbid	Chylorous fluid v. inflammation

- **Imaging**
  - On a standard upright CXR:
    - 75–100 mL of pleural fluid must accumulate in the posterior costophrenic sulcus to be visible on the lateral view
    - 175–200 mL must be present in the lateral costophrenic sulcus to be visible on the frontal view
  - Chest CT scans may identify as little as 10 mL of fluid
- **Labs to order**
  - Cell Count – levels >50k suggestive of parapneumonic effusion, empyema
  - pH – normal level is 7.60, if pH < 7.30 this suggests exudative (bacteria produce H+; less efflux of H+ in other exudative processes) ; 7.4-7.55 is more transudative
  - Protein – should be low in transudative source UNLESS patient is s/p Lasix administration
  - LDH – highly specific in differentiating transudative vs. exudative as elevated LDH in the pleural fluid is sugg. of exudative process (often empyema) as lysis of PMN ↑ LDH levels
  - Glucose – used to help differentiate type of exudative effusion (low levels are less likely infectious); can be seen with rheumatoid causes
  - Cytology
  - Culture
  - Additional: amylase (esophageal perf; pancreatitis), TG (↑ in chylothorax), cholesterol (↑ in exudative), AFB stain/culture, ADA (suspected TB source)
- **Treatment**
  - Antibiotics
    - Can be used for uncomplicated parapneumonic effusions (free-flowing, non-loculated)
    - Treat for anaerobic infection:
      - Clindamycin
      - Amoxicillin-Clavulanic Acid
      - Ampicillin-Sulbactam
      - Piperacillin-Tazobactam
    - Treat until there is resolution of the fluid on plain films (2-4 weeks)

- Thoracostomy
  - AKA: Chest tube drainage
  - Mostly indicated in:
    - Complicated parapneumonic effusions (loculation present)
      - Severe exudative effusions, pH <7.3 + glucose < 60
    - Empyema (+GS or culture and frank pus)
  - May require additional treatment: thoracoscopy with adhesion lysis and decortication
  - CT are continued until drainage falls below 50 mL/day AND the cavity has closed

PULMONARY EMBOLISM

- **Types**[286,287]
  - Low-Risk – no hemodynamic instability, no changes on EKG/CT/TTE
    - *Subsegmental PE*: poor data to recommend for or against treatment
  - Submassive/Intermediate-Risk – no hemodynamic instability but TTE/CT/EKG evidence of RV strain or dysfunction or TROP leak indicative of myocardial necrosis
    - TTE – look for RV dilatation, strain
    - CT – same as above
    - EKG – T wave inversions, ST depressions
  - Massive/High-Risk– hypotension (SBP<90 x 15min) +/- bradycardia
- **Risk Factors**
  - Age>70
  - Cancer
  - Symptoms of CHF
  - COPD
  - SBP<90
  - RR<20
  - RV hypokinesis on TTE
- **Scoring/Risk Systems**

PE Scoring/Risk	
Revised Geneva	
Age>65 (+1)	Low Risk: 0-3 Moderate Risk: 4-10 → consider d-dimer High Risk: 11+ → consider CT or US
Surgery or lower limb fx in last month (+2)	
Unilateral lower limb pain (+3)	
Tachycardia (75-94 is +3; >95 is +5)	
Hemoptysis (+2)	
Previous history of DVT or PE (+3)	
Active cancer (+2)	
Pain on limb palpation (+4)	

  - rGeneva
  - Pulmonary Embolism Severity Index
  - Shock Index (HR/SBP)
  - Wells Criteria
- **Treatment**
  - Supplemental oxygen should be administered if hypoxemia exists. Severe hypoxemia or respiratory failure should prompt consideration of intubation and mechanical ventilation

- Intravenous fluid administration is first-line therapy. It may improve hemodynamic performance, as illustrated by a series of 13 patients with acute PE and a cardiac index <2.5 L/min/m^2
- There are no randomized trials that definitively determine the optimal vasopressor for patients with shock due to acute PE
- Hemodynamically unstable: thrombolysis
- Hemodynamically stable:
  - UFH – not favored in treatment; used if GFR<30cc/min; BMI>40.
  - LMWH/Fondaparinux f/b Warfarin for INR 2-3 – once daily regimen has been favorable
  - DOAC – non inferior to above regimen
    - Apixaban (*AMPLIFY-EXTENSION)* – studied for use in first days of diagnosis
    - Rivaroxaban (*EINSTEIN-EXTENSION)* – studied for use in the first days of diagnosis; increased GIB
    - Pradaxa (only after 5 day bridge with LMWH; *REMEDY* – cannot be used without bridge; increased GIB
    - Edoxaban – cannot be used without bridge; increased GIB
- **Treat for:**
  - 6 months (first episode, unprovoked)
  - Lifelong (multiple episodes unprovoked
  - Check D-dimer in 1 month

Figure. Anticoagulation recommendations based on probability of PE

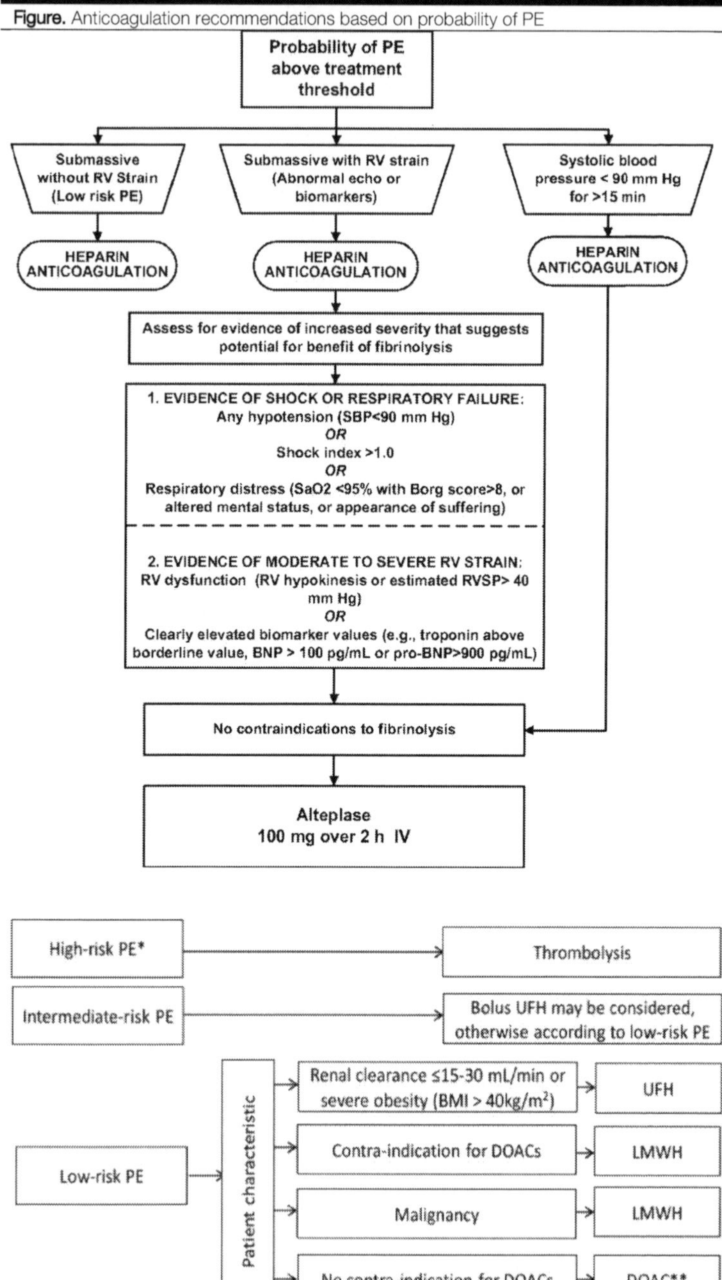

Use of NOACs in patients with VTE	
Patients to consider and discuss NOACs	Patients not to use NOACs
• NOACs are good choices in many patients with acute VTE or on long-term warfarin for VTE; the main reason to use a NOAC is one of patient • convenience, not of efficacy or safety • In patients on long-term warfarin, NOACs are particularly attractive in those with (a) fluctuating/unstable INRs, or (b) a high "warfarin hate factor"	• Patients with renal impairment when GFR is 30 mL/min. • Patients at high risk for bleeding because there is no antidote or known reversal strategy for the NOACs • Patients with cancer because LMWH is the treatment of choice in these patients; however, if the patient cannot afford LMWH, then either warfarin or • a NOAC are appropriate considerations • Significantly obese patients, such as those with a body mass index 40 kg/m2 or a body weight 140 kg because only a limited number of such • patients were studied in the phase 3 clinical trials • Underweight patients, such as those with a body weight of 50 kg or body mass index of 20 kg/m2 • Patients on interfering drugs • Patients with moderate to severe liver disease • Sick inpatients because they may need procedural interventions (central venous lines, etc) • Patients with high copays for NOACs for whom the existing financial drug support mechanisms do not apply

- Thrombolytic therapy/Fibrinolysis
    - Generally considered for patients with **massive PE .** PEITHO trial showed no mortality benefit in submassive PE patients.
- Embolectomy – **massive PE and thrombolytic therapy is contraindicated or** remain unstable after initiation of fibrinolysis
- Filter – patients with contraindications to anticoagulation or active bleeding or PE in setting of anticoagulation or patients who will likely die if they have another PE
    - After placement, if anticoagulation contraindication resolves, patients should be initiated on therapy
    - Most will get retrievable
    - Permanent are for those with long-term anticoagulation contraindications

SUPPLEMENTAL OXYGEN

- Nearly all oxygen is carried to the tissues by haemoglobin (hb). Each gram/dl of hb carries 1·3 ml oxygen when fully saturated. A negligible amount is dissolved in plasma. The oxygen content of blood can therefore be calculated:

Hb (g/dl) × oxygen saturation of Hb × 1·3 and × 10 to convert to litres

- In a 70 kg man a normal hb is 14 g/dl, normal saturation is above 95% and normal co is 5 liters per minute. Oxygen delivery is therefore: 14 x 0·95 x 1·3 x 10 x 5 = 864·5 ml o2 per minute.
- Low flow devices deliver oxygen at less than the inspiratory flow rate, for example nasal cannulae and simple face masks (including masks with a reservoir bag). Although they are low flow, they can deliver a high concentration of oxygen. The oxygen concentration is variable.
  - Nasal canula : fio2 ≈ 21% + (3 x lpm) (maximum 40%)
    - Are commonly used because they are convenient and comfortable. They deliver 2–4 liters per minute of 100% oxygen in addition to the air a person is breathing. Thus, nasal cannulae
    - Deliver a variable concentration of oxygen depending on how the patient is breathing → the person breathing slowly
    - Receives a large proportion of oxygen whilst the person breathing quickly receives much less.
  - Simple face mask = up to an fio2 of 50%
    - Deliver up to 50% oxygen when set to 15 liters per minute. Like nasal cannulae, the concentration is variable depending on the fit of the mask and how the patient is breathing.
  - Venturi face mask = based on color-coded adaptor, up to an FiO2 of 50%
    - High flow devices deliver oxygen at above the inspiratory flow rate, such as venturi masks. Although they are high flow, a low concentration of oxygen may be delivered. The oxygen concentration is fixed.
  - Nonrebreather face mask = always at an FiO2 of ~60%

ASTHMA

- **Background**[288]
  - Ask about family history
  - Allergies (seasonal or NSAIDs/ASA)
  - PM vs AM sx (PM more s/o dx)
  - F>M; AA>Caucasian
- **Definition** – chronic inflammatory disorder of the airways triggered by various sensitizing stimuli resulting in reversible airflow obstruction.
- **Classification**
  - Allergic
    - Most common form; peaking in the 2nd decade
    - Atopic (extrinsic)
    - Commonly associated with positive family history
    - Look for IgE+ to specific antigens such as dust, pollen, dander, mold
    - Treatment is commonly with immunomodulators
  - Non-Allergic
    - Less common; associated with later age of onset
    - Non-atopic (intrinsic)
    - Triggers are not really allergy related but more with exercise, cold exposure, smoke, viruses, fumes, medications
    - Treatment is with bronchial thermoplasty
- **Exam**
  - Nasal polyps (consider AERD)

- Nasal mucosal bogginess
- Sinus tenderness
- Wheezing (expiratory)

- **Diagnosis**
  - Look for the typical pattern of symptoms with the correct objective data on PFTs and appropriate response to therapy (beta agonists).
    - Symptoms - Combination of consistent symptoms (ie. cough, chest tightness, wheezing, SOB) with documented reversible airway obstruction (on PFTs or home peak-flow)
    - Data –
      - **Pulmonary Function Testing**
        - Reversible obstruction on PFTs showing FEV1/FVC < 70% with reversibility of 12% AND 200cc in FEV1 OR FVC with administration of SABA.
          - Ensure that bronchial hyperactivity is tested with methacholine challenge (drop in 20% of FEV1) if the initial PFTs are 'normal' and no reversibility is noted (80% SN, 96% SP)
          - If ratio is normal, but reversibility is still present, diagnosis is still made
      - **Labs**
        - Allergy testing and measurement of IgE levels may also help predict atopy and someone more likely to have asthma.
      - **Other Diagnostics**
        - CXR not necessary unless concerned for concurrent infection exists
        - FeNO – levels are often high due to ↑ eosinophils; can be used for long term monitoring
- **Treatment**
  - Treat to symptom control, not based on severity "levels"
    - Goal is for patient to have no limitations on physical activity, no night time awakenings, normal lung function, and 2x/week or less of daytime sx.
  - Pharmacologic
    - **Never provide LABA monotherapy without concurrent ICS treatment**
    - *Direct Bronchodilators*
      - B2 agonists –
        - Short acting: albuterol, levalbuterol
        - Long acting: salmeterol, vilanterol
      - Anti-cholinergics
        - Short acting: Ipratropium bromide
        - Long acting: Tiotropium bromide, glycopyrronium, aclidinium
      - Methylxanthines – aminophylline, theophylline
      - Adrenergic agonists - epinephrine
  - Anti-inflammatory medications
    - *Corticosteroids (inhaled, PO, IV, IM)*
      - Fluticasone
      - Prednisone
      - Beclomethasone
  - Mast cell stabilizers – cromolyn sodium, nedocromil
  - Leukotriene Antagonists – zileuton, montelukast
  - Immunomodulators
    - Should be started by Pulmonology; commonly used with severe allergic type asthma that is refractory to traditional therapy
    - Options include:
      - IgE – omalizumab

      - Anti-IL5 – mepolizumab, benralizumab, resilizumab
  - <u>Non-Pharmacologic</u>
    - Nonpharmacologic includes removal of allergens, patient education on how to use inhaler, physical training, smoking cessation, weight loss (if applicable).
    - Bronchial thermoplasty is an option in non-allergic asthma in patients with severe asthma but 40% reduction in symptoms seen in allergic asthma patients.

Long-term control medications for asthma			
Medication	Dosage Form	Adult Dose	Comments
Systemic Corticosteroids			
Methylprednisolone	2, 4, 6, 8, 16, 32 mg tablets	7.5-60 mg daily in a single dose in AM or every other day as needed for control	Administer single dose in AM either daily or on alternate days (alternate-day therapy may produce less adrenal suppression). Short courses or "bursts" are effective for establishing control when initiating therapy or during a period of gradual deterioration.
Prednisolone	5 mg tablets, 5 mg/5 mL, 15 mg/5 mL	Short-course "burst": to achieve control, 40-60 mg per day as single or 2 divided doses for 3-10 days	
Prednisone	1, 2.5, 5, 10, 20, 50 mg tablets; 5 mg/mL, 5 mg/mL		
Inhaled Long-Acting β_2-Agonists			
Salmeterol	DPI 50 mcg/blister	1 blister every 12 hors	Decreased duration of protection against EIB may occur with regular use.
Combined Medication			
Fluticasone/Salmeterol	DPI	1 inhalation twice daily; dose depends on severity of asthma	100/50 DPI or 45/21 HFA for patient not controlled on low- to medium-dose inhaled corticosteroids
	100 mcg/50 mcg		
	250 mcg/50 mcg, or		
	500 mcg/50 mcg		
	HFA		250/50 DPI or 115/21 HFA for patients not controlled on medium- to high-dose inhaled corticosteroids
	45 mcg/21 mcg		
	115 mcg/21 mcg		
	230 mcg/21 mcg		
Budesonide/Formoterol	HFA MDI	2 inhalations twice daily; dose depends on severity of asthma	80/4.5 for asthma not controlled on low- to medium-dose inhaled corticosteroids
	80 mcg/4.5 mcg		

	160 mcg/4.5 mcg		160/4.5 for asthma not controlled on medium- to high-dose inhaled corticosteroids
	Low Dose	Medium Dose	High-Dose
Inhaled Steroids			
Beclomethasone dipropionate (CFC)*	200-500	>500-1000	>1000
Beclomethasone dipropionate (HFA)	100-200	>200-400	>400
Budesonide (DPI)	200-400	>400-800	>800
Fluticasone propionate (HFA)	100-250	>250-500	>500
Mometasone furoate	110-220	>220-440	>440
Triamcinolone acetonide	400-1000	>1000-2000	>2000
Leukotriene Modifiers			
Montelukast	10mg	One tablet daily	
Zafirlukast	20mg	One tablet BID	
Zileuton	600mg	Two tablets BID within 1 hour of meals	

Step	Symptoms	PFT	Treatment
Intermittent	<1/week Waken <1/month	PEF/FEV >80% Variability <20%	SABA
Mild Persistent	<1/day >1/week Waken <2/month	PEF/FEV >80% Variability 20-30%	SABA +/- LABA/LAMA+ICS (low dose) *cannot give LABA alone* *consider adding leukotriene inhibitor, theophylline or cromolyn sodium
Moderate persistent	Daily Waken >1/week	PEF/FEV 60-80% Variability >30%	SABA+ICS (high/medium dose) +LABA/LAMA+leukotriene inhibitor Add tiotropium

Severe persistent	Continuous daily sx Waken frequently	PEF/FEV <60% Variability >30%	Low dose oral Steroid + ICS+LABA+LAMA Consider referring for add-on treatment (ie. tiotropium, omalizumab if IgE 30-700) Consider bronchial thermoplasty if non-allergic Triple therapy with LABA+LAMA+ICS has not been found to be beneficial

- **Refractory Asthma**
  - Represents a subgroup of patients (<5%) with high medication requirements to maintain good disease control or those with persistent symptoms despite high medication use
  - Most asthma patients are able to be controlled with use of beta-agonists and low dose anti-inflammatory agents
  - Assess inhaler technique
  - Encompasses asthma patients known to have 'severe' asthma or 'steroid-dependent' asthma
  - Severe asthma defined as steroid dependence with FEV1 < 50% predicted
  - Clinical Presentation
    - Widely varying peak flows
    - Copious phlegm production
    - Chronic airflow limitation
    - Rapidly progressive loss of lung function
  - 2 major, 7 minor criteria

Criteria for Diagnosis	
Major	Minor
Treatment with continuous or near continuous (>50%/year) oral steroids	Requirement for daily treatment with a controller medication in addition to inhaled steroids (ie. LABA, montelukast, theophylline)
Requirement for treatment with high-dose inhaled steroids	Asthma symptoms requiring SABA use on daily or near daily basis
	Persistent airway obstruction (FEV1<80%)
	One or more urgent care visits/year
	3+ oral steroid bursts/year
	Prompt deterioration with <25% reduction in oral or inhaled steroid dose
	Near fatal asthma event in the past

- **Evaluation**
  - Confirm reversible airflow limitation and quantify severity
    - FEV1, peak flow, and flow–volume loop before and after bronchodilator treatment
    - Total lung capacity and residual volume
    - Diffusion capacity (in adults—usually not indicated in children)
  - Consider other diagnoses
    - AF
    - COPD
    - Depression
    - Anxiety
    - Rhinosinusitis
    - GERD
    - VAD
    - OSA
  - Investigate co-comitant diseases
    - Allergin skin tests

        - CT sinus
        - 24 hour pH for GERD
        - Environmental diseases
            - Smoking
            - Viral Infections
            - Occupational agents (wood, birds, coal) → allergies
- **Therapy**
    - Controller Therapy – initial therapies include inhaled GA's, LABA with combination of 2+ controller agents
        - Oral Steroids – given in patients with frequent daytime or nocturnal sx, recent deterioration, or FEV1<60% of predicted for 2-3 weeks
        - Inhaled GAS – with increases to up to 1600-2000/day
        - LABA
        - Theophylline – not used as much, for rare cases
        - Anti-leukotriene agent – Zileuton, montelukast, and zafirlukast
            - Anti-IgE therapy – omalizumab (check IgE level), often takes 12 weeks minimum before response
    - Spirometry
        - Obtain in all patients with consideration for diagnosis of Asthma
        - Repeat after symptoms are under control on pharmacologic therapy to obtain true baseline
        - After this, repeat q1-2y or after episodes of poor control

Asthma Exacerbation

- Causes
    - Infection (viral vs bacterial)
    - Exposure (pollen, ozone, cold air, humidity, smoke)
    - Non-adherence to tx
- Clinical Exam
    - ↑HR, ↑RR, ↓SaO2, dyspnea, hyperresonance, ↓breath sounds
- Labs
    - CBC
    - CMP
    - TROP
    - Sputum Cx
    - ABG
    - Peak flows
- Imaging: **CXR**
- Categorization
    - Mild/Moderate (M)
        - Talks in phrases, not agitated, able to lie down
        - Normal RR, Pulse 100-120; O2 90-95%, PEF>50% predicted/or best
    - Severe (S)
        - Talks in words, agitated, must sit up
        - RR>30/m, Pulse>120, O2<90%, PEF<50%
- Acute Management
    - See table below
    - O2 to keep PaO2>92%
    - Bronchodilator
        - Neb treatment (albuterol 2.5 5.0mg NEB q6h +q1h prn + ipratropium 0.5mg NEB q6h)

- Steroids (prednisone 1mg/kg PO daily x 7-14d or methylprednisolone however PO = IV)
- Consider theophylline, $MgSO_4$ in refractory cases
- Hospital Admission Criteria
  - PaO_2<90% on supplemental oxygen
  - FEV1 <2.1L and PEF < 300 L/min

Asthma treatment options based on severity of attack

Cat	Treatment	Dosage
M/S	Oxygen	Maintain SpO_2>92%
M/S	Albuterol	2.5 mg by nebulization q20min or 4-6 puffs by MDI w/spacer q20min
S	Epinephrine	0.3 mL of a 1:1000 solution subcutaneously every 20 minutes x 3. Terbutaline is favored in pregnancy when parenteral therapy is indicated. Use with caution in patients > age 40 and in the presence of cardiac disease
M/S	Ipratropium bromide	0.5 mg combined with albuterol by nebulization every 20 minutes or 4-6 puffs by MDI with spacer combined with albuterol every 20 minutes
S	Methylprednisolone	60 mg IV every 6 hours or prednisone PO 40 mg Q6H
S	Magnesium sulfate	2 g IV over 20 minutes, repeat in 20 minutes if clinically indicated (total 4 g unless hypomagnesemic)
M/S	Theophylline	5 mg/kg IV over 30 minutes loading dose in patients not on theophylline, followed by 0.4 mg/kg per hour IV maintenance dose. Watch for drug interactions and disease states that alter clearance. Follow serum levels
M/S	montelukast	10 mg PO (the chewable formulation may have quicker onset of action)
S	Heliox	80:20 or 70:30 helium:oxygen mix by tight-fitting, nonrebreathing face mask. Higher helium concentrations are needed for maximal effect

SIRS → SEPSIS → SEVERE SEPSIS → SEPTIC SHOCK

Figure. Review of the sepsis bundle

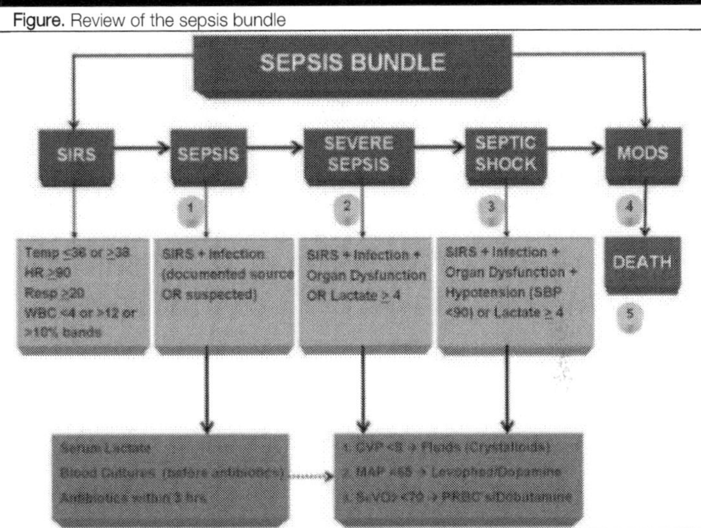

SEPSIS

- **Definition**[289]
  - Sepsis is defined as the presence (probable or documented) of infection together with systemic manifestations of infection:
    - SIRS
    - End organ dysfunction (AMS, hypoxemia, oliguria, ileus, thrombocytopenia, ↑lactate)
    - Significant edema
    - Hyperglycemia without hx of DM
    - ↑CRP (2SD above normal)
    - ↑PCT (2SD above normal)
    - Hypotension (SBP<90, MAP<70)

Severe sepsis
Sepsis + sepsis-induced organ dysfunction or tissue hypoperfusion
Sepsis-induced hypotension
Lactate above upper limits laboratory normal
Urine output < 0.5 mL/kg/hr for more than 2 hrs despite adequate fluid resuscitation
Acute lung injury with Pao2/Fio2 < 250 in the absence of pneumonia as infection source
Acute lung injury with Pao2/Fio2 < 200 in the presence of pneumonia as infection source
Creatinine > 2.0 mg/dL (176.8 μmol/L)
Bilirubin > 2 mg/dL (34.2 μmol/L)
Platelet count < 100,000 μL
Coagulopathy (international normalized ratio > 1.5)

- **Treatment**[290]
  - Hour-1 Bundle
    - Initiated within the **first hour** of presentation; this is highly debated as many feel it is unrealistic to meet such a time marker.
      - **Bundle consists of**:
        - Measurement of the lactate level; remeasure if >2 mmol/L
        - Obtaining blood cultures before giving antibiotics
        - Maintain MAP≥65
        - Administering antibiotics
        - Giving 30 mg/kg crystalloid for hypotension or lactate ≥4 mmol/L.
          - Some will extend this to within the first 3 hours
          - Worse outcomes (↑death) were noted in patients who received >5L total in the first day
        - Giving vasopressors if patient remains hypotensive despite fluid resuscitation.
  - Rapid fluid infusions
    - Initial fluid challenge should be 1L or more of crystalloid, and a minimum of **30 mL/kg** of crystalloid (2.1 L in a 70 kg or 154-pound person) in the first 4-6 hours.
      - Grade 2B recommendation for adding albumin as necessary (in patients who require "substantial amount" of fluid)
      - Monitor lactate every 2 hours for 8 hours, aiming for reduction in 20% every 2 hours (*LACTATE trial)*
    - Trials have found not benefit in crystalloid vs. colloid (SAFE, 6S; Grade 2C); **crystalloids are preferred**

Hemodynamic management of early septic shock		
Intervention	Recommendation	Considerations
MAP Target	≥65 mmHg	Permissive hypotension may be considered in cases of trauma
Fluid resuscitation	30 cc/kg at least within 1 hour	Consideration that large amounts may increase fluid overload and worsen outcomes
What fluids to give and for how long	Crystalloids for at least 1 hour, then re-assess clinically	Consider adding albumin with "substantial" fluid requirements
Pharmacologic vasopressor support	NE remains #1 choice with vasopressin as #2 to support NE. Add dobutamine only after #1 and #2 given to reach MAP goal	Should fluids always be given first then vasopressors?

- Vasopressors are next choice when fluids are not adequate
    1. First start should be norepinephrine (levophed) at 0.03U/minute (grade 2A)
    2. When additional pressor required: options should be **epinephrine or vasopressin** (0.03U/min) (grade 2B)
        - Patients at low risk for arrhythmias with low HR/CO can use dopamine otherwise avoided (grade 2C)
    3. **Dobutamine** should be added to above vasopressor if:
        - Signs of cardiac dysfunction (grade 1C) as evidenced by low CO or continued hypoperfusion with above pressors
        - Concern for cardiogenic shock (combine with dopamine, avoid PE, NE); add balloon pump if BP does not respond (acts to ↓ afterload); ↑survival if used after PCI

α_1 - vasoconstrictor effects, increases SVR
α_2 - inhibits pre-sympathetic release of NE thus no action on alpha1 receptors!
β_1 - think 1 heart, positive inotropic effects (↑Ca release at SR) from FS mech and ↑HR
β_2 - think 2 lungs, increases dilation of smooth muscle in arteries and bronchioles

Name	Recp/Hemo	Dose	Action	Use
Phenylephrine	α_1 ↑MAP ↑SVR ---HR	Continuous infusion for hypotension: Start at 0.1-0.5 mcg/kg/min, titrate to effect, range: 0.5-1 mcg/kg/min	Potent α vasoconstriction can cause significant distal tissue hypoxia; ensure appropriate volume resuscitation	Hypotension from low peripheral vascular tone. **Pressor of choice for septic patients** with cardiovascular disease, though patients likely have significant intrinsic sympathetic (and consequent) β1 stimulation anyway
Epinephrine	$\alpha_1\alpha_2\beta_1\beta_2$ ↑↑MAP ↑↑SVR ↑↑HR	0.01-0.05 mcg/kg/min (upper range 0.5-1 mcg/kg/min) titrated every 1-2 minutes <u>Anaphylaxis</u>: 0.1-0.5 mg SC/IM (usual dose is 0.3 mg, 1:1,000)	Highly arrhythmogenic, can cause myocardial ischemia/infarct; not for prolonged use, watch for unopposed α stimulation in patients on β-blockers	Cardiac arrest, refractory hypotension, status asthmaticus, anaphylaxis
Norepinephrine	$\alpha_1\alpha_2\beta_1$ ↑↑↑MAP ↑↑↑SVR ↑↑HR	<u>Continuous infusion for hypotension</u>: Start 0.1-0.5 mcg/kg/min, titrate to effect (~SBP>90, MAP>60), range: 0.5-3 mcg/min	Potent α vasoconstriction can cause significant distal tissue hypoxia; ensure appropriate volume resuscitation	Hypotension from low peripheral vascular tone, myocardial depression, or both **Convenient initial pressor choice** as it causes peripheral vasoconstriction, via α effect, and increased inotropy/chronotropy, via β1 effect
Dopamine	δ --MAP --SVR ↑HR	<u>Continuous infusion for hypotension</u>: Start 5-10 mcg/kg/min, titrate to effect: (0-2 mcg/kg/min <u>"renal dose"</u>, 2-5 mcg/kg/min β1 dose, >5 mcg/kg/min α1 dose)	Less potent α _vasoconstriction, but increased risk of tachyarrhythmias 2°/2 β activity vs. norepinephrine	At lower doses, hypotension from decreased myocardial contractility and at higher doses, from low peripheral vascular tone.

	β_1 ↑MAP ↑SVR ↑↑HR	2-10 mcg/kg/min	Positive inotropy, causes arrhythmias	
	α_1 ↑MAP ↑SVR ↑↑↑HR	10-20 mcg/kg/min	Vasoconstriction, causes arrhythmias	
Dobutamine	$\beta_1\beta_2$	Continuous infusion: Start at 2 mcg/kg/min, titrate to effect (usually Cardiac Index > 2), range: 2-20 mcg/kg/min	Expect hypotension, if needed support BP with dopamine first, and then start dobutamine - Risk of tachyarrhythmias, though less then epinephrine, dopamine, and isoproterenol; increased myocardial oxygen consumption, with resultant risk of ischemia	Low cardiac output states; produces significant inotropy/chronotropy, and "afterload" reduction with peripheral vasodilation.
Vasopressin	V_1 ↑↑↑MAP ↑↑↑SVR --HR	Start at 0.03U/min with upper limit of 0.06U/min	Antidiuretic hormone that causes vasoconstriction and works to supplement catecholamine therapy (NE) particularly (see *VASST Trial)*	Combine with NE to increase its effectiveness (can be secondary medication for septic shock)

- Antibiotics
  - Administration of effective intravenous antimicrobials **within the first hour** of recognition of septic shock
  - Obtain PCT level to assist in determining if a pt needs ABx but have no evidence of infection
  - Empiric combination therapy should not be administered for more than 3–5 days. De-escalation to the most appropriate single therapy should be performed as soon as the susceptibility profile is known (grade 2B).
  - Duration of therapy typically 7–10 days; longer courses may be appropriate in patients who have a slow clinical response, undrainable foci of infection, bacteremia with S. aureus; some fungal and viral infections or immunologic deficiencies, including neutropenia
- Neuromuscular blockers
  - The ACURASYS trial showed benefit of 48 hours of NM blockade in patients with ARDS
    - Studies have shown early severe ARDS may benefit from NMBA especially if elevated pressures are noted
    - 48-hour infusion of cisatracurium (Nimbex) with 15mg bolus f/b 37.5 mg/hr had lower 90-day mortality, morbidity, and quicker discharge from ICU than placebo
- Glucose
  - Upper limit should be 180 mg/dL
  - Initiate feeds 48 hours after dx of sepsis
- Steroids
  - If patient does not adequately respond (↓BP) to vasopressors, should add IV hydrocortisone gtt at 200mg/day (grade 2C)
  - Also add if patient has adrenal insufficiency
- Ventilation
  - ARDS patients should be kept at TV 0.6cc/IBW

IBW Males = 0.91 × (height [cm] – 152.4) + 50
IBW Females = 0.91 × (height [cm] – 152.4) + 45.5

- Transfusion
  - Target HGB 7-9 g/dL in absence of sx (tissue hypoperfusion, ischemic CAD, acute bleeding) (Grade 1B)

Physiologic effects of hemodynamic medications

Drug	Effect on HR	Effect on contractility	Arterial constriction effects
Dobutamine	+	+++	- (dilates)
Dopamine	++	++	++
Epinephrine	+++	+++	++
Norepinephrine	++	++	+++
Phenylephrine	0	0	+++
Amrinone	+	+++	-- (dilates)

SHOCK

- **Defined -** Inadequate tissue perfusion and oxygenation 2/2 circulatory abnormality
- **Pathophysiology**

- Remember CO = SV x HR and this is ultimately determined by preload, afterload, and contractility
- Preload itself is determined by volume status and venous capacitance. ↓venous return leads to decreased muscle stretch, leading to ↓frank-starling stretch, and thus less contractility. Afterload itself is separate and associated with vascular resistance towards the forward flow of blood
- Early compensation to blood loss is vasoconstriction to preserve flow to vital organs (kidney, brain, and heart) → seen as tachycardia
- Inadequately perfused tissues do not get oxygen and are deprived of completing normal aerobic metabolism thus the cells shift to anaerobic metabolism producing lactic acid → metabolic acidosis. Giving isotonic NS helps because it combats the lysosomes released and other enzymes that damage intracellular structures.

- **Assessment**
  - Initial treatment is aimed towards restoring organ perfusion and blood oxygenation
  - Vasopressors are C/I because they can worsen tissue perfusion d/t increasing vasoconstriction
- **Clinical symptoms**
  - Tachycardia
  - ↑RR
  - ↓skin circulation

Types of Shock

Types	CVP or RA (Preload)	PA	PCWP	CO (Pump fxn)	SVR	MAP
Hypovolemic	↓	↓	↓	↓	↑	↓
Cardiogenic	↑↓	↑	↑	↓	↑	↓
Tamponade	↑	↑	↑	↓	↑	↓
Constrictive Pericarditis	↑	↓	↑	↓/N	↑/N	↓
RV infarction	↑	↓/N	↑/N	↓/N	↑	↓/N
Acute MR	↑/N	↑	↑	↓	↑/N	↓/N
Massive PE	↑	↑	↓/N	↓	↑	↓
Acute LV Failure	N	↑	↑	↓	↑/N	↓/N
Early Sepsis	↓	↓	↓	↑	↓	↓/N

- **Types**
  - Hypovolemic
    - Most common type
    - Treatment based on EBL:
      - Class I - < 15% blood volume loss (750cc); tx with crystalloid
      - Class II – 15-30% blood volume loss (750-1500cc); treat with crystalloid
      - Class III – 30-40% blood volume loss (1500-2000cc); treat with crystalloid and blood
      - Class IV - >40% BVL (>2000cc); treat with crystalloid and blood
  - Neurogenic
    - Hypotension due to loss of sympathetic tone → hypovolemia/hypotension w/o tachycardia
    - Often, like hemorrhagic shock, see no response to fluid resuscitation
  - Cardiogenic
    - 2/2 myocardial dysfunction from blunt injury → tamponade, MI

        - Obtain EKG to detect injury patterns
        - Get new echo or look at prior TTE
        - R/O tamponade with FAST
        - Pressors: dobutamine + dopamine +/- IABP
    - Septic[291]
        - Due to infection leading to tachycardia, and cutaneous vasoconstriction
        - No hemodynamic response to 30cc/kg of fluid challenge
        - Look for warm, pink skin

OBSTRUCTIVE SLEEP APNEA

- **Screening[292,293]**
    - In patients who are dissatisfied with their sleep quality should undergo a questionnaire (STOP-BANG or Epworth)
    - Consider screening also in those with high risk occupations like bus drivers, truck drivers, surgeons, etc.
- **Clinical Symptoms / Risk Factors**
    - Daytime fatigue
    - Obesity
    - Family history of OSA
    - CHF
    - Stroke
    - AFib
    - Morning headaches
    - Snoring
    - Apneic episodes
    - Prior diagnosis of hypothyroidism
    - Concurrent metabolic syndrome is often found
- **Examination**
    - Obesity
    - Neck circumference (>16'' women; >17'' men)
    - Mallampati 3 or 4
    - Macroglossia
    - Tonsillar hypertrophy
- **Red Flags**
    - Excessive daytime fatigue
    - Morning headaches
    - Neck circumference of greater than or equal to 17 inches in males and 16 inches in females
    - Polycythemia
- **Pursuing sleep study**
    - STOP BANG $\geq$ 3
    - Epworth > 8 (however some studies recommend 10)
- **Diagnosis**
    - Home sleep testing (HST) – noninferior to traditional lab testing
    - In-lab sleep study – best for patients with significant cardiovascular disease, chronic opiate use, h/o stroke, h/o insomnia, neuromuscular disorders among others.
- **Severity/Grading (AHI)**
    - <u>Apnea-Hypopnea Index (AHI)</u> - number of times a patient has an episode of complete apnea (stops breathing for 10 or more seconds) + episodes of hypopnea (the definition of which varies) / hour.
        - < 5 – normal

        - 5-14 is - mild OSA
        - 15-29 - moderate OSA
        - 30+ - severe OSA
    - The number of times oxygen a patient's oxygen saturation drops from baseline by 4% or more / hour, or Oxygen Desaturation Index (ODI) and time spent with oxygen less than 90% (T90) are better markers for determining severity
- **Treatment**
    - Mild OSA may not require treatment if patients do not have excessive daytime sleepiness
    - Other levels can be treated with autoPAP, a mouth appliance (best for mild apnea and patients who are resistent to CPAP), BiPAP (in patients with high pressure requirements), and bariatric surgery

NEPHROLOGY

ACID BASE PHYSIOLOGY

STEP 1: Gather the necessary data (electrolytes and an ABG Make sure the HCO3 from the electrolyte panel and ABG are within 2 (if not the results are uninterpretable) **Understand the Normals** PaO2: 80-100mmHg PaCO2: 35-45mmHg HCO3: 22-28mEq/L SaO2: 95-100% SvO2: 60-80%	pH | CO2 | HCO3
STEP 2: Look at the pH If pH > 7.4, then pt is alkalemic (proceed to step 3a) If pH < 7.4, the pt is acidemic (proceed to step 3b)	Patient has primary: Acidosis / Alkalosis
STEP 3: Determine the primary etiology 3a Alkalemia: Increased HCO3 = Metabolic alkalosis (go to step 5); Decreased pCO2 = Respiratory alkalosis (go to step 4a) 3b Acidosis: Decreased HCO3 = Metabolic acidosis (go to step 5); Increased pCO2 = Respiratory acidosis (go to step 4b)	Primary process is: Respiratory / Metabolic
Respiratory Disorders — **STEP 4: If primary respiratory disorder, determine whether acute or chronic** (see table below)	Respiratory process: Acute / Chronic / Unknown

Respiratory Acidosis		Respiratory Alkalosis	
For each ↑ PCO2 of 10 above 40		For each ↓ PCO2 of 10 above 40	
Acute	**Chronic**	**Acute**	**Chronic**
HCO3 ↑ 1 mEq	HCO3 ↑ 4-5 mEq	HCO3 ↓ 2 mEq	HCO3 ↓ 4-5 mEq
pH ↓ 0.08	pH ↓ 0.03	pH ↑ 0.07	pH ↑ 0.02

All

STEP 5: Calculate the anion gap.

5a Na – (HCO3 + Cl) = ____________

If > 12 (or 3xalbumin) then pt has an anion gap metabolic acidosis (proceed to step 5b)
If <12, skip to Step 6b

Anion gap?
Yes / No

5b Calculate the excess anion gap

Calculated anion gap + 12 (or 3xalbumin) = ______________

Excess gap:
____

Metabolic Acidosis

STEP 6: Identify concomitant disorders.

6a Calculate the corrected HCO3. You must understand that this step essentially compares the decrease in measured HCO3 to the expected decrease in HCO3 based on the degree of anion gap.

Measured HCO3 + excess anion gap = ______

*If the corrected HCO3 is >30, then the patient has a concomitant metabolic alkalosis (more HCO3 than expected for the degree of gap acidosis).

*If the corrected HCO3 is <23, then the patient has a concomitant NAGMA (less HCO3 than expected for the degree of gap). See page 504 for more on this.

Metabolic alkalosis present:
yes / no

NAGMA present:
yes / no

6b Calculate the expected pCO2. Winter's formula shows what the pCO2 should be for the level of acidosis present (omit if primary disorder is respiratory).

Winter's formula = expected pCO2 = 1.5(HCO3) +8 +/- 2
pCO2 = (1.5)(______) + 8 +/- 2
*If the actual pCO2 > calculated pCO2 then pt has concomitant respiratory acidosis
*If the actual pCO2 < calculated pCO2 then pt has concomitant respiratory alkalosis

Respiratory disorder present:
yes / no

Metabolic Acidosis	Metabolic Alkalosis
For each ↓ HCO3 of 1 mEq...	For each ↑ HCO3 of 1 mEq...
PCO2 ↓ 1.25 mmHg Formula $Pa_{CO_2} = [HCO_3^-] + 15$ pCO2 = 1.5 x [HCO3] + 8 ± 2	PCO2 ↑ 0.75 mmHg Formula $Pa_{CO_2} = [HCO_3^-] + 15$ pCO2 = 0.7 x [HCO3] + 20 ± 5

STEP 7: Figure out what's causing the problem(s)

AGMA	NAGMA	ACUTE RESP ACIDOSIS	METABOLIC ALKALOSIS	RESPIRATORY ALKALOSIS
"MUDPILERS"	"HARDUPS"	Anything that causes hypoventilation	"CLEVER PD	"CHAMPS" Anything that causes hypervent.

Methanol Uremia DKA/ EtOH/ starvation Paraldehyde INH Lactic acid EtOH/ ethylene glycol Rhabdo/renal fail. Salicylates	Hyperalimentation Acetazolamide RTA Diarrhea Uretero-pelvic shunt Post-hypocapnia Spironolactone Normal saline	CNS depression Airway obstruction PNA PE Hemo/PTX Myopathy Chronic resp acid. Is caused by COPD and restrictive lung dz	Vomiting (↓U) Diuretics Hypokalemia Hyperaldosterone Licorice Conn's Cushing's Bartter's Hypercalcemia Refeeding Post-hypercapnia Laxative abuse	CNS dz Hypoxia Anxiety Mech ventilation Progesterone Salicylates/ sepsis

STEP 8: Fix it!

Figure. Flow chart interpretation of ABG

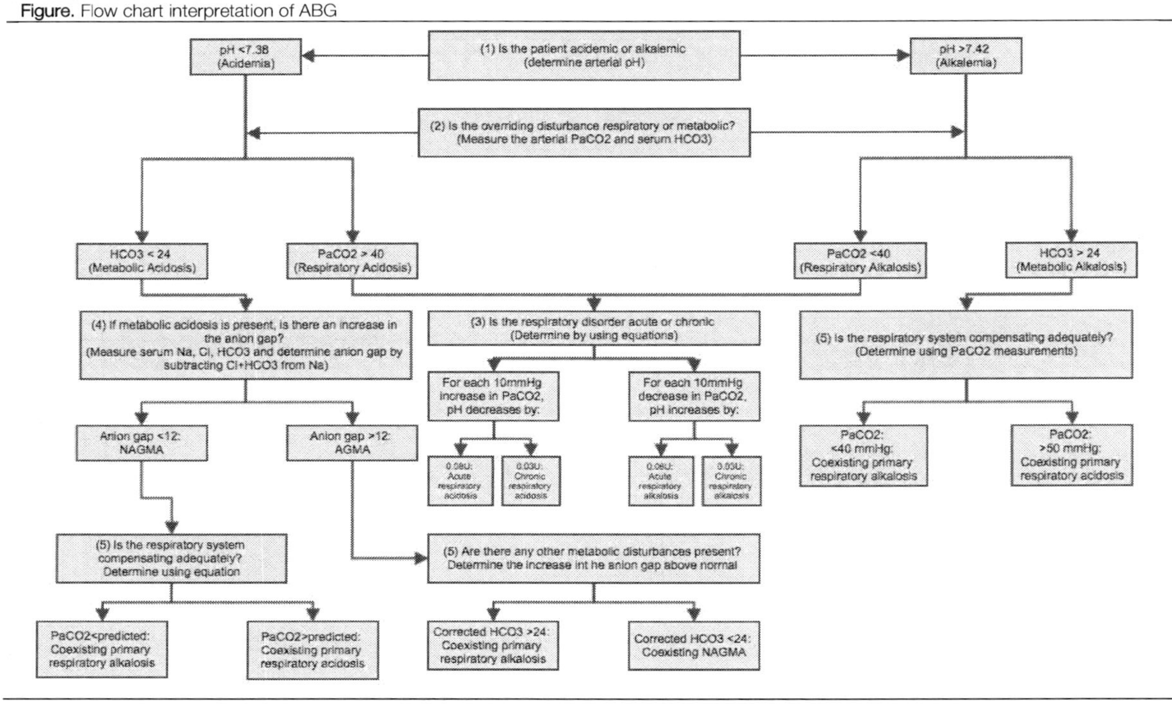

- **More on Delta Gap**
    - If there is an AG, determine whether this alone accounts for the change in HCO3. Calculate the gap-gap: (delta-gap) = patient's anion gap – 12 (normal anion gap).
    - Compensate for low albumin (for every 1 g/dl decrease from normal, increase AG by 2.5 mmol/L)
    - Add this to the measured HCO3. If the result is >30, then an additional metabolic alkalosis exists. If the result is <23, then an additional non-gap metabolic acidosis is present
    - Osmolar
      Done when considering concurrent toxic alcohols as cause
        - (2xNa)+(Bun/3)+Gluc/18
        - (+): methanol, ethanol, ethylene glycol
        - (0) or (-): other causes
    - <u>Urine AG</u>
        - Urinary Na + Urinary K - Urinary Cl
            - *The urinary anion gap can help to differentiate between GIT and renal causes of a NAG metabolic acidosis.*
        - (+): failure of kidneys to excrete NH4+ and retain HCO3 → RTA1 or RTA4
        - (-): appropriate increased renal NH4+ excretion (GI loss, dilutional, exogenous acid)
- **Differentials of Acidosis/Alkalosis**
    - <u>Respiratory alkalosis</u>
        - CNS disorders, hypoxia, pulmonary receptor stimulation (asthma, pneumonia, pulmonary edema, PE), anxiety, drugs (ASA, Theo), liver failure, sepsis, recovery phase of met acidosis
    - <u>Respiratory acidosis</u>
        - Respiratory center inhibition (opiates, myxedema, o2 in co2 retainer), neuromuscular disorder (Guillain–Barré, myasthenia gravis, botulism, hypokalemia), chest wall disorder, airway obstruction, acute and chronic lung disease
    - <u>Metabolic alkalosis</u>
        - Saline/chloride–responsive (urine Cl– <20 mEq/L): GI; due to low volume state vomiting, diarrhea, ng drainage, diuretics, post–hypercapnic, cystic fibrosis, villous adenoma
        - Saline/chloride–resistant (urine Cl– >20 mEq/L): ↑BP think primary aldosteronism, secondary aldosteronism (CHF, cirrhosis & ascites, Cushing's, Bartter's), if ↓BP think congenital adrenal hyperplasia, Liddle's, licorice
        - Miscellaneous: poorly resorbed anion (PCN, carbenicillin), refeeding alkalosis, administration of alkali (e.g. antacids, overshoot from rx of acidosis, massive transfusions with citrate anticoagulant, milk alkali)
    - <u>Metabolic acidosis</u>
        - **Gap**
            - Are ketones present?
                - Yes → diabetic ketoacidosis/starvation/EtOH ketoacidosis
                - No →
                    - There is an unmeasured anion
                    - Measure the serum osmolarity and compare to calculated osmolarity
                        - Increased – methanol, ethylene glycol
                        - Normal – uremia, paraldehyde, INH, iron toxicity, lactic acidosis, rhabdomyolysis / renal (esrd - uremic), salicylates
        - **Non-gap**

- Common causes: low albumin (cirrhosis, CKD), multiple myeloma, ↑Mg, ↑Ca, lithium, bromide
- Clinically, the major distinction is between renal and extrarenal (usually GI) causes.
  - To differentiate, calculate the urine anion gap (Uag) = sodium + potassium – chloride (some will subtract bicarb also if urine ph is >6.5)-

- UAG	(ie -30) - appropriate renal response → suggests GI loss of bicarbonate (eg diarrhea) with renal continuing to be able to acidify urine. However, if proximal RTA (type 2) can be negative as well.
+ UAG	(ie +25) -- suggests impaired renal distal acidification (ie renal tubular acidosis because kidney cannot excrete h).

- **Renal**
  - Renal tubular acidosis: NAGMA, ↑Cl, normal GFR

Evaluation of RTA Causes

	Type I	Type II	Type IV
Location	Distal	Proximal	Distal
Inability to...	H+ secretion	Hco3 resorption at proximal tubule	Produce nh3
Urine ph	>6	<5.5	<5.5
Urine K+	↓↓↓	↓	↑↑↑
Serum k	↓	↓	↑
Hco3	↓↓↓	↓↓	>17
Associated with	Autoimmune dz Hypercalcemia Nephrolithiasis	Osteomalacia Multiple myeloma Nephrotoxic mediations	Diabetic nephropathy Aids Hypertensive nephro Hyperaldosteronism

- Type I RTA: drugs (ampho), chronic pyelonephritis, obstructive uropathy, nephrocalcinosis, autoimmune (SLE, Sjogren's, thyroiditis, cryoglobulinemia, chronic active hepatitis, PBC), amyloidosis, myeloma
  - Positive UAG (alkalotic urine noted with attempt to acidify urine with NH3Cl via PO administration)
- Type II RTA: primary (hereditary), myeloma, amyloidosis, Sjogren's, PNH, acetazolamide, hyperglobulinemia, heavy metals (Pb, Cd, Hg, Cu, others)
  - ↑HCO3 with ↑Fractional excretion of HCO3
  - Negative UAG
- Type IV RTA: inadequate aldo activity
  - Low aldo levels with normal/increased renin levels: Addison's dz, isolated decreased aldo synthesis a/w heparin or LMWH, ACEi, ARB, critically ill patients
  - Low aldo levels with low renin levels: DM (most common), NSAIDS, HIV
  - Aldo antagonists: Aldactone, TMP, pentamidine, amiloride
  - DM patients with Type IV are sensitive to ACE inhibitors (↑K)
  - Positive UAG (acidic urine noted with attempt to acidify urine with NH3Cl via PO administration)

        - Miscellaneous: obstructive uropathy, sickle cell disease, amyloidosis, AIN
    - **Non-Renal**
        - Bicarb wasting: Gi: diarrhea, ileus, fistula, villous adenoma
        - Urinary tract diversions: ureterosigmoidostomy, ileal conduit
        - Administration of chloride-containing acid: NH_4Cl, HCl, TPN, cholestyramine
        - Normal saline
        - Spironolactone
        - Topiramate
        - Post hypercapnia (transient)

- **Treatment**
    - In general, severe acidosis (ph < 7.10) warrants the iv administration of 50–100 mEq of $NaHCO_3$, over 30–45 min, during the initial 1–2 h of therapy.
    - A reasonable approach is to infuse sufficient $NaHCO_3$ to raise the arterial pH to no more than 7.2 over 30–40 min.
    - It is essential to monitor plasma electrolytes during the course of therapy, because the [K^+] may decline as pH rises. The goal is to increase the [HCO_3^-] to 10 mEq/l and the pH to 7.20, not to increase these values to normal.

ACUTE RENAL INJURY

- **Etiology**
    - Occurs in about 10-25% of hospitalized patients → ATN is most common cause from ischemic or nephrotoxic injury
    - In hospital mortality of 23-80%
- **Risks**
    - Hyperkalemia
    - Metabolic acidosis (loss of bicarb)

Comparing AKI, AKD, and CKD

	AKI	AKD	CKD
Duration	< 7 days	≤ 3 months	> 3 months
Functional Criteria	↑ in SCr by ≥50% in 7 days -or- ↑ in SCr by ≥0.3 mg/dL within 2 days -or- Oliguria for ≥ 6h	AKI -or- GFR <60 -or- ↓ in GFR by ≥35%x baseline GFR -or- ↑ in SCr by ≥50%x baseline	GFR<60
Structural criteria	Not defined	Marker of kidney damage (albuminuria, hematuria, or pyuria is m/c)	Marker of kidney damage for >3 months (albuminuria, is m/c)

AKI = acute kidney injury *AKD = acute kidney disease* *CKD = chronic kidney disease*

- **Definition/Risk stratification**

- KDIGO consensus
  - Increase in the serum creatinine level of 0.3 mg per deciliter (26.5 μmol per liter) or more within 48 hours (>24 hours is sustained; over 48 hours is abrupt)
  - A serum creatinine level that has increased by at least 1.5 times the baseline value within the previous 7 days
  - A urine volume of less than 0.5 ml per kilogram of body weight per hour for 6 hours

- **Staging**

The worse the stage, the worse the prognosis for the patient

Acute Renal Injury Staging		
Stage	SCr	UOP
1	1.5-1.9x baseline within 1 week or ≥ 0.3 mg/dl ↑ within 48 hours	<0.5 cc/kg/h for 6-12h
2	2.0-2.9x baseline	<0.5 cc/kg/h for ≥ 12h
3	3.0x baseline	<0.3 cc/kg/h for ≥ 24h or anuria for ≥ 12 h

Lab associations with renal injury			
	Prerenal	Intrinsic	Postrenal
Labs	Urine Osmolality >500 U_{Na} <20 Urine/Plasma Cr >40 FE_{Na} <1 FE_{Urea} <35	Urine Osmolality <400 U_{Na} >40 Urine/Plasma Cr <20 FE_{Na} >2 FE_{Urea} >35	
Urine Sediment	Normal; occasional hyaline cast or fine granular cast	Renal tubular epithelial cells; granular and muddy brown casts	
DDx	Ischemia Toxins Hypotension	AIN AGN ATN SIADH ATN	BPH

- **Determine cause**
  - Labs
    - General
      - **Urinalysis**
      - Random urine electrolytes (will help for FENa)
      - Urine creatinine (will help for FENa)
      - Urine microscopy (↑casts/sediment suggestive of AIN)
      - CBC
    - *Others to consider if overt failure*
      - Glomerulonephritis/Vasculitis
        - ANCA (C-ANCA seen with Wegener's)
        - ANA
        - Anti-GBM

- Anti-dsDNA, ANA (SLE)
- ENA
- IgG, IgA
- Cryoglobulins
- Hepatitis B, C
- HIV
- Renal bx
- C3, C4 (low levels may be s/o SLE)
- Anti-SPO (UA: Coca-Cola color)

- Malignancy:
  - Urine cytology
  - Light chains
  - SPEP and UPEP
- Interstitial Nephritis
  - Eosinophils
  - Urine eosinophils
  - Renal bx
- TTP/HUS
  - LDH
  - Haptoglobin
  - PLT
  - Reticulocytes
  - Bilirubin

- <u>FENa</u> is the most accurate screening test to differentiate between prerenal disease and acute tubular necrosis.
  - Not beneficial if patient has received Lasix or iv contrast recently! If this is the case, get a FEUrea and look for a value <35% which indicates pre-renal etiology.

$$FEUREA = UREA \times P_{cr} / BUN \times UCR \times 100$$

  - The urine sodium concentration is usually above 40 mEq/l in intrinsic or post renal causes, and below 20 mEq/l in prerenal conditions. However, since the urinary sodium concentration is influenced by the urine output, there is substantial overlap due in part to variations in the urine volume.

$$FENA = UNA \times PCR / PNA \times UCR \times 100$$

  - A value below 1 percent suggests prerenal disease, where the reabsorption of almost all of the filtered sodium represents an appropriate response to decreased renal perfusion; in comparison, a value between 1 and 2 percent may be seen with either disorder, while a value above 2 percent usually indicates atn.
- <u>UA with electrolytes</u>
  - Pre-renal is suspicious on UA if you see high spec grav, low pH, hyaline casts, low urinary Na
  - Intra-renal is suspicious on UA if you see low spec grav with muddy brown casts, normal or elevated urinary Na >40 (urinary Na often elevated with ATN and SIADH due to lack of ability to reabsorb Na)

Urinary findings and associated renal disease	
Urinary pattern	Renal disease
Hematuria with red cell casts (>3 RBC on microscopy), dysmorphic red cells, heavy proteinuria, or lipiduria	Glomerular disease or vasculitis
Multiple granular and epithelial cell casts with free epithelial cells	Acute tubular necrosis in a patient with acute renal failure
White cell and granular or waxy casts and no or mild proteinuria	Tubular or interstitial disease or urinary tract obstruction
Hematuria and pyuria with no or variable casts (excluding red cell casts)	May be observed in acute interstitial nephritis, glomerular disease, vasculitis, obstruction, and renal infarction
Epithelial Cells	Normal
Renal tubular cells	Acute tubular injury
Non-dysmorphic red cells	Non-glomerular bleeding from anywhere in the urinary tract
Hyaline casts	Any type of renal disease
Leukocytes	Inflammation in urinary tract

- **Complications**
  - ↑K, ↑volume, acidosis, anemia, ↓immune response, myopathy, pleural effusion
- **Imaging**
  - Renal ultrasound
  - MAG3 scan – when considering post obstructive
  - Renal biopsy
    - Major indications include
      - Isolated glomerular hematuria with proteinuria
      - Nephrotic syndrome
      - Acute nephritic syndrome
      - Unexplained acute or rapidly progressive renal failure
    - Contraindications include:
      - Uncorrectable bleeding diathesis
      - Small kidneys which are generally indicative of chronic irreversible disease
      - Severe hypertension, which cannot be controlled with antihypertensive medications
      - Multiple, bilateral cysts or a renal tumor
      - Hydronephrosis
      - Active renal or perirenal infection
      - An uncooperative patient
- **Treatment**

  Remove the offending agent, improve hemodynamics, make non-oliguric, fix electrolytes, avoid nephrotoxins. Assess for indications for urgine dialysis (↑volume, uremia, electrolyte disorders, drug toxicity)
  - Pre-renal – fluids
  - Intrinsic
    - *Etiology*
      - Nephrotoxin
      - Ischemia from vasoconstriction
      - Obstruction
    - *Phases*
      - Initiation – acute drop in GFR and increase in SCr
      - Maintenance – sustained low GFR with continued elevation of SCr for 1-2 weeks

  - Recovery – tubular function restored leading to polyuria with ↓SCr
- CRRT – clears solutes that are not being filed through process of diffusion and convection. Main disadvantage is risk of hypotension (less so with CRRT than intermittent hemodialysis)
  - *Indications* - ↑K, metabolic acidosis, anuria, diuretic resistant volume overload, uremia
  - *Flow* – 20-25aa/kg/hr
  - *Anticoagulation* – citrate is recommended, if cannot be used, then UFH or LMWH

Figure. Differential diagnosis of different causes of ARF

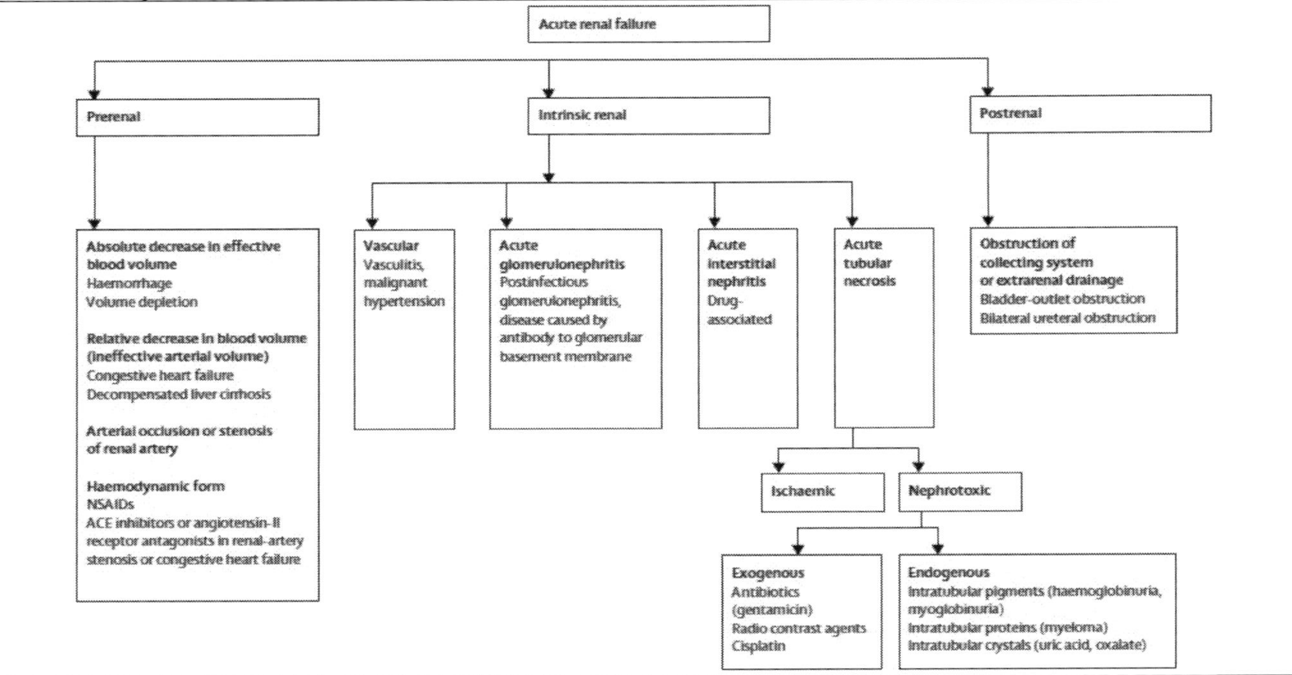

APPROACH TO CHRONIC KIDNEY DISEASE

- **Definition (any of the following:)** [295]
  - Kidney damage for three or more months based on findings of abnormal structure (imaging studies) or abnormal function (albuminuria > 30mg, hematuria, electrolyte issues)
  - GFR < 60 mL per minute per 1.73 m2 for ≥3 months with or without evidence of kidney damage

CKD Stages		
Stage	Damage	GFR
1	Kidney Damage	GFR≥90 mL/min
2	Kidney Damage	GFR 60-89 mL/min
3	Moderate	GFR 30-59 mL/min
4	Severe	GFR 15-29 mL/min
5	Failure	GFR<15 mL/min

KDIGO classification						
				Persistent albuminuria Categories		
				Normal to mildly ↑	Moderately ↑	Severely ↑
				<30 mg/g	30-300 mg/g	>300 mg/g
GFR Category	1	Normal	>90	1 if CKD	1	2
	2	Mildly decreased	60-89	1 if CKD	1	2
	3a	Mild-moderate decreased	45-59	1	2	3
	3b	Moderate to severe decreased	30-44	2	3	3
	4	Severely decreased	15-29	3	3	4+
	5	Kidney failure	<15	4+	4+	4+

- **Screening**
  - In general, anyone at higher risk of chronic kidney disease should be screened for it. This group includes US minorities and patients with hypertension, cardiovascular disease, and diabetes mellitus, among others. Screening includes an assessment of estimated GFR and urinalysis for proteinuria or hematuria.
  - SCr
    - Factors that alter SCr without changing GFR
      - Muscle mass
      - Dietary protein intake
      - Exercise
      - Cimetidine
      - Fibrates
      - Methyldopa
    - The serum creatinine concentration is directly dependent on muscle mass, which varies with sex (women tend to have less muscle mass as a percent of body weight than men), age (muscle mass decreases with age), and race (African

Americans have a higher serum creatinine level for the same GFR than other Americans). Thus, there is no "normal" value for serum creatinine that applies to all patients.

- Proteinuria on UA → if +1 then obtain Protein/SCr ratio → >200 should prompt nephrology referral but if <200 then repeat yearly for progression

Figure. Stages of CKD based on GFR

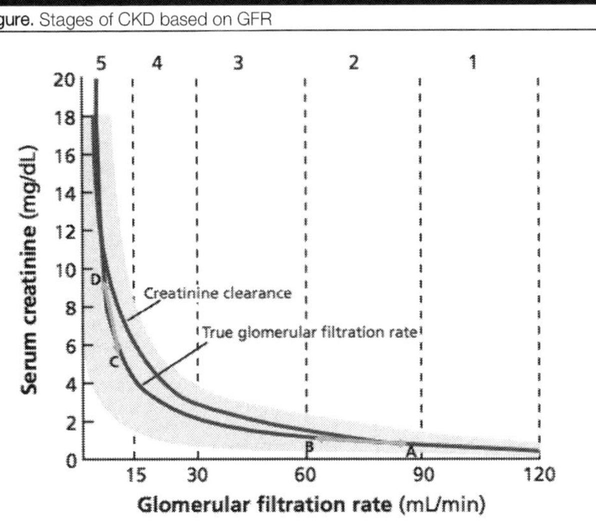

- **Etiologies**
  - DM (45%)
  - HTN (29%)
  - Glomerulonephritis (presence of dysmorphic RBCs) (5.5%)
  - C3/C4, anti-ASO, HIV, HepB, HCV, RPR
  - ANA, ANCA
  - SPEP/UPEP if age > 40
  - Interstitial nephritis (presence of WBC casts d/t medication s/e, fever, rash)
  - Ischemia/Hypovolemia (presence of hyaline casts (test for FENa, eosinophilia)
  - Chronic UTI
  - Malignancy
  - Tobacco use
  - RVD (doppler US)
  - Vasculitis (C3, C4, ANA, ANCA; HBsAg, HCV, cryoglobulins, ESR, RF, SS–A, SS–B, HIV)
- **Labs**
  - CMP (W/ Albumin)
  - Prot/SCr ratio (>300 = nephrotic range)
  - CBC (eval for normocytic anemia)
  - Vitamin D / PTH
  - UA
  - A1c and Lipid panel (eval. for risk factors)
  - <u>Other possible screening tests:</u>
    - SPEP/UPEP

        - Serum and urine free light chains
        - ANA, ds-DNA
        - C3/C4 (if concerned for glomerulonephritis based on presence of dysmorphic RBCs)
        - ANCA
        - Anti-GBM
        - HIV
        - Hepatitis B and C
        - Kidney biopsy
- **Imaging**
    - Renal US (eval. for hydronephrosis, medical renal disease)
- **Complications**
    - Poor calcium and phosphorus homeostasis
    - Vascular calcifications
    - Renal osteodystrophy
- **Treatment/Management**
    - Anemia: iron supplementation, particularly with intravenous iron, is known to enhance erythropoiesis and raise hemoglobin levels in CKD patients with anemia. ↑risk for hypotension but ↓GI s/e which is higher in oral iron supplementation (constipation)
        - Maintain transferrin saturation >30% and serum ferritin >500 ng/mL
        - EPO initiated if Hgb<9, stop when Hgb>11.5
    - Acidosis
        - Goal is HCo3 23-28
    - Electrolyte targets (mostly in ESRD)
        - Normalize Calcium (corrected): 8.4-9.5 mg/dL
        - Normalize Phosphate: 3.5-5.5 mg/dL
            - Restrict dietary phosphorus to 900mg/d
            - If remains high, test calcium level:
                - Calcium <9.5→ treat with calcium carbonate or calcium acetate
                - Calcium >9.5→ treat with sevelamer or lanthanum
        - Normalize PTH: 150-300 pg/mL
            - Correct vitamin D deficiencies and normalize Ca^{2+} and Phos
            - If despite above treatments, PTH is >300 pg/mL, test phosphorus level
                - Phosphorus <5.5 mg/dL
                    - And serum calcium <9.5
                        - Treat with vitamin D
                    - And serum calcium >9.5
                        - Treat with cinacalcet
                - Phosphorus >5.5 mg/dL
                    - Treat with cinacalcet
            - Tertiary hyperparathyroidism
                - Result of chronically elevated PTH, leads to ↑Ca levels and parathyroid hyperplasia with ↑PTH that will not respond to phosphate binders and calcitriol therapy
                - Requires parathyroidectomy

POLYURIA

- **Clinical Symptoms-**
    - Orthostatic hypotension
    - **Polyuria**

  - Polydypsia
  - Nocturia
  - ↓fluid intake
  - Ask about history of lithium use
  - PMHx of bipolar disorder
  - ↑HR, dry mucous membranes, ↓skin turgor
- **Differential**
  - Volume Depleted
    - Diabetes Insipidus (excess water loss by the kidney due to deficiency of ADH or renal resistance to ADH). Can be acquired due to medications, protein malnutrition, or metabolic abnormalities. Congenital causes of rarer.
      - Central (family history, head trauma)→ appropriate increase in urine osmolality after AVP challenge
      - Nephrogenic (chronic renal disease, ↑ca 2/2 malignancy such as MM, lithium, gentamycin) → no increase in urine osmolality after AVP challenge
    - Diuretic induced
      - Osmotic
      - Medication s/e
  - Euvolemic → primary polydypsia (h/o psychiatric disease; likely if water deprivation leads to increase in Urine osmolality of 1000-1200)
- **Labs**
  - Serum and urine osmolarity
    - Expect ↑serum Na (>143) and ↑serum osmolality (>295)
  - Urine sodium
  - Serum sodium
  - 24-hour urine
  - UPEP
  - SPEP
- **Testing**

1. Confirm hypotonic polyuria on 24 hour urine volume and osmolality
   - 24-hour urine volume is typically ≥3L in patients with DI
   - Urine osmolality is typically <300 mOsm/kg
2. Consider obtaining plasma vasopressin level (↑in nephrogenic DI) and plasma copeptin level (↑in nephrogenic DI)
3. If ↑Na and serum ↑osmolality → unlikely PP; perform vasopressin challenge test (good test for differentiating nephrogenic from central DI)
   - Water deprivation testing / Vasopressin challenge test
     To be done after vasopressin challenge test in patients with ↑Na (≥143) and ↑serum osmolality (≥295). Otherwise, perform before vasopressin challenge test in patients with normal Na and osmolality
     - Measure urine osmolality
     - Administer exogenous dose of ADH
     - Repeat urine osmolality measurement to evaluate response to ADH
4. If Na and serum osmolality are normal though, perform water deprivation testing **then** do to vasopressin challenge test

Water deprivation testing (WDT)

Protocol: varies by hospital, typically avoid alcohol, caffeine and tobacco 24 hours prior to test. STOP testing if body weight ↓ by 3-5%, significant orthostatic BP changes noted, urine osmolality plateaus (defined as <10% change over 3 consecutive measurements), urine osmolality normalizes (>750 mOsm/kg), plasma osmolality >295-300, or serum sodium is above 143. The following labs should be obtained during test:

plasma arginine vasopressin level at baseline; monitor body weight, BP, HR, serum sodium, plasma osmolality, urine osmolality, and urine volume **hourly** during water deprivation.
- If total daily urine volume is <3L in testing above, start testing at midnight
- If total daily urine volume is >3L in testing above, start testing 2 hours before test

- Interpretation
  - Little increase or no increase in urine osmolality (remaining below 300 mOsm/kg) during water deprivation → complete diabetes insipidus
  - Small increase in urine osmolality (increase to about 400-500 mOsm/kg) during water deprivation → partial diabetes insipidus or primary polydipsia
  - Increase in serum osmolality and urine osmolality → healthy response

Vasopressin challenge testing

Patient must be in a hyperosmolar state; if not, perform WDT above
- **Protocol**: varies by hospital, Administer arginine vasopressin (AVP) 5U or DDAVP 1-2 mcg SQ or IM. Check urine osmolality q30min for 2-4hours. If no change in urine osmolality, likely nephrogenic DI. If increase in urine osmolality by >50%, likely central DI. See table below.

Differentiating polyuric states: AVP stimulation test evaluation				
Condition	Uosm Max dehydration	Uosm Max after AVP	Percent change	Uosm Increase
Normal	1068±69	979±79	-9±3	<9%
Psychogenic polydypsia	738±53	780±73	-5±2	<9%
Partial central DI	438±34	549±28	28±5	>9%<50%
Complete central DI	168±13	445±52	183±41	**>50%**
Nephrogenic DI	124	174	42	**<50%**

- **Treatment/Management**
  - Ensure adequate water intake to prevent dehydration
  - Stop lithium if patient taking; consider starting amiloride
  - Low Na diet (<500mg/d)
  - Nephrology and endocrinology consultation

Figure. Algorithm for the differential diagnosis of polyuria

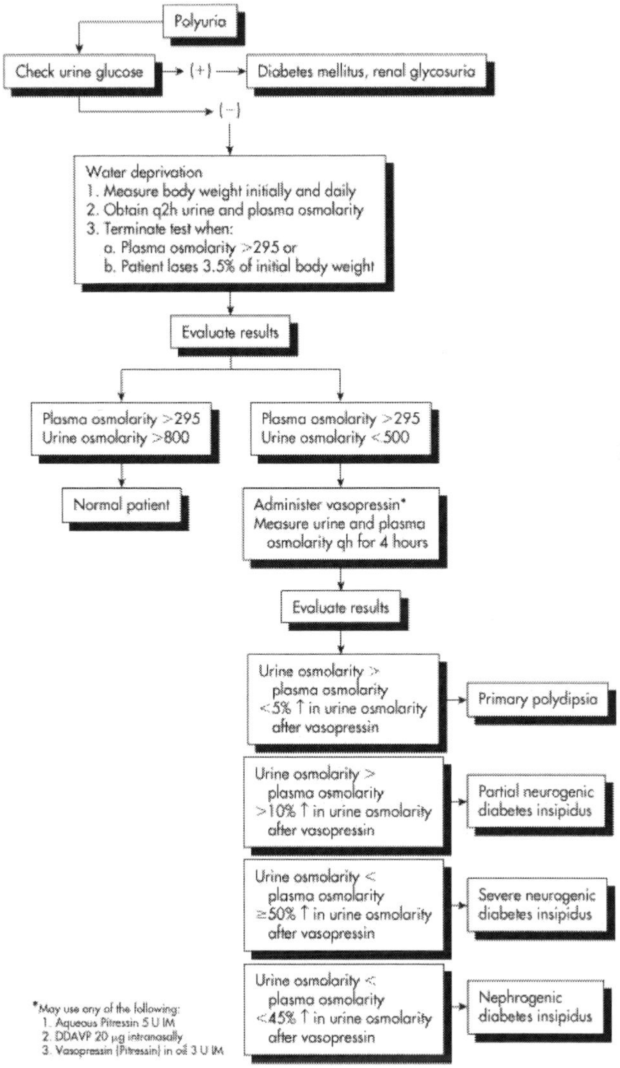

Polyuria

Check urine glucose → (+) → Diabetes mellitus, renal glycosuria

Check urine glucose → (−)

Water deprivation
1. Measure body weight initially and daily
2. Obtain q2h urine and plasma osmolarity
3. Terminate test when:
   a. Plasma osmolarity >295 or
   b. Patient loses 3.5% of initial body weight

Evaluate results

Plasma osmolarity >295
Urine osmolarity >800
→ Normal patient

Plasma osmolarity >295
Urine osmolarity <500
→ Administer vasopressin*
Measure urine and plasma osmolarity qh for 4 hours

Evaluate results

Urine osmolarity > plasma osmolarity
<5% ↑ in urine osmolarity after vasopressin → Primary polydipsia

Urine osmolarity > plasma osmolarity
>10% ↑ in urine osmolarity after vasopressin → Partial neurogenic diabetes insipidus

Urine osmolarity < plasma osmolarity
≥50% ↑ in urine osmolarity after vasopressin → Severe neurogenic diabetes insipidus

Urine osmolarity < plasma osmolarity
<45% ↑ in urine osmolarity after vasopressin → Nephrogenic diabetes insipidus

*May use any of the following:
1. Aqueous Pitressin 5 U IM
2. DDAVP 20 μg intranasally
3. Vasopressin (Pitressin) in oil 3 U IM

Figure. Alternative algorithm for the differential diagnosis of polyuria

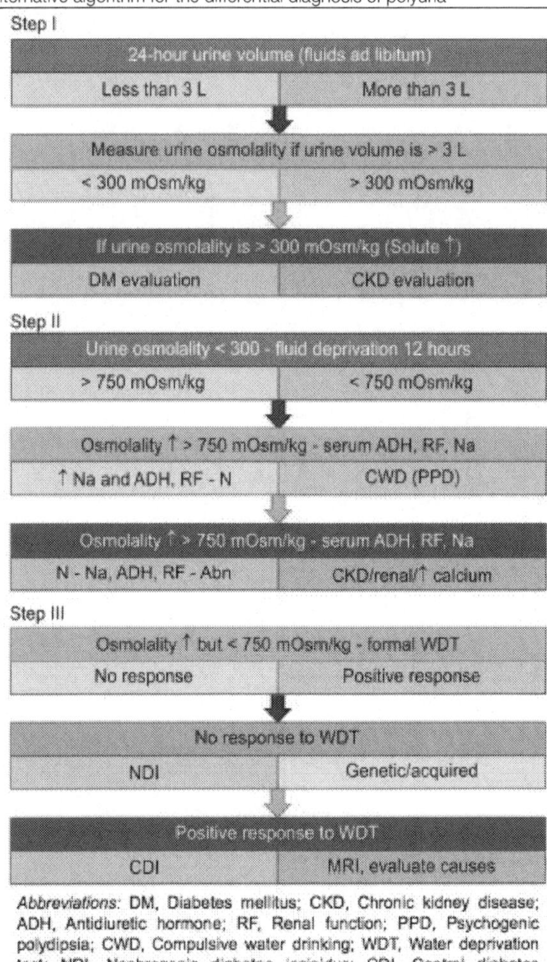

Abbreviations: DM, Diabetes mellitus; CKD, Chronic kidney disease; ADH, Antidiuretic hormone; RF, Renal function; PPD, Psychogenic polydipsia; CWD, Compulsive water drinking; WDT, Water deprivation test; NDI, Nephrogenic diabetes insipidus; CDI, Central diabetes insipidus; MRI, Magnetic resonance imaging

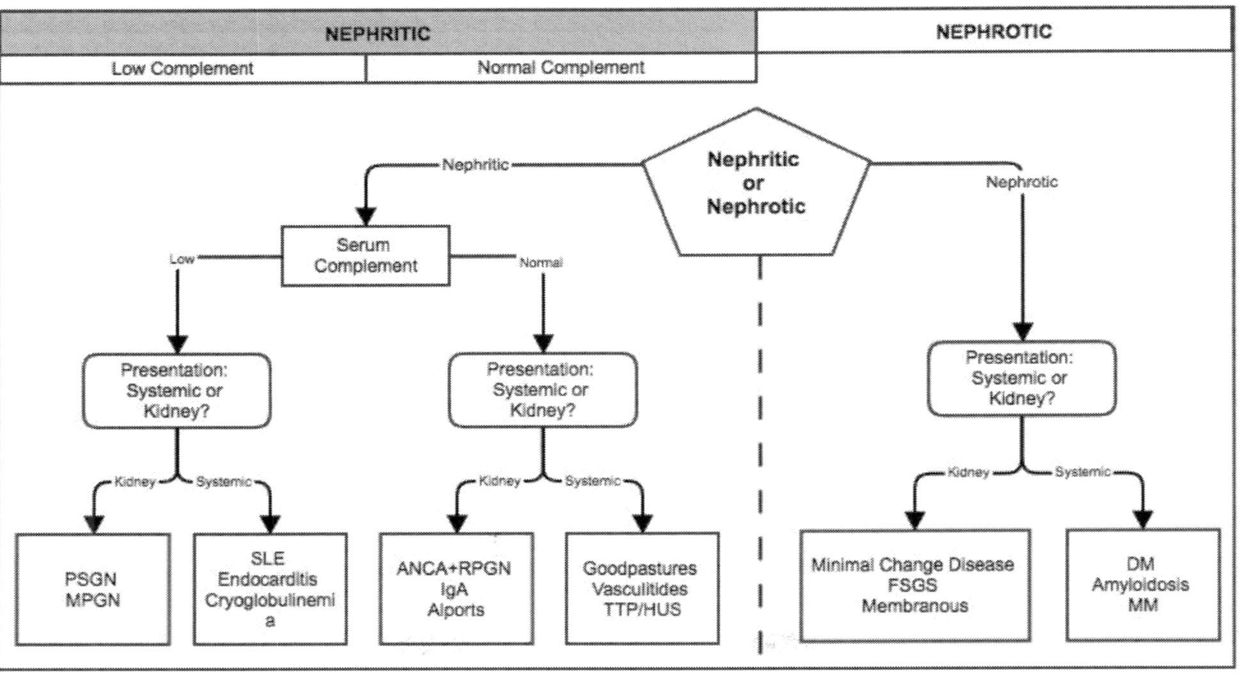
NEPHRITIC
NEPHROTIC
Low Complement
Normal Complement
Nephritic or Nephrotic
Nephritic
Nephrotic
Serum Complement
Low
Normal
Presentation: Systemic or Kidney?
Presentation: Systemic or Kidney?
Presentation: Systemic or Kidney?
Kidney
Systemic
Kidney
Systemic
Kidney
Systemic
PSGN
MPGN
SLE
Endocarditis
Cryoglobulinemi
a
ANCA+RPGN
IgA
Alports
Goodpastures
Vasculitides
TTP/HUS
Minimal Change Disease
FSGS
Membranous
DM
Amyloidosis
MM

GLOMERULAR DISEASE

- **Types**[297]
  (see chart on prior page)
  - Nephritic
    - *Features*
      - HTN
      - Hematuria
      - Oliguria
    - *Examples*
      - MGN
      - MPGN
      - IgA nephropathy
      - Anti-GBM disease
      - PSGN
      - HSP
      - SLE
      - Wegener's
      - Orthostatic proteinuria (young adults) → dx with split 24-hour urine protein collection
  - Nephrotic
    - *Features*
      - Massive proteinuria (>3g)
      - ↓albumin
      - edema
      - hyperlipidemia
    - *Examples*
      - Primary Causes
        - Membranous (most common overall)
        - FSGS (think African Americans)
        - Minimal change disease (most common in children)
        - Membranoproliferative Glomerulonephritis (MPGN)
      - Secondary Causes
        - Tumor (lymphoma) → MN
        - Heroin (FSGS)
        - Infection (HepB, C)
        - Systemic
        - Lupus
        - Amyloidosis
        - Sarcoidosis
        - DM
        - Hepatitis B, C (B=MN, C=MPGN)
        - AIDS
        - Syphilis (MN)

Lab findings in nephritic vs. nephrotic range proteinuria	
Nephrotic	Nephritic
Bland without casts Severe proteinuria (Spot prot/creat ratio >3.5 mg/dl or albumin/creatinine ratio >300 mg/dL) Lipiduria Associated hypoalbuminurea, hyperlipidemia Edema	Active sediment (casts, RBCs, dysmorphic) Sterile pyuria Spot prot/creat ratio <3

Differential of glomerulonephritis based on complement levels	
Low complement	Normal compliment
PSGN (↓C3) Endocarditis SLE (↓CH50, ↓C3/4, +ANA +anti-SM +anti-dsDNA) Cryoglobulinemia (+HepC commonly) MPGN (+HepC commonly, ↑monoclonal proteins)	Positive ANCA MPA (+P-ANCA/MPO, no lung granulomas) GPA (+C-ANCA/PR3, saddle-nose, pulm nodules) EGPA (asthma, atophy, ↓eosinophils) Renal limited ANCA Negative ANCA Goodpastures (hemoptysis common) Anti-GBM renal dz Immune Complex HSP/IgA vasculitis (palpable purapura, age<20) IgA nephropathy (gross hematuria post URI)

- **Labs**
  - C3, ANCA, Hepatitis C, Hepatitis B, anti-GM
  - ABG to determine pH
  - UA – presence of hematuria is often always seen with glomerulonep**hritis** whereas it is rarely seen with nephrotic syndrome. Also, nephritis is associated with more active sediment (RBC/WBC/Glomerular casts). Presence of heavy proteinuria (4+ which equals album of 1000 mg/dl) and lipiduria is classic of nephritic syndrome
  - Measure a spot urine Prot/SCr ratio from first morning void
    - Normal is <0.2 mg/mg
    - Ratio >3.5 = nephrotic range
  - Glomerulonephritis
    - Anti-SPO (r/o PSGN)
    - ANA/anti-DNA (r/o SLE)
    - C3/C4/CH50 (r/o PSGN and MPGN)
    - ANCA (r/o Wegener's)
    - IgA level (HSP, IgA nephropathy)
    - Anti-GBM antibody
  - Nephrotic Syndrome
    - Hypoalbuminurea (<3 g/dl)
    - Hyperlipidemia
- **Biopsy**

  - Determines diagnosis, amount of injury, and future
- **Medications/Management**
  - Consult nephrology
  - Consider medications to control elevated PO4 (Renvela 1-2 tabs TID), low HCO3 (Bicitra 30cc/TID if NAGMA; HCO3 drip (D5W+150mEQ) if low pH)

NEPHROLITHIASIS

- **Causes**[298]
  - Genetics – familial hypocalcemic hypocalciuria, homocystinuria, xanthine
  - Low water intake
  - RTA type 1
  - Hyperuricemia
  - M>F in 2:1 ratio
  - UTIs (staghorn calculi)
  - Hyperparathyroidism
- **Diagnosis**
  - Labs
    - SCr, Uric Acid, Ionized Calcium, Na, K, Cl, PTH, CBC, CRP, Coagulation Panel (for future surgery)
    - UA (red cells, white cells, nitrite, pH, volume, spec grav)
    - Urine calcium, oxalate, uric acid, citrate, Mg
    - Urine culture and microscopy
    - **Multiple Episode Patient**
      - 24hr urine collection for oxalate, calcium, citrate, sodium, and uric acid
      - Serum Mg, PO4
      - 24hr cysteine level
      - PTH and VIT D
  - Imaging
    - CT renal without contrast
    - US used to detect dilatation of ureters (upper) and stones at UVJ – imaging of choice if pregnant
  - Stone analysis
    - Calcium oxalate stones occur in 2 forms
      - dihydrated calcium oxalate crystals - pyramidal (squares with X's) and fragile
      - monohydrated calcium oxalate crystals - modular and very hard
    - Uric acid stones - yellow, smooth surface, very hard, occur in acidic environment
    - Phosphate stones (apatite) - whitish powder (appears as micro-bubbles if in contact with hydrochloric acid), occur in alkaline environment
    - Calcium phosphate stones - may appear as brushite, occur in acidic environment
    - Phosphor-ammonium-magnesium stones (struvite) - whitish, prismatic crystals, occur in alkaline environment, usually with infection

Kidney Stone Make-up			
Stone	Metabolic Abnormality	Clinical Setting	Urine Findings
Calcium oxalate	↑calciuria	Hyperparathyroidism Immobilization ↑vitamin d Cushing Genetic	Envelope-shape
	Hyperoxaluria	Increased oxalate uptake IBD High dietary VitC	
Calcium phosphate	Hypocitraturia Hypercalciuria High urine pH (>7)	Similar to calcium oxalate Distal RTA	
Struvite	High urinary ammonium and Bicarb levels	UTI w/ urease splitting organisms	Staghorn calculi Coffin-lid crystals
Uric Acid	Low urine pH (<5.5) Hyperuricosuria	Metabolic syndrome Insulin resis T2DM	Rhomboid crystals Radiolucent Stone
Cystine	Cystinuria	Genetics	Hexagonal green/yellow Large branched calculi

- **Treatment**
  - Urology Consultation – recommened in the following situations
    - Stones ≥ 10mm
    - AKI
    - Sepsis
    - Complete ureteral obstruction
    - Uncontrolled pain
    - Nausea
  - Fluids
  - Pain control
    - NSAID – ketorolac, diclofenac, indomethacin, Toradol IM injection all remain the first line treatment options
    - Morphine (hydromorphone, pentazocine, tramadol) 3mg prn q2h
+
Dilaudid 0.2mg q2h
    - Antispasmodics – metamizole sodium
  - Facilitate passage (for stones >5mm)
    - Alfuzosin 10mg/d, tamsulosin 0.4mg/d
  - Ureteral stone
    - Upper < 1cm – ESWL
    - Upper > 1cm/resistant to ESWL/any stone >2cm – percutaneous nephrolithotomy
    - Distal < 1cm – ESWL
    - Distal > 1cm – Ureterorenoscopy
  - Kidney
    - < 2cm – ESWL
    - > 2cm – percutaneous nephrolithomy
- **Prevention**

- Pain: diclofenac sodium 100-150 mg/day for 3-10 days
- >2.5L water/day
- ↓ salt & protein diet
- ↑dietary calcium intake
- ↑fruits/veggies
- Thiazide diuretics unless calcium stone composition

OTOLARYNGOLOGY

ALLERGIC RHINITIS

- **Diagnosis**[299]
  Diagnosis is made through clinical and physical exam; can confirm with allergy testing (skin or IgE)
  - Intermittant: <4 days a week or less than 4 weeks
  - Persistent: >4 daysa week and for more than 4 weeks
  - Mild: none of the following are present: sleep disturbance; impairment of daily activities, leisure, and/or sport; impairment of school or work; troublesome symptoms.
  - Moderate to severe: one or more of the following symptoms are present: sleep disturbance; impairment of daily activities, leisure, and/or sport; impairment of school or work, troublesome symptoms.
- **Causes**
  - Allergic rhinitis is most common cause
  - Non-allergic rhinitis
  - Congestion
  - PND
  - Rhinorrhea
  - Vasomotor
  - Gustatory - common causes being smoking, perfume, car exhaust, medications, hormone changes, idiopathic.
  - Drug-induced rhinitis (recent use of afrin, NSAIDs, ACEi)
  - Nasal polyps
  - Adenoid hypertrophy
- **Exam**
  - Sneezing
  - Nasal itching
  - Rhinorrhea
  - Nasal congestion
- **Management/Treatment**

Figure. Management options in allergic rhinitis based on severity

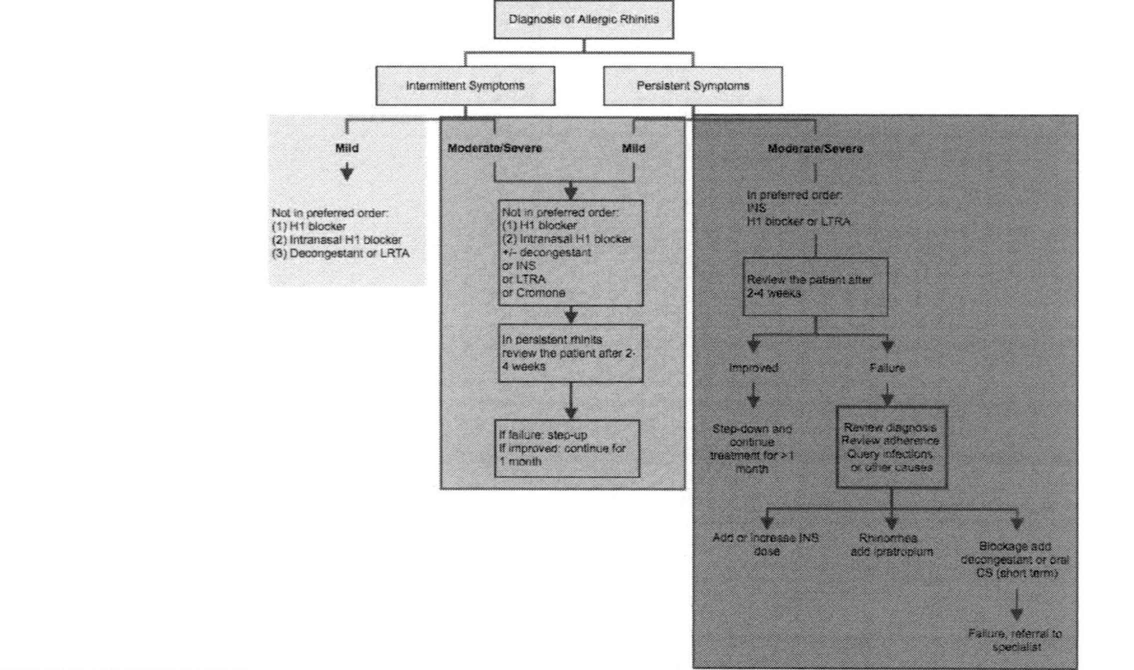

- Intranasal Corticosteroid
  - Treat nasal congestion and ocular symptoms
  - The combination with a second-generation antihistamine intranasal preparation has also been found to be effective
  - Rhinocort Aqua (good for pregnancy)
  - Flonase 2 sprays each nostril daily
  - Nasarel 2 sprays each nostril BID
  - Nasacort 1-2 sprays each nostril daily
  - Triamcinolone Acetate
  - Azelastine 137mcg/spray 1-2 sprays per nostril BID
  - Olopatadine 665mcg/spray 2 sprays per nostril BID
- Oral Antihistamines
  Treat sneezing, purities, and rhinorrhea
  - Allegra 60mg/BID or 180mg/d
  - Claritin 10mg/d or 5mg/BID
  - Clarinex 5mg/d
  - Zyrtec 5-10mg
- Decongestants
  - Afrin 2 sprays into each nostril BID for < 3 days
  - Phenylephrine
  - Pseudoephedrine
- Intranasal Antihistamines
  - Azelastine 0.15% 2 sprays/BID
- Combination Therapy
  - Dymista (Azelastine+Fluticasone)
- Acute
  - Afrin BID x 3 days
  - NEILmed saline rinse
  - ipratropium nasal spray 0.03% 2 sprays each nostril BID-TID
- Chronic
  - Flonase (most effective)

RHINOSINUSITIS[300]

- **Types**
  - Acute rhinosinusitis: Sudden onset, lasting less than 4 weeks with complete resolution. Most commonly due to viruses and is usually self-limiting. Approximately 90% of patients with colds have an element of viral sinusitis.
  - Subacute rhinosinusitis: A continuum of acute rhinosinusitis but less than 12 weeks.
  - Recurrent acute rhinosinusitis: Four or more episodes of acute, lasting at least 7 days each, in any 1-year period.
  - Chronic – presence of at least two of the following cardinal symptoms for at least 12 consecutive weeks:
    - Nasal obstruction
    - Nasal drainage
    - Facial pain/pressure
    - Hyposmia/anosmia
    - -And-
    - Objective evidence on PE (mucopurulent d/c, edema, polyps in the middle of the meatus or XR/sinus
- **Symptoms** - nasal discharge, cough, congestion, headache, fever, facial pain
- **Treatment**

- Acute Rhinosinusitis
  - ABx indicated for:
    - Symptoms >10 days
    - Facial pain > 3 days +/- purulent discharge
    - Worsening symptoms after initial improvement
    - Temp>102.2F
  - Treatment (if no improvement in >7 days)
    - ***Mild Disease:***
      - Amoxicillin 500mg q8h x5-10d or 875mg BID x5-10d
      - Augmentin 500/125 q8h x5-10d or 875/125 BID x5-10d recommended
      - *High S.pneumonia risk due to child at daycare:*
      - Amoxicillin 1g Q8H x5-10d or 1g QID x5-10d
    - ***Mod/Severe Disease/Treatment Failure***
      - Augmentin XR 2g/125 BID x10d
      - PCN Allergy:
      - Levaquin 500mg/d x10-14d
      - Doxycycline 200mg/d x5-10d
- Chronic Rhinosinusitis
  - Treatment consists of medical mgmt. and endoscopic sinus surery if meds are not successful
  - Options
    - Isotonic nasal saline rinse/irrigation (low pressure high volume 240cc)
    - Topical intranasal corticosteroids (ie. Flonase) injected laterally away from septum while leaning forward
    - Anti-histamines (Claritin, Allegra, Zyrtec)
      - Can lead to impaired drainage.
      - They are only of benefit in early allergic sinusitis
    - Ipratropium 2 sprays of the 0.06% solution in each nostril 4 times daily
    - Decongestants: oxymetolazone 2-3 sprays each nostril BID (no more than 3d), pseudoephedrine 60mg q4-6h, nasal saline rinse, guaifenesin, Flonase (intranasal steroids), Afrin
    - Zinc 25mg/d
    - Humidification

PHARYNGITIS

- **Cause**[301]
  - Non-infectious (smoking, workplace inhalation exposure to chemicals, foreign body, GERD, allergic rhinitis
  - Viral vs. Bacterial
    - Viruses
      - Viral causes are most common (rhinovirus)
      - Others (adenovirus, HSV, Coxsackie)
    - Atypical (Mycoplasma, Chlamydophila pneumoniae
    - Remember prodrome of early HIV can present as pharyngitis/mono like symptoms (look for patients that participate in high risk sexual activity, IVDA)
      - R/o with HIV RNA testing or p24 antigen in serum
    - Bacterial
      - Bacterial m/c caused by GAS (pyogenes) → remember can lead to RF and PSGN

Pharyngitis Etiologies		
Cause	Statistics	Facts/Findings
Strep	5-15% of cause	Group A Sudden onset sore throat Tonsillar exudates Fever No Cough Risk of progression to scarlet fever Group C/G Similar symptoms to GAS but negative rapid strep screen
EBV	Most Common (viral)	Can lead to infectious mono Malaise/Headache Low grade fever Prolonged course Rarely has exudates Severe pharyngotonsillar inflammation, which can be obstructive and require intensive anti-inflammatory treatment. Tonsillar exudates in 50% of cases. Inflammation of cervical lymph nodes. Takingantibiotics can result in a maculopapular rash on the trunk and extremities
CMV	Less common than EBV	Prolonged fever Less likely to have LAD Mild if any pharyngitis
HIV	Less Common	Mucosal ulcerations Febrile Pharyngeal edema WITHOUT exudates
Fusobacterium necrophorum	Less Common	Suspect in patients with negative RADT and not improving Cause in severe cases of Lemierre' s syndrome

- **Signs/Symptoms**
  - Bacterial
    - Sore throat
    - Fever
    - Headache
    - N/V/abdominal pain
    - Cervical adenitis
  - Viral
    - Conjunctivitis
    - Cough
    - Diarrhea
    - Hoarseness
    - Rash
    - Presentation in winter
- **Serious Symptoms**
  - Stridor
  - Drooling
  - Respiratory Distress

- Recent travel
- Cases lasting over 2 weeks with poor outcome
- Suspicion of lingual pharyngitis with obstruction
- Concern for Lemierre's Syndrome – thrombphlebitis of the internal jugular vein (worsening sx with chills, fever, pain, and ipsilateral cervical swelling at the angle of the jaw and along the SCM and stiff neck)

- **Evaluation (Scoring System)**
  - Centor criteria (GABHS)
    - Fever (subjective or measured >100.5° F): 1 point
    - Absence of cough: 1 point
    - Tender anterior cervical lymphadenopathy: 1 point
    - Tonsillar exudates: 1 point
    - **Analysis**
      - 0-1 points: low risk therefore does not require treatment; probability 2.5-10%
      - 2-3 points: assess for GAS with rapid strep testing (RADT) without reflex culture for negative tests; probability 10-35%
      - 4+ points: empirical treatment; probability 39-57%
  - McIsaac criteria (modified Centor)
    - Fever (subjective or measured >100.5° F): 1 point
    - Absence of cough: 1 point
    - Tender anterior cervical lymphadenopathy: 1 point
    - Tonsillar exudates: 1 point
    - Age
      - 3–14 years: 1 point
      - 15–44 years: 0 point
      - 45 years or older: –1 point
    - **Analysis**
      - 0-1 points: low risk therefore does not require treatment
      - 2-3 points: assess for GAS with rapid strep testing (RADT) without reflex culture for negative tests
      - 4+ points: empirical treatment
- **Complications**
  - Epiglottitis
  - Peritonsillar abscess
  - Cervical lymphadenitis
  - Sinusitis
  - Mastoiditis
  - ARF
  - PSGN
- **Diagnostic Testing**
  - RADT (if CENTOR 3+) but do not get reflex culture if negative
- **Treatment**
  - Self-limited illness; viral pharyngitis resolves in 3-7 days
  - If ABx are indicated, resolution noted within 24-48 hours of initiation
  - Supportive therapy
    - Analgesics
      - NSAIDS to ↓ fever and pain
      - Tylenol 325mg for pain
    - Nasal congestion
      - Combination antihistamine+decongestant is best (ie. Claritin+Sudafed)
        - Acute – Afrin BID x 3 days, NEILmed saline rinse, sodium cromoglycate dry powder (20mg/INH) q2h

    - Chronic – Flonase, sinus rinse, Sudafed IR 60mg q4-6h or ER 120mg q12h / 240mg daily
- Cough (see page 431 for more details)
  - Tessalon Pearls
  - Robitussin (guaifenesin with codeine)
  - Mucinex
- Sneezing/Rhinorrhea
  - ipratropium nasal spray 0.03% 2 sprays each nostril BID-TID
- Sore Throat
  - Chloraseptic Spray 1 spray PO Q 2-hour prn sore throat
    - Leave in place x 15 sec then spit
  - Benzoate 100-200mg prn TID max 600 mg/day
  - Guaifenasin+Codeine
    - Capsule: G (200mg) and C (9mg) q4h max 12cap/24hr
    - Liquid: 15mL q4-6h max 45ml/day
    - Tablet G (400 mg) and C (10-20 mg): One tablet q4-6h (maximum: 6 tablets/24 hours)
  - Hurricane Spray
  - Benmalid (diphenhydramine/Maalox/lidocaine viscous) suspension 30ml swish and swallow Q2H prn.

Antibiotic Treatment		
Antibiotic	Dose	Duration
Penicillin V	250 mg QID or 500 mg BID	10 days
	1.2M I.U. /oral/12h	8-10 days
Penicillin G	1.2M I.U. I.M	1 dose
Amoxicillin	500mg BID	8-10 days
Cefadroxil	500mg BID	8-10 days
Recurrence		
Clindamycin	300mg Q8H	10 days
Augmentin	500mg/125mg Q8H	10 days

Figure. Evaluation of acute pharyngitis

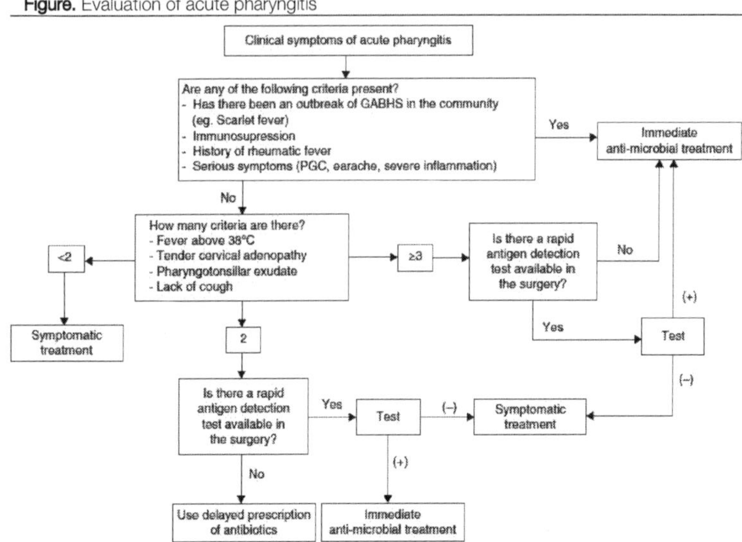

EPISTAXIS

- **Background**[302]
  - Nasal bleeds are either anterior, posterior, or a combination of the two.
  - About 5% of nasal bleeding originates in the posterior nasal cavity. Such bleeds are more commonly associated with atherosclerotic disease and hypertension.
- **Cause**
  - Digital trauma, a deviated septum, dry air exposure, rhinosinusitis, neoplasia, or chemical irritants such as inhaled corticosteroids or chronic nasal cannula oxygen use.
  - Systemic factors that increase the risk of bleeding include chronic renal insufficiency, alcoholism, hypertension, vascular malformations such as hereditary hemorrhagic telangiectasia, or any kind of coagulopathy, including warfarin administration, von Willebrand's disease, or hemophilia.
- **History**
  - Ask about prior or recurrent epistaxis, duration and severity of the current episode, and laterality.
  - Ask specifically about nonsteroidal anti-inflammatory drugs, warfarin, heparin, or aspirin use. Alcohol or cocaine abuse, trauma, prior head and neck procedures, and a personal and family history of coagulopathy should be assessed.
- **Tools**
  - Create an epistaxis kit containing nasal speculum, bonyet forceps, headlamp, suction catheter, cotton pledgets, 0.05% oxymetolazone an 4% lidocaine solutions, silver nitrate ($AgNO_3$) swabs, petroleum jelly
- **Diagnosis/Testing**
  - The division between anterior and posterior bleeding is often based on the ability to visualize the site of bleeding with a light source and a nasal speculum.

- Generally, the diagnosis of posterior hemorrhage is only once measures to control anterior bleeding have failed.
- Clinical features suggestive of a posterior source include: elderly patients with either inherited or acquired coagulopathy, a significant amount of hemorrhage visible in the posterior nasopharynx, hemorrhage from bilateral nares, or epistaxis uncontrolled with either anterior rhinoscopy or an anterior pack.
  - Posterior, bilateral, or large-volume epistaxis should be triaged immediately to a specialist in a critical care setting.
- Laboratory evaluation or other ancillary studies are not required unless management of comorbid illness requires it, or the hemorrhage is poorly controlled. In the latter case, collect blood for CBC, type and cross-match, and coagulation studies if coagulopathy is suspected.

- **Treatment**
  - Anterior Bleed
    - Direct Nasal Pressure
    - Instill a topical vasoconstrictor such as oxymetazoline or phenylephrine.
    - The patient should lean forward in the "sniffing" position and pinch the soft nares between the thumb and the middle finger for a full 10 to 15 minutes, breathing through the mouth.
      - If the patient is uncooperative, fashion a hands-free pressure device made from two tongue depressors that are taped together between halfway and two thirds of the way up the depressors. Place the device on the nose and leave it undisturbed for 10 to 15 minutes. These initial measures are often sufficient to achieve hemostasis and facilitate further examination by anterior rhinoscopy.
  - Chemical Cauterization
    - If two attempts at direct pressure have failed, chemical cauterization with silver nitrate is the next appropriate step for mild bleeding.
    - Before cautery, anesthetize the nasal mucosa using three cotton pledgets soaked in a 1:1 mixture of 0.05% oxymetazoline and 4% lidocaine solution.
      - Do not attempt chemical cautery unless the bleeding vessel is visualized. Electrical cautery should be left to the otolaryngologist due to the risk of septal perforation.
    - After visualizing the (anterior) bleeding site, silver nitrate sticks may be judiciously placed just proximal to the bleeding source on the anterior nasal septum. Silver nitrate requires a relatively bloodless field, as the chemical reaction leading to precipitation of silver metal and tissue coagulation cannot proceed in the setting of amative hemorrhage due to washout of substrate. Once a relatively bloodless field is achieved, gently and briefly (a few seconds) apply silver nitrate directly to the bleeding site. Chemical cautery should never be attempted on both sides of the nasal septum. Subsequent attempts on the same side of the nasal septum should be separated by 4 to 6 weeks to avoid perforation.
  - Iced Lavage
      - If neither vasoconstrictors nor direct external pressure stops the bleeding, try an iced normal saline lavage of each nostril, with the patient leaning forward. This may help decrease or stop the bleeding and allow better assessment of bleeding sites.
      - Have the patient seated during both the examination and the therapeutic procedures; this will lower his or her blood pressure.
  - Packing
    - Lubricating a vaginal tampon and slipping it into the nose can make an improvised “prepackaged” anterior pack.
      - As with anything else inserted into or through the nose, insert the tampon straight back along the floor of the nose.

        - May need to start oral antibiotics

HEARING LOSS

- **Overview**
  - Sudden hearing loss is defined as a rapid onset, occurring over a 72-hour period, of a subjective sensation of hearing impairment in one or both ears.
  - Approximately 1 in 8 individuals aged 12 years or older in the United States have a bilateral hearing loss, and 1 in 5 have a unilateral hearing loss.1
  - Disorders anywhere along the auditory pathway from the external auditory canal to the central nervous system may result in diminished hearing.
  - Patients presenting with sudden hearing loss, however, demand a more urgent and vigilant approach
- **Evaluation**
  - In a patient with auditory complaints, the goals in the evaluation are to determine: (1) the nature of the hearing impairment (conductive or sensorineural)
    (2) the severity of the impairment (mild, moderate, severe, profound)
    (3) the anatomy of the impairment (external ear, middle ear, inner ear, or central auditory pathway pathology)
    (4) the etiology.
  - <u>Onset</u>
    - **Sudden**
      - A sudden onset of unilateral hearing loss, with or without tinnitus
      - May represent an inner ear viral infection or a vascular accident
      - Patients with unilateral hearing loss (sensory or conductive) usually complain of reduced hearing, poor sound localization, and difficulty hearing clearly with background noise.
    - **Gradual**
      - Gradual progression in a hearing deficit is common with otosclerosis, noise-induced hearing loss, vestibular schwannoma, or Meniere disease.
      - People with small vestibular schwannomas typically present with any or all of the following conditions: asymmetric hearing impairment, tinnitus, and imbalance (although rarely vertigo).
      - Cranial neuropathy, especially of the trigeminal or facial nerve, may accompany larger tumors.
      - In addition to hearing loss, Meniere disease or endolymphatic hydrops may be associated with episodic vertigo, tinnitus, and aural fullness.
      - Hearing loss with otorrhea is most likely due to chronic otitis media or cholesteatoma.

Source of Hearing Loss Based on Weber / Rinne Testing			
Type	Rinne	Weber	DDx
Conductive	Bone>air	Localized to affected ear	Cerumen Otitis Media Otitis Externa Otosclerosis TM rupture Cholesteatoma
Sensorineural	Air>bone	Localizes to unaffected ear	Meniere Acoustic Neuroma Presbycusis Ototoxic Rx
Normal	Air=bone	No localization	N/a

- **Testing**
  - Weber/Rinne - The combined information from the Weber and Rinne tests permits a tentative conclusion as to whether a conductive or sensorineural hearing loss is present. However, these tests are associated with significant false-positive and -negative responses and therefore should be used only as screening tools and not as a definitive evaluation of auditory function.
    - **Weber**
      - The Weber tuning fork test may be performed with a 256- or 512-Hz fork.
      - The stem of a vibrating tuning fork is placed on the head in the midline
      - The patient is asked whether the tone is heard in both ears or in one ear better than in the other.
        - With a unilateral conductive hearing loss, the tone localizes to the affected ear.
        - With a unilateral sensorineural hearing loss, the tone is perceived in the unaffected ear (the ear that is not localized to)
    - **Rinne**
      - Sensitive in detecting conductive hearing losses.
      - A Rinne test compares the ability to hear by air conduction with the ability to hear by bone conduction.
      - Place vibrating tuning fork (256 or 512 Hz) over the mastoid bone of one ear, then move the tuning fork to the entrance of the ear canal (not touching the ear)
      - The sound should be heard better via air conduction (at the entrance to the ear canal).
      - If the sound is heard better by bone conduction, then there is a CHL in that ear.
      - Repeat for the other ear
- **Types**
  - Sensorineural hearing loss
    - Decrease in hearing of 30 dB or greater across at least 3 consecutive frequencies
    - Etiology in up to 90% of cases remains elusive.
    - 10% or so of cases have been associated with neoplastic, autoimmune, infectious, circulatory, coagulation, and demyelinating disorders
    - **Weber/Rinne**
      - Weber tuning fork test lateralizes to the unaffected side
      - Rinne tuning fork test demonstrates air conduction greater than bone conduction

        - Speech discrimination testing less than 90% correct.
        - **Differential**
            - Age-related (presbycusis) - symmetric, high-frequency hearing loss that eventually progresses to involve all frequencies. The hearing loss is associated with a significant loss in clarity.
            - Alport
            - Otitis Media
            - Labyrinthitis
            - S/e of medication (ie. aminoglycosides)
            - Head trauma
            - MS
            - Vestibular schwannoma
        - **Treatment**
            - Sudden onset
                - Hydrocortisone (1mg/kg/d max 60mg/d x 7-14d f/b taper for same time period with repeat audiogram after)
                - Hyperbaric O2
    - <u>Conductive hearing loss</u>
        - Results from dysfunction of the external or middle ear.
        - There are four mechanisms, each resulting in impairment of the passage of sound vibrations to the inner ear:
          (1) obstruction (eg, cerumen impaction)
          (2) mass loading (eg, middle ear effusion)
          (3) stiffness effect (eg, otosclerosis)
          (4) discontinuity (eg, ossicular disruption).
        - Conductive losses in adults are most commonly due to cerumen impaction or transient eustachian tube dysfunction associated with upper respiratory tract infection.
        - Persistent conductive losses usually result from chronic ear infection, trauma, or otosclerosis. Conductive hearing loss is often correctable with medical or surgical therapy—or in some cases both.

OTITIS EXTERNA

- **Overview**[303]
    - 90% of cases unilateral; peaks at age 7 to 12 yr; tends to decline after age 50 yr
- **Risk factors**
    - High humidity; warm weather; swimming; local trauma; hearing aids; hearing protection
- **Symptoms** — mild pain or itching to severe pain; pain worsens with motion and chewing; discharge; hearing loss if ear canal swollen; discharge
- **Causes**
    - Bacterial causes associated with scant, white, often thick discharge; chronic bacterial infection can cause discharge of bloody granulation tissue
        - Bacterial otitis externa — associated with more intense pain; commonly due to Pseudomonas and Staphylococcus; topical treatment preferred after thorough cleaning of ear canal
    - Fungal causes associated with white to off-white fluffy discharge or green, black, or gray discharge (sign of Aspergillus)
- **Treatment**
    - Topical agents: 2% acetic acid; risk for ototoxicity

  - Neomycin — effective; 15% develop contact dermatitis; others
  - Polymyxin B can miss Staphylococcus
  - Aminoglycosides less irritating, but potentially ototoxic and costly
  - Quinolones — highly effective against Pseudomonas; no risk for ototoxicity; can be used twice daily with no irritation or sensitization; expensive; potential for resistance
- **Prevention**
  - Acidifying drops or alcohol drops during risk periods; hair dryer at low setting; avoid cotton swabs

CERUMEN IMPACTION

- Debrox
- Almond-oil
- Earex
- Cerumenex
- Colace
- Hydrogen Peroxide
- Referral to ENT for cleaning

RHEUMATOLOGY

GOUT

- **Background**[304,305]
  - Along with pseudogout, one of the most common crystal-induced arthropathies
  - Uric acid (UA) produced by purine metabolism
  - Risk Factors: older age, males, red meat consumption, shell fish, EtOH, ASA, loop diuretics, HTN, IV contrast
- **Symptoms**: sudden onset pain, warm and erythematous joint, often one joint but can become polyarticular, resolves spontaneously in days to weeks. Patients may have systemic symptoms of fever, chills, ↑WBC but often resolved spontaneously in a few days if untreated.
  - Joints affected often are 1· MTP, ankle, or knee
- **Labs**
  - Check LFTs if on allopurinol
  - Synovial fluid with 2k-100k WBC
  - Crystals during joint aspiration (needle shap, negative birefringent, **monosodium urate**)
  - Uric Acid level (may be normal during acute flare) but monitored monthly during prevention therapy titration
  - HLA-B*5801 – consider testing in certain Asian ethnic groups who may have predisposition to allopurinol hypersensitivity.
- **Treatment**
  - Acute Gouty Arthritis
    - The acute phase is self-limited and characterized by recurrent attacks of synovitis that presents with pain, erythema, and swelling, most frequently in the large toe but other joints, tendons, bursae or other areas may be involved.
    - Primary treatments for acute gout attacks have included non-steroidal anti-inflammatory agents (NSAIDs), corticosteroids (intraarticular), colchicine. See below.
    - If the patient does not have an adequate response to initial therapy with a single drug, ACR guidelines advises that adding a second appropriate agent is acceptable.
      - Using combination therapy from the start is appropriate for an acute, severe gout attack, particularly if the attack involves multiple large joints or is polyarticular. Acceptable regimens include any of the following, in full or prophylactic doses as appropriate:

- Colchicine plus NSAIDs
  - ***NSAIDs*** (unless CKD) such as Indomethacin 50–75 mg, followed by 50 mg every 6–8 hours, with a maximum dose of 200 mg in the first 24 hours. Indomethacin should be continued for an additional 24 hours after attack resolution, then tapered to 50 mg every 6–8 hours for the next 2 days to prevent relapse.
  - ***Colchicine*** 1.2 mg at the first sign of a flare or in the earliest phase of a flare (e.g. within the first 12 hours of onset), followed by 0.6 mg one hour later
    - Doses should be limited to 0.5–0.6 mg/d in patients with moderate renal insuffi- ciency (eGFR from 30 to 60 mL/min) and to 0.5–0.6 mg every 2 or 3 days in those with eGFR from 15 to 30 mL/min.
    - The drug should be stopped promptly with the onset of side effects, usually gastrointestinal, including nausea, vomiting, and diarrhea. The drug is contraindicated in patients taking clarithromycin and should be used cautiously in those with severe renal or hepatic impairment.
- Oral corticosteroids plus colchicine
  - *PO steroids* – prednisone 30mg daily x1w then 10mg daily for 1 week in patients with multiple joints involved
- Intra-articular steroids plus colchicine or NSAIDs
  - *Intra-articular joint injection* (Triamcinolone 10mg with Lidocaine and Marcaine; inject up to 3x/year)

Gout Treatment Options

Treatment	Indications	Contraindications	S/E
NSAID	First line	PUD CKD CHF	GIB AKI Edema Sodium retention
Colchicine	NSAID intolerance	CKD	Diarrhea Abdominal pain Neuromyopathy
Intraarticular Steroids	1-2 inflammed joints NSAID/colchicine contraindications	Drug hypersensitivity	No major systemic s/e
Systemic Steroids	>2 joints involved NSAID/colchicine intolerance	Drug hypersensitivity	Rebound attacks ↑BP ↑Glucose Fuid retention

- Chronic Gout
  - Although initial episodes may be brief and rare, acute episodes may increase in frequency and duration over time and lead to the development of chronic gout.
  - In addition to more frequent attacks, chronic gout may be associated with deposits of uric acidcrystals known as tophi. Tophi may develop in joints, cartilage, bone, and auricular or other cutaneous tissues.
  - The average interval between the onset of gout and appearance of tophi, in the absence of treatment, is approximately 10 years.

    - Increase hydration, decrease red meats and EtOH
    - Pharmacotherapy
        - Therapy to control the underlying hyperuricemia generally is contraindicated until the acute attack is controlled.
        - **Starting chronic therapy to control hyperuricemia during an acute attack may intensify and prolong the attack. As a result, always concurrently treat with Colchicine or NSAID.**
        - If the patient has been on a consistent dosage of probenecid or allopurinol at the time of the acute attack, however, the drug **should be continued** at that dosage during the attack and **not stopped**.
        - Goal UA level is <6 if no tophi present or 5 in the presence of tophi
        - Medications considered if $\geq$ 2 attacks/year, erosive disease on radiograph, nephrolithasis, CKD stage 2, tophi, or urinary UA >1.1g/dL
        - **Colchicine should be co-administered** to ensure decreased risk of flare during initiation of therapy for at least 6 months or 3 months after achieving goal UA (increase to 6 months if tophi present)
        - **Allopurinol** 100 mg/day x 2w then 200mg daily x 2w; titrate to goal decrease in UA by 1mg/dL/wk with typical doses of 300-800mg/d
            - May ↓ progression to CKD, patients with underlying renal disease should be considered for early Allopurinol administration.
        - **Febuxostat**: 40 mg/d starting dose, up to 80 mg/d
        - **Probenecid**: appropriate for pts w/ ↓ renal UA secretion. May help reverse tophaceous changes over time.
        - **Pegloticase** indicated in pts who have contraindications to or who are refractory to above

MONOARTHRITIS

- **Etiology**[306]
    - Infection
        - Septic: RF include prosthesis, recent surgery, RA, overlying infection). Organisms include MRSA, GBS, Lyme disease, Gonorrhea (suspect if other joints previously affected) is the most common cause!
            - Consider in patients with prosthetic hip/knee, overlying skin infection, age>80, DM
        - Crystal (mc causes include monosodium urate, calcium pyrophosphate)
    - Trauma (fractures, ligament tears) → hemarthrosis
    - Osteonecrosis (chronic steroid use, alcoholism)
    - OA
    - Crystal Induced
        - Gout
        - Pseudogout
    - Reactive Arthritis
- **Presentation**
    - Isolated swollen joint(s)
    - Hot/warm to touch
- **Assessment**
    - Synovial Fluid Analysis
    - Clarity and color (clear = non inflammatory; yellow = inflammatory; red = traumatic vs hemarth)
    - Viscosity = ↓ with inflammatory etiology
- **Labs**

  - Cell count
  - Differential
  - Suspect infection:
  - Gram stain
  - Culture
  - Crystal analysis
  - Cell Count
- **Assessment**
  - Class I - < 2000; Non-inflammatory
    - OA
    - Trauma
    - AVN
  - Class II - 2,000-75,000; Inflammatory
    - Crystal-induced
    - RA
    - SLE
    - Stills, Dermatomyositis, Vasculitis
  - Class III - Septic; >75,000
    - SA, GN, Mycobacterium
  - Class IV
    - Hemorrhagic
    - TB, Charcot's

POLYARTICULAR ARTHRITIS

- **General**[307]
- **Clinical/Evaluation**
  - Determine chronicity (acute vs. chronic)
    - *Acute* – hours to two weeks
    - *Chronic* - >2 weeks
  - Duration, Triggers
    - Intermittant or Constant
  - Symmetric vs Assymetric
  - Number of joints involved
    - *Pauciarticular* – 2 to 4 joints (ie. spondyloarthropathies such as psoriatic, inflammatory, ankylosing, reactive)
    - *Polyarticular* – 5+ joints (ie. RA)
  - Types of Joints Involved (see table below)
    - Spine, SI, hips, shoulder, knees – can be seen with OA, spondyloarthropathies
    - First digit – consider gout
    - Smaller joints (wrists, fingers, toes) – consider RA, SLE
  - Rule Out
    - Should rule out other causes of "joint" pain → depression, fibromyalgia, hypothyroidism, bursitis, metabolic factors (Ca), neuromuscular disease
- **Differential/Types**
  - Inflammatory – suggestive in patients with joint swelling, erythema, morning stiffness >1hr, symmetric, pain at rest, ↑C-RP, ↑ESR
    - Rheumatoid arthritis
    - Infectious arthritis (ie. septic, lyme)
    - Anklylosing spondylitis
    - Reactive arthritis

        - Psoriatic Arthritis
    - <u>Non-Inflammatory</u> – worse with weight bearing, asymmetric, morning stiffness for <1 hr, no pain rest, pain ↓ with activity, nml C-RP and ESR
        - Osteoarthritis (most often involves weight bearing joints such as the spine, hips, and knees along with distal finger joints such as the DIP)
    - <u>Crystal-Associated</u>
        - Gout
        - Calcium pyrophosphate arthropathy
    - <u>Immune-Mediated</u>
        - SLE
- **Labs**
    - ANA
    - ESR
    - C-RP
    - RF and anti-CCP
    - Uric acid
    - Hepatitis B, C, parvovirus
    - Synovial fluid aspiration (see page 541 for evaluation of aspirate)
    - Crystal analysis
- **Imaging**
    - Plain films – evaluate for erosive disease, calcium deposition, fractures, pencil-in-cup
- **Treatment/Management**
    - Treatment is based on ultimate diagnosis as above, this is beyond the scope of this book to list all individual treatment modalities

Joint involvement pattern and suggested diagnoses

	Autoimmune / CTD			Spondyloarthropathies				Infectious		Crystal		Other
Characteristic	RA	SLE	Vasculitis	AS	PA	RA	IBD	Bacterial	Viral	Gout	CPPD	OA
Symmetry												
>symmetric	X	X	X						X			
>asymmetric	X			X	X	X	X	X		X	X	X
Inflammatory	X	X	X	X	X	X	X	X		X	X	
Noninflammatory									X			X
Number												
>pauciarticular				X	X	X	X	X		X	X	X
>polyarticular	X	X	X						X			
Joints												
>Spine	X			X	X	X	X	X				X
>SI	X			X	X	X	X					X
Joints/Small												
>Wrist	X	X	X				X	X	X			X
>Carpo											X	X
>Metacarpoph	X	X							X		X	
>PIP	X	X	X		X				X			
>DIP					X							X
>Ankle	X			X	X	X	X		X	X	X	X
>Metatarsoph	X				X	X			X	X		X
Joints/Medium												
>Shoulders	X	X		X	X	X	X				X	X
>Elbows	X	X		X	X	X	X	X				
>Hips/Knees	X		X	X	X	X	X	X			X	X

COMMON RHEUMATOLOGIC LABS

- **Common Generic Rheumatologic Labs**
  - CBC, CMP, CK, UA
  - RF
  - ANA
  - Cryoglobulins
  - HBV (HBsAg with PAN)
  - HCV (Cryogobulinemia, PAN)
  - CH50, C3, C4
  - HSV, HIV, CMV (r/o vasculitis)
  - Parvovirus IgM (GPA, PAN)
  - C-ANCA (PR3; GPA or MPA)
  - P-ANCA (MPO; MPA and CSS)
  - BCx (rules out SBE)
  - SPEP, UPEP (rule out MM)
- **Inflammatory Arthritis**
  - Rheumatoid Arthritis
    - ESR (normals: male = age/2; female = age+10/2)
    - C-RP (normals: male = age/50; female = age / 50 + 0.6)
    - RF (frequenc of false positives ↑ with age; incidence of disease ↑ with ↑ titer)
    - CCP (can be diagnostic in RF negative dz, better predictor of erosive dz)
    - 1433 (presence is associated with worse dz)
- **ANA**
  - Seen in 5-30% of normal individuals

Significance of ANA Pattern

Pattern	Nature of Antigens	Antibody	Associated Dz
Homogenous/diffuse	Histone (H1, H2a)	Histone	SLE, DIL
Rim/Peripheral/Shaggy	Double or single stranded DNA	dsDNA	SLE
Speckled	Proteins A-G, snRNAs, U1-6	ENA-RNP & Smith SS-A, SS-B	SLE, MCTD, Sjogrens
Centromere	Kinetochore	Centromere	CREST
Nucleolar	nRNA	Jo-1	Myositis

ANA Profiles in ANA Positive DIsease

Antibody	SLE	MCTD	PSS	CREST	Sjogrens	RA	DIL
ANA	>95%	>95%	70-90%	60-90%	>70%	40-50%	100%
Anti-dsDNA	60%	Neg	Neg	Neg	Rare	Rare	Neg
Anti-Smith	30%	Neg	Neg	Neg	Neg	Neg	Neg
Anti-RNP	30%	>95%	Comm	Neg	Rare	Rare	10-20%
Anti-Centromere	Rare	Rare	10-15%	60-90%	Neg	Neg	Neg
Anti-Ro (SSA)	30%	Rare	Rare	Neg	70%	10-15%	Neg

Anti-La (SSB)	15%	Rare	Rare	Neg	60%	Rare	Neg
Anti-nucleolar	Occ	Neg	Comm	Neg	Occ	Rare	Neg
Anti-SCL-70	Rare	Neg	10-20%	Neg	Neg	Neg	Neg
Anti-Histone	24-95%	Occ	Occ	Occ	Occ	20%	Neg

- **Myopathies**
  - Commonly will have +ANA and +anti-cystoplasmic Ab (synthetase and anti-SRP)
- **Vasculitis**
  - Differential
    - *Large* – Takayasu, GCA
    - *Medium* – Kawasaki, PAN, Central Angiitis
    - *Small* –
      - Immune complex (Hypersensitivity, cryoglobulinemic, HSP)
      - Pauci Immune (GPA, microscopic polyangiitis, Churg-Strauss)
  - Labs
    - Systemic Inflammation
      - CBC
      - ESR
      - C-RP
      - ↓Albumin
    - Organ involvement
      - SCr, UA
      - LFT
      - CK
      - Occult blood
      - CXR
      - Brain MRI/MRA
      - Abdominal CTA

PSYCHIATRY

CAPACITY

- Made by physician, not a lawyer or judge, often by neuropsychologist or forensic psychologist. You can consider getting specialists involved if, after performing the ACE below, you feel the patient is **incapable** of consenting to a procedure.[308]
- (1) Capacity is imbedded in informed consent, one of a **triad** of factors that also includes: (2) disclosure and (3) voluntariness.
  - Capacity – consists of four criteria, to have capacity, paients must demonstrate the following:
    - Have understanding of their situation and care options
    - Have appreciation of how information presented applies to their situation
    - Have reasoning consistent with their goals, preferences and values
    - Have ability to communicate a choice
    - Evaluation of capacity can be done with the ACE bedside test by answering yes or no to the following questions:

      Is the patient...

      1. Able to understand medical problem
      2. Able to understand proposed treatment
      3. Able to understand alternative to proposed treatment (if any)
      4. Able to understand option of refusing proposed treatment (including withholding or withdrawing treatment)
      5. Able to appreciate reasonably foreseeable consequences of accepting proposed treatment
      6. Able to appreciate reasonably foreseeable consequences of refusing proposed treatment (including withholding or withdrawing proposed treatment)

      7a. The person's decision is affected by depression

      7b. The person's decision is affected by delusions/psychosis
  - Disclosure - discussing the risks and benefits of available tests and treatments, including of declining care.

    - Voluntariness - the patient's decision isn't being forced or coerced by others.
- All three—capacity, disclosure, voluntariness—must be present to meet ethical and legal muster
- **2 point test:**
    1. Understands procedure action
    2. Understands consequences of decision—they say it out to you
        - Level of capacity increases the higher the risk of the procedure, i.e. demented patient doesn't need much capacity to agree to IV Fluids but does require higher level of capacity to agree to open heart surgery.

DELIRIUM

- **Definition**
    - Disturbance of consciousness with ↓ ability to focus or maintain attention
    - No pre-existing or established dementia
    - Occurs over short period of time (hours/days) and fluctuates, sometimes lasting for months
    - Ultimately caused by a medical condition or substance intoxication
- **Risk Factors**
    - Underlying dementia, hx of stroke, or parkinson's disease
    - Post-operative
    - age >70, comorbidities, male, dementia, history of alcohol use, malnutrition, polypharmacy
    - Admission risk factors
        - Infection, dehydration, severe pain, fracture, heart failure, abnormal blood pressure
- **Presentation**
    - Disturbed Consciousness – inability to focus or maintain attention; "mother just isn't acting right."; patient may appear more lethargic, or if undergoing withdrawal will be hypervigilant
    - Change in Cognition - ↓memory, disoriented (confirm A&O' s); perceptual disturbances (see objects or shadows in room); hallucinations
    - Look for initial daytime fatigue, sleep disturbances which will then erupt into full on delirium
- **Causes**
    - Highest causes are seen in the hospital (ICU, ER)
    - Fluid and electrolyte disturbances (dehydration, hyponatremia/hypernatremia)
    - Infections (urinary tract, respiratory tract, skin and soft-tissue, meningitis)
    - Drug toxicity (Opioids, sedatives, anti-psychotics, NSAIDs; Withdrawal from EtOH or Benzodiazepines, use of Antihistamines)
    - Metabolic disorders (hypoglycemia, hypercalcemia, uremia, liver failure, TSH)
    - Low perfusion states (shock, heart failure)
    - Immobility (restraints)
    - Malnutrition
    - Organ failure (liver, renal)
- **Stepwise evaluation**[309]
    - Initial evaluation
        - History with special attention to medications (including over-the-counter and herbals)
        - Short onset of symptoms
        - Inability to focus when asking questions during initial examination
        - Tangential and disorganized speech

- General physical examination and neurologic examination
- Nonrhythmic, asynchronous muscle jerking (metabolic abnormality)
- Flapping motion of outstretched hands (hepatic encephalopathy)
- Nystagmus, ataxia (consider Wernicke's)
- Complete blood count
- Electrolyte panel including sodium, calcium, magnesium, phosphorus
- Liver function tests, including albumin
- Renal function tests

Common symptoms in delirium	
Feature	Assessment
Acute onset and fluctuating course	Usually obtained from a family member or nurse and shown by positive responses to the following questions: "Is there evidence of an acute change in mental status from the patient's baseline?"; "Did the abnormal behavior fluctuate during the day, that is, tend to come and go, or increase and decrease in severity?"
Inattention	Shown by a positive response to the following: "Did the patient have difficulty focusing attention, for example, being easily distractible or having difficulty keeping track of what was being said?"
Disorganized thinking	Shown by a positive response to the following: "Was the patient's thinking disorganized or incoherent, such as rambling or irrelevant conversation, unclear or illogical flow of ideas, or unpredictable switching from subject to subject?"
Altered level of consciousness	Shown by any answer other than "alert" to the following: "Overall, how would you rate this patient's level of consciousness?" Normal = alert Hyper alert = vigilant Drowsy, arousable = lethargic Difficult to arouse = stupor Unarousable = coma

** *The diagnosis of delirium requires the presence of features 1 AND 2 plus either 3 OR 4.*

- First-tier further evaluation guided by initial evaluation
  - Systemic infection screen
    - Urinalysis and culture
    - Chest radiograph
    - Blood cultures
  - Electrocardiogram
  - Arterial blood gas
  - Serum and/or urine toxicology screen (perform earlier in young persons)
  - Brain imaging with MRI with diffusion and gadolinium (preferred) or ct
  - Suspected CNS infection: lumbar puncture after brain imaging

    - Suspected seizure-related etiology: electroencephalogram (eeg) (if high suspicion, should be performed immediately)
    - Tools
      - AWOL (**A:** Age is 80 years or older; **W:** Inability to spell "world" backwards; **O:** Not oriented to name, city, county, state, hospital, and floor; **L:** Nursing illness severity assessment moderately to severely ill
      - MOCA
      - CAM
  - Second-tier further evaluation
    - Vitamin levels: $b12_{12}$, folate, thiamine
    - Endocrinologic laboratories: thyroid-stimulating hormone (TSH) and free t_4; cortisol
    - Serum ammonia
    - Sedimentation rate
    - Autoimmune serologies: antinuclear antibodies (ana), complement levels; p-anca, c-ANCA
    - Infectious serologies: rapid plasmin reagin (RPR); fungal and viral serologies if high suspicion; hiv antibody
    - Lumbar puncture (if not already performed)
    - Brain mri with and without gadolinium (if not already performed)
    - EEG (r/o Non-convulsive Status Epilepticus; look for nystagmus and anisocoria on exam; MRI may show frontal/parietal atrophy)
- **Diagnostics**
  - Labs
    - Electrolyte panel (ICU panel)
    - CBC
    - UA
    - Urine culture
    - LFTs (if history of cirrhosis)
    - TSH/FT4
    - Drug levels if appropriate (digoxin in AM assuming dose given in PM, lithium)
    - ABG (respiratory alkalosis is early sign of sepsis)
    - LP (older patients; suspecting bacterial meningitis)
  - Imaging
    - CXR
    - CT head (if no cause is identified)
- **Types**
  - Hyperactive – restlessness, rapid mood changes, hallucinations, will not cooperate with medical care
  - Hypoactive – inattention, reduced activity, drowsiness
  - Mixed – combination of above; patients may switch back and forth between the two
- **Treatment**
  - **Treat underlying cause**
  - Behavior: sitters, family, reorientation, bed rails, minimize restraints

Medications for agitation based on demographic		
Context[310]	RX	Dosage
Severe violence	Droperidol	0.625-5mg IM/IV
	Midazolam	2.5-5mg IM/IV
	Haldol PLUS	2.5mg PO/IV
	Lorazepam	0.5mg IM/IV

	Generally want to avoid benzodiazepines, but in conjunction with haloperidol can be useful. Haldol can be given 0.5-2.5mg IV prn (TID for example) then 1-2mg IV QHS short term with a quick taper.	
Undifferentiated	Lorazepam	2-4mg IM/IV
	Midazolam	2.5-5mg IM/IV
	Haldol PLUS Lorazepam	5mg IM/IV 2mg IM/IV
Known psych	Haldol	2.5-5mg IM/IV
	Droperidol	2.5-5mg IM/IV
	Haldol PLUS Lorazepam	5mg IM/IV 2mg IM/IV
Intoxication	Lorazepam	2-4mg IM/IV
	Midazolam	2.5-5mg IM/IV
Cooperative	Olanzapine	5-10mg IM/SL/or PO
	Ziprasidone	20mg IM
	Lorazepam	2-4mg IM/IV
	Risperidone	0.25mg PO
Elderly *(all anti-psychotics are black-box)*	Seroquel	15mg prn q6h
	Oxazepam	10mg BID-TID; ↑ to total 30-45mg/d
	Buspirone	5mg BID; ↑ by 5mg q2-3d up to 20-30/d
	Haldol AND Ativan	0.5mg to 1mg IM & 1 mg Q 8 hours prn; hold if BP<100/60
	Haldol	1mg po/IV Q30min prn
	Quetiapine	12.5mg PO (elderly dose) 25-100mg PO (all other ages)
	Olanzapine	2.5mg
Alternative	Divalproex sodium	500-1500 mg/d
	Carbamazepine	300-600 mg/d
	Olanzapine	2.5mg IM/PO
Sun downing (give at 1500)	Olanzapine	2.5mg - 5mg IM/PO (up to 10 mg po daily)
	Quetiapine	12.5mg po prn (elderly) up to BID 25-100mg PO prn (other ages)
	if no response in 6h then give additional 12.5 mg p.o. May ↑ dose by 25 mg q2 days	
	Risperidone	0.5mg po BID (max 2mg q12h)
	May be ↑ x 1 mg q 2 days. Max dose is 6 mg in 24 hours	

** *Risperdal or Haldol*: Caution if prolonged QT

1. Try having a 1:1 sitter in the room, move pt to room by nursing station, and/or decrease noise/light
2. Agitation in elderly may be first manifestation of an illness: new infection, MI, dyspnea/hypoxia, CVA, pain, etc
3. Consider adding Cogentin to ↓ risk of EPS
4. Check vitals, Pulse Ox, Na/K, glucose, Fever, meds, sources of infection (UA, CXR)

5. Check EKG (esp if post-operative patient)
6. Treatment
   - Agitation in context of non-acute psychosis
     - Risperidone (Risperdal) 0.25–1.5 mg/d
     - Olanzapine (Zyprexa, Zydis) 2.5–10mg/d
     - Quetiapine (Seroquel) 12.5–200 mg/d
     - Aripiprazole (Abilify) 2.5–12.5 mg/d
   - Acute in context of acute psychosis:
     - Haloperidol (Haldol) 0.5–2 mg/d
   - Agitation in context of depression
     - SSRI, eg, citalopram (Celexa) 10–30 mg/d

- **Delirium prophylaxis**[311]
  - General
    - When a consult is placed for altered mental status, it is important to determine the affected domain that has changed from the patient's normal state. Changes can include alterations in consciousness, attention, behavior, cognition, language, speech, and praxis and can reflect varying degrees of cerebral dysfunction.
  - Orientation: accurately assess baseline, provide orientation clues, perception aids (hearing aids, glasses), regulate sleep-wake cycle, active involvement of family/caregivers
  - Minimize iatrogenesis: stop inappropriate/unnecessary medications, minimize urinary catheters, minimize restraints
  - Housekeeping measures: oxygen delivery, hydration, monitor electrolytes/glucose
  - Prophylaxis: bowel regimen, nutrition, early mobilization, pain control
  - Red Flag: an isolated alteration in speech, language, behavior, or praxis should suggest an underlying neurologic or psychiatric substrate in the early evaluation for delirium

Compare and Contrast Delirium and Dementia	
Delirium	Dementia
Onset: over hours to days	Onset: over months to years
Disturbance of consciousness such as reduced Awareness, inability to sustain attention	Level of attention not initially compromised
Altered cognition: memory, language, Disorientation, perceptual disturbance	Multiple cognitive impairments: language, motor Activities, agnosia, executive function
Caused by medical condition	Not explained by any medical condition
Evaluation: check medications, infections, cbc, Electrolytes, creatinine, glucose, liver function panel, cardiac enzymes, ua, cxr, ekg, pulse oximetry and/or abg. Consider head ct and lp.	Evaluation: obtain thorough history from the patient and family members, physical exam (with focus on neurologic testing), mmse, functional status, cbc, tsh, vitamin b12, electrolytes, vdrl, hiv. Consider neuroimaging and lp if onset <60, abrupt onset or rapid decline, or history of cancer or anticoagulant use

For more information on dementia, see page 281

INSOMNIA / SLEEP AIDS

- **Define**: inadequate sleep despite opportunities (3 episodes/week **for 3 months**) to obtain full sleep causing daytime impairment and there is no other disorder that is likely the cause. Has been associated with the development of CVD, T2DM, HTN (↑SBP during sleep, non-dipper).
- **Types**
  - Short Term: <3 months
  - Chronic: >3 months of symptoms, 3x/week
  - Primary: present the whole life of patient
  - Secondary: developed, p/w sleepiness
- **Treatment**
  - **Inpatient**
    - You are not obligated to give a sleep aid if you think the patient is at high risk of becoming confused or altered. If you decide they can have one:
      - **Elderly**
        - Trazodone (Desyrel) 25-50 mg (max 150mg)
        - Mirtazepine 7.5mg PO x1
      - **Any Age**
        - Temazepam (Restoril) 15-30 mg
        - Zolpidem (Ambien) 5-10 mg
        - Diphenhydramine (Benadryl) 25-50 mg (not a first-line choice)
        - Lorazepam (Ativan) IV 0.5-1 mg can be given to patients who are NPO.
        - Be cautious in elderly patients > 65. Would choose trazodone 25-50 mg in the elderly or Ambien. Avoid benzodiazepines and Benadryl.
        - If someone is delirious and agitated do not give sleep aid.
  - **Outpatient**
    - Acute (<3 months) vs. Chronic (>3 months)
      - Rule out comorbid conditions (2/2 insomnia) such as depression, PTSD, anxiety, etc.
      - Rule out other causes of insomnia:
        - OSA (30-70%, more common in F), most validated tool is ESS
        - RLS
        - PLMS
        - Stress (psychological insomnia)
      - Medication should also be used in conjunction with CBT (sleep hygiene, sleep restriction, stimulus control, etc.)
        - Behavioral Treatment
          CBT has been shown to have sustained beneficial effects up to 6 months past treatment per AHRQ.
          - *Sleep Hygiene* – maintain regular sleep schedule, avoid naps, avoid caffeine after lunch, avoid alcohol/tobacco/large meals near bedtime, adjust bedroom environment to be quiet, dark and cool.
          - *Stimulus control* – use bed only for sleep and sexual activity, go to bed only when sleepy, leave bed when unable to sleep and go to another room
          - *Relaxation* – progressive muscle relaxation, relaxation response
          - *Sleep restriction* – restrict time in bed to hours when actually sleeping, increase time in bed by 15-30m increments when sleep efficiency is >90%
    - Types
      - *Sleep Onset (SO)*:

    - Ramelteon 8mg (30 min prior to bed-time)
    - Zaleplon 10mg QHS
    - Zolpidem 5-10 mg PO QHS prn insomnia
        - If hepatic impairment or elderly give 5 mg
    - Triazolam 0.25mg QHS (0.125mg if geriatric)
    - Lorazepam (Ativan) IV 0.5-1 mg can be given to patients who are NPO
- *Sleep Onset and Maintenance (SO/SM):*
    - Suvorexant 10mg (5mg if other meds on board)
    - Lunesta 1mg PO QHS
    - Zolpidem ER 6.25mg
    - Temazepam (Restoril) 15 (7.5mg if geriatric)
    - Estazolam (ProSom) 1mg (0.5mg if low body weight)
    - Flurazepam 30mg (15mg if geriatric)
    - Vistaril 25-50 mg po or im q HS prn
- *Middle-of-Night Awakenings:*
    - Zolpidem SL 3.5mg male/1.75mg female
- *Sleep Maintenance (SM):*
    - Doxepin 6mg (3 mg if geriatric)
    - Zolpidem SL 3.5 male/ 1.75 female
- *Safe in Elderly:*
    - Trazodone 25-50 mg QHS prn insomnia
    - Nefazodone 100mg QHS
    - Chloral hydrate 500-1000 mg PO QHS PRN
    - Restoril 15 mg po QHS prn
- *Safe For Long-Term Use[313]:*
    - Trazodone
    - Zolpidem
    - Zaleplon
    - Eszopiclone
    - Ramelteon
    - Doxepin
    - Suvorexant
- *Off-Label:*
    - Antidepressants: trazodone, mirtazapine
    - Antipsychotics: quetiapine, olanzapine
    - Antihistamines: diphenhydramine, doxylamine
    - Herbs: melatonin

The medication classes with the strongest benefits have been eszoplicone, zolpidem, and suvorexant in the general adult population for global and sleep outcomes. Doxepin was shown to have the strongest evidence of <u>effectiveness</u> for global and sleep outcomes in adults >55. Ramelteon and benzos did very poorly.

Types and Treatment		
SO		
Zolpidem IR	Initial: 5mg	Take immediately before bedtime. Do not use unless have 7-8 h time in bed
Zolpidem SL	Initial: 5mg	
Zolpidem PO spray	Initial: 5mg (1 spray)	
Triazolam	Initial: 0.125mg Max:	
SO/SM		
Lunesta	Initial: 1mg	Take immediately before bedtime.

	Maximum: 2mg	
SM		
Suvorexant	Initial: 10mg Maximum: 20mg	Take 30 min before bedtime. Starting dose 10 mg in elderly and maximum is 20 mg. It is contraindicated in narcolepsy patients. Concentration levels in elderly are higher by 15% compared with nonelderly
Doxepin	Initial: 3mg Maximum: 6mg	Take 30 min before bedtime. Do not take within 3 h of a meal it is contraindicated in untreated narrow-angle glaucoma, severe urinary retention
Middle of Night Awakenings		
Zolpidem ZST	Initial: 1.75mg	Must have at least 5 hrs of sleep left before taking
Zaleplon	Initial: 5mg	Take immediately before bedtime A high fat/heavy meal can delay absorption

SEDATION OF THE VIOLENT PATIENT

- **General**
  - Always call the police / hospital security in any Insafe situation
  - Pharmacologic restraints should be considered last resort

Pharmacologic management of a violent patient		
Oral	IM	IV (not recommended)
Lorazepam 1-2mg PO	Lorazepam 2-4mg IM	Benzodiazepine
Lorazepam 1-2mg PO + Haldol 1.5-3mg PO (if psychiatric context)	Lorazepam 2-4mg IM + Haldol 5-10mg IM (if psychiatric context)	Haldol

DEPRESSION

- **Work-up**[314,315, 316, 317]
  - TSH
  - OSA
  - Vitamin D
  - Bipolar depression
  - Medications: steroids, dopaminergic agents
  - EtOH
  - B12/folate
  - Post concussive symptoms
- **Screening**
  - PHQ-9
    - Interpretation:
      - 1-4: none
      - 5-9: mild
      - 10-14: moderate
      - 15-19: moderately severe
      - 20+: severe
  - Hamilton Depression Rating Scale
- **Co-Existing Anxiety**

- Harder to treat depression with co-existing anxiety (STAR*D trial)
  - See page 565.
- **Treatment (see table on following pages)**
  - Phasic approach advised
    - ***Acute phase* (first 3 months)**
      - CBT +/- Rx
      - Continue to ↑ dosage q3-4wk until sx in remission. Full medication effect is complete in 4 to 6 weeks. Augmentation with second medication may be necessary.
      - F/u with patient within 2-4wof starting medication and q2wk until improvement and then monthly to monitor medication changes.
    - ***Continuation phase* (4-9 months)**
      - Regular visits to monitor for signs of relapse, q3-6mo if stable; depression rating scales should be used for objective data.
      - Once remission achieved, dosage should be continued for at least 6-9m to reduce relapse; CBT is also effective in reducing relapse (visits typically q2wk).
      - If/when drug discontinuation is considered, medications should be tapered gradually (weeks to months).
    - ***Maintenance phase* (9 months-d/c)**
      - Same as continuation phase above
  - Pharmacotherapy
    - *Based On Side Effect Profile*
      - Fatigue, amotivation: SNRI, buproprion
      - Anxiety: SSRI
      - Insomnia: trazodone, mirtazapine
    - *Augmentation with Benzodiazepine*
      - See page 565.
    - *Options*
      - Watchful waiting
      - Psychopharmacology (see table on following page)
        - SSRI - Get baseline sodium and PLT
        - SNRI
          - ↑risk for HTN
        - Mirtazapine good for patients with both depression and insomnia
      - Psychotherapy
      - Referral to Psychiatrist
- **Combining Antidepressants**
  - Combining two antidepressants is not supported by high-level evidence.
  - Rationale is that targeting different receptors will have a synergistic effect.1
  - Combinations of SSRI or SNRI (venlafaxine) with bupropion or mirtazapine have the best evidence of efficacy.
  - See table below for options
- **Switching Between Anti-Depressants**[318]
  - Multiple techniques exist, there is no consensus best option
  - Gradual antidepressant withdrawal reduces the risk of complications. If the washout period is not long enough (defined by half-life of the drug), introducing a new antidepressant can cause drug interactions leading to toxicity, particularly serotonin syndrome.
  - Conservative switch:
    - The first antidepressant is gradually reduced and stopped

    - There follows a drug-free washout interval of five half-lives of the first antidepressant
    - The new antidepressant is started according to its dose recommendation
  - <u>Moderate switch:</u>
    - The first antidepressant is gradually reduced and stopped
    - There follows a drug-free washout interval of 2–4 days
    - The new antidepressant is started at a low dose
  - <u>Cross-taper switch:</u>
    - The first antidepressant is gradually reduced and stopped
    - The second antidepressant is introduced at a low dose at some stage during the reduction of the first antidepressant, so that the patient is taking both antidepressants simultaneously
    - The dose of the second antidepressant is increased to the therapeutic dose when the first antidepressant has been stopped
- **Treatment Resistent Depression**
  - Approximately 50% of patients experience no response to treatment with a first-line antidepressant.
  - Clinicians have 4 broad pharmacologic strategies to choose from for treating antidepressant non responders:
    - Increasing the dose of the antidepressant
    - Switching to a different antidepressant
    - Augmenting the treatment regimen with a non antidepressant agent:
      - Antipsychotic agents: aripiprazole, olanzapine, quetiapine, andrisperidone
      - Other agents: mirtazapine, mianserin, and omega-3 fatty acids
      - Not well studied: bupropion, desipramine, mecamylamine, and testosterone
    - Combining the original antidepressant with a second antidepressant.
      - For patients with mild to moderate treatment resistant major depression, augment initial antidepressant with a second drug and/or psychotherapy
  - Advanced option includes ketamine drip
    - Research has shown it to be a rapidly effective within hours of administration
      - Doses varied; m/c was 0.5mg/kg IV/IM
      - Patients with quickest response had a positive family history of alcohol dependence
    - Should only be administered by psychiatry
- **Discontinuation**
  - Treatment discontinuation is as high as 40% in the first 3 months
  - Longer tapers required for those medications with short half life
    - No official guidelines on the best taper method, options include:
    - Decreasing dose by 25% per week until DC of the medication
    - Decreasing dose by 25% per month or 12.5% per week to complete a 4 month w/d period
- **Acute Withdrawal Management**[320]
  - Symptoms start within 3 days and may last up to 3 weeks
  - Discontinuation Syndrome (DCS) symptoms are more likely after at least 5-8 weeks of therapy or those with a short half-life (such as paroxetine)
  - Those with short half-life may require 6-12 month tapers
    - Symptoms include: dizziness, nausea, vomiting, fatigue, muscle aches/twitches, chills, anxiety, sensory abnormalities, and irritability
    - Symptoms may last 1-2 weeks
- **Monitoring**
  - PHQ-9
  - Follow up every 3 weeks for the first 3 months (first follow up should be a week later)

Pharmacologic treatment options for depression

Drug or Drug Class	Dosing	Side Effects	Precautions	Clinical Use
Selective serotonin reuptake inhibitors		Platelet dysfunction, GI side effects, xerostomia, insomnia, anxiety, agitation, asthenia, drowsiness, headache, sexual dysfunction, hyponatremia, rare serotonin syndrome or NMS. S/e typically resolve within the first week.	Suicidality, particularly in young adults. Avoid abrupt discontinuation, other serotonergic drugs and MAOI therapy. Drug interactions due to CYP450 metabolism	An option for first-line therapy. Use side effects to choose a specific agent
Citalopram (Celexa)	Initial:10mg Therapeutic:20-40mg Max: 60mg <55 YO: Maximum 40 mg qd >55 YO: Maximum 20 mg qd	Dose-dependent QT prolongation	Avoid if patient has active heart disease. Avoid with drugs that prolong QT interval. Maximum dose 20 mg qd with hepatic disease, age >60 years, poor metabolizers of CYP2C19 or receiving a CYP2C19 inhibitor. Caution with CrCl <20	Low rate of anxiety and activation (however co-existing anxiety does ↓ effectiveness of treatment as in STAR*D trial). EKG monitoring for doses > 40mg/d.
Escitalopram (Lexapro)	Initial: 10 mg qd. Therapeutic:10-20mg Max: 20 mg qd	CNS depression	Avoid if patient has active heart disease. Maximum dose 10 mg qd with hepatic disease, elderly. Caution with CrCl < 20	Low risk for drug interactions. Low rate of anxiety and activation. Better response than citalopram (iSPOT-D trial)
*Fluoxetine (Prozac, Prozac Weekly)	Initial: 10mg x1week Therapeutic: 20-60mg Max: 80mg Weekly: 90 mg once weekly		May need to decrease dose with hepatic disease. Significant inhibitor of CYP isoenzymes	Long half-life. Highest rate of anxiety and agitation. Good for teenagers.
*Paroxetine (Paxil, Paxil CR, Pexeva)	Paxil Initial: Start at 10mg x1week		Avoid with pregnancy. Decrease starting dose and	More anticholinergic side effects than other agents; high

	Therapeutic: 20-40mg Max: 60mg Controlled-release Initial: 12.5 mg qd in AM. Therapeutic: 5-62.5 mg qd		maximum dose with hepatic disease, elderly, CrCl <60. Potent inhibitor of CYP2D6. May decrease efficacy of tamoxifen	rate of drowsiness; highest association with weight gain of SSRIs
*Sertraline (Zoloft)	Initial: 25mg Therapeutic: 50-200mg (50-150 is normally the target) Max: 200mg		May need to decrease dose with hepatic disease. Mild inhibitor of CYPs 2D6 and 3A4	Higher rate of diarrhea and headache but lowest incidence of weight gain among SSRIs Low risk for drug interactions.
Serotonin-norepinephrine reuptake inhibitors		Platelet dysfunction, nausea, constipation, anorexia, weight loss, xerostomia, insomnia, anxiety, asthenia, dizziness, drowsiness, headache, hypertension, tachycardia, hyperhidrosis, sexual dysfunction, hyponatremia, serotonin syndrome, rare NMS	Suicidality, particularly in young adults. Avoid abrupt discontinuation. Avoid other serotonergic drugs and MAOI therapy	
Venlafaxine (Effexor, Effexor XR)	Immediate-release: 37.5 mg. Goal: 150mg-225mg. Extended-release: 37.5mg to start; goal 75-300mg.		Decrease initial dose by 50% with moderate hepatic disease. Decrease dose by 25%-50% if CrCl <70. Caution with CYP2D6 inhibitors	High rate of nausea and vomiting. May increase HR and BP
Desvenlafaxine (Pristiq)	Initial: 50 mg qd Therapeutic: 50-100mg Max: 100mg		Maximum dose 100 mg qd with hepatic disease. If CrCl <50, maximum dose 50 mg qd. If CrCl <30, maximum dose 50 mg qod	May increase BP
Duloxetine (Cymbalta)	Start at 30mg (goal 30-90 mg total daily dose, dosed qd-bid)	Urinary retention, hepatotoxicity,	Avoid with hepatic disease, severe CKD, closed-angle	May increase BP

	Max: 120mg	musculoskeletal pain, muscle spasms	glaucoma. Substrate and moderate inhibitor of CYP2D6. Caution with diabetics	
Tricyclic antidepressants	Due to sedation, bedtime dosing may be preferred	Drowsiness and other CNS side effects, anticholinergic side effects (such as constipation, xerostomia, urinary retention, visual impairment), orthostatic hypotension, ECG abnormalities, tremor, nausea, weight gain, sexual dysfunction	Suicidality, particularly in young adults. Avoid abrupt discontinuation, MAOI therapy. Decrease dose with hepatic disease, elderly. Caution with decreased GI motility, cardiac disease, closed-angle glaucoma, BPH, urinary retention, seizure disorder, thyroid disease, diabetes, sunlight	
Amitriptyline	25-50 mg qhs, up to 100-300 mg total daily dose, qhs or in divided doses			Most anticholinergic effects: -Constipation: ↑hydration, laxative -Delirium: assess other causes -Dry mouth: sugarless gum -Hesitancy: bethanechol -Visual chg: pilocarpine gtt -Orthostasis: fludrocortisone
Other			Suicidality, particularly in young adults. Avoid abrupt discontinuation, MAOI therapy	
Bupropion (Wellbutrin)	Immediate-release: 100 mg bid-tid. Sustained-release (SR): 150 mg qd-bid. Maximum 400 mg/d. Extended-release (XL): 150-300 mg qd. Maximum 450	Dose-dependent seizures. Insomnia, dizziness, tremor, agitation, anxiety, confusion, weight loss, hyperhidrosis	Avoid with seizure disorder, eating disorder. Decrease dose with severe hepatic disease, moderate-severe CKD. Caution with mild-moderate hepatic disease.	Commonly augmented with SSRI to ↓ fatigue, sexual s/e from SSRI (300mg dose req' d) Lowest rates of sexual side effects and weight gain

	mg qd. Aplenzin: 174-348 mg qd. Maximum 522 mg qd. Forfivo XL: Not for initial use. 450 mg qd		Inhibitor of CYP2D6 and substrate of CYP2B6	-Dry mouth: sugarless gum
Mirtazapine (Remeron)	Initial: 7.5mg qhs. Therapeutic: 15-30 mg/d Maxium dose: 45mg/d	Drowsiness, dizziness, nausea, vomiting, increased appetite, weight gain, constipation, xerostomia, rare agranulocytosis or severe neutropenia	Decrease dose with elderly, CrCl <40. Caution with seizure disorder, inhibitors of CYPs 2D6, 1A2, or 3A4	Can be augmented with SSRI to help ↓ sexual s/e and to help combat insomnia (↑sedation), and helps ↑ appetite. **Be aware of serotonin syndrome risk** More drowsiness; can **stimulate appetite** and cause weight gain (↑cholesterol reqd statin tx), quickest onset of action! Good in geriatric population for depression, weight loss, and insomnia symptoms
Trazodone (Oleptro)	Immediate-release: 150 mg total daily dose, given in divided doses. Maximum 400 mg total daily dose. Extended-release: 150 mg qhs, on an empty stomach. Maximum 375 mg qd	Drowsiness, dizziness, hypotension, anxiety, insomnia, xerostomia, constipation, nausea, blurred vision, priapism	Decrease dose with elderly, hepatic disease, potent CYP3A4 inhibitors. Caution with cardiac disease, CKD	Can be augmented with SNRI to ↑sedation but high risk for priaprism Priaprism Drowsiness

SSRI Side Effect Profile					
Side Effects	Citalopram	Escitalopram	Fluoxetine	Fluvoxamine	Paroxetine
Sexual d/f	++	++	++	++	+++
Weight Gain	+	+	+	+	++
GI toxicity	+	+	+	+	+
QTC prolong	+	+	+	+	+
Insomnia	+	+	++	+	+
Drowsiness	±	±	±	+	+
Side Effects	Desvenlafaxine	Duloxetine	Milnacipran	Venlafaxine	Sertraline
Sexual d/f	+++	+++	±	+++	++
Weight Gain	±	±	±	±	+
GI toxicity	++	++	++	++	++
QTC prolong	±	±	±	±	+
Insomnia	++	++	±	++	++
Drowsiness	+	±	+	+	±
Orthostasis	±	±	±	±	

Others Side Effect Profile			
Side Effects	Wellbutrin	Mirtazapine	Trazodone
Sexual d/f	±	+	+
Weight Gain	±	+++	+
GI toxicity	+	±	+++
QTC prolong	+	+	++
Insomnia	++	±	±
Drowsiness	±	+++	±
Orthostasis	±	±	+++

Neuroleptic Malignant Syndrome Vs. Serotonin Syndrome		
	NMS[321]	SS[322]
Mental State	Confusion → Coma	Confusion → Coma
Vitals	Fever (>104), ↑HR, ↑BP	↑BP
Muscles	Rigid**	Unaffected
Neuro	Autonomic instability w/sweating, tremor	Sweating, Tremor, more GI symptoms of n/v/d**; ↑reflexes**
Labs	↑WBC	Nml WBC**
CPK	↑↑↑	Nml

ALCOHOLIC PATIENT

- **Banana Bag**[323]
  - Not all patients need a banana bag; especially be weary of providing this in a patient with alcoholic cardiomyopathy
  - Thiamine 100 mg IV + Folate 1 mg+ MVT 1 mg in 1 L NS. Continue this for 3-4 days.
    - Important to give Thiamine before giving any other IV Fluids with *glucose*
- **Labs**
  - Monitor PO4, Mg, and K for low levels
  - At risk for refeeding syndrome-, see page 632
- **Delirium Tremens**[325]
  - Risk Factors: hx of DT, age>30, prolonged EtOH history, ↑ amount of days since last drink
  - Sx: hallucinations, disorientation, tachycardia, hypertension, low-grade fever, agitation, and diaphoresis

Progression of DT		
Phase	Last drink	Duration
Early *Tremulous* *Anxiety* *Palpitations* *Nausea* *Anorexia*	6-8 hours	1-2d

W/D seizure *Tonic/clonic*	6-48 hours	2-3d
Hallucinations *Visual* *Tactile* *Auditory*	12-48 hours	1-2d
DT *↑HR* *HTN* *↑Temp* *Delirium* *Agitation*	48-96 hours	1-5d

- Labs to follow: Mg, K, PO4
- Nursing: CIWA, seizure precautions

- **Treatment**
  - Hydration: Plasmalyte or LR basal rate
  - Supplementation**: Thiamine** (50-100mg IV x 3d then 100mg PO), folate, MVI, replete electrolytes (K, Mg, PO4), fluids
    - Chronic thiamine deficiency can cause Wernicke's Encephalopathy and eventually Korsakoff if not replaced prior to giving any glucose.
      - Other than EtOH, other causes of WE include: chronic nausea/vomiting, malnutrition, bariatric surgery patients
  - Medications**:**
    - *Calculate Ativan requirement by this conversion (1mg Ativan for every 1 shot/beer day) is total requirement over 24-hour period*
    - While trials have showed benefit in symptom triggered vs standing doses, patients with CIWA>15 +/- hx of complicated withdrawal may benefit from standing doses
      - Ativan 2-4mg IV q1h or q2h with CIWA for breakthrough; shorter half-life; slower onset and preferred in COPD patients
      - Diazepam 5-10 mg slow IV push q3-4h until calm, awake state (preferred choice esp for rapid titration)
        OR
      - Chlordiazepoxide (Librium) 25-100mg IV q3h (avoid in patients with marked liver disease) or 50-100mg PO. Longer duration of action, can ↓ rate of breakthrough symptoms.
      - Haldol 3-5mg q1h prn severe agitation/hallucinations/delirium (double q30min for max 100-480mg)
    - Drips:
      - Versed
      - Propofol
      - Precedex[326]
      - Avoid Ativan given risk for polyethylene glycol accumulation
    - Tapering
      - After stability for 24 hours; convert to PO dosing and taper dose by 25% every day over 3-day period
- **Placement:**
  - Admit to telemetry
  - ICU referral:
    - Age >40 with medical comorbidities

    - Electrolyte deficiencies with EKG changes
    - Hemodynamic instability
    - Hyperthermia
    - Rhabdomyolysis
    - Need for IV benzodiazepines or drips

PTSD

- **Diagnosis**[327] - consists of re-experiencing trauma with distressing recollections, dreams, flashbacks, and/or psychological/physical distress; persistent avoidance of stimuli that might invite traumatic memories or experiences; and increased arousal.
- **Screening**
  - Obtain trauma history
  - DREAMS
    - Detached - With each event, the examiner should determine if the patient appears emotionally detached (called alexithymia), either from the event or in relationships with others. It may also manifest as a general numbing of emotional responsiveness.
    - Reexperiences - The patient reexperiences the event in the form of nightmares, recollections or flashbacks.
    - Event - The event involved substantial emotional distress, with threatened death or loss of physical integrity, and feelings of helplessness or disabling fear.
    - Avoids - The patient avoids places, activities or people that remind the patient of the event.
    - Month - The symptoms have been present longer than one month
- **Treatment**
  - Nonpharmacologic therapy should always be initiated, many patients treated with psychotherapy will improve or recover.
  - If pharmacologic therapy required, SSRI are considered first line therapy
    - Options include fluoxetine, paroxetine, sertraline, escitalopram, and fluvoxetine
      - Help with ↓rexperiencing, avoidance/numbness, and hyperarousal
      - Consider combining with trazodone 50-200mg to counteract the insomnia s/e of SSRI
  - Anti-adrenergic Agents
    - Help with nightmares, autonomic hyperactivity, hypervigilance, and startle reactions
    - Monitor BP
    - Prazosin 1mg/qhs x3d then ↑ 1mg/q3d until nightmares improve (max ~ 10mg)
    - Clonidine 0.2mg TID titrated from 0.1mg qhs
    - Propranolol and guanfacine also options
  - Second generation anti-psychotics may be needed to treat comorbid psychotic-like features or anxiety refractory to other agents. Options include:
    - Clozapine (least often used, ↑weight), risperidone, olanzapine (↑weight, ↑DM risk), quetiapine, ziprasidone (weight neutral), and aripiprazole (weight neutral)
    - Patients started on 2nd generations should be monitored for the following (interval in parentheses)
      - BP (q12w, q1y)
      - BG (q12w, q1y)
      - Lipids (q12w, q1y)
      - Weight Check (q4,8,12,18,24w)

SUBSTANCE ABUSE

- **History**
  - Intoxicated patients should be monitored for overt and covert overdoses
  - Severe withdrawal states can present as an overdose with delirium and psychosis

Evaluation						
Substance	Temp	HR	RR	BP	Complaints	Mental Status
Opiates	↓	↓	↓↓	↓	Euphoria when high N/V constipation later signs	Slurred speech Nodding off
	Dosing: - IV/SQ: Narcan 0.4mg (can do 0.2mg initially if patient is opiate naïve) repeated q3-5 minutes - Intranasal: 4.0mg intranasal repeated q3-5 minutes until effect. - Drip: often done in patients on methadone; use 2/3 of total effective dose of naloxone per hour (typically 0.25-6.25mg/hr) and provide ½ of that bolus dose about 15 minutes after starting the drip to prevent a drop in naloxone levels					
Benzo	NC	NC	↓	↓	Talkative Sedation with ↑↑ dose	Irritable Emotional disinhibition Confusion Stupor
	Tx: Intoxication: Flumazenil 0.2mg IV over 15s repeated after 45s and again each subsequent minute until sedation reversed (max 1mg) Overdose: Flumazenil 0.2mg IV over 30s, 0.3mg after 30s if no response and up to 0.5mg each subsequent 30s interval to total dose 3mg					
Barbituates	NC	NC	↓↓	↓	Talkative Slow speech + think	Disinhibtion Confusion Innatentive Slurred speech
	Tx: supportive measures					

ANXIETY DISORDER

- **Screening**
  - PRIME-MD
  - SDDS-PC
  - CES-D

Treatment (recommended for 6-12 months)[328]			
Treatment	Prescription	Use	More Information
SSRI+BZD[329]	Fluoxetine 20mg + Clonazepam 0.5mg qhs (↑ to 1mg, split as 0.5 BID, after day 3) for 3 weeks then taper over 7 days	Fluoxetine daily for prescribed duration of MDD treatment + Clonazepam augmentation to increase compliance	In practice, combining a benzodiazepine with an SSRI can offer the patient the following benefits: (1) more rapid control of anxiety (2) reduction of SSRI-induced anxiety or agitation that can occur early in the course of therapy (3) improved adherence to antidepressant therapy, and (4) improved control of episodic or situational anxiety that occurs in response to certain stimuli. *See below for more on tapering.*
Remeron	15-30mg initial; target 30-60mg	N/A	Sedation, weight gain, dry mouth
Buspirone	7.5mg BID	Dose may be increased q2d in increments of 2.5mg/BID to max 30mg BID	Buspirone has a role in treating GAD in patients who cannot tolerate, or fail to respond to, an SSRI or SNRI. It may have limited efficacy in patients with chronic GAD who have successfully been managed on a benzodiazepine. Buspirone is better suited for benzodiazepine-naive patients, especially if "on-demand" relief of anxiety is not a major therapeutic goal.
Gabapentin	600mg initial; target 900-3600mg	N/A	Side effects include sedation, ataxia, dizziness, dry mouth, nausea, flatulence, decreased libido

As Needed Treatment for Anxiety[330]			
Rx	Dosage	Onset	Pearls
Atarax	50-100mg QID	Fast	Good for elderly
Diphenhydramine	50mg	Fast	Good for elderly
Alprazolam (Xanax)	0.25-0.5mg PO TID (therapeutic at 2-9mg)	Intermediate	C/I Liver Dz
Ativan	2 mg PO/IV Q 4-6 hours	Intermediate	
Oxazepam	15mg	Fast	Elderly Liver dz
Diazepam	2mg	Very Fast	Long duration
Librium	5-10mg TID	??	
Trazodone	50-100mg		3rd line agent
Clonazepam	0.25-1 mg po QHS (increase to 0.5mg prn after 3 days)		

- **Pre-Procedure Anxiety**
  - <u>Overview</u>[331]
    Patients may experience anxiety in anticipation of or during procedures. In mild acute procedure anxiety, providing information on outcomes and realistic evaluations of the risks is often enough to decrease anxiety. Moderate to severe anxiety may require medications or psychotherapy to reduce distress and allow completion of the procedure.
  - <u>Pharmacologic Treatment</u>
    Give 30 to 90 minutes prior to surgery/procedure, benzodiazepines are preferred due to rapid onset and duration. Midazolam is IV preferred therapy, whereas diazepam is the PO preferred option. Some patients experience nonspecific symptoms for up to 24 hours after the administration of sedative meds. Advise the patient on this risk.
    <u>Patients 60 should have a 50% reduction in the doses below.</u>

Medications for pre-procedural anxiety management			
	PO	IV	Description
Midazolam		0.07 mg/kg 0.5-2mg IV	Best if IV will be established; rapid onset and short duration of action with amnestic properties
Diazepam	2-10mg	0.03-0.1 mg/kg	<u>Onset</u>: 15 min <u>IV</u>: 2-5 min Has rapid onset, short duration
			15min prior to procedure; ↓by 50% if age>60 or on opioids
Lorazepam	1-2mg	0.02-0.04 mg/kg (1-4 mg per dose) PO: 2mg IV:2-4mg	<u>PO Onset</u>: 15-30 min <u>IV Onset</u>: <10-15 min Favored if want to take well before procedure (>2 hrs prior) and has intermediate onset and duration of action DOC if liver failure

			** repeat with PO dose after 30 min if no effect
Alprazolam	0.05mg	N/A	Onset: 15-30 min

- **Augmentation with Benzodiazepines**[332]
  - Best to use longer acting benzodiazepines.
  - Patients will likely experience rebound anxiety, insomnia, restlessness, tremor, sweating, agitation. These are more commonly seen if they were on the medication for >8 weeks.
    - Ensure patients are not concurrently using EtOH or stimulants
    - If withdrawal symptoms are noted, stay on current dose (or ↑ dose for 1-2 weeks longer) then continue taper at slower rate
  - The slower the taper, the better the adaptation to change will be tolerated
  - Avoid using for longer than 1 month, physiologic dependence can develop in 2 months.
  - Abrupt withdrawal is not recommended due to ↑ risk for seizures +/- delirium
  - Moderate reductions are done with high doses, and smaller reductions with lower doses
  - Recommended taper durations

Example long taper		
Duration of use	Taper Length Recommendation	Comment
<6-8 weeks	May not be required	Depends on patient and their preference; may consider short taper if high-dose was required or if you prescribed benzo with a short/intermediate half life such as alprazolam or triazolam
8 weeks - 6 mo	Slow over 2-3 weeks	Go slow during latter half of taper
6 mo - 1 year	Slow over 4-8 weeks	
>1 year	Slow over 2-4 months	

  - Taper Reigmens
    - **Slow (6 months)**

Alternate example of long taper	
Week	Dosage (mg/d)
1	Starting dose (ie. diazepam 15mg/d)
2	↓ to 11mg
3	↓ to 8.5mg
4	↓ to 6mg
5	↓ to 4.75mg
6	↓ to 3.5mg
7	↓ to 2.5mg
8	↓ to 2mg
9	↓ to 1.5mg

10	↓ to 1mg
11	↓ to 0.75mg
12	↓ to 0.5mg
13	↓ to 0.25mg
14	Stop

- For patients who have been on the medication for >1 year, consider even slower taper by 10% a week
- **Fast (2-6 weeks)**
  - *Example* #1 – decrease dose in half (1mg→0.5mg) for 7 days then QOD for 5 days then stop.
  - *Example* #2 - calculate the total daily dose. Switch from short acting agent (alprazolam, lorazepam) to longer acting agent (diazepam, clonazepam) if necessary.
    - To start, decrease dose by 25% for first 2 weeks; continue decreasing by 25% q2w until lowest dose is reached
  - *Example* #3 - decrease daily dose by 25% on weeks 1 and 2 then decrease by 10% a week until stopped.

Benzodiazepine Comparison for Oral Preparations

Drug	Usual Dose (mg)	Peak onset (h)	Duration
Clonazepam	**0.25-1**	**1-4**	**Intermediate**
Diazepam	2-10	0.25-2.5	Long
Lorazepam	1-2	~2	Intermediate
Oxazepam	10-15	~3	Intermediate

FDA approved indications for SSRI and Atypical Antidepressants[334]

	Depression			Anxiety				
Medication (initial-target)	MDD	Sea AD	PMDD	Panic	SocAD	PTSD	OCD	GAD
Fluoxetine	X	X		X			X	
Sertraline 50-200mg	X		X	X	X	X	X	
Paroxetine 10-60mg	X		X	X	X	X	X	X
Citalopram	X							X
Venlafaxine 75-375mg	X			X	X			X
Mirtazapine 15-60mg	X							
Buproprion	X	X						

PERIOPERATIVE CARE

PERIOPERATIVE MANAGEMENT OF WARFARIN

Warfarin Management Based on Stroke Risk

Risk[335]	Mechanical heart valve	Chronic AF	VTE	Bleeding risk	Recommendations
High	At least 1 of the following: Aortic valve prosthesis Mitral valve prosthesis (any) with risk factors for thromboembolism** Stroke or tia within past 6 months May also include: Patients with a history of stroke or tia more than 3 months before surgery and a CHA2DS2-VASc score < 5 Patients undergoing surgeries with high risk of thromboembolism	At least 1 of the following: Chad2 score of 5 or 6 Rheumatic mitral valve disease Stroke or tia within past 3 months May also include: Patients with a history of stroke or tia more than 3 months before surgery and a CHA2DS2-VASc score < 5 Patients undergoing surgeries with high risk of thromboembolism	At least 1 of the following: Severe thrombophilia Vte within past 3 months May also include: Previous thromboembolism during temporary vitamin k antagonist interruption Patients undergoing surgeries with high risk of thromboembolism	Very low	Dental: continue warfarin with an oral pro hemostatic agent or stop warfarin 2 to 3 days before procedure; inr of 2.0 dermatologic: continue warfarin and optimize local hemostasis cataract: continue warfarin
				Low	Stop warfarin 5 days before surgery and restart 12 to 24 hours postoperatively Vte prophylaxis and Therapeutic dose of LMWH before the procedure and beginning approximately 24 hours after the procedure
				High	Stop warfarin 5 days before surgery and restart 12 to 24 hours postoperatively vte prophylaxis and therapeutic dose of lmwh before the procedure and beginning 48 to 72 hours after the procedure

Moderate	Aortic valve prosthesis (bileaflet) and at least 1 of the following: Age > 75 years AF CHF DM HTN Prior stroke or TIA	CHA2DS2-VASc 3-4	At least 1 of the following: Active cancer Non severe thrombophilic condition Recurrent vte VTE within past 3 to 12 months	Very low	Dental: continue warfarin with an oral pro hemostatic agent or stop warfarin 2 to 3 days before procedure dermatologic: continue warfarin and optimize local hemostasis cataract: continue warfarin
				Low	Stop warfarin 5 days before surgery and restart 12 to 24 hours postoperatively Therapeutic dose of lmwh before the procedure and beginning approximately 24 hours after the procedure
				High	Stop warfarin 5 days before surgery and restart 12 to 24 hours postoperatively Vte prophylaxis and Therapeutic dose of lmwh before the procedure and beginning 48 to 72 hours after the procedure
Low	Aortic valve prosthesis (bileaflet) without thromboembolism risk factors**	No prior stroke or tia and CHA2DS2-VASc Score ≤ 2	Single vte occurred > 12 months ago and No other risk factors	Very low	Dental: continue warfarin with an oral pro hemostatic agent or stop warfarin 2 to 3 days before procedure Dermatologic: continue warfarin and optimize local hemostasis Cataract: continue warfarin

				Low	Stop warfarin 5 days before surgery and restart 12 to 24 hours postoperatively Do not bridge
				High	Stop warfarin 5 days before surgery and restart 12 to 24 hours postoperatively Do not bridge

** Atrial fibrillation, recent thromboembolism, LVEF<30%, hypercoagulable state, older generation thrombogenic valve, mechanical tricuspid valve, multiple mechanical valves

Management of NOAC[336]	
Standard Risk Bleeding	Stop 24-36 hours before surgery
High Risk Bleeding	Stop 2-4 days before surgery

Anti-coagulation based on device		
Characteristics	Annual Risk of VTE	Recommendation
No valvular prosthesis	Low (dental, colo)	Hold warfarin for 4-5 days before the procedure without bridge (grade 2C)
	Low (cataract, derm)	Continue warfarin perioperatively (grade 2C)
Mechanical heart valve, AF, or hx of VTE	High	Bridging with heparin or Lovenox (grade 2C) during cessation of warfarin 5 days prior to surgery (grade 1C) with last dose given 24 hours prior to surgery and resumption of Lovenox 12-24 hours after surgery (grade 2C) unless high bleeding risk surgery (see below) in which it should be delayed to 48-72 hours
	Moderate	
	Low	No bridging recommended (grade 2C)
Bare metal coronary stent	High (within 6 months of placement)	Recommend deferring surgery for at least 6 weeks after placement of a bare-metal stent instead of undertaking surgery within these time periods however if absolutely necessary (grade 1C), continue ASA and Plavix (grade 2C) or delay for 30 days minimum
DES	High (within 12 months of placement)	Recommend deferring surgery for at least 6 months (ideally 1 year) after placement of a drug-eluting stent instead of undertaking surgery within these time periods however if absolutely necessary (grade 1C), continue ASA and Plavix (grade 2C) and wait minimum of 3 months
CAD	High/Moderate	Suggest continuing ASA around the time of surgery instead of stopping ASA 7-10 days before surgery (Grade 2C).
	Low	Suggest stopping ASA 7-10 days before surgery instead of continuation of ASA (Grade 2C).

Bridging *means enoxaparin, 1 mg/kg BID or 1.5 mg/kg QD, dalteparin 100 IU/kg BID or 200 IU/kg QD, | tinzaparin 175 IU/kg QD, IV UFH to attain aPTT 1.5- to 2-times the control aPTT*

Thromboembolism Risk stratification		
Mechanical Heart Valve	High	*Any mitral valve prosthesis, caged-ball AV prosthesis, stroke/TIA <6mo ago*
	Medium	*Bileaflet aortic valve with hx of any of: AF/CVA/TIA/HTN/DM/CHF/75y*
	Low	*Bileaflet aortic valve without hx of above*
Atrial Fibrillation	High	CHA2DS2VASC ≥7,
	Medium	CHA2DS2VASC 5-6
	Low	CHA2DS2VASC ≤4
VTE	High	VTE<3m ago, severe thrombophilia
	Medium	VTE 3-12m ago, heterozygous thrombophilia, recurrent VTE, active cancer
	Low	VTE>12m ago

High Risk For Bleeding

- Urologic surgery/procedures: TURP, bladder resection or tumor ablation, nephrectomy or kidney biopsy (untreated tissue damage after TURP and endogenous urokinase release)
- Pacemaker or ICD implantation (separation of infraclavicular fascia and no suturing of unopposed tissues may lead to hematoma)
- Colonic polyp resection, especially >1-2 cm sessile polyps (bleeding occurs at transected stalk after hemostatic plug release)
- Vascular organ surgery: thyroid, liver, spleen
- Bowel resection (bleeding may occur at anastomosis site)
- Major surgery involving considerable tissue injury: cancer surgery, joint arthroplasty, reconstructive plastic surgery
- Cardiac, intracranial or spinal surgery (small bleeds can have serious clinical consequences)

OVERALL MANAGEMENT

- **Qustions to ask**
  - Last meal
  - Family History - There is a rare, but serious disorder known as malignant hyperthermia that affects susceptible patients under anesthesia and is heritable. Another heritable disorder is pseudocholinesterase deficiency which affects succinylcholine duration and may require extended postoperative ventilation.
  - Allergies – be aware of any that may be important from an anesthesia standpoint
  - Smoking - Currently smoking? Airway and secretion management can become more difficult in smokers.
  - Alcohol Consumption or Drug Abuse? - Drinkers have an increased tolerance to many sedative drugs (conversely, they have a decreased requirement if drunk), and are at an increased risk of hepatic disease, which can impact the choice of anesthetic agents.
- **Diabetes**
  - Hospital
    - *Before Surgery*
      - Hospital BS goal 140(pre-meal)-180 (random) mg/dL
        - All sugars should be <200 mg/dL

    - A1c<8
  - *Evening before surgery*
    - If insulin-dependent → reduce evening glargine by 20%
  - *Morning of Surgery*
    - <u>If surgery <2 hours</u>
      - Patient on oral diabetes medications only → simply hold the day-of medication and plan for morning surgery
    - <u>If surgery >4 hours</u>
      - Use continuous IV insulin with rate = current glucose / 100
      - Monitor glucose hourly
      - Always have D51/2NS running concurrently with insulin (separate IV) at 100cc/hr
      - If on 70/30 give half the total morning dose the day of surgery as intermediate acting
      - Start D51/2NS with 40meQ of K at 100cc/hr
  - *Day of Surgery*
    - <u>If surgery <2 hours</u>
      - Patient on oral diabetes medications only → simply hold the day-of medication and plan for morning surgery
    - <u>If surgery >4 hours</u>
      - Use continuous IV insulin with rate = current glucose / 100
      - Monitor glucose hourly
      - Always have D51/2NS running concurrently with insulin (separate IV) at 100cc/hr
      - Continue IV insulin post operatively for 1-2 hours after initiation of aspart or 2-3 hours after lantus given
  - *Post Operatively*
    - Continue lantus/glargine at 80% of home dose and use scheduled aspart q6h until eating and then provide with meals and at bedtime
    - If unknown insulin dose, then use the 50/50 rule for long/short acting but calculate based on 0.5U/kg *(RABBIT-2)*
- **Steroids**
  - Only will suppress if taking for > 2-3 weeks at >20mg/d
  - If patient was on suppressive doses (as above) and came off the steroid <1 year from surgery, consider cosyntropin stim testing
    - Can also obtain fasting cortisol (<5 concening for suppression)
  - <u>If steroids will be continued, keep home dose and…</u>
    - Minor surgery: no additional steroid
    - Moderate surgery: 50 HCT IV pre operatively and 25mg IV q8h for 24 hr
    - Major surgery: 100 HCT IV and 50mg IV q8h for 24 hours
- **Cardiac Device**
  - Patients with a cardiovascular implantable electronic device should consult a cardiologist to determine best management preoperatively (ie. change to asynchronous mode or inactivating ICD)
- **Pulmonary**
  - Patients with chronic but not active COPD do not require further therapy
  - Therapies for pulmonary hypertension should not be discontinued preoperatively
- **DVT Prophylaxis (focusing on THA, TKA, HF)**
  - Use SCDs
  - Enoxaparin 30mg SQ BID starting 12-24h post operatively x 5 weeks
  - Rivaroxiban 10mg/d starting 6-8h post operatively or can do only 5 days and then replace with ASA 81mg/d for 30 days

- Dabigatran 220mg/d with first dose given as 110mg 4 hours post op
- Apixaban 2.5mg BID 12 hours post op
- **Hypertension**
  - Hold ACE-I for 24 hours before non-cardiac surgery (reduced composite death/stroke/MINS) due to risk for refractory hypotension. (*VISION*)
- **Anticoagulation**
  - DOAC – hold most 2 days prior to surgery, resume 24 hours after
  - When to Bridge Warfarin
    - CHADS2VASC score >7

BRIDGING ANTICOAGULATION

- **Questions to ask**[337]
  1) Determine thrombo-embolic risk of patient via CHADS2VASC score
  2) Determine bleeding risk via HAS-BLED/ORBIT score
  3) Determine timing of stopping DOAC before an invasive procedure
  4) Consider any special considerations for invasive procedures such as neuroaxial anesthesia and AF with ablation
  5) Consider when bridging therapy with heparin required
     *Heparin bridging has no clinical benefit in patients with a short period of perioperative DOAC interruption. If high thromboembolic risk and patient will require prolonged interruption however (>3 days), consider heparin bridge. See below for bridging for Warfarin (in most cases, it is **not** recommended).*
  6) Resume a DOAC after invasive procedure or surgery
     Almost all guidelines recommend resumption after 24-72h; consider restarting the night after surgery with a reduced dose (see table below).
- **Indications**
  - See tables below
- **Warfarin Management**
  - No Bridging
    - Warfarin should be withheld 5 days before the procedure to allow the INR to fall below 1.5.
    - Warfarin is restarted 24 hours after the procedure.
  - Bridging
    - **Bridging due to warfarin cessation not required in majority of patients as it unnecessarily ↑ risk fo bleeding without benefit.**
    - Warfarin should be withheld 5 days before the procedure.
    - LMWH:
      - Bridging begins 3d prior to surgery at therapeutic dose of 1mg/kg BID or dalteparin 200U/kg daily
        - BID dosing: hold evening dose prior to surgery
        - Daily dosing: ½ dose is giving the morning of surgery
      - Stop 24 hours prior to surgery and resume 48-72 hours after if high risk for bleeding, otherwise 24 hours.
    - UFH:
      - goal aPTT of 1.5-2x control
      - Started when the INR falls below 2 (usually 48 hours before the procedure).
      - Stop 4-5 hrs prior to surgery
      - Heparin is stopped 4 to 6 hours before the procedure.
      - Restarted as soon as bleeding stability permits, goal 12-24 hours
        - Heparin is discontinued when the INR reaches therapeutic levels.

Bleeding risk stratification for invasive procedures		
Minimal risk of bleeding	Low to moderate risk of bleeding	High risk of bleeding
▪ Tooth extraction (1-3 teeth) ▪ Periodontology ▪ Simple endoscopy without biopsy ▪ Superficial surgery (e.g. abscess incision or minor dermatologic procedures (small superficial excision) ▪ Cataract procedure ▪ Double J stent insertion	• Endoscopy with simple biopsy • Prostate or bladder biopsy • Coronary angiography • Simple abdominal hernia repair • Anal surgery • Gynecologic surgery: simple total laparoscopic hysterectomy • Orthopedic surgery: hand surgery, arthroscopy • Pace-maker or cardioverter-defibrillator implantation	• Neuraxial anesthesia Intracranial surgery • Thoracic surgery • Cardiac surgery • Complex abdominal or gynecological cancer surgery • Major orthopedic surgery • Ear/Nose/Throat complex cancer surgery or specific surgery requiring good hemostasis (e.g. cochlear implant or thyroid surgery) • Liver and kidney biopsy • Transurethral prostate or bladder resection • Extracorporeal shockwave lithotripsy Infected pace maker lead extraction (increased risk of cardiac tamponade) • Robotic surgery

ACC Recommendations on Anticoagulation in AF		
Bridging Advised	Uncertain	No Bridging Advised
• Mechanical aortic valve with any risk factor (atrial fibrillation, previous thromboembolism, left ventricular dysfunction, a hypercoagulable state, older generation thrombogenic valves, a mechanical tricuspid valve, or multiple valves) • Any mechanical mitral valve • Atrial fibrillation and multiple stroke risk factors (eg, $CHADS_2$ ≥4, CHA_2DS_2-VASc ≥5)	• Mechanical heart valve with AF or VTE history with moderate risk for thromboembolism	• Bileaflet aortic valve with no risk factors (see column to right) • Dental procedures (stop warfarin 2-3 days prior to procedure) • Continue warfarin without cessation in dermatology and cataract procedures

Thromboemoblism Risk Categories

	High	Moderate	Low
Mechanical Heart Valve	• Cardiac valve replacement surgery • CHADS<5 but prior stroke >3mo prior to surgery • Carotid endarterectomy • Major vascular surgery • Any mitral valve prosthesis • Caged-ball or tilting disc aortic valve • Recent stroke or TIA (<6 mo)	• Bileaflet aortic valve prosthesis **and** one or more of the of following risk factors: atrial fibrillation, prior stroke or transient ischemic attack, hypertension, diabetes, congestive heart failure, age >75)	• Bileaflet aortic valve prosthesis without atrial fibrillation and no other risk factors for stroke
Atrial Fibrillation	• CHADS ≥6 • Recent (<3 mo) stroke or TIA • Rheumatic valvular heart disease	• CHAD 4-5 • Prior stroke or TIA > 3 mo ago	• CHAD 2-3 • No prior stroke or TIA
VTE	• Recent (within 3 mo) VTE • Severe thrombophilia	• Nonsevere thrombophilia (heterozygous factor V, prothrombin) • VTE in last 3-12 mo • Active cancer	• VTE > 12 mo previous and no other risk factors

Anti-coagulation Management				
	High Bleeding Risk Procedure	Warfarin • Give last dose 6 days prior to operation and bridge with LMWH or UFH. • Resume 24 hours post operatively DOAC • Give last dose 3 days prior (extend to 4-5 days if high risk bleeding procedure) to operation and resume 2-3 days after	Warfarin • Give last dose 6 days before operation, determine need for bridging by clinician judgment and current evidence, resume 24 hours postoperatively DOAC • Give last dose 3 days prior to operation*, resume 2-3 days postoperatively	Warfarin • Give last dose 6 days before operation, bridging not recommended, resume 24 hours postoperatively DOAC • Give last dose 3 days prior to operation*, resume 2-3 days postoperatively
	Low Bleeding Risk Procedure	Warfarin • Give last dose 6 days before operation, bridge with LMWH or UFH, resume 24 hours postoperatively DOAC • Give last dose 2 days prior to operation*, resume 24 hours postoperatively	Warfarin • Give last dose 6 days before operation, determine need for bridging by clinician judgment and current evidence, resume 24 hours postoperatively DOAC • Give last dose 2 days prior to operation*, resume 24 hours postoperatively	Warfarin • Give last dose 6 days before operation, bridging not recommended, resume 24 hours postoperatively DOAC • Give last dose 2 days prior to operation*, resume 24 hours postoperatively

Example propositionsfor perioperative management of DOACs

DOAC		Dabigatran		Rivaroxiban-Apixiban		Edoxaban	
Bleeding risk of invasive procedure		Low bleeding risk	High bleeding risk	Low bleeding risk	High bleeding risk	Low bleeding risk	High bleeding risk
Preoperative interruption No bridging (except patients with high risk of TE)	CrCl ≥50 ml/min	Last dose 2 days before surgery	Last dose 3 days before surgery	Last dose 2 days before surgery	Last dose 3 days before surgery	Last dose ≥ 24 h before surgery	Last dose 3 days before surgery
	CrCl 30-50 ml/min	Last dose 3 days before surgery	Last dose 4-5 days before surgery				
	For very high risk procedure (neuraxial anaesthesia)	Last dose 5 days before surgery					
Resumption after invasive procedure or surgery		Resume on day after surgery at 150mg BID	Resume 2 days after surgery at 150mg BID	Resume on day after surgery at 10mg/d	Resume 2 days after surgery at 10mg/d		
		Prophylactic dose of LMWH, UFH or fondaparinux minimum 6 h after invasive procedure or surgery if venous thromboprophylaxis is indicated For neuraxial anesthesia with indwelling catheter: Resumption with LMWH or UFH until indwelling catheter is out					

GIHP (Groupe d'Intérêt en Hémostase Péri-opératoire)

ACC Recommendations on Warfarin Management in AF		
Thromboembolic Risk Category	Bleeding Risk Category	Recommendation
Low (CHA2DS2VASC < 4)	All levels	Stop Vit K antagonists without bridging
Moderate (CHA2DS2VASC 5-6)	High Risk	Stop Vit K antagonists without bridging
	No significant bleeding risk (no h/o stroke or TIA)	Stop Vit K antagonists without bridging
	No significant bleeding risk **with history of stroke or TIA**	Bridging should be considered
High (CHA2DS2VASC > 7)	All levels	Bridging should be considered
	High bleeding risk	Clinical judgement

ASA CLASSIFICATIONS

1. Assess the degree of a patient's "sickness “or "physical state" prior to selecting the anesthetic or prior to performing surgery. [338]
2. The grading system is not intended for use as a measure to predict operative risk.

ASA	Physical status	Functional status	Examples	Risk status	Mortality
1	Healthy, no disease outside surgical process	Can walk up one flight of stairs or two level city blocks without distress		Little or no risk Green flag for treatment	<0.03 percent
2	Mild to moderate systemic disease, well controlled, no functional limitation	Can walk up one flight of stairs or two level city blocks stop after completion of the exercise	Well controlled disease states diabetes, hypertension, obesity, epilepsy, asthma or thyroid prob.	Minimal risk Yellow flag for treatment	0.2 percent
3	Severe systemic disease that results in functional limitation	Can walk up one flight of stairs or two level city blocks but will have to stop enroute	H/O angina MI, CVA, CHF, COPD, DM - complications, uncontrolled HTN, morbid obesity	Yellow flag for treatment	1.2 percent
4	Severe incapacitating disease process that is a constant threat to life	Unable to walk up one flight of stairs or two level city blocks. Distress is present even at rest	H/O unstable angina, MI or CVA within 6 months; severe COPD; uncontrolled DM, CHF, HTN, epilepsy	Red flag for treatment The risk may be too great for elective surgical procedure Medical consultation	8 percent

5	Moribund patient not expected to survive 24 hours without an operation		Ruptured AAA, PE, head injury with increased intracranial pressure	Red flag for treatment Elective contraindicated, emergency-may be necessary	34 percent
E	Suffix to indicate emergency surgery for any class	Any patient in whom an emergency operation is required	Healthy young woman requiring D&C for persistent vaginal bleeding		Increased risk

CARDIAC PREOPERATIVE EVALUATION

- **General**[339]
  - Goal is to assess and optimize risk (or lower the risk as much as possible)
  - Not needed for: emergency surgery, patients without active cardiac conditions undergoing a low risk surgery, or those with no active cardiac conditions or symptoms with good exercise capacity.
  - Duke Activity Score Index (DASI) > METS assessment in predicting postoperative events
  - Can use any surgical calculator (RCRI, ACS-NSQIP, or MICA)
    - ACS-NSQIP best for **medically complex patients**
    - RCRI is the oldest and has been externally validated for predicting major adverse cardiac events. It may **overestimate** the risk for low risk surgical procedures and **underestimate** the risk for major vascular surgeries. Best for high-risk procedures.
    - MICA may perform best at identifying **high risk** patients
  - Evaluate for risk of OHS and RH failure
  - The essential elements of a preoperative evaluation include reviewing overall health and underlying conditions, including pregnancy; exercise tolerance; reaction to previous anesthesia and surgery; and use of medications, tobacco, alcohol, and illicit drugs from the patient's history and physical examination. These results should guide laboratory testing, and healthy patients having minor procedures may need no testing. In patients at elevated cardiac risk with poor functional status, noninvasive cardiac testing should be considered only if the results are likely to change management.
- **Cardiology Consult**
  - Recent coronary stenting
  - Severe AS
  - Valve dysfunction
  - Recent MI (within 60 days)
  - Decompensated HF
  - High-grade arrythmias (think CHB, second degree type 2 AVB)
  - Unstable angina

Evaluation[340] **(see tables on following pages and flow charts)**

If emergency surgery, then proceed no matter what

If it is not an emergency, then you have time to evaluate the patient:

- If patient has acute coronary syndrome, then treat appropriately
- If patient does not have ACS then calculate surgical risk based on NSQIP/RCRI
  - Low Risk (NSQIP shows MACE <1%) → proceed to surgery
  - Moderate/High risk (NSQIP shows MACE >1%)...
    - If METS≥4 → proceed to surgery
    - If METS unknown or <4 → If further testing will impact decision making then do stress test otherwise proceed to surgery

Overall Management[341]

Step 1: Establish the urgency of surgery. Many surgeries are unlikely to allow for a time-consuming evaluation

Step 2: Assess for active cardiac conditions

- Unstable coronary syndromes including severe angina
- Recent MI (b/w 7-30 days ago)
- Decompensated CHF
- Significant arrhythmia
- Severe valvular disease (esp. AS)
- Clinical risk factors for coronary artery disease (CAD)
- Preexisting, stable CAD
- Diabetes mellitus
- Prior CVA or TIA
- CKD
- Poorly controlled HTN (SBP<180+DBP<110 are acceptable)
- Abnormal ECG (ie. LVH, LBBB, ST-T wave abnormalities)
- Age >70 years
- CHF

Reschedule Surgery if....

Recent MI (7-30d) with ischemia, class 3-4 angina, decompensated CHF, high grade AV block, critical AS with symptoms.

Step 3: Determine the surgery-specific risk

High (Reported cardiac risk often greater than 5%)
Emergent major operations, particularly in the elderly
Aortic and other major vascular surgery
Peripheral vascular surgery
Anticipated prolonged surgical procedures associated with large fluid shifts and/or blood loss
Major abdominal surgery and prolonged procedures with large fluid shifts or blood loss (duodenopancreatic, liver resection, bile duct surgery, perforated bowel, total cystectomy)
Esophagectomy
Pneumonectomy
Adrenal resection
Intermediate (Reported cardiac risk generally 1-5%)
Carotid endarterectomy surgery
Endovascular aneurysm repair (stents/coils)
Neurologic or orthopedic, major (hip and spine surgery)
Urologic (prostate) or gynecologic, major
Head and neck surgery
Intraperitoneal and intrathoracic surgery
Orthopedic surgery
Renal transplant
Low (Reported cardiac risk generally less than 1%)
Endoscopic procedures
Superficial procedure
Cataract surgery
Breast surgery
Dental
Orthopedics, minor
Urologic, minor (TURP, TURBT)
Thyroid
Reconstructive, cosmetic

Step 4: Assess the patient's functional capacity

Poor functional capacity (<4 METs) is associated with an increased risk of perioperative cardiac events. Exercise testing is the gold standard but functional capacity can be estimated by patient self-report. Examples of activities that are at least of moderate functional capacity (>4 METs) include: climbing one to two flights of stairs or walking a block at a brisk pace.

Patients with a functional capacity of >4 METs without symptoms can proceed to surgery with relatively low risk.

Can use the website whyiexercise.com to estimate METS

Step 5: Estimate the patients perioperative risk.

The history, PE, and ECG will help identify risk factors and can be used to determine/estimate the perioperative risk of adverse cardiac events. Example facors include history of: ischemic heart disease, heart failure, CVA/TIA, IDDM, SCr$\geq$2. The risk will determine whether surgery should proceed without further cardiovascular testing or not. You can use one of the following calculators to determine this risk:

RCRI	NS-QIP	MICA
Indication - MI/cardiac arrest, CHB, pulmonary edema **during admission (do not use for post operative risk)**	*Indication - MI/cardiac arrest* ***within 30 days*** *after surgery and can predict length of stay.*	*Indication* - MI/cardiac arrest **within 30 days** after surgery
When to use - Best for higher risk procedures *Pearls -* May over-estimate risk of post operative cardiac events. Easier to use.	*When to use -* Best to use this when patients are undergoing a low-risk procedure or those with an expected LOS of $\leq$ 2 days. *Pearls -* Made specifically for surgeons. As with the MICA, very good at predicting cardiac event within 30 days of surgery. Underestimate cardiac events in patients at **elevated** risk per ACC/AHA. Did not perform well specifically wih head and neck surgery patients.	*When to use -* Best to use for high risk patients (can use RCRI to determine) who are undergoing a low or intermediate-risk procedure or those with an expected LOS of $\leq$ 2 days. *Pearls -* Most reliable in selecting **higher risk patients**. Incorporates newer laparoscopic surgeries. Uses same variables as the NS-QIP. Underestimate cardiac events in patients at **elevated** risk per ACC/AHA.

Step 6: Now based on the risk you calculated, determine if you need to do any further evaluation:

Patients with 0 clinical risk factors are at low risk (<1% risk of cardiac events) and may proceed to surgery without further testing.	Patients with 1-2 clinical risk factors are generally at intermediate risk (1-6%) and may proceed to surgery, although stress testing might help refine risk assessment in selected cases.	Patients with $\geq$3 clinical risk factors are at high risk of adverse cardiac events (11%), particularly when undergoing vascular surgery. In this population, stress testing may provide a better estimate of cardiovascular risk and may be considered if knowledge of this increased risk would change management.

- **Considerations**
  - Stable CAD - *COURAGE Trial* – PCI can safely be deferred in pts with stable CAD even in those with significant inducible ischemia and MV involvement provided medical tx is instituted and maintained
  - Positive Stress Test
    - Need to intervene with CABG/PCI:

        - Angioplasty only: 1 week delay of surgery
        - CABG: delay surgery 2 weeks
        - BMS: 6 week minimum, ideal 12 months if low risk bleed; ASA lifetime delay surgery 2 weeks
        - DES: 6 month minimum; ideal 12 months if low risk bleed; lifelong ASA; delay surgery 3-6 months
    - Cardiac Stents – see page 575
    - Repair of hip fractures should be done within 48 hours if possible
- **Diagnostics**
    - Labs

Guideline–directed labs to consider prior to elective noncardiac surgery	
Hgb	Major blood loss or symptoms of anemia
PLT	h/o bleeding diathesis, myeloproliferative dz, liver dz
PT	h/o bleeding diathesis, liver dz, malnutrition, recent or long term abx, warfarin use
PTT	Heparin use, bleeding diathesis
Electrolytes	Renal insufficiency, CHF, diuretics
BUN/SCr	CKD, HTN, DM, cardiac dz
Glucose	DM, obesity
LFT	Cirrhosis
UA	UTI sx, instrumentation of the GU tract
EKG	Known CAD, DM, uncontrolled HTN, CKD
CXR	Sx of active pulmonary disease
T&S	If large amount of blood loss expected

    - Pacemaker Management
        - If patient is pacemaker dependent, the device should be reprogrammed to an asynchronous mode (e.g., VOO, DOO) for the surgery. If no cardiologist available, consider applying a magnet.
        - Anti-tachycardia functions of an ICD will typically need to be programmed off for surgical procedures in which electrocautery may cause interference with device function, leading to the potential for unintentional discharge.
        - Consultation with an EP is recommended if there is uncertainty regarding the perioperative management of a device.
    - Who needs TTE
        - Current CHF symptoms
        - Prior CHF with worsening sx
        - Dyspnea of unknown cause
        - Murmur on examination suggestive of severe valvular disease
    - Who needs EKG
- **What if I have a patient undergoing major vascular surgery?**
    - Use the AHA/ACC guidelines, which feature a complex algorithm that is based on functional capacity, clinical predictors, and procedure-specific risks (see reference below).
    - Delay surgery and proceed to direct treatment/risk reduction if patient has a major clinical predictor of postoperative cardiac complication. Noninvasive testing may not be helpful here because of the high rate of false negatives. Major clinical predictors are defined as:
        - Unstable coronary syndromes (recent MI, unstable or severe angina)
        - Decompensated CHF
        - Symptomatic or uncontrolled arrhythmias (such as symptomatic ventricular arrhythmias, SVT with uncontrolled rate, high grade AV block)

    - Severe valvular disease
- **What are defined as cardiac complications?**
  - Hard end-points: MI, cardiovascular death (by MI, arrhythmia, heart failure).
  - Soft end-points: non-fatal arrhythmia, CHF/pulmonary edema, ischemia.
- **Perioperative MI**
  - Usually presents atypically (without chest pain). Look for hypotension, pulmonary edema, altered mental status (especially in elderly patients), and arrhythmia.
  - Usually occurs within the first 2 days of surgery and carries a high mortality.
- **How can you reduce cardiac risk?**
  - Consider a lower risk alternative to the planned type of operation.
  - Consider using epidural or spinal anesthesia.
  - Correct, modify, and optimize the management of co-morbid medical conditions.
  - Recent MI: delay surgery for 6 months; if the surgery is semi-elective, fully evaluate/optimize from cardiac standpoint and wait at least 6-12 weeks.
  - CHF: optimize and avoid over-diuresis (patient should not be orthostatic)
  - Aortic stenosis: in general, go with symptoms (syncope, CHF, angina). If the patient has symptoms, evaluate fully (obtain echocardiogram, rule out other causes of symptoms). However, if the patient has no symptoms (make sure they are active enough to produce symptoms), then proceed with surgery. This even applies to patients who have severe AS. Patient with critical AS and without symptoms should only undergo procedures that are truly necessary.
  - Use perioperative beta-blockers - Only use if: pt already using β-Blocker, Pt with known CAD, need additional tx for HTN, RCRI>1
  - Consider adding statin if using beta-blocker
  - Only control hypertension if >180/110
- **Medications**
  - *Essential medications*: beta blockers, clonidine, CCB
  - *Medications to withhold*: ACEi, ARB, diuretics AM of surgery. NSAIDs stopped 1 week prior to surgery
  - Stop ASA/Plavix 7 days prior to surgery
  - NSAIDS: 3-5 days prior to surgery
  - HRT: ok if DVT ppx used post-op
  - The decision to hold diuretics/ARB/ACEi in AM of surgery due to risk of refractory hypotension should be made on a case by case basis. However, in some studies, worse outcomes were noted in patients who experienced perioperative hypotension.
  - Continue beta blockers
  - Continue statins; those not on them but at-risk, and undergoing vascular or intermediate risk surgery (with RFs) may benefit from starting statin perioperatively
- **Take home points**
  - When to do stress test:
    - 1) poor/unknown fxl status
(2) >=3 risk predictors
(3) major vascular surgery
(4) results will change management
    - Chest pain in past week and symptoms are class 3/4
  - When to skip stress test:
    - Pt had stress test in past 2 years and asymptomatic
    - PCI/CABG in past 5 years and remains asx
  - If patient is cleared state: **"Pt is optimized medically and there are no further additional recommended tests necessary"**

- It is often helpful to give an estimate of the percentage risk of cardiac complications (see above, by risk class) so that the surgeons can make the most educated decision regarding whether or not to proceed with surgery.

Figure. Perioperative evaluation of patient with possible CAD risk

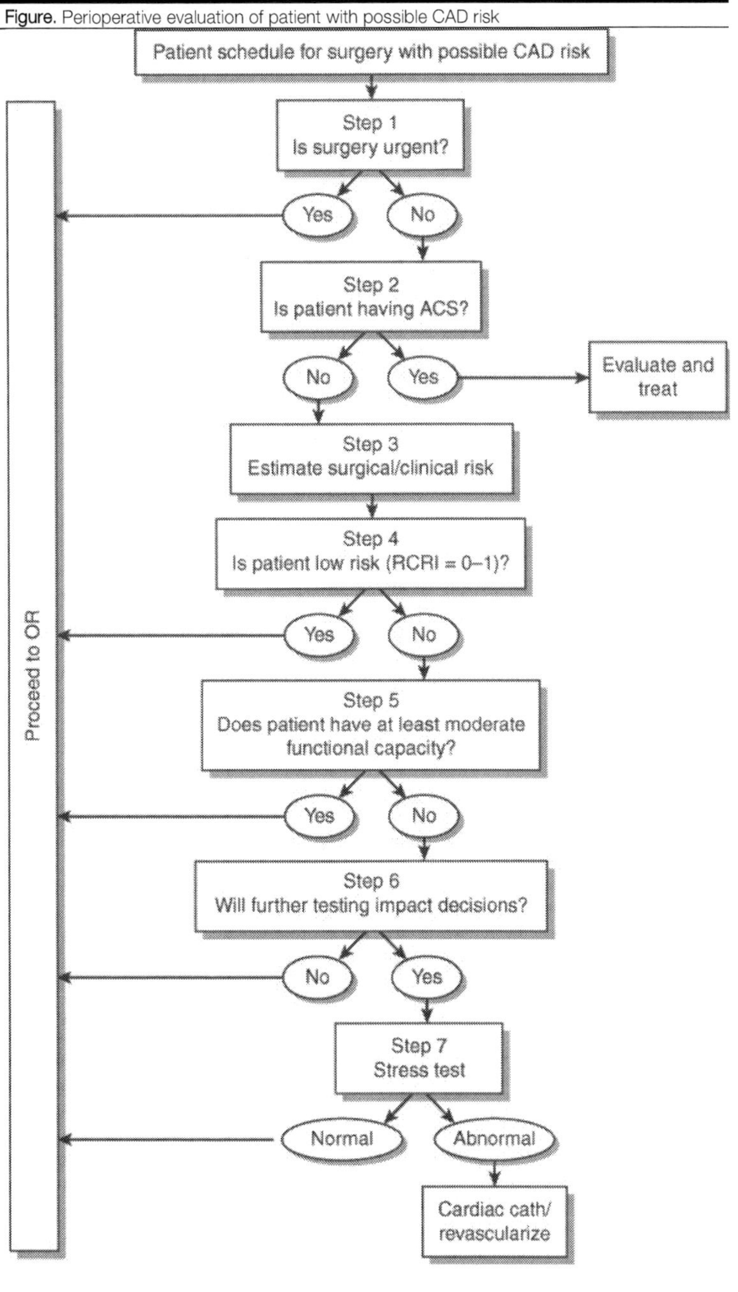

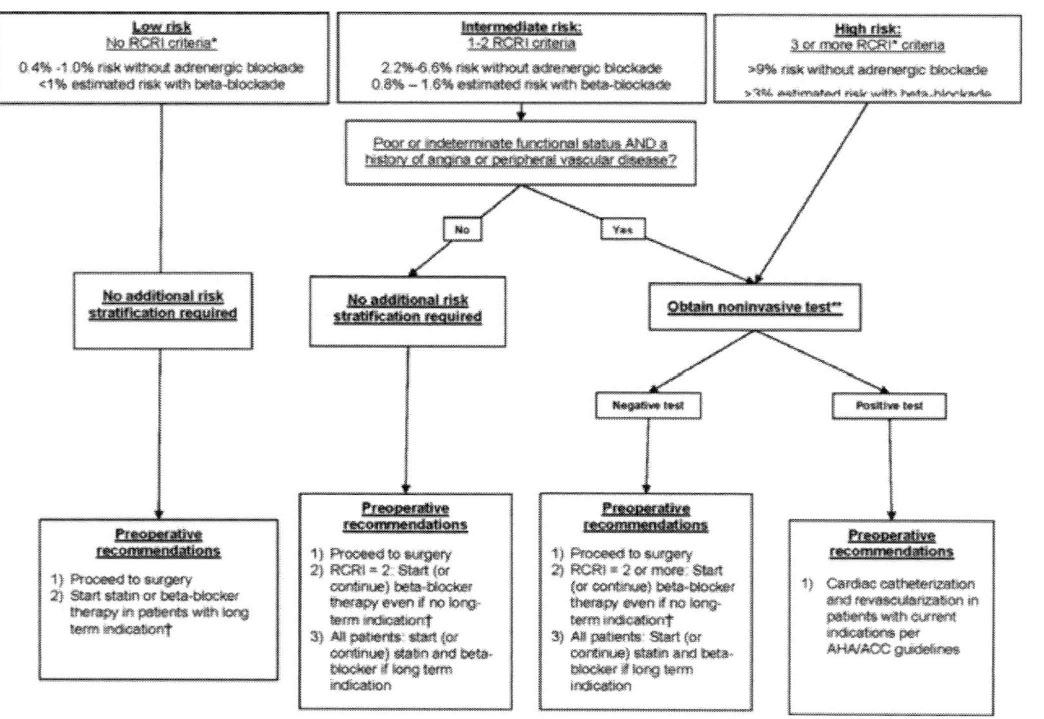

Low risk
No RCRI criteria*
0.4% -1.0% risk without adrenergic blockade
<1% estimated risk with beta-blockade
Intermediate risk:
1-2 RCRI criteria
2.2%-6.6% risk without adrenergic blockade
0.8% – 1.6% estimated risk with beta-blockade
High risk:
3 or more RCRI* criteria
>9% risk without adrenergic blockade
Poor or indeterminate functional status AND a history of angina or peripheral vascular disease?
No
Yes
No additional risk stratification required
No additional risk stratification required
Obtain noninvasive test**
Negative test
Positive test
Preoperative recommendations
1) Proceed to surgery
2) Start statin or beta-blocker therapy in patients with long term indication†
Preoperative recommendations
1) Proceed to surgery
2) RCRI = 2: Start (or continue) beta-blocker therapy even if no long-term indication†
3) All patients: start (or continue) statin and beta-blocker if long term indication
Preoperative recommendations
1) Proceed to surgery
2) RCRI = 2 or more: Start (or continue) beta-blocker therapy even if no long-term indication†
3) All patients: Start (or continue) statin and beta-blocker if long term indication
Preoperative recommendations
1) Cardiac catheterization and revascularization in patients with current indications per AHA/ACC guidelines

PULMONARY EVALUATION

Contributor: Jorge Samaniego, MD. [342,343]

- Pulmonary complications are defined as: pneumonia, respiratory failure, need for mechanical ventilation, bronchospasm, atelectasis, or exacerbation of underlying lung disease.
- **Risk factors:**
  - Smoking: RR 1.4-4.3 for post-op pulmonary complications; risk declines only if patient quits smoking 4 weeks or earlier prior to surgery.
  - COPD: RR 2.7-4.7. Treat COPD aggressively prior to surgery with inhalers, physical therapy, smoking cessation, and steroids and antibiotics when indicated. Strongly consider delaying surgery if possible in COPD patients with active URI, bronchitis, or pneumonia.
  - Asthma: RR ~2 though recent studies have not supported this risk. In the preoperative period, aim for no wheezing and a peak flow > 80% predicted; can use short course of oral steroids (prednisone 60 mg PO QD) prior to surgery to reach these goals.
  - OSA – requires evaluation and continued treatment if already diagnoses, if new diagnosis, no guidelines on empiric treatment with CPAP
  - Poor functional status: ask about exercise tolerance preoperatively → this correlates with risk of post-op pulmonary complications.
  - Current medical health: the Goldman Risk Index as well as the ASA classification both predict post-op pulmonary complications.
  - Age: not a proven independent risk factor for post-op pulmonary complications.
  - Obesity: not a proven independent risk factor for post-op pulmonary complications.
  - Procedure-related risk factors: primarily based on how close the surgery is to the diaphragm (i.e. upper abdominal and thoracic surgery are the highest risk procedures).
  - Length of surgery (> 3 hours) and general anesthesia (vs. epidural or spinal) are also risk factors for post-op pulmonary complications.
- **Not considered risk factors**
  - Obesity
  - Asthma
    - Surprisingly, asthma that is well controlled can proceed to surgery at average risk
    - General recommendation: avoid elective surgery if not controlled; should be wheeze free
- **Pre-op pulmonary evaluation**
  - Ask about decreased exercise tolerance, chronic cough, and dyspnea and consider delaying surgery until these symptoms (if present) can be explained or treated.
  - On physical exam, look for prolonged expiratory phase and any abnormal lung findings to guide further testing and evaluation.
  - Routine pre-op PFT, ABG, and/or CXR are not warranted. Only perform these tests if the history and/or physical exam guide you to do so (e.g. unexplained dyspnea in a patient undergoing upper abdominal surgery).
    - PFT mostly for those undergoing intrathoracic or upper abdominal surgery with unexplained dyspnea
- **Risk-reduction strategies**
  - Preoperative: quit smoking > 8 weeks pre-op, treat COPD or asthma exacerbation, treat respiratory infection and delay surgery if possible, and begin patient education about lung expansion maneuvers.

- Intraoperative: limit surgery to < 3 hours, use spinal or epidural anesthesia, opt for laparoscopic procedure when possible, and try to limit upper abdominal or thoracic surgery when possible.
- Postoperative: control pain, consider epidural anesthesia for pain control, use deep breathing exercises and incentive spirometry in all patients, and use CPAP or similar ventilatory support when needed.

Predictors of post-operative complications		
Risk Factors	Strength of Recommendation	Odds ratio
Advanced age 60-69	A	2.09 (1.66-2.64)
Age is an independent predictor: even healthy older patients at higher risk vs. revised cardiac risk index in which age is not included as a risk factor		
Advanced age 70-79	A	3.04 (2.11-4.39)
ASA class > II	A	4.87 (3.34-7.1)
CHF	A	2.93 (1.02-8.43)
Functionally depend-total	A	2.51 (1.99-3.15)
Functionally dependent-partial	A	1.65 (1.36-2.01)
COPD	A	1.79 (1.44-2.22)
Weight loss	B	1.62 (1.17-2.26)
Impaired sensorium	B	1.39 (1.08-1.79)
Cigarette use	B	1.26 (1.01-1.56)
Alcohol use	B	1.21 (1.11-1.32)
Abnormal chest exam	B	5.8 (1.04-32.1)
Asthma	D	

TOXICOLOGY

ALCOHOL WITHDRAWAL

Effects of various concentrations of alcohol	
Concentration (mg/100cc = mg/dL)	Effect
30-50	Measurable impairment of motor skills
50-100	Reduced inhibitions, excitant effect
100-150	Loss of co-ordination and control
150-200	Drunkeness; nausea, ataxia
200-350	Vomiting, stupor, possible comoa
350+	Respiratory paralysis, ?death

- **General**[344,345,346]
  - Symptoms that occur due to abrupt cessation of EtOH in a patient who has previous heavy use. Symptoms often start within 6-24h, peak at 72h, and diminish within 5-7d of abstinence.
- **Physical Exam/Diagnosis**
  - Initial Withdrawal Symptoms (minor withdrawal; onset 6-8 hours after last drink):
    - Tachycardia, hypertension, increased body temperature, tremulousness, anxiety, nausea/vomiting, headache, diaphoresis, and palpitations
      - Patients taking beta blockers or alpha-2 agonists may display blunted vital signs.
    - Alcohol Hallucinations (onset 12-24 hours after last drink):
    - 7–8% of patients with AWS
    - Tactile hallucinations common, visual less likely
    - Auditory hallucinations possible (sometimes persecutory)
    - May present with tremors and other withdrawal symptoms, though some do not
    - Normal sensorium
  - Withdrawal Seizures (12-48h after last drink)
    - Generalized tonic-clonic, though often isolated, short in duration, short post-ictal period
    - 1/3 of patients with withdrawal seizures will progress to delirium tremens
  - Delirium Tremens (begins 3 days after withdrawal symptoms start; lasts up to 8 days):

- Criteria for DTs include ≥2 of the criteria for AWS and rapid-onset, fluctuating disturbances in orientation, memory, attention, awareness, visuospatial ability, or perception.
  - Diagnosis requires autonomic instability

Example CIWA Protocol

CIWA Score	Lorazepam IV	Oxazepam (Serax) IV
	Recommended for patients with compromised hepatic function/hepatic encephalopathy, geriatric, high risk for respiratory depression/oversedation	For patients with history of withdrawal seizures or seizure disorder, need for a smoother withdrawal (fewer withdrawal symptoms, less breakthrough or rebound symptoms), or if withdrawal symptoms are not controlled on lorazepam
0-9	None	None
10-15	2mg	2.5mg
16-21	2mg	2.5mg
22-30	4mg	5mg
31-45	4mg	7.5mg
>45	Continuous IV Ativan	10mg
PRN breakthrough	1mg between scheduled doses	5mg between scheduled doses

- **Labs**
  - Carbohydrate Deficient Transferase (can detect EtOH use in past 2 weeks)
  - CBC, CMP, LFTs, Coags, ETOH level, Urine Tox
- **Imaging**
  - CNS imaging should be considered in patients with AMS
- **Orders**
  - **CIWA order set available**
    - CIWA Score
      - < 8 = not yet in withdrawal
      - > 8 = withdrawing
      - > 25 = needs monitoring
    - When To Start The CIWA-Ar:
      - What the client's history indicated a likelihood of withdrawal reaction-large amounts over a long period of time, history of withdrawal symptoms, last drink within the past 12 hours. If history not evident, observe informally until symptoms occur-not all people develop withdrawal symptoms.
    - When To Stop The CIWA-Ar/Discharge Criteria:
      - When the score is <10 after 3 consecutive assessments.
  - Elevate HOB > 30 degrees
  - Suction PRN orally
  - Thiamine 200mg (if DTs, then 500mg BID for 3 days) until resuming normal diet
  - MgSO4 2gm
  - VS q15min

- **Supportive Treatment**
  - NS+Banana Bag initially
  - Vitamin Supplements: Thiamine 100mg IV, Folic Acid 1mg, & MVI PO when tolerating
  - Promethazine 12.5mg IV Q4H for nausea/vomiting
  - Benzodiazepines Regimens
    - Diazepam 10-20mg IV or PO q1h or q4h prn
    - Diazepam 5mg IV (if prn, repeat 10min later, then 10mg 10min later prn, etc.)
    - Ativan 8mg IV/IM/PO q15m prn, after 16mg administered and if delirium is still severe, administer 8mg bolus IV then 10-30mg/hr
    - Ativan 1-4mgIV q5-15m prn –or- 1-40mg IM q30-60m prn
  - Haldol (for uncontrolled agitation or hallucinations)
    - 0.5-5.0mg IV or IM q30-60m prn for severe agitation NOT TO EXCEED 20mg
    - 0.5-5.0mg PO q4h up to 30mg
  - **Schedule** Ativan/Serax if hx of complicated withdrawals (Serax 15mg IV Q6H)
- **Treatment**
  - **Calculating Ativan Requirement**
    - Total # mg's in a day = # shots/beer
    - Use above to then calculate requirement per hour
  - Long-Acting
    - *Best for preventing seizures (pt's with known DT's, seizures)*
      - Serax
      - Chlordiazepoxide [Librium]) – avoid if known marked liver disease

  - Short-Acting
    - *Used in elderly or when other conditions make you fearful of having prolonged sedation*
    - *Preferable in patients with known hepatic disease*
    - Serax 15-45 mg PO with Ativan 2mg Q6-8 hr
      - If in acute w/d, order Serax **scheduled** AND PRN to be given for CIWA > 8
      - If only h/o abuse without acute w/d symptoms, can order Serax PRN for CIWA >8
    - Valium 10mg PO Q6-8 hr x 24h, then 5mg PO TID-QID
  - Delirium Tremens
    - Thiamine 100mg IV BID for 3 days (if known Wernicke's, then 500mg IV qd or TID for 3 days)
    - MVI

Figure. Algorithmic approach to alcohol withdrawal treatment

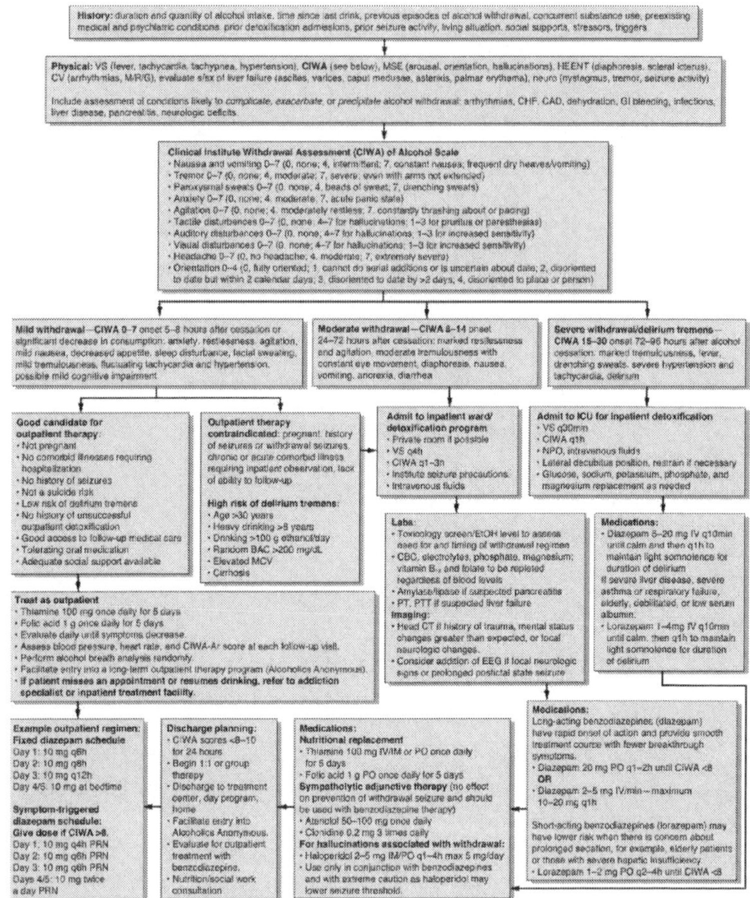

- **Long term management**
  - Consider d/c to outpatient treatment facility for further management
  - Available medication-assisted treatments for EtOH cessation include acamprosate (666mg PO TID), naltrexone (50mg/d PO; 380mg IM q4w), and disulfiram (250mg daily PO)

URINE DRUG TESTING

- **Pearls**
  - Fentanyl does not show up on standard 5-item UDS testing
- **General Information**[347,348]

  - Specimens collected in the early morning have the highest concentration and therefore will contain higher levels of the drug.
  - Adulteration or dilution of the urine specimen should be suspected if the pH is less than 3 or greater than 11 or the specific gravity is less than 1.002 or greater than 1.030.
  - Urine drug testing for marijuana is based on THC's main metabolite 11-nor-delta-9-tetrahydrocannabinol-9-carboxylic acid.
    - Detection of marijuana can occur in the urine for greater than 30 days after cessation among chronic users, whereas single exposure to marijuana in nonusers typically can be detected in the urine only up to 72 hours.
    - Medications reported to cross-react with cannabinoid immunoassays include proton pump inhibitors (PPIs), nonsteroidal anti-inflammatory drugs (NSAIDs), and efavirenz.
- **Confirmatory Testing**
  - The basic principle of confirming a positive drug test is to retest the same urine sample with a different type of test. Gas chromatography / mass spectrometry (GC / MS) is the procedure generally accepted by the scientific community for the confirmed identification of drugs of abuse.

Figure. Duration of drug levels in different lab test-able portions of the body

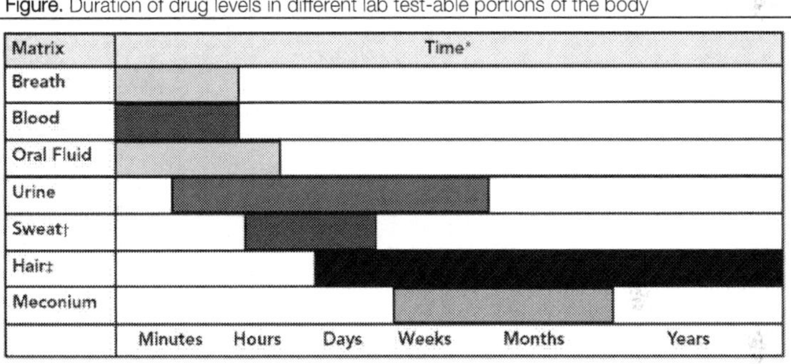

Approximate Drug Detection Time in the Urine				
Drug	Urine	Hair	Saliva	Sweat
Alcohol	10-12 h	N/A	24h	N/A
Amphetamine	2-4d	Up to 90d	1h-2d	7-14d
Methamphetamine	48 h	Up to 90d	1h-2d	7-14d
Barbiturate				
Short-acting (eg, pentobarbital)	24 h	Up to 90d	N//A	N/A
Long-acting (eg, phenobarbital)	3 wk			
Benzodiazepine				
Short-acting (eg, lorazepam)	3 d	Up to 90d	N//A	N/A
Long-acting (eg, diazepam)	30 d			
Cocaine metabolites	2-4 d	Up to 90d	1-36h	7-14d
Marijuana				
Single use	3 d	Up to 90d	Up to 24h	7-14d
Moderate use (4 times/wk)	5-7 d			

Chronic use (daily)	10-15 d			
Chronic heavy smoker	>30 d			
Opioids				
Codeine	2-4d	Up to 90d	1-36h	7-14d
Heroin (morphine)	2-3d	Up to 90d	1-36h	7-14d
Hydromorphone	2-4 d	Up to 90d	1-36h	7-14d
Methadone	3 d			
Morphine	48-72 h	Up to 90d	1-36h	7-14d
Oxycodone	2-4 d			
Synthetic cannabinoids				
Single use	72 h			
Chronic use	>72 h			
Synthetic cathinone	Variable			

ANTIDOTES

- Poison control hotline: 1-800-222-1222
- Charcoal 1g/kg with sorbitol for unknown exposures, coma cocktail (see page 412)

Overdose Medication	Treatment
Tylenol	NAC 140mg/kg PO then 70mg/kg x17
Anticholinergics	Physostigmine 0.5-2.0mg slow IV push
Cholinergics	Atropine 0.5-2mg IV up to 5mg IV q15min if severe Pralidoxime 2g at 0.5g/min
Benzodiazepine	Flumazenil 0.2mg IV
Beta Blocker	Glucagon 0.05mg/kg IV bolus for BP<90 then infusion of 75-150mg/kg/h
Carbon Monoxide	High Flow O2
Calcium Channel Blocker	Calcium Chloride 10-20cc/kg of 1% solution then 20mg/kg/h
Cyclic antidepressants	NaHCO3 3 amps (50 mg/50 mL) in 1 L D5W at 2-3 mL/kg/h
Ethylene glycol	Fomepizole 15 mg/kg slow infusion

OVERDOSE

<table>
<tr><th colspan="4">Medications associated with overdose</th></tr>
<tr><td>Substance</td><td>Symptoms</td><td>Labs</td><td></td></tr>
<tr><td rowspan="3">Acetaminophen</td><td>N/V with asymptomatic period with abdominal pain, n, v, and jaundice</td><td>>150 ug/dl after 4 hours
LFTs ↑ @ 12 hours, peak 4-6 hours (AST and ALT > 10,000)

Obtain acetaminophen levels 4 hours post-acute ingestion to plot below

Use Rumack-Matthews nomogram to dictate treatment in patients with acute treatment when time of ingestion is <u>known</u> and has been validated for use only up to 24 hours after ingestion</td><td></td></tr>
<tr><td colspan="3">Treatment</td></tr>
<tr><td colspan="3">Charcoal if within 30 minutes of presentation

NAC
<u>Time Known Ingestion</u>
1. Plot the APAP concentration onto the Rumack-Matthew nomogram.
2. If the level will not return before 8 hours from the time of ingestion, begin NAC pending the level.
3. If the level plots above the 150 (mg/mL) treatment line, begin NAC.
4. Two regimens equally effective and if patient is above the treatment line in R-M nomogram within 8 hours of ingestion:
a. 140 mg/kg load then 70 mg/kg q4h x 15-20 doses
b. 150 mg/kg IV over 15min followed by 50 mg/kg over the next 4 hours @ 12.5 mg/kg/h and then 100mg/kg over the next 16 hours (@ 6.25 mg/kg/h)

Time Unknown Ingestion
1. Obtain serum APAP level and serum AST and ALT levels.</td></tr>
</table>

	2. If APAP is less than 10 mg/mL and the AST and ALT are normal, no treatment is necessary. 3. If either the APAP level is detectable more than 10 mg/mL or either the AST or ALT are elevated more than the reference range and not otherwise explained, begin NAC treatment. 4. Continue NAC until APAP is less than 10 mg/mL and the AST and ALT have peaked and are improving and there are no other signs of hepatic dysfunction, including INR of 1.3 or less.		
			TREATMENT
ASA	n/v, tinnitus, GI bleed	Anion gap metabolic acidosis ↑ serum salicylate	Activ. charcoal NaHCO3 to goal pH 7.4-7.5 Hemodialysis
Lithium	Altered MS, tremor, hyperreflexia, vomiting, diarrhea	↑lithium level	NaHCO3 to urine Volume replacement Dialysis if level >4 mEq/L
SSRI	Somnolence, agitation	--	Supportive
TCA	Dilated pupils, dry mouth, tachycardia, ileus, urinary retention	Widened QRS AV block	Activated charcoal Alkalization to prevent cardiac toxicity Lidocaine
Methanol	Altered MS Seizures Visual disturbance, Blindness	Anion gap metabolic acidosis with elevated osmolar gap	Within 1-2 hours = gastric lavage >50mg/dL = immediate hemodialysis (>50 mg/dl) IV fomepizole Folic acid 50-100mg q4-24h
Ethylene Glycol	Oxalate crystals in urine Fluorescence of urine in woods lamp	Anion gap metabolic acidosis Elevated osmolar gap	Within 1-2 hours = gastric lavage Severe = immediate hemodialysis (>20 mg/dl) IV fomepizole
Beta Blocker	Bradycardic Hypotensive	↓glucose	Glucagon 2-5mg slow IVP

WOMENS HEALTH

ABNORMAL UTERINE BLEEDING

Contributor: Loren Walwyn-Tross, MD

- **Overview**[349]
  - Normal Menstrual Cycle
    - 5 Days: average duration of menstrual flow
    - 21-35 days: duration of avg menstrual cycle
    - 5- 80cc
  - Physiology Review
    - Anterior pituitary release LH and FSH → FSH leads to ovarian production of estrogen and proliferation of the endometrium while LH surge leads to ovulation.
    - The corpus luteum produces progesterone which stabilizes the endometrium
    - The loss of estrogen leads to sloughing of the endometrium
- **Types**
  - Acute – heavy bleeding warranting intervention to prevent further loss
  - Chronic – abnormal volume of bleeding, regularity, or timing present for 6 months
- **Causes**
  - Non-pregnant vs. Pregnant
    - Non-pregnant: menses, DUB, leiomyoma, polyp, trauma
    - Pregnant: threatened abortion, spontaneous abortion, ectopic pregnancy
  - Structural – polyps, adenomyosis, leiomyoma, malignancy, ovarian cyst, PCOS, liver dz
  - Non-structural – coagulopathy, ovulatory dysfunction, endometrial, iatrogenic, unknown, eating disorder, thyroid d/o, medications (antiepileptics, antipsychotics)
- **Evaluation/History**
  - Age of menarche
  - Menstrual bleeding pattern
  - Bleeding severity
  - Pain
  - Medical conditions
  - Surgical hx
  - Medications
- **Exam**
  - Pelvic exam

- **Labs**
  - HCG, TSH, PRL
  - CBC, COAG, G/C
- **Imaging**
  - TV ultrasound
  - Saline infused sonohysterography
  - MRI
- **Management**
  - Ovulatory
    - Levonorgestrel-releasing intrauterine system 20mcg per 24 hours
    - Medroxyprogesterone acetate 10mg PO TID for 21 days/month
    - TXA 1.3g PO TID for 5 days/month
    - Ibuprofen 600-1200mg/d 5 days
    - Naproxen 550-1100mg/d 5 days
  - Anovulatory
    - Combined OCP with 20-35mcg of ethinyl estradiol-monophasic
    - Medroxyprogesterone 10mg/d x14d
  - **Acute AUB (choose either)**
    - Sronyx TID x7d
    - Provera 20mg PO TID x7d
    - TXA 1.3g TID x5d

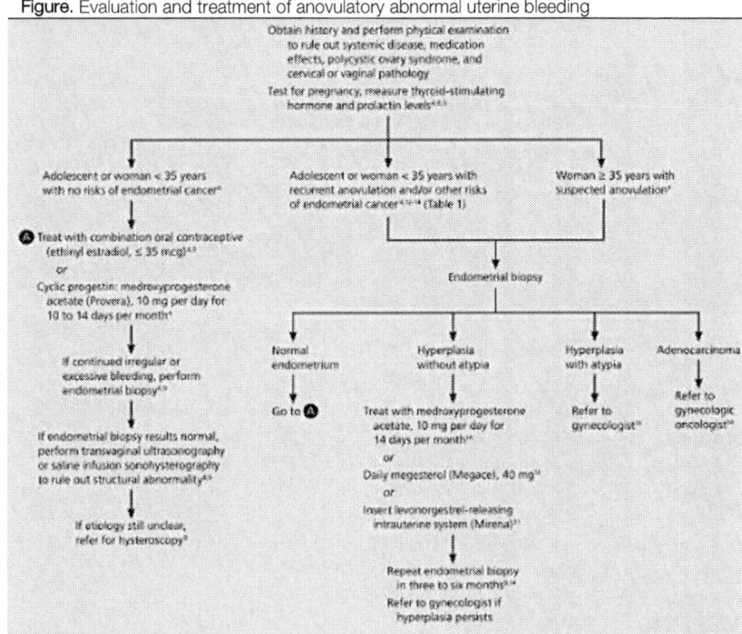

Figure. Evaluation and treatment of anovulatory abnormal uterine bleeding

POLYCYSTIC OVARIAN SYNDROME (PCOS)

- **Pearls**[350]

  - Etiology is unknown
  - Associated with hirsutism, obesity as well as an increased risk of diabetes mellitus, cardiovascular disease, and metabolic syndrome
  - Affects 5–10% of women of reproductive age
  - Usually presents with menstrual irregularities and hyperandrogenism
  - Pelvic US is not required to make the diagnosis but is recommended in patients with high suspicion for androgen-secreting tumors
  - OCPs and weight loss is the preferred treatment
- **Clinical Exam**
  - Pts often present with menstrual disorder (amenorrhea to menorrhagia) and infertility
  - May have associated hirsuitism and acne along with male pattern blood loss
- **Differential**
  - Hypothalamic amenorrhea 2/2 stress, weight loss, exercise
  - Obesity
  - ↓T4
  - ↑PRL
  - Cushings
- **Diagnosis**
  - Clinical or biochemical evidence of hyperandrogenism
  - Anovulation or oligoovulation
  - PCO on US
- **Labs**
  - FSH, LH, TSH, DHEAS
  - Fasting glucose
  - A1c
  - Lipid panel
- **Initial Evaluation of Hirsuitism**
  - R/O common causes of hirsuitism
    - s/e to medication
  - If only mild, consider cosmetic treatment or OCP
  - If moderate/severe, perform AM testosterone
- **Treatment for PCOS**

  Dictated by whether the patient desires pregnancy or not
  - Wishes to become pregnant
    - Clomiphene or other drugs can be used for ovulatory stimulation
      - Clomiphene is the first-line therapy for infertility
    - Metformin can improve menstruation but has little or no benefit in treating infertility; it is beneficial for metabolic or glucose abnormalities
    - Weight loss
  - Does not desire pregnancy
    - Medroxyprogesterone acetate, 10 mg daily orally for the first 10 days of each month
    - If contraception is desired, a low-dose combination oral contraceptive can be used
  - Weight loss
- **Treatment of Hirsuitism**
  - OCP
  - Anti-androgens
    - CPA 50-100 mg/d on menstrual cycle on day 5-15 with ethinyl estradiol 20-35 mcg on day 5-25
    - Spironolactone 100-200mg/d (divided BID)
    - Finasteride 2.5-5mg/d

MENOPAUSE

- **Defined** - physiologic event characterized by loss of ovarian activity and permanent cessation of menses, diagnosed after **12 consecutive months** of amenorrhea.[351]
- **Symptoms** (typically last 4-10 years)
  - Hot flashes
  - Night sweats
  - Insomnia
  - Vaginal atrophy
  - Sexual dysfunction
- **Labs**
  - Not typically obtained but can be used to stage menopause
  - Estradiol (<20 pcg/mL may indicate menopause)
  - FSH (>30-40 miu/mL)
- **Treatment**
  - Vasomotor symptoms best treated with systemic therapy; genitourinary symptoms (vaginal atrophy) can be treated with topical therapy
    - Mild symptoms may respond to CBT or behavioral modification
    - More moderate symptoms may require pharmacologic intervention (SSRI if contraindication to systemic estrogen (ie. h/o breast CA, CVD, endometrial CA, liver dz, h/o clots); systemic hormones if no contraindication)
      - Intact uterus → use estrogen+progesterone
      - S/p hysterectomy → can use estrogen alone
  - Unopposed estrogen should never be used in women with an intact uterus (add progestin)
  - Vasomotor Symptoms
    - Conjugated estrogen 0.625mg/day (Premarin) or micronized 17-beta-estradiol 1mg/day (can give transdermal as well)
    - Medroxyprogesterone acetate 2.5mg/day or micronized progesterone 100mg/day
    - When stopping therapy, no taper required
  - Genitourinary Symptoms
    - If no systemic symptoms, can use topical lubricants only (water or silicone based)

CONTRACEPTION

Contributor: Dr. Natasha Pyzocha

- **Pearls**[352,353]
  - Breastfeeding – progestin only is safe; avoid restarting combined hormone pills until 6 weeks post-delivery (alternative option is barrier method)
  - Start PNV at visit if patients are sexually active and in child-bearing age
  - Decrease estrogen content if want to decrease bleeding amount during periods
- **PMHx That May Alter Management**
  With the below conditions, if present, consider non-hormonal options or progestin-only contraception
  - Liver disease
  - Migraines with aura (will worsen)
  - Uncontrolled HTN
  - Active smoker (↑risk for thrombosis)
  - Breast/Endometrial/Cervical cancer history
  - Recent surgery
  - DM

- **Permanent Contraception**
  - Vasectomy vs tubal ligation (not necessarily 100%)
  - Hysterectomy
    - 99% effective with side effects including scrotal pain/epididymitis
  - Neither is easily reversed
- **Initiating Contraception**
  - Quick Start Method
    - First day of LMP <5 days ago → start today
    - First day of LMP >5 days ago → do HCG and initiate therapy with condom use concurrently for 1 week

Contraception Options Based on MOA

	Combined OCP	Progestin Only	Vaginal Ring	Patch	Nexplanon	IUD	Depo-Provera
MOA	Inhibits ovulation with estrogen and progestin	Thickens mucus in cervix to prevent sperm from attaching, may stop ovulation	Prevents ovulation with estrogen and progestin	Prevents ovulation with estrogen and progestin	Prevents ovulation Progestin only	Copper: spermicide and disrupts implantation Mirena: progestin and disrupts implantation	Prevents ovulation as a progestin only
Efficacy	92%	92%	92%	92%	**99%**	**99%**	97%
S/E	Blood clots, MI, CVA	**Irregular bleeding**	Blood clots, MI, CVA Vaginal discharge	Blood clots, MI, CVA	Irregular bleeding Headaches Weight gain Mood changes	Irregular bleeding Migration possible ↑ risk for PID	Irregular bleeding ?weight gain (5#)
Notes	Needs to be taken every day to be effective!	Good for breastfeeding moms Needs to be taken daily	3 weeks on, **1 week off** Good if can't remember to take pills	New patch qweek then no patch on 4th week Not effective if >200#	Lasts 3 years Reversible Expensive $$$ Good if can't remember to take pills	Mirena: lasts 5 years Copper: lasts 10 years Best for stable monogamous relationships	Lasts 12 weeks May take up to 18 months for fertility to return Reversible osteopenia
Example Options	**Sronyx** Yaz Ortho Tri Cyclin **Seasonique** Loestrin	Minipill Nor-QD Nexplanon (see right)	NuvaRing	Ortho evra		Copper Mirena	Depo-Provera

EMERGENCY CONTRACEPTION

- Refer patients to not-2-late.com[354,355]
- Regimen should be used as soon as possible after sex but appear to have some efficacy through at least 4 to 5 days after sex (some studies say no more than 72 hours).
- Neither regimen has any contraindications.
- The most commonly used oral emergency contraceptive regimen is the **progestin-only pill,** which consists of 1.5 mg of levonorgestrel (see table below).
- The levonorgestrel regimen is labeled for use for up to 72 hours after unprotected sex but is best used as soon as possible after unprotected sex
- 98% effective
- Patients should have STI screen
- Pregnancy test if no menses in 3-4 weeks
- The most effective method of emergency contraception is the copper intrauterine device, which almost eliminates the risk of pregnancy resulting from recent unprotected sex and can be used for ongoing contraception for at least 10 years. It is contraindicated if active cervicitis or PID is present.
- If starting routine contraception after, start after the next menstrual period and use a barrier method in the interim
- You can also use a different dose of a number of brands of regular birth control pills. While these are not sold specifically as emergency contraceptive pills, they have been proven safe and effective for preventing pregnancy in the few days after sex. You take the first dose as soon as possible (up to 120 hours after you have sex without using birth control, your birth control failed, or you were made to have sex against your will. You take the second dose **12 hours later**.

Name	Formulation	Timing Of Use From Intercourse Date	Access	FDA
Aftera	1 tablet	Up to 3 days	OTC	Y
After Pill	1 pill	Up to 3 days	OTC	Y
Copper IUD (most effective)	N/A	Up to 5 days (? up to 10)	Office visit	N
OCP	Variety	Up to 5 days	Office visit	Y
Ulipristal acetate	1 tablet	Up to 5 days	Office visit	Y

Contraception Options Explained[356]

IUD

- Very effective, no maintenance; good option for women who desire to avoid pregnancy for >3 y; avoids estrogen exposure

- <u>Contraindications</u>: Uterine distortion, active pelvic infection (wait 3 mos before insertion), women w/ ↑risk for STIs, pregnancy, unexplaineduterine bleeding, active cervical/endometrial CA; not contraindicated in adolescents/young adults or nulliparous women					
Name	Dosing	Info	Side Effects/C/I	Effectiveness	Pearls
Paraguard	N/A	Stable monogamous relationship with low risk for STD; <1% failure rate	Heavy or painful periods, iron deficiency anemia, severe distortion of uterine cavity, copper allergy or Wilson disease, active pelvic infection	10 years	Heavier menses Contains copper Can be used for 10 years
Mirena				5 years (3 years if Skyla)	Lighter bleeds/Amenorrhea Irregular bleeds and spotting in first month is common Risk for ectopic pregnancy **place during start of menses because cervical os is largest**
Copper				10 years	Releases copper continuously into uterine cavity;interferes w/ sperm transport, prevents fertilization;
Injectable					
Nexplanon	N/A		Overweight Psych history Hx of HA **Planned pregnancy in the next year (~delayed return of fertility)**	3 years	Reversible with rapid return of fertility upon removal Placed @ start of menses S/E: irregular bleeds, weight gain, HA, depression, emotional lability

Oral					
-Combined pill: stops ovaries from releasing egg/monthly; small chance of blood clots, CVD. Should not be used if >30YO+smoke. May cause irreg. bleeds -Progestin only: thickens mucous and may stop ovarian release of egg; may cause irregular bleeding <u>*Initiation:*</u> *-Quick start – preferred method; take first dose as soon as prescription filled* *-1st day start – take first pill on 1st day of period* *-Sunday start – take first pill on Sunday after period begins* <u>*Pattern of use:*</u> *-Cyclic (21 active pills → 7 hormone free pills)* *-Extended cycle regimen (e.g., 84 active pills → 7 hormone-free pills)* *-Continuously*					
Sesonique *20 mcg E/0.1mcg P*	1 tab/d	Only 4 periods/year		N/A	Q3M periods
Lybrel *20 mcg E/90mcg P*	1 tab/d	Continuous so **no** periods			No breakthrough period, used continuously
Sronyx					
Yaz					
Micronor (Minipill)	1 tab/d				-Safe for women who are breast-feeding (should not reduce milk supply). Patients should start taking the pill two weeks after delivery.
Patch					
Ortho-Evra	20 μg EE, 150 μg norelgestromin;apply q1wk		Hx of skin pathology Wt>195lb Hx of CVA/TIA	1 week	92% effective 1x each week x 3 weeks and stop on 4th week

IM					
Depo-Provera	N/A	N/A	Hx of osteoporosis Desire to become pregnant quickly (delay in 18 months after cessation)	3 months	97% effective Irregular bleeds in first few months; amenorrhea common after 1 year of use
Ring					
Nuvaring	15 μg EE, 150 μg etonogestrel; flexibleplastic ring inserted by pt; intravaginal × 3 wk, removed × 1 wk	Patient desires low doses of hormones	Hx of vaginal discharge or UTI	3 weeks	92% effective 1 ring q 3 weeks Higher risk for UTI
Barrier					
Condom	N/A	Revsible; STD prevention	N/A	85% effective in males 80% effective in females	
Diaphragm with spermicide		*See above*		80% effective	

- **Common side effects from contraception**
  - HA/nausea/mastalgia – likely due to estrogen excess; try dosing QHS vs. using a low estrogen pill (understand this ↑↑ risk for breakthrough bleeding)
  - Hirsutism/acne/weight gain – likely due to progestin and/or androgen excess; try changing to 3rd generation progestin
  - Mood changes or ↓ libido – due to progestin excess; as above, change to 3rd gen progestin
  - Breakthrough bleeding – often multifactorial in causes; first rule out other causes such as polyps or infxn, consider changing to continuous cycle treatment or chest to triphasic preparation
  - Amenorrhea – get a pregnancy test and if negative, reassure patient but if they desire a period then ↑ estrogen content or chose a progestin with ↑endometrial activity such as 1mg norethindrone to 5mg

MENORRHAGIA

- **Defined**[357] - widely defined as menstrual blood loss (MBL) of 80 mL or more per cycle based on the research undertaken by Hallberg et al. in the 1960s
- **Risks** – ↑↑ risk for iron deficiency anemia; 20% of patients will have underlying coagulation disorder (ask if family history of heavy bleeding, ask if heavy bleeding since menarche)
- **Assessment**
  - Menstrual History – cycle length, duration of menses, passage of clots or flooding, how frequently changing tampons, symptoms of anemia. History of irregular bleeding should ↑ suspicion for uterine pathology
  - Quality of life – limitations at work, exercise, social functions
  - Bleeding history
- **Causes** – those that are underlined can be distinguished through imaging/visualization or histology
  - Polyps
  - Adenomyosis
  - Leiomyoma
  - Malignancy
  - Hyperplasia
  - Coagulopathy
    - Von Willebrand disease (13% prevalence) – ask about bleeding with brushing teeth, tooth extraction, post-partum, epistaxis, bruising, excessive bleeding with minor lacerations
    - Platelet Function Disorders (PFD)
  - Ovulatory dysfunction
  - Endometrial
  - Iatrogenic
  - Other/Not classified
- **Labs**
  - Obtain HCG to r/o pregnancy, ectopic, etc.
  - CBC
  - Iron panel
  - PT/PTT
  - TSH/PRL
  - HFP if suspecting liver disease
- **Imaging**
  - Pelvic US to r/o lesions
- **Treatment Options**

Treatment modalities for menorrhagia

Other	Hormonal	Hemostatic	Surgical
NSAIDS - first line therapy with success in up to 46% of patients by directly acting on prostaglandin levels. Treatment should only be for 5 days. Options include naproxen and diclofenac	*Oral progestin's are most commonly prescribed for menorrhagia. Oral therapy for 21 continuous days (starting on day 5 of cycle) can reduce menstrual related blood loss. Higher satisfaction scores in patients are seen with the levonorgestrel-releasing IUD* • Progestin-releasing IUD - the most common is levonorgestrel-releasing IUD which is a good option if females want to maintain a form of contraception. Major s/e are spotting, pain. • Combined Hormonal Contraception - another good option if form of contraception remains desired. Major s/e were related to the hormones themselves. The only FDA approved form is estradiol valerate and dienogest (Natazia). This form is contraindicated in women with a h/o migraines w/aura, VTE, breast cancer.	• TXA - effective in stopping bleeding but does not affect the actual cycle itself. • DDAVP - specifically indicated for heavy bleeding in women with mild history of inherited coagulopathy.	Endometrial ablation

	• Cyclic oral Progestogens - short-phase which are administered for <14 days; poor evidence.		

UROLOGY

HEMATURIA

- **Diagnosis**[358]
  - Amount
    - Gross
      - Females, consider menses
      - Confirm with urine dipstick testing
      - Seen with ARF and can be confirmed with renal biopsy; etiology often ATN, IgA nephropathy, and lupus nephritis
      - Recommend cystoscopy (see below)
    - Microscopic
      - ≥3 RBC/HPF
      - Always repeat dipstick finding
      - If confirmed, do microscopic analysis
        - Look for dysmorphic RBCs, casts, proteinuria → glomerular disease
        - If above not found, continue to next line.
  - Type
    - Painless/Asymptomatic
      - R/O benign causes: infection, menstruation, exercise, trauma
      - Obtain good history → tobacco use, chemical exposures (aniline dye)
      - Obtain CMP to measure GFR → r/o intrinsic kidney disease
      - Next step is to do urology consult for cystoscopy (ages 35+) to r/o malignancy
        - May obtain multiphase CT urography w/w-o contrast to evaluate renal parenchyma to r/o mass (MRI alternative if CT contraindicated d/t dye)
        - Alternative is renal US with retrograde pyelogram
      - If workup so far is negative, may need to obtain cytology
      - If workup is completely negative, do yearly UA
    - Painful
      - Consider kidney stone
- **Imaging**
  - CT Urography – unexplained persistent hematuria (no infection or glomerular source)
  - Cystoscopy – done with gross hematuria unless active UTI
- **Etiologies**
  - Prostatitis
  - Glomerulonephritis
  - Kidney stone

- Urinary tract malignancy (confirmed with IVP)
- BPH
- Bladder cancer

Figure. Hematria algorithm

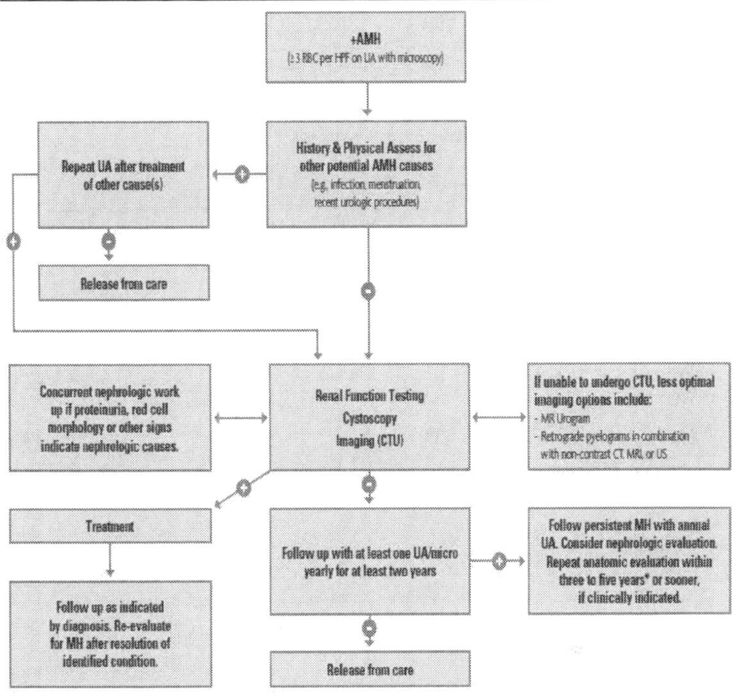

BPH

- **PSA**[359]
  - <3 → routine f/u
  - 3-7 ng/dl → repeat PSA weeks later and if remains >3 then TRUS
  - >7 ng/dl → TRUS and Urology consult
- **Indications for Urology Referral**
  - Moderate to severe sx
  - PSA>7 (for TRUS-guided prostate biopsy without further testing)
  - Persistent gross hematuria
  - Urinary retention
  - Renal insufficiency 2/2 to BPH
  - Recurrent UTI
  - Bladder calculi

Treatment			
	Drugs	Time req'd	S/E
α_1-adrenergia antagonists *Works quickly to relax prostate and the bladder neck smooth muscle tone*	Selective Tamsulosin 0.4-0.8mg Silodosin 8mg Nonselective Terazosin 1-20mg Doxazosin 1-8mg Alfuzosin 10mg	2-4 weeks	Nonselective have highest risk of orthostatic hypotension ED Dizziness Syncope
After one year of combined alpha and 5a therapy, can consider stopping alpha-blocker[360]			
5α-reductase Inhibitors *Work gradually to reduce prostate size over multiple months*	Finasteride 5mg Dutasteride 0.5mg	2-6 months	Act on anatomic component by reducing conversion of testosterone→DHT which ↓growth ED Abnormal ejaculation
Anti-muscarinic	Selective Darifenacin 7.5-15mg Solifenacin 5-10mg Nonselective Trospium 20mg BID Oxybutynin 2.5-20mg Tolterodine 2-4mg	12 weeks	Constipation Dry mouth/Dry eyes Headache

- **Non-pharmacologic**
  - Scheduled voiding q3h
  - Avoid excessive evening fluid intake

TESTICULAR PAIN

Differential Diagnosis				
Diagnosis	Description	Clinical features	Risk Factors	Treatment
Acute epididymitis	Infection from retrograde spread of organism (chlamydia or gonorrhea) via the vas deferens; gradual onset of pain and swelling	Marked scrotal swelling and pain, urethral discharge, irritative symptoms; heaviness; pain into spermatic cord and flank (posterior testes); +Prehn sign; +/- fever, chills	Sexually active men younger than 35, heavy physical strain	<35: Ceftriaxone 250mg IV x1 + Doxycycline 100mg PO BID x10d >35: Levofloxacin 500mg/d x10d or Ofloxacin 300mg/d x10d

Cellulitis	Non-necrotizing infection, inflammation of skin and SQ tissue; expands over 6-36 hours	Local erythema, pain, swelling; no fluctuance; usually lower extremity; +/- fever, chills, malaise	H/o venous insufficiency, IVDA, open wounds, DM, trauma, obesity	PCN
Fournier's gangrene	Necrotizing fascitis of perineal, perianal, genita areas; can spread up to 3cm/h; high mortality	Sudden, intense pain out of proportion to PE; severe swelling, erythema, bullae, tissue crepitus, eventual necrosis	Males 5-70; impaired immunity, esp DM; urogenital trauma	IV fluids ER transfer for possible surgerical intervention; initiate ABx such as ciprofloxacin and clindamycin or amp/sulb or zosyn. Consider vanco to cover MRSA
Scrotal abscess	Collection of pus in dermis and deeper tissues; often at hair follicle; grows over 4-14d; +/- multiple in one area	Local swelling, pain, warmth, erythema; round or conical nodule; fluctuance; +/- drainage; +/- fever, chills, malaise	H/o DM, shaving, IVDA, therapeutic injections, HIV, immunosuppres sion	
Testicular torsion	Testicule rotates, twisting the spermatic cord and reducing blood flow to the scrotum	Sudden, severe pain; high-riding testicle, erythema, swelling; +/- nausea, vomiting; painful urination; absent cremasteric reflex	Prepubertal boys (12-16); direct trauma; h/o cryptorchism	ER transfer for surgical intervention

OVERACTIVE BLADDER

- **Diagnosis**[361,362]
  - Overactive bladder (OAB) is a clinical diagnosis characterized by the presence of bothersome urinary symptoms. OAB symptoms consist of four components: urgency, frequency, nocturia and urgency incontinence.
  - Urgency is defined as the complaint of a sudden, compelling desire to pass urine which is difficult to defer." Urgency is considered the hallmark symptom of OAB.
  - Urinary frequency; traditionally, up to seven micturition episodes during waking hours has been considered normal
  - Nocturia is the complaint of interruption of sleep one or more times because of the need to void.
  - Urgency urinary incontinence is defined as the involuntary leakage of urine, associated with a sudden compelling desire to void.
- **Mimickers**

  - OAB also must be distinguished from other conditions such as polydipsia. In OAB, urinary frequency is associated with many small volume voids. Frequency that is the result of polydipsia and resulting polyuria may mimic OAB; the two can only be distinguished with the use of frequency-volume charts. In polydipsia, urinary frequency occurs with normal or large volume voids and the intake is volume matched.
  - Cystitis
  - Bladder pain syndrome
  - Endocrine: DM, CDI, Cushing's syndrome
  - Renal: CRF, relief of urinary tract obstruction, chronic pyelonephritis, NDI, Fanconi syndrome
  - Iatrogenic: Diuretic therapy, alcohol, lithium, tetracyclines
  - Metabolic: Hypercalcemia, potassium depletion
  - Psychological: PPD or CWD
  - Other causes: Sickle cell anemia, pulmonary and systemic venous thromboembolism (PSVT).
- **History**
  - Rule out co-morbid conditions such as neurologic disease (stroke, MS), mobility deficits, DM, fecal motility disorders, h/o recurrent UTIs, pelvic cancer
- **Questionnaires**
  - Urogenital Distress Inventory
  - UDI-6 Short Form
  - Incontinence Bladder Questionnaire
- **Exam**
  - Abdominal exam (look for suprapubic distention)
  - LE edema
  - GU exam to r/o pelvic floor dysfunction or prolapse
  - Perianal skin breakdown
- **Diagnostics**
  - Urinalysis (r/o UTI and hematuria)
  - Urine culture (r/o infection; need at least 100k CFU)
  - Post-void residual volumes (want <300cc; that or more is defined as urinary retention)
- **Advanced**
  - Urodynamics
  - Cystoscopy
  - Diagnostic renal and bladder US
- **Treatments**

  Most treatments can improve symptoms but will not always eliminate them
  - Behavioral Therapy
  - Bladder training
  - Bladder control strategies
  - Pelvic floor muscle training
  - Fluid management
  - <u>Second Line Therapy</u>
    - Anti-muscarinic (avoid in patients with glaucoma, impaired gastric emptying, h/o urinary retention)
    - Oral β-3 adrenoreceptor agonists
  - <u>Therapies</u>
    - Oxybutynin
    - Tolterodine
    - Fesoterodine

    - Solifenacin
    - Mirabegron

URINARY INCONTINENCE

- **Types**
    - Urge
    - Stress
    - Mixed
- **Differential Diagnosis**
    - Atrophic vaginitis
    - Prolapse
    - Bladder cancer
    - Dysfunctional voiding
    - Diabetes
    - Urethral obstruction
    - Interstitial cystitis
    - Urinary tract infection
    - Neurogenic bladder
    - Vulvodynia/vestibulitis
- **Transient Causes**
    - Delirium (UI can be secondary to acute delirium)
    - Infection
    - Atrophic vaginitis
    - Pharmacologic
    - Psychological (depression)
    - Excessive urine production (diabetes, hypercalcemia, CHF, peripheral edema ? polyuria ? incontinence)
    - Restricted mobility (patient cannot get to toilet fast enough)
    - Stool impaction (can cause UTI, overflow UI, fecal incontinence)
- **Exam**
    - Women → pelvic
    - Men → digital rectal
    - Also do neurologic exam to r/o MS, PD
- **Labs**
    - UA, culture, VB12, Ca, glucose
- **Orders**
    - Postvoid residual volume
        - Postvoid residual (pvr) testing, by catheterization or ultrasound, is recommended in current guidelines for evaluation of incontinence
        - High quality evidence from randomized trials is not available to support this recommendation, which is based on expert opinion
        - A PVR of less than 50 ml is considered adequate emptying, and a pvr greater than 200 ml is considered inadequate and suggestive of either detrusor weakness or obstruction
        - Treatment of coexisting conditions (eg, treatment of constipation, stopping medications with antimuscarinic action) may reduce PVR
    - Timed voids

Treatment	
Type	Treatment
Urge	Bladder training for urge, stress, and mixed incontinence in cognitively intact patients involves timed voiding and urgency suppression, which may be combined with biofeedback. Behavior modification: ↓fluid intake by 25%, pelvic floor muscle training (Kegel), ↓caffeine intake, scheduled voids (q2-3hr) Antimuscarinic therapy for patients with urge and mixed urinary incontinence provide a small benefit over placebo; aim to use er formulations to ↓se Duloxetine 20mg bid x 2 weeks then 40mg bid; caution: nausea Oxybutynin ir 2.5mg bid-tid Tolterodine ir 1-2mg tid
Stress	Pelvic muscle exercises (Kegel exercises) are recommended for urge, stress, and mixed incontinence. The following regimen can be performed: 3 sets of 8 to 12 slow-velocity contractions sustained for 6 to 8 seconds each, performed 3 or four 4 a week and continued for at least 15 to 20 weeks.

NUTRITION / DIET

INPATIENT DIETS

Diet	Guidelines	Indications
Regular	Adequate in all essential nutrients All foods are permitted Can be modified according to patient's food preferences	No diet restrictions or modifications
Mechanical Soft	Includes soft-textured or ground foods that are easily masticated and swallowed	Decreased ability to chew or swallow. Presence of oral mucositis or esophagitis. May be appropriate for some patients with dysphagia
Pureed	Includes liquids as well as strained and pureed foods	Inability to chew or swallow solid foods. Presence of oral mucositis or esophagitis. May be appropriate for some patients with dysphagia
Full Liquid	Includes foods that are liquid at body temperature Includes milk/milk products Can provide approximately: 2500-3000 mL fluid 1500-2000 Cal 60-80 g high-quality protein <10 g dietary fiber 60-80 g fat per day	May be appropriate for patients with severely impaired chewing ability. Not appropriate for a lactase-deficient patient unless commercially available lactase enzyme tablets are provided
Clear Liquid	Includes foods that are liquid at body temperature Foods are very low in fiber Lactose free Virtually fat free Can provide approximately: 2000 mL fluid	Ordered as initial diet in the transition from NPO to solids. Used for bowel preparation before certain medical or surgical procedures. For management of acute medical conditions warranting minimalized biliary contraction or pancreatic exocrine secretion.

	400-600 Cal <7g low-quality protein <1g dietary fiber <1g fat/day This diet is inadequate in all nutrients and should not be used >3d without supplementation	
Low-fiber	Foods that are low in indigestible carbohydrates Decreases stool volume, transit time, and frequency	Management of acute radiation enteritis and inflammatory bowel disease when narrowing or stenosis of the gut lumen is present
Carbohydrate controlled diet (ADA)	Calorie level should be adequate to maintain or achieve desirable body weight Total carbohydrates are limited to 50-60% of total calories Ideally fat should be limited to ≈30% of total calories	Diabetes mellitus
Acute renal failure	Protein (g/kg DBW) 0.6 Calories 35–50 Sodium (g/day) 1-3 Potassium (g/day) Variable Fluid (mL/day) Urine output + 500	For patients in renal failure who are not undergoing dialysis
Renal failure/hemodialysis	Protein (g/kg DBW) 1.0-1.2 Calories (per kilogram DBW) 30-35 Sodium (g/d) 1-2 Potassium (g/d) 1.5-3 Fluid (mL/d) Urine output + 500	For patients in renal failure on hemodialysis. Confirm placement on CXR at R atrium
Peritoneal dialysis	Protein (g/kg DBW) 1.2-1.6 Calories (per kilogram DBW) 25-35 Sodium (g/d) 3–4 Potassium (g/d) 3-4	For patients in renal failure on peritoneal dialysis

	Fluid (mL/d) Urine output + 500	
Liver failure	In the absence of encephalopathy do not restrict protein In the presence of encephalopathy initially restricted protein to 40-60 g/d then liberalize in increments of 10 g/d as tolerated Sodium and fluid restriction should be specified based on severity of ascites and edema	Management of chronic liver disorders
Low lactose/lactose free	Limits or restricts mild products Commercially available lactase enzyme tablets are available on the market	Lactase deficiency
Low fat	<50 g total fat per day	Pancreatitis Fat malabsorption
Fat/cholesterol restricted	Total fat >30% total calories Saturated fat limited to 10% of calories <300 mg cholesterol <50% calories from complex carbohydrates	Hypercholesterolemia
Low-sodium	Sodium allowance should be as liberal as possible to maximize nutritional intake yet control symptoms "No-added salt" is 4 g/d; no added salt or highly salted food; 2 g/d avoids processed foods (ie, meats) <1 g/d is unpalatable and thus compromises adequate intake	Indicated for patients with hypertension, ascites, and edema associated with the underlying disease

BODY WEIGHT CALCULATIONS

- Males: 106lb for the first 5ft + 6lb for each additional inch
- (48kg for the first 152.4cm + 1.1kg for each additional cm)
- Females: 100lb for the first 5ft + 5lb for each additional inch
- (45kg for the first 152.4cm + 0.9kg for each additional cm)

K/CAL ENERGY NEEDS

- High stress trauma/burn patient - 25-30 kcal/kg/day dry weight
- Mechanically Ventilated – 20-25 kcal/kg/day dry weight
- Obese (BMI>30) - 15 kcal/kg/day dry weight

PROTEIN NEEDS

- ICU/Stable: 1.0-1.5 g/kg
- Hepatic Encephalopathy: 0.6 g/kg
- Protein Intolerant: 0.6-0.8 g/kg
- Hemodialysis patient: 1.1-1.4 g/kg
- Obese critically ill patient: 1.5-2.0 g/kg
- ward catabolic patient (mult wounds, high trauma): 1.5-2.0 g/kg

ADULT FAT NEEDS

30% of calories (only 15-20% in burn patients)

ADULT WATER NEEDS

1 mL/kcal

LABS ASSOCIATED WITH NUTRITION

- **BUN: reflects protein intake and hydration**
- **SCr: reflects muscle breakdown**
- **Albumin, Prealbumin (goal > 17), Transferritin, CRP**
- **General Recommendations**
  - Provide calories of 30-35 cal/kg current weight (adjust if obese)
    - ↑ calorie foods: butter, sour cream, etc.
  - Provide a high protein diet (1.5-2.0 g/kg)
  - ↑fluid to promote wound healing (30-40 cc/kg) → should match caloric intake
- **Vitamins**
  - MVI
  - Wound Healing
    - Vitamin C
    - Arginine (general, C/I if patient septic) and Glutamine (GI) → Juven supplement here at Tripler
    - Zinc 220mg x 14d

- **Tube Feeds**
  - Start at 20-30 mL/hr and advance 10-20 mL/hr x 4-6hrs or as tolerated to goal rate
  - Types
    - Pivot 1.5 – high protein with arginine and glutamine
    - Two Cal HN – high calorie may require additional fluids
    - Nepro – good for dialysis patients
  - Goal rate
    - (Total calories needed per day / 24 hours) / calories per mL of formula
  - Flushing
    - Determine the patient's total fluid needs (free water deficit: see pg 655)
    - Determine the amount of free water provided by tube feeding formula (free water content x total volume of tube feeds = free water provided)
    - This gives you:
      Fluid needs – Free water from formula = volume of free water flushes required
    - Divide the above into 3-4 boluses per day
- **Oral Supplements**
  - Ensure Plus 8oz
  - ProCel (1 scoop)
  - ProMod
  - Supershake
  - Juven
  - Carnation Instant Bfast 8oz
- **TPN**
  - Indication – patient unable to use gut at goal feeds within 5 days of admission
  - Risks
    - Trauma, hematoma, pneumothorax when inserting PICC
    - Hyperglycemia
      - BS should be monitored q4h for first 48hrs then daily
      - Do a UA BID
      - Should be started at slow rate (40-60cc/hr) due to the risk of hyperglycemia (if occurs with glycosuria, should be suspicious for underlying sepsis)
    - Sepsis from line infection
    - Refeeding syndrome – electrolyte abnormalities seen in a patient with severe protein malnutrition (↓PO4, ↓K, and ↓Mg), see page 632.
  - Labs
    - Ca/Mg/PO4
    - LFT weekly
    - INR weekly
    - UA and BS as above
  - Initiating
    - Start enteral tube feeding at full strength formula at 20 cc/hr
    - Increase rate by 10-20 cc/hr every 6-8 hours to get to goal rate
  - Estimating Needs
    - Ideal Body Weight (IBW)
      - Energy: 25-30 kcal/kg (aim for 25 cals/kg)
      - Protein: 1.0-1.8 g/kg (aim for 1.5)
      - Lipids: 30-70 g/day
  - Weaning Off
    - Enteral feeding → If patient receiving TF at 50% goal then ↓TPN to 50% and continue weaning as tolerated
    - PO intake → once patient tolerating 50% of needs then ↓TPN to 50% goal and wean off

HYPERTRIGLYCERIDEMIA

- It is often caused or exacerbated by uncontrolled diabetes mellitus, obesity, and sedentary habits
- **Causes/Types**
  - Type I
    - Rare disorder
    - Severe elevations in chylomicrons and extremely elevated triglycerides, always reaching well above 1000 mg/dL and not infrequently rising as high as 10,000 mg/dL or more.
    - Caused by mutations of either the lipoprotein lipase gene (LPL), which is critical for the metabolism of chylomicrons and very low-density lipoprotein (VLDL)
  - Type IIb
    - Classic mixed hyperlipidemia (high cholesterol and triglyceride levels), caused by elevations in low-density lipoprotein (LDL) and VLDL.
  - Type III
    - AKA dysbetalipoproteinemia,
    - Typically, patients with this rare condition have elevated total cholesterol (range, 300 600 mg/dL) and triglyceride levels (usually >400 mg/dL; may exceed 1000 mg/dL),
  - Type IV
    - Abnormal elevations of VLDL, and triglyceride levels are almost always less than 1000 mg/dL.
    - Serum cholesterol levels are normal.
  - Type V
    - Triglyceride levels are invariably greater than 1000 mg/dL, and total cholesterol levels are always elevated.
    - The LDL cholesterol level is usually low.
- **Symptoms**
  - Hypertriglyceridemia is usually asymptomatic until triglycerides are greater than 1000-2000 mg/dL (ie. pancreatitis).
  - Signs and symptoms may include the following:
    - GI: Pain in the mid-epigastric, chest, or back regions; nausea, vomiting
    - Respiratory: Dyspnea
    - Dermatologic: Xanthomas
    - Ophthalmologic: Corneal arcus, xanthelasmas
- **Diagnostics**
  - Lipid analysis
  - Chylomicron determination
  - Fasting blood glucose level
  - TSH level
  - Urinalysis
  - Liver function studies
- **Management**
  - Nonpharmacologic – diet, exercise, Mediterranean diet, smoking and EtOH cessation, consider stopping any estrogen containing OCP
  - Pharmacologic - many physicians use drugs to reduce the triglyceride level only when the level exceeds 866 mg/dL. Main indications for pharmacologic therapy are prevention of pancreatitis and lowering of cardiovascular risk; goal is TRIG < 500.
    - **Fenofibrate – preferred to be combined with statin due to least reported s/e**
      - Nanocrystal formulation (145 mg daily taken without regard to meals)

    - Micronized capsules (200 mg daily taken with dinner)
  - Gemfibrozil – more side effects when compared to fenofibrate; 50
  - Fenofibric acid (also called choline fenofibrate; 145 mg daily without regard to meals)
  - Niacin – not as potent as fenofibrate; rarely used as sole therapy; high doses (>1500mg) can decrease TRIG by 40% and raise HDL by 40%; can cause chemical hepatitis
  - Omega-3-fatty acids – high doses required (>4g/d) and most beneficial if TRIG is between 200-500 mg/dL
  - **Statins – recommend high dose such as atorvastatin 80mg and rosuvastatin 20mg; best if TRIG<500 and LDL is elevated. Should be taken at bedtime**
    - Takes up to 2 weeks to see result, maximum 8 weeks. Safe to re-test lipid results in 2 months.

REFEEDING SYNDROME

- **High risk**
  - Wt loss, poor PO intake, prolonged NPO, alcoholic
- **Physiology**
  - Seen in chronically malnourished patients who develop ↓PO4 due to IV dextrose being given which stimulates insulin release and drives PO4 into the cells
  - Depletes ATP which can lead to ↓strength, cardiac abnormalities, and neurologic dysfunction
- **Overview**
  - Body at state of glucose deficit but high intake of glucose is provided which causes phosphate to bind intracellularly along with Mg and K.
  - All three (PO4, Mg, and K) become deficient
  - Check electrolytes q6h and replace prn with TPN regiment (rather than ↑TPN)
- **Treatment**
  - Careful introduction of ↑ caloric intake (200 kcal q24-48h
  - Implement supplemental PO4 PO or IV+NS
  - Sodium Phosphate Salt @ 0.08mmol/kg infused over 8 hours

NUTRITIONAL REQUIREMENTS

- Caloric needs can be determined by one of two means: the Harris–Benedict BEE and the "rule of thumb" method.
- A patient's caloric needs can be calculated by the following methods:
- **Harris–Benedict BEE**
  - For men:
    - BEE = 66.47 + 13.75 (**w**) + 5.00 (**h**) – 6.76 (**a**)
  - For women:
    - BEE = 655.10 + 9.56 (**w**) + 1.85 (**h**) – 4.689 (**a**)

  *where **w** = weight in kilograms; **h** = height in centimeters; and **a** = age in years.*

  - After the BEE has been determined from the Harris–Benedict equation, the patient's total daily maintenance energy requirements are estimated by multiplying the BEE by an activity factor and a stress factor.

Total energy requirements = BEE x Activity factor x Stress factor

Use the following correction factors:

Activity Level	Correction Factor
Bedridden	1.2
Ambulatory	1.3
Minor operation	1.2
Skeletal trauma	1.35
Major sepsis	1.60
Severe burn	2.10

- **"Rule of Thumb" Method**
  - Maintenance of the patient's nutritional status without significant metabolic stress requires 25–30 Cal/kg body weight/d.
  - Maintenance needs for the hypermetabolic, severely stressed patient or for supporting weight gain in the underweight patient without significant metabolic stress requires 35–40 Cal/kg body weight/d.
  - Greater than 40 Cal/kg body weight/d may be needed to meet the needs of severely burned patients.

IDENTIFYING A MALNOURISHED PATIENT

Parameters	Measurement	Usefulness
Anthropometric Measurement		
Actual body weight (ABW) compared with ideal body weight (IBW)	"Rule-of-thumb" method to determine IBW Step 1 For men: IBW (lb) = 106 lb for 5 ft of height, plus 6 lb for each inch of height over 5 ft For women: IBW (lb) = 100 lb for first 5 ft of height plus an additional 5 lb for each inch over 5 ft Step 2 % IBW = ABW / IBW X 100 %IBW: 90-110 Normal nutritional status 80-90 Mild malnutrition 70-80 Moderate malnutrition <70 Severe malnutrition	

Actual body weight compared with usual body weight (UBW)	% UBW = ABW / UBW X 100 % of UBW: 85-95% Mild malnutrition 75-84% Moderate malnutrition <75% Severe malnutrition	
Biochemical Measurement		
Serum albumin	3.5-5.2 g/dL Normal 2.8-3.4 g/dL Mild depletion 2.1-2.7 g/dL Moderate depletion <2 g/dL Severe depletion	Routinely available Valuable prognostic indicator: depressed levels predict increased mortality and morbidity. Inexpensive Large body stores and relatively long half-life (approximately 20 d) limit usefulness in evaluating short-term changes in nutritional status
Carbohydrate controlled diet (ADA)	Calorie level should be adequate to maintain or achieve desirable body weight Total carbohydrates are limited to 50-60% of total calories Ideally fat should be limited to ≈30% of total calories	Diabetes mellitus
Acute renal failure	Protein (g/kg DBW) 0.6 Calories 35-50 Sodium (g/day) 1-3 Potassium (g/day) Variable Fluid (mL/day) Urine output + 500	For patients in renal failure who are not undergoing dialysis
Renal failure/hemodialysis	Protein (g/kg DBW) 1.0–1.2 Calories (per kilogram DBW) 30-35 Sodium (g/d) 1-2 Potassium (g/d) 1.5-3 Fluid (mL/d) Urine output + 500	For patients in renal failure on hemodialysis
Peritoneal dialysis	Protein (g/kg DBW) 1.2-1.6 Calories (per kilogram DBW) 25-35 Sodium (g/d) 3–4 Potassium (g/d) 3-4 Fluid (mL/d) Urine output + 500	For patients in renal failure on peritoneal dialysis
Liver failure	In the absence of encephalopathy do not restrict protein In the presence of encephalopathy initially restricted protein to 40-60 g/d	Management of chronic liver disorders

	then liberalize in increments of 10 g/d as tolerated Sodium and fluid restriction should be specified based on severity of ascites and edema	
Low lactose/lactose free	Limits or restricts mild products Commercially available lactase enzyme tablets are available on the market	Lactase deficiency
Low fat	<50 g total fat per day	Pancreatitis Fat malabsorption
Fat/cholesterol restricted	Total fat >30% total calories Saturated fat limited to 10% of calories <300 mg cholesterol <50% calories from complex carbohydrates	Hypercholesterolemia
Low-sodium	Sodium allowance should be as liberal as possible to maximize nutritional intake yet control symptoms "No-added salt" is 4 g/d; no added salt or highly salted food; 2 g/d avoids processed foods (ie, meats) <1 g/d is unpalatable and thus compromises adequate intake	Indicated for patients with hypertension, ascites, and edema associated with the underlying disease

FLUIDS

FLUID CALCULATIONS

- **Body fluid composition:**
  - Total Body Water = 0.6 x wt (kg) for males|0.5 x wt (kg) for females
    - Extracellular fluid (ECF) = 0.2 x wt (kg)
    - *Intravascular* = 1/3ECF
      - Interstitial = 2/3ECF
      - Intracellular fluid (ICF) = 0.4 x wt (kg)
- **Maintenance Fluids**
  - Generic
    - Weight in kg + 40 = hourly rate
  - 24HR Requirements
    - **100/50/20 RULE**
      - Administer 100 mL/kg/day for the first 10 kg of weight
      - Add 50 mL/kg for the next 10 kg
      - Add 20 mL/kg for each kg over 20kg
  - Hourly Requirements
    - **4/2/1 RULE**
      - Administer 4 mL/kg/hr for the first 10 kg
      - Add 2 mL/kg/hr for the next 10 kg
      - Add 1 mL/kg/hr for each kg over 20
      - Maintenance Fluids
- **Fluid deficit ml/hr**
  - (Pre-illness weight in kg- illness weight in kg)/24
  - 1 kg of weight lost = 1 L of fluid lost
- **Figure out IV rate:**
  - Maintenance dose + Fluid deficit to get Total Deficit in ml/hr
  - Give ½ of Total deficit over 1st 8 hours
  - If gave any boluses, subtract them from this number.
  - Give 2nd ½ of Total Deficit over next 16 hours
- **Decide what IV fluid to give:**
  - Hypovolemic: NS
    - Postural hypotension, dry mucous mems, flat neck veins, skin tenting
  - Euvolemic: NS
    - Hypervolemic: D5W at KVO or Hep lock
    - Tachypnea, moist MM, crackles, JVP >3cm above sternal angle, taut skin, S3,
  - **Look at BUN: Cr ratio:**
    - Ratio less than 12 =volume depletion
  - Check Ins/Outs

- Human: 140 mEq/L Na^+, 103 mEq/L Cl^-, 4 mEq/L K^+, 5 mEq/L Ca^{++}, 2 mEq/L Mg^{++}, 25 mEq/L $HCO3^-$, pH 7.4, Osmolality 290 mOsm/L

IV Solutions				
Solution	pH	Contents (1L)	Osmolarity mOsm/L (nml 240-340)	Type
D5W	5	5g dextrose	252	Isotonic - hypotonic in body
0.9NaCl	5.7	154 mEq Na 154 mEq Cl	308	Isotonic
Ringers Lactate	5.8	147 mEq Na 4 mEq K 4 mEq Ca 155 mEq Cl	308-324	Isotonic
Lactated Ringers	6.6	130 mEq Na 4 mEq K 3 mEq Ca 109 mEq Cl 28 mEq NaLa	273	Isotonic
0.45 NaCl	5.6	77 mEq Na 77 mEq Cl	154	Hypotonic
3% NaCl	5.0	513 mEq Na 513 mEq Cl	1026	Hypertonic
5% NaCl	5.8	855 mEq Na 855 mEq Cl	1710	Hypertonic
10% Dextose	4.3	10g dextrose	505	Hypertonic
D51/4NS	4.4	5g Dextose 34 mEq Na 34 mEq Cl	406	Hypertonic
D51/2NS	4.4	5g Dextose 77 mEq Na 77 mEq Cl	406	Hypertonic
D5NS	4.4	5g Dextrose 154 mEq Na 154 mEq Cl	560	Hypertonic
D5LR	4.9	5g Dextrose 130 mEq Na 4 mEq K 3 mEq Ca 109 mEq Cl 28 mEq NaLa	525	Hypertonic
0.9NS + 150 mEQ NAHCO3		Na 308 K 0 Cl 0 HCO3 50	616	Very hypertonic

*** 50g of dextrose is rapidly metabolized therefore does NOT contribute to tonicity*

IV FLUIDS

- **For Most Patients**
  - Maintenance Fluids*: "4/2/1 Rule" = [4 ml/hr for first 10 kg wt] + [2 ml/hr for next 10 kg] + [1 ml/hr for every 1 kg over 20 kg]

- Deficit: (Hrs NPO x Maintenance)
- Insensible Loss: 3-15 cc/hr
- Trauma: Replace 1 cc of EBL with 3 cc of isotonic IVF
- **Parkland Formula*** for burn patients: wt (kg) x TBSA% x 4cc LR over 24 hr. Give 1/2 first 8 hours, second 1/2 over next 16 hours.
  *Common: (wt) (% TBSA) (3cc LR) over 24 hours

Electrolyte Requirements		
	Adults	Children
Na	80-120 mEq/day	3-4 mEq/kg/day or per 100 ml fluid
K	50-100 mEq/day	2-3 mEq/day or per 100 ml fluid
Cl	80-120 mEq/day	3 mEq/day or per 100 ml fluid
Glucose	100-200 g/day	100-200 mg/kg/hr
	The protein-sparing effect is one of the goals of basic IV therapy. The administration of at least 100 g of glucose/d reduces protein loss by more than one-half. Virtually all IV fluid solutions supply glucose as dextrose (pure dextrorotatory glucose).	
PO4	7-10 mmol/1000kcal	
Mg	20 mEq	
Ca	1-3 gm/d	

Specific Replacement Fluids	
Gastric Loss (Nasogastric Tube, Emesis):	D51/2NS with 20 mEq/L (mmol/L) potassium chloride (KCl)
Diarrhea:	D5LR with 15 mEq/L (mmol/L) KCl. Use body weight as a replacement guide (about 1 L for each 1 kg, or 2.2 lb, lost)
Bile Loss:	D5LR with 25 mEq/L (1/2 ampule) of sodium bicarbonate mL for mL
Pancreatic Loss:	D5LR with 50 mEq/liter (1 amp) HCO3 mL for mL
Burn Patients:	Use the Parkland: (% body burn) x (body weight in kg) x 4 mL or "Rule of Nines" Formulas:

PAIN MANAGEMENT

PHARMACOLOGIC PAIN MANAGEMENT

1. **Risk Stratify**
   - SOAPP-R score is a system used to rate patient as high risk for addiction

Pain Management by Adminstration Type		
Method	Type	Medication
IV/IM	Opioids	Fentanyl 25-100 mg/kg q30-60 min Hydromorphone 0.2-2 mg q4-6h Meperidine 25-50 mg q3-4h Morphine 1-10 mg q2-6h
	NSAIDs	Ketorolac 30-60 mg loading then 15-30 mg IV q6h MAX 5 days Rofecoxib 50mg MAX 5 days
	Mixed	Butorphanol 20 mg/kg Nalbuphine 0.25 mg/kg
Oral	Acetaminophen	Acetaminophen 325mg-650g q4-6h max 3250mg/day
	NSAIDs	Ibuprofen 600mg PO QID Ketorolac 10-20 mg q4-6h Naproxen 500 mg q6-8h Rofecoxib 50mg QDx5d then 25mg QD
	Cox-2 inhib	Celecoxib 400 mg x1 then p12h 200mg BID
	Opioid/non Combination	Acetaminophen/propoxyphene Napsylate (Darvocet) q4-6h Acetaminophen/oxycodone (Percocet) q4-6h Acetaminophen/codeine (Tylenol with codeine) q4-6h Acetaminophen/hydrocodone (Vicodin) q4-6h
	Opioids	Hydrocodone 5-10 mg q4-6h Morphine 10-30 mg q3-4h Oxycodone 5 mg q3-6h
	Other	Acetaminophen 325-1000mg q4-6h

Transdermal	Opioids	Fentanyl patch 25-100 mcg/h ql2h
Intranasal	Opioids	Fentanyl Meperidine Butorphanol
Local	N/a	Neuraxial anesthesia Regional nerve block Local infiltration by surgeon Continuous subcutaneous catheter
Non Pharm	N/a	Heat/cold therapy, massage, TENS relaxation, hypnosis, acupuncture, biofeedback

Example options for opiate prescribing (inpatient)		
Long acting	+	Breakthrough
Percocet 5/325 1-2 tabs PO q3h PRN (1 tab for mild-mod pain < 5/10; 2 tabs for mod-severe pain > 5/10) Hydrocodone/Acetaminophen (Norco) 5/325mg 1 tab PO q4h PRN mild to moderate pain (< 5/10) Hydrocodone/Acetaminophen (Norco) 5/325mg 2 tabs PO q4h PRN moderate to severe pain (> 5/10)		Morphine Sulfate 4-8mg IV q1-2h PRN Dilaudid .5-1.5mg IV q2h PRN

Pain Management by Pain Type	
Type	Prescription
Neuropathic Pain	• Gabapentin 300 mg PO BID prn pain • Start at 100 mg tid • Lyrica 75-300 mg PO BID • Capsaicin 0.075% topical QID • Lidocaine patch 4% - Apply patch to painful area. Patch may remain in place for up to 12 hours in any 24-hour period. No more than 1 patch should be used in a 24-hour period.
Muscle pain/Spasm	• General o Flexeril IR 5mg TID x 3 weeks o Flexeril ER 15mg daily o Baclofen 5mg TID o Robaxin 500mg 1-2 q6h prn • Acute/Severe Pain o Valium IM 5-10mg q4h x 2 o Zanaflex 4mg daily→TID q6h
Cancer related pain	• Mild → Tylenol, NSAID • Moderate → Codeine, Hydrocodone, or Tramadol + above • Severe → Short acting (Morphine or Hydromorphone) and calculate to long acting (fentanyl patch or oxycodone) and give short acting for break through • Fentanyl Patch Conversion o Morphine 2mg PO/day = Fentanyl 1mag/hr TSD

	○ Percocet (9 tabs/day) = Fentanyl 25mag TSD ○ Lortab (9 tabs/day) = Fentanyl 25mag TSD ○ Tylenol #3 (9 tabs/day) = Fentanyl 25mag TSD

Options in the Pharmacologic Management of Generic Pain

	Name	Dosage	Onset	Duration	Timing/Interval	Other
Mild	Tylenol	650mg-1g *(Max 3250mg/day (2 g per day in patients with liver disease)*	30min-1hour		PO q4-6h prn mild pain	*Check LFTs*
	ASA (Bayer)	325-650 mg			PO q4h (max 3.9 g/day)	
	Ibuprofen (Advil, Motrin)	600mg PO			Q6h (max 1.2g/day)	
	Naproxen (Aleve)	220-440 PO initially then 220			Q8-12h (max 600mg/day)	
	Tramadol (Ultram)	50-100mg			q6 hrs max 400 mg/day	
Moderate	Opioid+NSAID/Acetaminophen					
	Toradol (IV/IM NSAID)	15-30mg IV/IM	10 min		q6h MAX 5d (120mg/day)	
	Hydrocodone 5mg/acetaminophen 325mg (Vicodin)	1-2 tab po			Q4 hours prn	
	Neurontin	300-1200mg			TID	
	Morphine	15-30 mg PO q3-6h	30 min	4 hours		
		2-10 mg iv/im/SQ	5-10min	3-6 hours	q3-4h	
	MS Contin	15-30 mg			q8-12h	

	Percocet	Mild: 1 5/325 tab PO q3h prn			q6 hours PO	
	Percocet	Severe: 2 10/325 tab PO q3h				
	Norco	Mild: 5/325 Mod: 10/325	10-20 min	3-4 hours	q3-4h	
	Codeine	RR: 120mg q4-6h CR: 50-300mg q12h	1-1.5 hours	4-6 hours		
	Topical Agents					
	Lidoderm	1 patch for 12 hours daily				*Apply to intact skin, cover most painful area*
	Capsaicin cream	3-4x/day x 2 months				
	Opioid/Epidural/Periph Nerve Block					
	Fentanyl	25-100 mcg IV	TD: 6 h IV: immed	TD: 12 hour IV: 30m-1 h	q1-2h	
	Demerol	0.5mg IV			q2-3 hours	*5x stronger than morphine and can lower seizure threshold*
	Oxymorphone SR	20/40/60mg		48 hours		
Severe	Dilaudid	IV: 0.2-1.5mg PO: 2-7mg	IV: 5-15min PO:	4-5 hours	Q1-2H PRN severe pain	*5-6x stronger than morphine*

		30m-1 hour			
Vicodin	2 tab			Q6H	
Meperidine	25-100 mg iv/im/subq (1-1.8mg/kg)	2 hours	2-4 hours	Q4H	*Max 150mg*
Methadone	2.5-10 mg IM/IV	1-2 hours	4-8 hours	q4-8h 5-20 mg	*Can accumulate in adipose → delayed toxicity*
Oxycodone IR 5/325	Mild pain - 5 mg Mod pain - 10 mg	30m-1 hour		4 hours	
Oxycodone CR 5/325	10-20 mg			q12h	
Oxycontin	10-30mg PO	4-5 hours	<12 hours	q4-6h	
Morphine	0.1mg/kg (up to 15mg) IM/SQ/slow IV	PO: 30 min IV: 5-10min	O: 4 hours IV: 3-4 hours	Q4H prn	
Fentanyl IV	0.35-0.5 mcg/kg	IV: 1-2min	IV: 2-4 hours	Q30min - q1h	
Fentanyl	50mcg		72hrs	Q2H	
Ketamine	IV Initial: 0.1 to 0.5 mg/kg bolus; followed by 0.83 to 6.7 mcg/kg/minute (equivalent to 0.05 to 0.4 **mg**/kg/**hour**)				

OPIOID PRESCRIBING

- Morphine is first line opioid of choice
- Initiate sustained release morphine (Morphine SR or Oxycontin) 10-15mg daily
- At the same time prescribe PRN Morphine IR 2.5-5mg q6h
- Review after 24 hours, add up total daily dose of morphine given.
- Calculate how many mg of opioid pt is using in 24 hrs → convert that amt to Opioid (SR) by 1/2
- Add a rescue doses (IR) of same opioid if possible - should be~10-20% of total daily opioid dose
- **Example**
  - 10mg oxycodone 6 times/day = 60mg oxycodone in 24 hrs
  - Equivalent SR Oxycodone = Oxycontin 30mg q12h
  - Add opioid rescue dose – Oxycodone 5- 10 mg q4h prn

CONVERSION FACTORS FOR OPIOIDS

Opioid Strength
Demerol<Codeine<Morphine=Hydrocodone<Oxycodone<Oxymorphone<Hydromorphone< Fentanyl

Drug 1		Drug 2
Morphine po	⇔	Oxycodone po
1mg iv morphine	⇔ ⇔ ⇔	3 mg po morphine 10 mcg iv fentanyl 100mcg fentanyl lollipop 0.1mg epidural morphine 0.01mg intrathecal morphine
1mg/hr iv morphine	⇔	25 mcg/hr fentanyl patch
5 mg po morphine	⇔	1mg po dilaudid
1 mg iv dilaudid	⇔	4- 5 mg po dilaudid
10mg po morphine	⇔	1mg po methadone (average)
IV	⇔	Sq (morphine and dilaudid)

Long Acting Opioids		
Drug	Duration	Dose
Buprenorphine Patch 5/10/20mcg/hr	72 HRS	120 mcg 240 mcg 480 mcg
Fentanyl ER 25mcg/hr	72 HRS	600 mcg
Hydromorphone SR 8/12/16 mg	24 HRS	8/12/16 mg
Methadone 5/10 mg	72 HRS	15/30 mg
Morphine ER 15/30/6080/90/100 mg	48 HRS	30/60/90...
Oxymorphone SR 10/15/20/40 mg	48 HRS	20/40/60
Oxycodone SR 10/20/40/80	48 HRS	" "

- **PCA**
  - Dilaudid PCA: Adult naive: load 0.2mg; demand 0.2mg, lockout 10min, 4hr limit 4.8mg

- **Pain Contract**
    - Medication is for patient only
    - Will take as directed
    - Will only fill at one pharmacy
    - Will not accept controlled substances from any other physician
    - Will come to office for monthly refills
    - Will be held to random drug testing

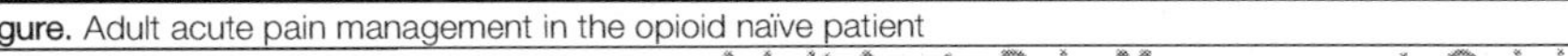

Figure. Adult acute pain management in the opioid naïve patient

Adult Acute Pain Management: Opioid Naïve

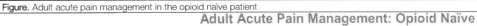

PCA Dose = Patient Push dose
Basal = Continuous infusion
Bolus = Large dose for breakthrough pain

Severe or increased pain *

Not taking opioids for at least 7 days around the clock (Opioid Naïve)

IV:

Give stat dose 2-4 mg IV** morphine or morphine equivalent (see pain card). Repeat every 15 minutes as needed until PCA started

Begin PCA at 1 mg morphine or morphine equivalent every 6 minutes IV or every 15 minutes subcutaneously **and** Bolus 2-4 mg SQ/IV every hour as needed
Use no basal infusion

PO:

If taking by mouth, give 5 – 15 mg of immediate release morphine or equivalent every 3 hours around the clock while awake; patient may refuse, hold for sedation

Reassess at 1 hour; initiate 1-2 senna tablets every night at bedtime when tolerating orally

If excessive sedation notify provider

If patient reports inadequate pain relief → Double PCA dose and bolus, or increase oral opioid by 50% (Tylenol Free Product) → Reassess every 1-2 hours; if pain still uncontrolled consider pain consult

If patient states pain relief is adequate (and medicine tolerated) → Continue current dosing → Reassess and continue to adjust as needed

At 48 hours, if pain expected to last > 4 weeks (i.e. chronic), calculate the total morphine equivalent (PCA, bolus IV or PO) used in the past 24 hours convert **and** add 50% of it to a basal infusion/long acting opioid.

Continue PCA or as needed oral dosing; reassessment and dose adjustment as needed

- 1mg IV morphine = 3 mg oral morphine
- oral morphine = oral oxycodone = oral hydrocodone
- 1 mg IV dilaudid = 5 mg IV morphine
- 1 mg PO dilaudid = 5 mg PO morphine
- 25 mcg Fentanyl patch = 1 mg IV Morphine an hour
- 10 mcg IV fentanyl = 1 mg IV morphine
- 200 mcg fentanyl lozenge = 2 mg IV morphine
- 1 mg PO methadone = 10 mg PO morphine
- 1 mg IV methadone = 2 mg PO methadone

Notes: * Any sudden increase in pain scores with change in vital signs requires immediate assessment. ***Monitor levels of sedation closely; notify provider for increased sedation.***

** If no IV access available, consider SQ

Consider Palliative Care Consult for ongoing Pain/Side Effect Issues

Cerner

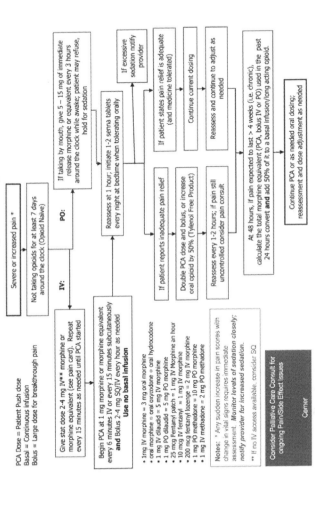

Property of VCU Massey Cancer Center, July, 2010

Figure. Adult acute pain management in the opioid tolerant patient

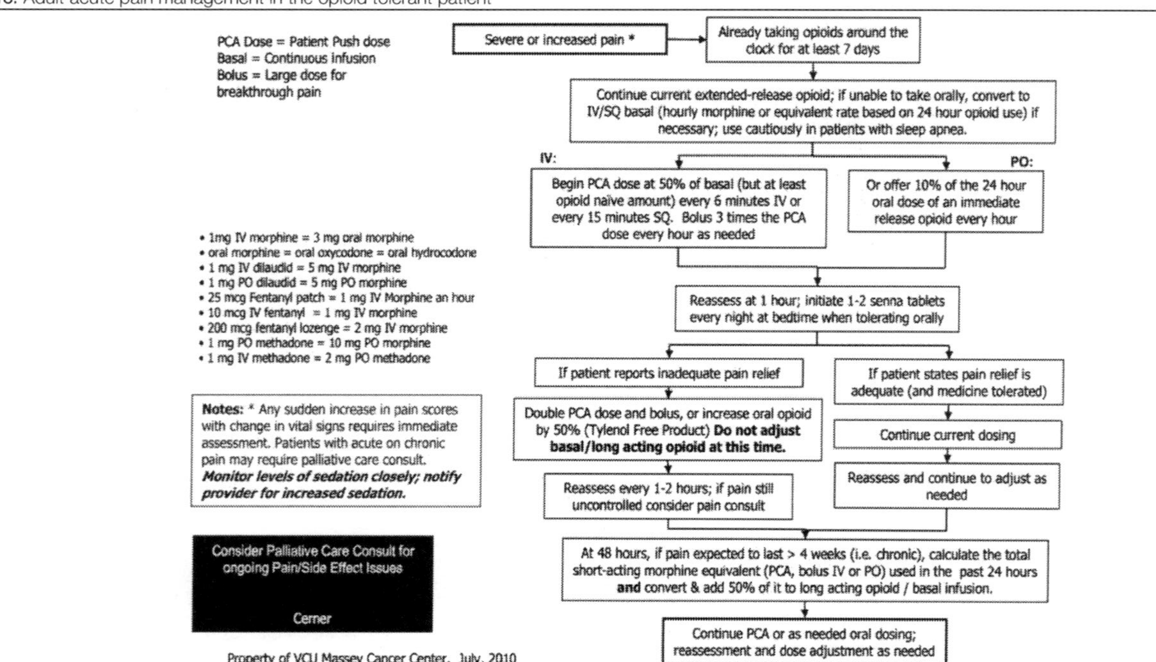

EQUIANALGESIC OPIOID CHART

Drug Name	Equianalgesic Dose		Oral→Parental Ratio	Dosing Interval (Hrs)	Strength (Cr, Ir) Btp = Break Through Pain Cr = Chronic Release Ir = Immediate Release
	ORAL (MG)	IV (MG)			
<u>Morphine</u>	30	10	3:1	CR 12	MS Contin 15, 30, 60, 100, 200mg tab Oramorph 15, 30, 60, 100mg tab
	30	10	3:1	IR 4	MSIR, Roxanol, RMS - tab, liq, supp
<u>Hydromorphone</u>	7.5	1.5	5:1	IR 4	Dilaudid 1,2,3,4 mg tab, liq, sup
<u>Oxycodone</u>	30	N/A	N/A	CR 12	Oxycontin 10,20,40,80mg q8h or q12h Roxicodone, OxyIR, OxyFast (brand names) Percocet and Roxicet contain Oxy+Acetominphen (BTP) All available in tab/liq form
<u>Hydrocodone</u>	30	N/A	N/A	N/A	Vicodin (hydrocodone, acetaminophen) Vicodin 5 (5/500) Vicodin 7.5 (7.5/750) Vicodin 10 (10/660)
<u>Codeine</u>	200	130	1.5:1	N/A	15,20,60mg Tabs Doses exceeding 65mg not recommended d/t ↑ constipation

Meperidine	300	75	4:1	N/A	Demerol 50,100mg tabs, syrup Not recommended for use >48hrs or cancer mgmt.
Levorphanol	4	2	2:1	6-8	Levo-Dromoran 2mg tabs Long half-life: caution for accumulative s/e
Methadone			N/A	VARIABLE DURING TITRAT	5,10,40mg tabs, liq Very good for **neuropathic** pain, long ½ life
Fentanyl	Refer to conversion	Refer to conversion	N/A	72 HRS	Duragesic 25, 50, 75, 100 mcg Patch It is necessary to also use breakthrough medication

OPIOID CONVERSION

$$\frac{\text{CURRENT OPIOID (MG)}}{\text{24HR DOSE OF CURRENT}} = \frac{\text{DESIRED NEW OPIOID DOSE}}{\text{24 DOSE OF DESIRED OPIOID}}$$

OR

X RATIO ABOVE

IV-to-PO equivalents are approximations. Thus, the calculated PO equivalent may be too high, and the actual dose given to the patient should be reduced to 1/2 to 2/3 of the calculated PO dose. For instance, if a patient has received effective analgesia with 120 mg/d IV morphine, the equivalent dose of oral oxycodone is 240 mg/d PO. 2/3 of this amount is 180 mg/d PO. This amount can be given in divided doses in q3h intervals and use of sustained-release oxycodone for 1/3 to 1/2 of the total daily dose may be considered. Further dose adjustment should be made based on patient response

WOUND CARE

- **Skin/Wound Care**[4]
  - Overview of Anatomy
    - *Epidermis*
    - *Dermis* – goal to maintain sebum layer (acts as acid mantle); avascular in nature
    - *Adipose tissue*
  - Risk Factors
    - *Advanced Age* – thinning of dermal layer; loss of rete ridges; ↓sebum production
    - *DM*
    - *Smoking* (vasoconstriction inhibits delivery of healing products to site of injury)
    - ↓*Nutrition* (albumin, prealbumin, transferritin)
  - Stages of Infection
    - Wound considered contaminated if left open for >24 hours → leads to colonization which will compete with host for O2, nutrients → infection (tissue biopsy > 100,000 organisms)
      - To obtain culture, clean wound thoroughly and compress tissue to express drainage then culture that drainage
      - Look for change from healthy pink granulation tissue to pale, white
  - Surgical Healing
    - Primary
    - Secondary – keep open to air, let heal from bottom up
    - Tertiary – keep open, delayed primary closure

Wound closure timelines

Location	Suture type	Technique	Timeline for Removal
Scalp	3-0/4-0 nylon or polypropylene	Interrupted in galea, tight single layer in scalp, use horizontal mattress to control bleeding	7-12 d
Ear	5-0 vicryl/dexon in perichondrium	Close perichondrium with interrupted Vicryl; use nylon for skin	3-5 d
Eyebrow	4-0/5-0 vicryl (SQ) 6-0 for skin	Layered	3-5 d
Eyelid	6-0 nylon	Single-layer horizontal mattress or simple interrupted	3-5 d
Lip	4-0 vicryl (mucosa) 5-0 vicryl (muscle) 6-0 nylon (skin)	Must close three layers if involving lip; all others do 2 layers	3-5 d
Perioral	4-0 vicryl	Single interrupted or horizontal mattress if muscularis of tongue involved	N/A
Face	6-0 nylon (skin) 5-0 vicryl (SQ)	Simple interrupted for single layer but use layered closure for full-thickness lac	3-5 d

Trunk	4-0 vicryl (SQ, fat) 4-0/5-0 nylon (skin)	Single or layered closure	7-12 d
Extremity	3-0/4-0 vicryl (SQ, muscle) 4-0/5-0 nylon (skin)	Single-layer interrupted or vertical mattress Use a splint if over a joint	10-14 d
Hand/Foot	4-0/5-0 nylon	Single-layer closure Use simple interrupted or horizontal mattress sutures Use a splint if over a joint	7 -12 d
Nail	5-0 vicryl	Ensure you maintain even edges Allow sutures to dissolve	N/A

- Wound Healing
    - *Principles*
        - Balance Moisture (use dressing to prevent excessive saturation)
            - ↑ hydration with hydrogel, amorphous gels, sheets
            - ↑ absorption with alginates, foams, gauze
        - Thermoregulation (warm environment)
        - Manage bacteria load through debridement
            - Silver, honey
        - Protect peri-wound skin (edges→6cm) to ↓ excessive moisture
    - *Partial*
        - Painful
        - Partial regeneration healing
    - *Full*
        - Involves subcutaneous layer and beyond
        - Scar will form
        - Takes 4-12 weeks
- Principles of Topical Therapy
    - D = debride
    - I = identify and treat infection
    - P = lightly pack dead space
    - A = absorb excess exudates
    - M = moist wound surface
    - O = open wound edges
    - P = protect from infection and trauma
    - I = insulate
- Treatment
    - *Skin Tear*
        - **Category 1** (<=1mm between edges): appx edges from R→L with moisten cue tip and keep appx with Mepitel contact layer; keep on for 14 days
        - **Category 2** (>1mm between edges): epidermal flap still viable thus do not trim edges; place mepilex lite (if ↑drainage then go for mepilex)
        - **Category 3** (loss of epidermal flap): use mepilex borderline (can cut in half) vs. mepilex border (integrated therefore do not cut in half!) → keep in place for 7 days or if >75% saturated

- **Pressure Ulcers**
    - *Information Source: AHRQ, NDNQI training, woundsource.com*
    - Localized injury over bony prominent of the skin as a result of pressure as a combination of shear and friction

- Pathophysiology - Tissue load exceeds capillary closing pressure → ischemia → ↑O2 deprivation → trapping of metabolic waste leading to inflammatory reaction and necrosis
- Actual wound is larger as you get closer to bone/muscle (cone shape area of damage)
- Shear is the biggest factor leading to pressure ulcers (friction + gravity). Most prominent if HOB>30 degrees because it forces body to slide down (↑friction against bed)
- Documentation
  - Length (head→toe), Width (hip→hip), Depth
  - Wound Bed (color, adipose tissue)
- Points
  - Back of Head (occiput)
  - Shoulder
  - Base of spine
  - Inner Knees
  - Elbow
  - Buttocks (sacrum, coccyx)
  - Heal
  - Toes
- At Risk For Pressure Ulcers
  - Use Braden Scale (<18 → at risk)
- Types
  - "Pressure Ulcer Stage (I-IV)"
  - "Deep Tissue Injury"
  - "Incontinent Associated Dermatitis"
  - "Moisture Associated Skin Damage"
  - "Eschar/Necrosis C/W Partial (or Full) Thickness Wound"
- Treatment
  - *Debridement*
    - Autolysis
    - Biological (maget)
    - Hydrotherapy (used in the OR)
    - Chemical (collagenase, Skintegrity Hydrogel)
    - Mechanical (wet→dry, ultrasonic mist)
    - Sharp
    - Hyperosmolar (Medihoney)
- Prevention
  - ReadyBath Wipes
  - Trapeze bar
  - Optimize hydration
  - Specialized bed
  - Prevalon Boot (confirm you can see heal through opening)
  - Use foam wedges to prop patient at 30 degree angles
  - Daily walking
  - Patient Education (Krames, WiredMd, NPP 40-23)
- Tips for Wound Care Options
  - **Eschar:**
    - If on heel and no infection, leave on→biologic dressing
    - If on sacrum or has pus under it→debride
  - **Venous Stasis Ulcers:** Adaptic with Kerlix or nonadhesive foams, consider compression (ace wraps)
  - **Incontinence Assoc Dermatitis:** Calmoseptine, add antifungal (Microgaurd) if needed
  - **Friction Rub/Skin Tears:** Tegaderm Absorbent or Adaptic with Kerlix
  - **Diabetic/Arterial Ulcers that are dry/calloused:** SoloSite Wound Gel (adds moisture)
  - **Necrotic Tissue:** Mechanical/chemical debridement (sharp, wet-to-dry, whirlpool) to remove biofilm and dead tissue

    - **Whirlpool:** Mechanical debridement, stop when necrotic tissue gone, and pink appears
    - **Wound Vacc:** placed by PT, wound care or surgery; very expensive
- **Staging of Pressure Ulcers**
  - **DTI:** Deep Tissue Injury, soft, intact, purple/maroon, painful
  - **Stage I:** intact skin, non-blanching erythema, painful
  - **Stage II:** Partial thickness, loss of dermis, pink wound bed, ruptured blister, no depth
  - **Stage III:** Full thickness, Subcutaneous fat visible, has depth
  - **Stage IV:** Full thickness tissue loss with exposure of bone or muscle
- **Lower Extremity Ulcers**
- **Nutrition**
- **Consult**
  - Inpatient and Outpatient consults available, through Dept of Surgery
- **Products**
  - <u>Dressing Selection</u>
    - Absorption (Alginate) – made from seaweed, highly absorptive, forms a gel to easily remove
    - Protective (Ionic Silver, Mepilex Border) – act as mechanical barriers, remove after 70% saturation, remove after 7 days
    - Wet to dry – not standard therapy, high moisture transmission with no bacterial protection.
  - **Wound VAC** – creates negative pressure environment to ↑ wound contraction and approximation, cannot have >20% necrotic tissue in wound bed
  - **Calmoseptine Ointment:** Moisture barrier, good for stool incontinence (add Micro guard) good around PEG tubes; less expensive
  - **Micro guard Powder:** Antifungal, mix with Calmoseptine; less expensive and easier to use than Nystatin
  - **Santyl:** Chemical debrider
  - **Curasalt/Aginate:** Hypertonic solutions for Wet-to-Dry with absorbent properties
  - **Tegaderm Absorbent:** Good for skin tears, Stage II, can see through it to monitor wound
  - **Replicare:** Same as Duoderm; Stage II, opaque, can't see through it
  - **Adaptic & Kerlix:** Skin tears, weeping, venous stasis ulcers, needs changed daily
  - **Allevyn Adhesive Foam:** Absorbent; for moist ulcer/ Stage II
  - **Vasolex/Xenaderm:** Ointment, moisture barrier from urine; more expensive than Calmoseptine
  - **Sage Barrier Wipes:** Used to clean pt, has protective moisture barrier ingredients
  - **Solosite would gel:** Adds moisture to dry, calloused areas
  - **Unna Boot:** For compressions such as venous stasis ulcers; watch for compromised circulation, avoid in PAD, only use MWF (not every day)
  - **Tubifast** compression stockings to help prevent/treat skin tears
- **Outpatient Products**
  - Honey
  - Desitin: for irritation d/t stool
  - Sween Cream: Good OTC moisture barrier, not expensive
  - Calmoseptine Samples: Call 800-800-3405

FORMULAS

Electrolytes

Na+ (corrected for hyperglycemia):
Corrected Na+ = measured Na+ + [(glucose - 100) x 0.024].

Ca++ (corrected for hypoalbuminemia):
Corrected Ca++ = [(4 - serum albumin) x 0.8] + measured Ca++.

Free Water Deficit:
Water deficit = wt (kg) x k x [(plasma Na+ / 140) - 1];
where k = 0.5 for males and 0.4 for females.

Osmolality:
Calculated Osm = (2 x Na+) + (glucose / 18) + (BUN / 2.8) + (EtOH / 4.6)
{normal 270-290}

Osm gap = measured Osm - calculated Osm {normal < 10}.
>10 is abnormal: caused by renal failure, methanol, ethylene glycol, sorbitol, mannitol, isopropanol, radiocontrast dye.

<u>Creatinine Clearance</u>

- Medications are dosed based on creatinine clearance, not GFR.
- To calculate CrCl:

$$\frac{(140-age)\times IBW}{72\times SCr}$$ = ml/min (if female, multiply by 0.85)

<u>Anion Gaps</u>

- Serum AG = [Na+] - [Cl-] - [HCO3] {normal 10-14}.
  - Corrected AG (for hypoalbuminemia):
    Corrected AG = serum AG + [(4 - serum albumin) x 2.5]   OR   albumin x 3
- Delta Gap (DAG) = (AG - 12) + HC03 {normal 23-30}.
  - DAG >30: concomitant metabolic alkalosis (excessively high HCO3).
  - DAG <23: concomitant non-AG metabolic acidosis (excessively low HCO3).
- Urine AG = U[Na+] + U[K+] - U[Cl-]
  NH4+ is the major unmeasured cation, so a strongly negative UAG suggests high urine NH4+.
  - Urine AG <0: GI HCO3 loss.
  - Urine AG >0: Renal HCO3 loss (RTA).

Critical Care

- Oxygenation Index
  Calculates oxygenation index, useful for predicting outcome especially in pediatric patients.
  (F_iO_2 * Mean Airway Pressure) / P_aO_2
- King's College Criteria for Acetaminophen Toxicity
  Provides lab-based recommendations for who should be immediately referred for liver transplant after acetaminophen overdose.
  - Lactate > 3.5 mg/dL (0.39 mmol/L) 4 hrs after early fluid resuscitation?
  - pH < 7.30 or lactate > 3 mg/dL (0.33 mmol/L) after full fluid resuscitation at 12 hours
  - INR > 6.5 (PTT > 100s)
  - Creatinine > 3.4 mg/dL (300 µmol/L)
  - Grade 3 or 4 Hepatic Encephalopathy?
  - Phosphorus > 3.75 mg/dL (1.2 mmol/L) at 48 hours

Nephrology

- CrCl
  [(140-age) x Wt in kg] / (Serum Cr x 72) (For ♀: result x 0.85)
- FeNa
  [(UrineNa x PlasmaCr) / (PlasmaNa x UrineCr)] x 100
  - <1% = prerenal; >2% = intrinsic renal etiology (ATN)
  - for FeUrea (pts on diuretics), substitude Urea for Na in equation
  - FeUrea <30% = prerenal; >50% = intrinsic (ATN)

ELECTROLYTES

POTASSIUM CHLORIDE

Etiology[363]

U_K Gradient = Urine Potassium (meq/L) × 100 [(mg × L)/(dL × g)] ÷ Urine Creatinine (mg/dL)

>20: kidney potassium wasting (ie. Lasix)

<20: extrarenal losses (ie. diarrhea, obstruction)

IV Replacement

Central line: 20 mEq/hr max rate

Peripheral line: 10 mEq/hr max rate

Hyperkalemia

- Etiology - acidosis, ↓insulin, beta-blockers, digoxin, ARF, heparin, K-sparing diuretics, NSAIDS, ACE-i
- Workup - EKG (peaked T waves, ↑PR interval, ↑QRS, sine wave), ABG, CK, digoxin level, review meds
- Treatment
  - Calcium gluconate 1-2 amps
  - Bicarb 1-3 amps bolus over several minutes or in D5W
  - Insulin 10-15U regular insulin
  - Glucose 1 amp D50
  - Kayexalate 40g in 25-50cc 70% sorbitol q2-4h
  - Lasix 40mg IV
  - Albuterol 10-20mg nebulizer

K>4 mEq/L	Give Nothing
K 3.5-4.0 mEq/L	Peripheral: 20 mEq KAl over 2 hours Central: 20 mEq KAl over 1 hours
K 3.1-3.4 mEq/L	Peripheral: 40 mEq KAl over 4 hours Central: 40 mEq KAl over 2 hours
K 2.5-3.0 mEq/L	Peripheral: 60 mEq KAl over 6 hours Central: 60 mEq KAl over 3 hours
K <2.5 mEq/L	Peripheral: 80 mEq KAl over 8 hours Central: 80 mEq KAl over 4 hours
Enteral Replacement (KAl)	
K>4 mEq/L	Give Nothing
K 3.5-4.0 mEq/L	20 mEq KAl
K 3.1-3.4 mEq/L	40 mEq KAl
K 2.5-3.0 mEq/L	40 mEq KAl now then 20mEq in 2 hours
K <2.5 mEq/L	40 mEq KAl now then another 40mEq in 2 hours, consider IV replacement

MAGNESIUM

Infuse each gram over 1 hour; Milk of Magnesia provides the most elemental Mg then MgCl is the second best option. PO options include MgOH tablet 400-800mg daily or MOM 24% concentrate susp 10cc (1001 mg of elemental Mg/82 mEq)

>= 1.5 mEq	Do Nothing
1-1.5	2gm MgSO4 IV in 100cc of D5W or NS over 2 hours
<1	4gm MgSO4 IV in 250cc of D5W or NS over 4 hours

CALCIUM

>7.5mmEq	Do Nothing
0.85-1	Check iCa... <u>IV Replacement</u> - If >0.8mMol/L → Do Nothing - If <0.8, give 1gm Calcium Gluconate in 50aa D5W over 30 minutes or 2g in 100cc over 1 hour in D5W <u>Oral Replacement</u> - Calcium carbonate 1250-2500mg (500-1000mg elemental Ca) PO TID-QID
<0.85	3 grams Calcium Gluconate IV in 100 mL of D5W or NS over 2 hours

PHOSPHATE

If K+ <4.0 mEq/L	
<u>PO_4 1-2 mg/dl</u>	Peripheral: 30 mmol KPO4 (contains 44mEq of K+) in 500aa NS over 6 hrs
	Central: 30 mmol KPO4 (contains 44mEq of K+) in 100aa NS over 6 hrs
	Enteral: Use equivalent neutraphos packets (1 packet = 8mmol PO4; 7mmEq Na, 7mmEq K+) → 3 packets
<u>PO_4 <1 mg/dl</u>	30 mmol KPO_4 (contains 44mEq of K+) q6h x 2 Check labs 1 hour after completion of last bag
If K+ >4.0 mEq/L	
<u>PO_4 1-2 mg/dl</u>	30 mmol $NaPO_4$ (contains 44mEq of K+) in 250aa NS over 6 hrs
<u>PO_4 <1 mg/dl</u>	30 mmol $NaPO_4$ (infused over 6 hrs) q6h x 2 Check labs 1 hour after completion of last bag
	Enteral: Use equivalent neutraphos packets (1 packet = 8mmol PO4; 7mmEq Na, 7mmEq K+)

HYPERPHOSPHATEMIA IN DIALYSIS PATIENTS

Steps to follow	
<u>1</u>	Restrict dietary intake by 900mg/d
	If Ca < 9.5: calcium carbonate or acetate
	If Ca > 9.5: Sevelamer or Lanthum
<u>2</u> (if PO4 remains high despite #1)	Check PTH and If PTH>300pg/mL then
	PO4<5.5 & Aa <9.5: Vitamin D analog
	PO4<5.5 & Aa >9.5: Cinacalcet

	PO4>5.5: Cinacalcet

- **Goals In Dialysis Patients:**
  - Ca: 8.4-9.5 mg/dL
  - PO4: 3.5-5.5 mg/dL
  - PTH: 150-300

ABBREVIATIONS

Ab ......antibody
AACG......acute angle closure glaucoma
ABC ......airway, breathing, and circulation
ABG .....arterial blood gas
ACEi .....angiotensin-converting enzyme inhibitor
ACS ....acute coronary syndrome
ADH .....antidiuretic hormone
AF ....atrial fibrillation
AFB ......acid-fast bacillus
Ag ....antigen
AIDS ....acquired immunodeficiency syndrome
AKI ....acute kidney injury
ALKP ......alkaline phosphatase
ANA .....antinuclear antibody
ANCA ...antineutrophil cytoplasmic antibody
APTT ....activated partial thromboplastin time
ARB .....angiotensin II receptor blocker
ARDS ...acute respiratory distress syndrome
AS ....aortic stenosis
AST ......aspartate transaminase
ATN ......acute tubular necrosis
AV ....atrioventricular
BAL ......bronchoalveolar lavage
BKA .....below-knee amputation
BNP ......brain natriuretic peptide
BP ....blood pressure
BPH ......benign prostatic hyperplasia
CA ....cancer
CABG ...coronary artery bypass graft
CI ....contraindications
CKD ......chronic kidney disease
CMV .....cytomegalovirus
CNS ......central nervous system
COPD ....chronic obstructive pulmonary disease
CPAP ....continuous positive airway pressure
CPR ......cardiopulmonary resuscitation
CRP ......c-reactive protein
CSF ......cerebrospinal fluid
CT ....computed tomography
CVA ......cerebrovascular accident
CVP ......central venous pressure
CXR ......chest x-ray
D/C......discharge
DM ....diabetes mellitus
DVT ......deep venous thrombosis
EKG/ECG......electrocardiogram
EEG ......electroencephalogram
EMG .....electromyogram
ERCP ....endoscopic retrograde cholangiopancreatography
ESR ......erythrocyte sedimentation rate
FEV1 .....forced expiratory volume in 1st sec
FiO2 ....partial pressure of O2 in inspired air
FFP ......fresh frozen plasma
FLQ ......fluoroquinolone
FSH ......follicle-stimulating hormone
FVC ......forced vital capacity
g ....gram
G6PD ....glucose-6-phosphate dehydrogenase
GCS ......Glasgow Coma Scale
GFR ......glomerular fi ltration rate
GGT ......gamma-glutamyl transferase
Hb ....haemoglobin
HbA1c .glycated haemoglobin
Hct ......hematocrit
HCV ......hepatitis C virus
HDL ......high-density lipoprotein
HIV ......human immunodefi ciency virus
HSV ......herpes simplex virus
IBD ......inflammatory bowel disease
ICD ......implantable cardiac defi brillator
ICP ....intracranial pressure
ICUP....ICU panel / Metabolic Panel
IDDM ...insulin-dependent diabetes mellitus
INR ......international normalized ratio
IVC ......inferior vena cava
JVP ......jugular venous pressure
K ....potassium
kg ....kilogram
L ....liter
LA.......left atrium of the heart
LAD ....left axis deviation on the ECG
LBBB ....left bundle branch block
LDH ......lactate dehydrogenase
LDL ......low-density lipoprotein
LFT ......liver function test
LH ....luteinizing hormone
LMN .....lower motor neuron
LMWH ..low-molecular-weight heparin
LOC ......loss of consciousness
LP ....lumbar puncture
LUQ ......left upper quadrant
LV ....left ventricle of the heart
LVH ......left ventricular hypertrophy

MAP .....mean arterial pressure
MCV .....mean cell volume
mg ......milligram
MI ....myocardial infarction
mmHg... millimetres of mercury
MRCP ...magnetic resonance cholangiopancreatography
MRI ......magnetic resonance imaging
MRSA ...meticillin-resistant Staph. aureus
MS ....multiple sclerosis
MSM ....men who have sex with men
NA........not applicable
NIDDM .non-insulin-dependent diabetes mellitus
NSAID ..non-steroidal anti-infl ammatory drug
OCP ......oral contraceptive pill
PaCO2 ...partial pressure of CO2 in arterial blood
PaO2 .....partial pressure of O2 in arterial blood
PCR ......polymerase chain reaction
PE ....pulmonary embolism
PEEP ....positive end-expiratory pressur
PET ......positron emission tomography
PMH .....past medical history
PRN......as needed
PSA ......prostate-specifi c antigen
PTH ......parathyroid hormone
PTT ......prothrombin time
PTX......pneumothorax
PUD.....peptic ulcer disease
PVD ......peripheral vascular disease
RA.......right atrium of the heart
RAD .....right axis deviation on the ECG
RBBB ...right bundle branch block
RBC ......red blood cell
RCT ......randomized controlled trial
RDW ....red cell distribution width
RUQ .....right upper quadrant
R/O ......rule out
RTA......renal tubular acidosis
RV ....right ventricle of heart
RVF ......right ventricular failure
RVH ......right ventricular hypertrophy
S1, S2 ....fi rst and second heart sounds
SC ....subcutaneous
SE ....side-effect
SIADH ..syndrome of inappropriate anti-diuretic hormone secretion
SL ....sublingual
SLE ......systemic lupus erythematosus
SOB ......short of breath
SpO2 ....peripheral oxygen saturation (%)
STD/I ...sexually transmitted disease/infection
SVC ......superior vena cava
SVT ......supraventricular tachycardia
T3 ....tri-iodothyronine
T4 ....thyroxine
TFT ......thyroid function test
TIA ......transient ischaemic attack
TIBC ....total iron-binding capacity
TPN ......total parenteral nutrition
TSH ......thyroid-stimulating hormone
TTP ......thrombotic thrombocytopenic purpura
U ....units
UC ....ulcerative colitis
UMN .....upper motor neuron
URT ..upper respiratory tract
US....ultrasound
UTI ......urinary tract infection
VF ....ventricular fibrillation
V/Q ....ventilation/perfusion scan
VTach ....ventricular tachycardia
VTE ......venous thromboembolism
WBC ....white blood cell

APPENDIX

COMMON OUTPATIENT CONDITIONS AND TREATMENT

Bloating

- Nexium 20mg daily
- Simethicone 40-360 mg after meals and qhs prn
- Dicyclomine
- Probiotics (Lactobacillus)

Indigestion

- Maalox 30 ml PO Q 4 hours prn indigestion
- Avoid in dialysis pts
- $CaCO_3$ (Tums) 2 tablets PO
- Safe in dialysis pts
- Zantac 150 mg PO BID prn indigestion
- GI Cocktail (Benmalid 15cc; combo of Maalox, viscous lidocaine, Benadryl), give with Toradol 15mg

Dry Eyes

- Liquitears (1-2 drops into eye(s) prn to relieve sx)
- HCMP (1-2 drops per eye prn q6h or qhs)
- Tears Naturale (1-2 drops into eye(s) prn to relieve sx)
- Fish oil
- Polyvinyl alcohol 1.4% 1 drop OU q4h prn
- PEG/PG 0.4/0.3% (Systane) 1 drop OU q4h prn
- Lacri Lube ophthalmic ointment thin ribbon to both eyes Q6H

Hiccups

- Baclofen10mg po Q8H prn.
- Chlorpromazine 25mg po Q6H prn.
- Metoclopramide 10mg PO or IV Q6H prn

Mucolytics

- Mucomyst
- Pulmozyme

Nausea/Vomiting

- Alcohol pads (smelling)
- Zofran 4 mg IV Q 4 hours prn nausea
- Phenergan 25 mg IV/IM or 50mg PO Q 4 hours prn N/V
  - Use lower doses in elderly d/t increase side effects
  - Watch for dystonic reactions and restlessness
- Reglan 10 mg IV/PO Q 6 hours prn N/V
  - Avoid in bowel obstruction or diarrhea b/c stimulates gut motility
  - Consider risk of Extrapyramidal Symptoms

- Given Benadryl concurrently to ↓ risk
  - Document you discussed risk with patient
  - If EPS develops, give Cogentin
- Tigan 250 mg po tid/qid or 200 mg im/pr q 6-8h
- Compazine 10 mg IM/IV/PO/PR Q 6 hours prn Nausea
- Scopolamine 1.5mg patch behind ear q3d
- Meclizine 25 mg PO 4 times daily
  - For N/V d/t motion sickness & vertigo
- Zyprexa 10mg QHS - used by heme/onc

Oral Ulcers

- Triamcinolone 0.1% dental paste

Pruitis

- Benadryl 25-50 mg PO/IV Q 4 hours
  - Avoid or reduce dose in elderly
- Hydroxyzine 25-100 mg PO/IM Q 6 hours
  - Avoid in elderly, can't be given IV
- Cholestyramine 4g BID-TID
- Ursodiol

Secretions

- Atropine ophthalmic solution 1% 2gtts SL Q4H prn
- Glycopyrrolate (Robinul) 0.4mg IV Q6H prn
- Scopolamine patch 1.5mg behind the ear Q3days

QUALIFYING FOR HOME OXYGEN

- **Conditions**
  - Physician determines patient suffers from severe lung disease or hypoxia-related symptoms that may improve with oxygen.
  - Patient's arterial blood gas indicates a need for oxygen:
    - Continuous Oxygen
      - PaO2 < 55 mmHg or O2 sat < 88% at rest
      - PaO2 56-59 mmHg or O2 sat ≥ 89% AND dependent edema suggesting CHF OR pulmonary hypertension/cor pulmonale (measured PA pressure, echocardiogram, P pulmonale on EKG→P wave > 3 mm in leads II, III, or aVF)
    - Nocturnal oxygen therapy only if
      - PaO2 < 55 mmHg or O2 sat < 88% while asleep AND PaO2 > 56 mmHg or O2 sat > 89% while awake
      - PaO2 ↓ > 10 mmHg, Resting PaO2 ≤ 59 mmHg or O2 sat ↓ > 5% from waking to sleeping or SaO2 ≤ 89% AND cor pulmonale or erythrocytosis (HCT>55%)
    - Exercise oxygen therapy only if:
      - PaO2 < 55 mmHg or O2 sat < 88% during activity for a patient with PaO2 > 56 mmHg or O2 sat > 89% during the day at rest, and it is documented that use of oxygen improves hypoxemia with exercise
    - Alternative treatment measures have been tried or considered and have failed

CERVICAL CANCER SCREENING

- **Pap Smear Procedure**
  - Sampling – when using the *broom-like device*, place central bristles into the endocervical canal and *rotate clockwise 5 times.* Then, if using the *endocervical brush*, place brush so that the bristles closest to the examiner are inserted to the level of the external cervical os. Then *rotate in 180 degrees in one direction*.

TOBACCO ABUSE

- **General**
  - Quitting smoking by age 50 cuts the risk of a smoking-related death in half and quitting by age 30 almost completely negates it.
  - Nicotine patches are contraindicated at the time of acute coronary syndrome, malignant arrhythmia, CHF exacerbation, pregnancy.
- **Treatment Options By Success Rate**[364,365]
  - Highly nicotine-dependent smokers may require initial therapy for 6 months or longer. Some individuals may require low-dose maintenance therapy for years.

Smoking Cessation Options			
Therapy	Prescription	Other Info	Side Effects
Chantix	• Days 1-3: 0.5 mg/day. Days 4-7: 0.5 mg twice a day. • Day 8+: 1 mg twice a day. • Use 3-6 months.	• Start 1-4 weeks before quit date. • Take with food and a tall glass of water to minimize nausea. • Quit date can be flexible, from 1 week to 3 months **after** starting drug. • Dual action: relieves nicotine withdrawal and blocks reward of smoking.	Nausea, insomnia, abnormal dreams, neuropsych sx?
Patch	Starting dose • 21 mg for ≥10 cigarettes per day. • 14 mg for <10 cigarettes per day. • After 6 weeks, option to taper to lower doses for 2-6 weeks. • Use ≥3 months. • After 6 weeks, continue original dose or taper to lower doses (either option acceptable).	• Apply a new patch each morning to dry skin. • Rotate application site to avoid skin irritation. • May start patch before or on quit date. • Can add prn gum, lozenge, inhaler, or nasal spray to patch to cover situational cravings.	• Skin irritation • Trouble sleeping • Vivid dreams (patch can be removed at bedtime to manage insomnia or vivid dreams)
Patch+Nortryptiline	(OFF LABEL) 75-100mg/d for 12-14wk	Good if co-morbid depression present	↑QT interval, drowsiness, dry mouth
Wellbutrin	• 150 mg/day for 3 days, then 150 mg twice a day. • Use 3-6 months.	Start 1-2 weeks before quite date: May lessen post-cessation weight gain while drug is being taken.	Insomnia, dry mouth, seizures, neuropsych sx?
Transdermal Patch	• If smoke more than 10 cigarettes/day	21mg: >10 cig/d 14mg: ≤10 cig/d	skin irritation, insomnia

	○ 21-mg/day patch for the first 4-6 weeks then taper by 7mg at 2wk intervals • <u>If smoke less than 10 cigarettes/day</u> ○ 14-mg/day patch for the first 4-6 weeks then taper by 7mg at 2wk intervals		
<u>Gum</u>	• If 1st cigarette is ≤30 minutes of waking: 4 mg. • If 1st cigarette is >30 minutes of waking: 2 mg. • Use ≥3 months. • Patients are instructed to use 1 piece of gum every 1-2 hours for the first 6 weeks and then reduce their use to 1 piece every 2-4 hours for the next 3 weeks and finally to 1 piece every 4-8 hours for the 3 weeks after that. • In highly dependent smokers, the 4-mg gum is superior to the 2-mg gum. • Because about 50% of the nicotine in gum is absorbed, a smoker who is on a fixed schedule of 10 pieces per day will receive a daily nicotine dose	• Chew briefly until mouth tingles, then 'park' gum inside cheek until tingle fades. Repeat chew-and-park each time tingle fades. Discard gum after 30 minutes of use. • Use ~ 1 piece per hour (Max: 24/day). • Can damage dental work and be difficult to use with dentures. • No food or drink 15 minutes prior to use and during use.	Mouth soreness, dyspepsia

	of about 10 mg with the 2-mg gum and 20 mg with the 4-mg gum.		

INDEX

4

A

B

C

D

E

F

H

I

L

N

O

P

R

S

T

U

---

[1] Kane RL. Finding the Right Level of Posthospital Care: "We Didn't Realize There Was Any Other Option for Him". *JAMA.* 2011;305(3):284-293. doi:10.1001/jama.2010.2015

[2] Baile et al. "SPIKES-A six-step protocol for delivering bad news: application to the patient with cancer." Oncologist. 2000;5(4):302-11.

[3] Wijdicks EF. The diagnosis of brain death. N Engl J Med. 2001 Apr 19;344(16):1215-21.

[4] Mills, Crystal. "Night Call Survival Guide."

[5] Von Gunten, Charles F. "Discussing Do-Not-Resuscitate Status."THE ART OF ONCOLOGY: WHEN THE TUMOR IS NOT THE TARGET. Journal of Clinical Oncology, Vol 19, No 5 (March 1), 2001: pp 1576-1581

[6] Zaenglein, A. L., Pathy, A. L., Schlosser, B. J., Alikhan, A., Baldwin, H. E., Berson, D. S., ... Bhushan, R. (2016). Guidelines of care for the management of acne vulgaris. Journal of the American Academy of Dermatology, 74(5), 945–973.e33. doi:10.1016/j.jaad.2015.12.037

[7] Titus et al. "Diagnosis and Treatment of Acne." Am Fam Physician. 2012;86(8):734-740.

[8] Leyden et al. "Why Topical Retinoids Are Mainstay of Therapy for Acne." Dermatol Ther (Heidelb): 25 APR 2017.

[9] Wolff K, Johnson R, Saavedra AP. *Fitzpatrick's Color Atlas and Synopsis of Clinical Dermatology, 7e.* New York, NY: McGraw-Hill; 2013

[10] Alguire PC, Mathes BM. Skin biopsy techniques for the internist. J Gen Intern Med. 1998;13(1):47

[11] Silen W. (2012). Chapter 13. Abdominal Pain. In D.L. Longo, A.S. Fauci, D.L. Kasper, S.L. Hauser, J.L. Jameson, J. Loscalzo (Eds), *Harrison's Principles of Internal Medicine*, 18e. Retrieved April 29, 2012

[12] Runyon, Bruce. Management of Adult Patients with Ascites due to Cirrhosis: An Update. AASLD Practice Guidelines. 2009

[13] Bambha et al. "Model for End-stage Liver Disease (MELD)" UpToDate.com

[14] Rifai et al. "Bleeding esophageal varices: Who should receive a shunt?" *Cleveland Clinic Journal of Medicine*. 2017 March;84(3):199-201.

[15] ASGE. "The role of endoscopy in the management of variceal hemorrhage." Gastrointestinal Endoscopy. 80(2). 2014.

[16] Runyon BA; AASLD Practice Guidelines Committee. Management of adult patients with ascites due to cirrhosis: an update. Hepatology. 2009;49(6):2087-2107.

[17] Schneiderhan et al. "Targeting gut flora to treat and prevent disease." J Fam Pract. 2016 January;65(1):34-38.

[18] Ford et al. "American College of Gastroenterology Monograph on the Management of Irritable Bowel Syndrome and Chronic Idiopathic Constipation." Am J Gastroenterol 2014; 109:S2 – S26.

[19] Ruepert L Quartero AO de Wit NJ van der Heijden GJ Rubin G Muris JW Bulking agents, antispasmodics and antidepressants for the treatment of irritable bowel syndrome. Cochrane Database Syst Rev 2011 CD003460.

[20] Jamshed N, Lee ZE, Olden KW. "Diagnostic approach to chronic constipation in adults." Am Fam Physician. 2011 Aug 1;84(3):299-306.

[21] Wilkins T, McMechan D, Talukder A. "Colorectal Cancer Screening and Prevention." Am Fam Physician. 2018 May 15;97(10):658-665.

[22] Diarrhea, Acute. In: Papadakis MA, McPhee SJ, Bernstein J. eds. Quick Medical Diagnosis & Treatment 2018 New York, NY: McGraw-Hill; . http://accessmedicine.mhmedical.com/content.aspx?bookid=2273§ionid=178292926. Accessed March 13, 2018.

[23] MMWR. "Diagnosis and Management of Foodborne Illnesses." January 26, 2001 / 50(RR02);1-69.

[24] Diarrhea, Chronic. In: Papadakis MA, McPhee SJ, Bernstein J. eds. Quick Medical Diagnosis & Treatment 2018 New York, NY: McGraw-Hill; . http://accessmedicine.mhmedical.com/content.aspx?bookid=2273§ionid=178292959. Accessed March 13, 2018.

[25] Surawicz, Christina M. "Guidelines for Diagnosis, Treatment, and Prevention of Clostridium difficile Infections." Am J Gastroenterol 2013; 108:478–498; doi:10.1038/ajg.2013.4; published online 26 February 2013.

[26] McDonald et al. "Clinical Practice Guidelines for Clostridium difficile Infection in Adults and Children: 2017 Update by the Infectious Diseases Society of America (IDSA) and Society for Healthcare Epidemiology of America (SHEA)." Clinical Infectious Diseases: An Official Publication of the Infectious Diseases Society of America 2018 February 15.

[27] Shen NT et al. Timely use of probiotics in hospitalized adults prevents clostridium difficile infection: A systematic review with meta-regression analysis. Gastroenterology 2017 Feb 10; [e-pub].

[28] Roberts, M. A., Md, W. H., & Manian, F. A. (2018, November 02). How do you evaluate and treat a patient with C. difficile–associated disease? Retrieved from https://www.the-hospitalist.org/hospitalist/article/178718/gastroenterology/how-do-you-evaluate-and-treat-patient-c-difficile

[29] Jacobs, Danny. "Diverticulitis." N Engl J Med 2007;357:2057-66

[30] Gralnek et al. "Acute Lower Gastrointestinal Bleeding." N Engl J Med 2017; 376:1054-1063.

[31] Stanley AJ, Laine L, Dalton HR, Ngu JH, Schultz M, Abazi R, et al; International Gastrointestinal Bleeding Consortium. Comparison of risk scoring systems for patients presenting with upper gastrointestinal bleeding: international multicentre prospective study. BMJ. 2017;356:i6432.

[32] Chey WD, Wong BC; Practice Parameters Committee of the American College of Gastroenterology. American College of Gastroenterology guideline on the management of Helicobacter pylori infection. Am J Gastroenterol. 2007;102(8):1808-1825.

[33] Barkun et al. "International Consensus Recommendations on the Management of Patients With Nonvariceal Upper Gastrointestinal Bleeding." Ann Intern Med. 2010;152:101-113

[34] Kilgore et al. "Bowel preparation with split-dose polyethylene glycol before colonoscopy: a meta-analysis of randomized controlled trials." Gastrointest Endosc. 2011 Jun;73(6):1240-5.

[35] Clinical Practice and Economics Committee. "AGA Institute Medical Position Statement on Acute Pancreatitis." GASTROENTEROLOGY 2007;132:2019 –202162

[36] Baron, Todd. "Managing severe acute pancreatitis." CCJM. 80(6) June 2013

[37] Tenner at al. "American College of Gastroenterology Guideline: Management of Acute Pancreatitis." Am J Gastroenterol. July 2013.

[38] Conwell DL, Banks P, Greenberger NJ. Acute and Chronic Pancreatitis. In: Kasper D, Fauci A, Hauser S, Longo D, Jameson J, Loscalzo J. eds. *Harrison's Principles of Internal Medicine, 19e* New York, NY: McGraw-Hill; 2014. http://accessmedicine.mhmedical.com/content.aspx?bookid=1130§ionid=79749276. Accessed February 08, 2018.

[39] Trikudanathan et al. "Current Controversies in Fluid Resuscitation in Acute Pancreatitis." Pancreas. 41(6). August 2012

[40] Wu et al. "Lactated Ringer's Solution Reduces Systemic Inflammation Compared With Saline in Patients With Acute Pancreatitis." Clinical Gastroenterology And Hepatology 2011;9:710 –717

[41] De Waele et al. "Intra-abdominal Hypertension and Abdominal Compartment Syndrome." Am J Kidney Dis. 57(1):159-169.

[42] Tintinalli JE, Stapczynski JS, Cline DM, Ma OJ, Cydulka RK, Meckler GD. Chapter 86. Bowel Obstruction and Volvulus. In: Tintinalli JE, Stapczynski JS, Cline DM, Ma OJ, Cydulka RK, Meckler GD, eds. *Tintinalli's Emergency Medicine: A Comprehensive Study Guide*. 7th ed. New York: McGraw-Hill; 2011.

[43] AGA Institute. "American Gastroenterological Association Medical Position Statement on the Management of Gastroesophageal Reflux Disease." GASTROENTEROLOGY 2008;135:1383–1391.

[44] Katz et al. "Diagnosis and Management of Gastroesophageal Reflux Disease." *Am J Gastroenterol* 2013; 108:308–328.

[45] Davies et al. "Diagnosis and Management of Anorectal Disorders in the Primary Care Setting." Prim Care. 2017 Dec;44(4):709-720.

[46] Lanas, Angel et al. "Peptic ulcer disease." The Lancet , Volume 390 , Issue 10094 , 613 - 624

[47] Crowe et al. "*Treatment regimens for Helicobacter pylori.*" In: UpToDate, Basow, DS (Ed), UpToDate, Waltham, MA, 2012.

[48] Osama Siddique, Anais Ovalle, Ayesha S. Siddique, Steven F. Moss, Helicobacter Pylori Infection: an Update for the Internist in the Age of Increasing Global Antibiotic Resistance., The American Journal of Medicine (2018), https://doi.org/10.1016/j.amjmed.2017.12.024.

[49] Giannini et al. Liver enzyme alteration: a guide for clinicians. CMAJ. 2005 February 1; 172(3): 367–379.

[50] Oh, Robert C et al. "Mildly Elevated Liver Transaminase Levels: Causes and Evaluation." Am Fam Physician. 2017 Dec 1;96(11):709-715.

[51] Calderon et al. "Statins in the Treatment of Dyslipidemia in the Presence of Elevated Liver Aminotransferase Levels: A Therapeutic Dilemma." Mayo Clin Proc. 2010;85(4):349-356.

[52] Kopec, K. L., & Burns, D. (2011, October). Nonalcoholic fatty liver disease: A review of the spectrum of disease, diagnosis, and therapy. Retrieved from https://www.ncbi.nlm.nih.gov/pubmed/21947639

[53] Montgomery Family Practice Residency Program, Intern Guide 2005-6

[54] Mangrum JM, DiMarco JP. The evaluation and management of bradycardia. N Engl J Med 2000; 342:703-9.

[55] The Antimicrobial Stewardship Program. UCLA Health System.

[56] Roth et al. "Approach to the Adult Patientwith Fever of Unknown Origin." Am Fam Physician 2003;68:2223-8.

[57] Berthold, Jessica. "It's all about the history: Diagnosing fever of unknown origin." ACP Hospitalist. May. 2014.

[58] Baddour et al. "Cellulitis and Erysipelas." UpToDate.com

[59] Swartz, Morton N. Cellulitis. N Engl J Med 2004;350:904-12.

[60] Keller et al. "Distinguishing cellulitis from its mimics." CCJM. Vol 79 (8). 547-552.

[61] Thomas KS, Crook AM, Nunn AJ, et al; U.K. Dermatology Clinical Trials Network's PATCH I Trial Team. Penicillin to prevent recurrent leg cellulitis. N Engl J Med. 2013 May 2;368(18):1695-703. PMID: 23635049

[62] Lin et al. "The Evaluation and Management of Bacterial Meningitis Current Practice and Emerging Developments." The Neurologist 2010;16: 143–151.

[63] Johnson JR, Russo TA. "Acute Pyelonephritis in Adults." N Engl J Med. 2018 Jan 4;378(1):48-59.

[64] Baddour LM, Wilson WR, et. al. "Infective endocarditis: diagnosis, antimicrobial therapy, and management of complications: a statement for healthcare professionals from the Committee on Rheumatic Fever, Endocarditis, and Kawasaki Disease, Council on Cardiovascular Disease in the Young, and the Councils on Clinical Cardiology, Stroke, and Cardiovascular Surgery and Anesthesia, American Heart Association: endorsed by the Infectious Diseases Society of America." Circulation. 2005;111:e394.

[65] Infectious Diseases Society of America, Society of Critical Care Medicine, Society for Healthcare Epidemiology of America. Guidelines for the Management of Intravascular Catheter-Related Infections. Clinical Infectious Diseases. 2001;32:1249.

[66] DeSimone et al. Mayo Clin Pro. 2018.

· Haji, Showkat. Right Ventricular Infarction—Diagnosis and Treatment. Clin. Cardiol. 23, 473–482 (2000)

· Emergency Nurses Association (ENA). "Translation into Practice: Right-sided and Posterior ECGs." December 2012.

[69] Edhouse J, Brady WJ, Morris F. ABC of clinical electrocardiography: Acute myocardial infarction-Part II. BMJ. 2002; 324: 963-6.

· EKGS Made Simple: Bundle Branch Blocks" < https://sites.google.com/site/ekgsmadesimple/h-bundle-branch-blocks>

· MacKenzie, Ross M.D. "Poor R-Wave Progression" J Insur Med 2005;37:58–62

· American College of Physicians "In the Clinic: Heart Failure." Annals of Internal Medicine 1 June 2010

· Aurigemma, Gerard P. Diastolic Heart Failure. N Engl J Med 2004; 351:1097-1105September 9, 2004

[74] Nicklas et al. Heart Failure: Clinical Problem and Management Issues. Prim Care Clin Office Pract 40 (2013) 17–42

[75] Brown, Jennifer. "Acute Decompensated Heart Failure." Cardiol Clin 30 (2012) 665–671

[76] Cullington D, Goode KM, Clark AL, Cleland JG. Heart rate achieved or beta-blocker dose in patients with chronic heart failure: which is the better target? Eur J Heart Fail. 2012 May 22

[77] American College of Physicians "In the Clinic: Heart Failure." Annals of Internal Medicine 1 June 2010

[78] The American College of Cardiology and the American Heart Association Stages of Heart Failure

[79] Epocrates Online

[80] Evidence from the randomized, placebo- controlled CHARM (Candesartan Cilexitil [Atacand] in Heart Failure Assessment of Reduction in Mortality and Morbidity)- Alternative trial showed that the ARB candesartan decreased a combined end point of death from cardiovascular causes or hospitalization due to heart failure when compared with placebo in patients with left ventricular dysfunction who could not tolerate ACE inhibitors

[81] The CAPRICORN (Carvedilol Post-Infarct Survival Control in Left Ventricular Dysfunction) trial showed that the B-blocker carvedilol significantly reduced mortality in patients with left ventricular dysfunction with or without heart failure after MI and who also received ACE inhibitors, revascularization, and aspirin

[82] The MERIT-HF (Metoprolol CR/XL Randomized Intervention Trial-Heart Failure) randomly assigned 3991 patients with NYHA class II to IV heart failure to metoprolol CR/XL, up to 200 mg/d, versus placebo. All-cause mortality was reduced 34% (P < 0.001), and sudden death was reduced 59% (P < 0.001) for patients receiving metoprolol versus placebo

[83] Feenstra J et al. Association of nonsteroidal anti-inflammatory drugs with first occurrence of heart failure and with relapsing heart failure: The Rotterdam Study. Arch Intern Med 2002 Feb 11; 162:265-70.

[84] A-HeFT (African American Heart Failure Tri- al), which compared isosorbide plus hydralazine with placebo in African Americans with heart failure, showed that adding this therapy increased survival in those who were already taking other neurohormonal blockers, including ACE inhibitors and B-blockers

[85] ALES (Randomized Aldosterone Evaluation Study), a large, randomized, placebo- controlled trial involving 1663 patients with NYHA class III to IV heart failure on appropriate therapy with or without spironolactone, was halted 18 months early by the Data Safety Monitoring Board because there were significantly fewer deaths in the spironolactone group than in the placebo group (284 vs. 386 deaths; 35% reduction; P < 0.001)

[86] The CARE (Cholesterol and Recurrent Events) trial found that pravastatin significantly reduced the incidence of heart failure, subsequent cardiovascular events, and mortality.

[87] ACC/AHA/HRS 2008 Guidelines for Device-Based Therapy of Cardiac Rhythm Abnormalities: Executive Summary

[88] Falk, Erling. "The SHAPE Guideline: Ahead of Its Time or Just in Time?" Curr Atheroscler Rep 2006.

[89] Grundy SM et al. AHA/ACC/AACVPR/AAPA/ABC/ACPM/ADA/AGS/APhA/ASPC/NLA/PCNA guideline on the management of blood cholesterol: A report of the American College of Cardiology/American Heart Association Task Force on Clinical Practice Guidelines. J Am Coll Cardiol 2018 Nov 10; [e-pub].

[90] Raff et al. "SCCT guidelines on the use of coronary computed tomographic angiography for patients presenting with acute chest pain to the emergency department: A Report of the Society of Cardiovascular Computed Tomography Guidelines Committee." Journal of Cardiovascular CT. (2014). 254-271.

[91] Parikh et al. "Coronary artery calcium scoring: Its practicality and clinical utility in primary care." Cleveland Clinic Journal of Medicine. 2018 September;85(9):707-716.

[92] Lloyd-Jones DM, et al. J Am Coll Cardiol. 2017;70(14)1785-1822.

[93] Tota-Maharaj R, Defilippis AP, Blumenthal RS, Blaha MJ. A practical approach to the metabolic syndrome: review of current concepts and management. Curr Opin Cardiol. 2010;25(5):502-512

[94] Sharma M, Ansari MT, Abou-setta AM, Soares-Weiser K, Ooi TC, Sears M, et al., Systematic
Review: Comparative Effectiveness and Harms of Combinations of Lipid-Modifying Agents and High-Dose Statin Monotherapy. Ann. Int. Med. 2009;151.

[95] Gotto AM Jr. Management of lipid and lipoprotein disorders. In: Gotto AM Jr, Pownall HJ, eds. Manual of lipid disorders. Baltimore: Williams & Wilkins, 1992.

[96] Ahmed SM et al. Management of Dyslipidemia in Adults. Am Fam Physician. 1998 May 1;57(9):2192-2204, 2207-8.

[97] Yebyo et al. Ann Intern Med. 2019.

[98] Kang JH, Nguyen QN, Mutka J, Le QA. Rechallenging statin therapy in veterans with statin-induced myopathy post vitamin D replenishment. J Pharm Pract. 2016 Oct 24. pii: 0897190016674407. [Epub ahead of print]

[99] Snow V, Barry P, Fihn SD, et al. Primary care management of chronic stable angina and asymptomatic suspected or known coronary artery disease: A clinical practice guideline from the American College of Physicians. Ann Intern Med. 2004;141(7):562-567.

[100] Graham, Ian. "Diagnosing coronary artery disease—the Diamond and Forrester model revisited." Eur Heart J (2011)

[101] Stub D et al. Air versus oxygen in ST-segment–elevation myocardial infarction. *Circulation* 2015 Jun 16; 131:2143.

[102] O'Gara et al. "2013 ACCF/AHA Guideline for the Management of ST-Elevation Myocardial Infarction: Executive Summary: A Report of the American College of Cardiology Foundation/American Heart Association Task Force on Practice Guidelines." Circulation. 2013;127:529-555

[103] Spaulding CM, Joly LM, Rosenberg A, et al. Immediate coronary angiography in survivors of out-of-hospital cardiac arrest. N Engl J Med 1997; 336:1629-33.

[104] The ESPRIT Investigators. Novel dosing regimen of eptifibatide in planned coronary stent implantation (ESPRIT): a randomized, placebo-controlled trial. Lancet 2000;356:2037-44.
The PURSUIT trial investigators. Inhibition of platelet glycoprotein IIb/IIIa with eptifibatide in patients with acute coronary syndromes. N Engl J Med 1998;339:436-43.
Cohen M, Demers C, Gurfinkel E et al for the ESSENCE Trial. A comparison of lowmolecular-weight heparin with unfractionated heparin for unstable coronary artery disease. N
Engl J Med. 1997;337:447-52.
Grines CL, Browne KF, Marco J et al. A comparison of immediate angioplasty with thrombolytic therapy for acute myocardial infarction. (PAMI-1). N Engl J Med 1993;328:673-9.
Antman EM, Cohen M, Bernink PJ, McCabe CH, Horacek T, Papuchis G, Mautner B, Corbalan R, Radley D, Braunwald E. The TIMI risk score for unstable angina/non-ST elevation MI: A method for prognostication and therapeutic decision making. JAMA. 2000;284:835-842.).
Braunwald E, Antman EM, Beasley JW, Califf RM, Cheitlin MD, Hochman JS, Jones RH, Kereiakes D, Kupersmith J, Levin TN, Pepine CJ, Schaeffer JW, Smith EE III, Steward DE, Theroux P. ACC/AHA guideline update for the management of patients with unstable angina and non-ST-segment elevation myocardial infarction: a report of the American College of Cardiology/American Heart Association Task Force on Practice Guidelines (Committee on the Management of Patients with Unstable Angina). 2002. Available at: http://www.acc.org/clinical/guidelines/unstable/unstable.pdf.).
Tcheng JE. Clinical challenge of platelet glycoprotein IIb/IIIa receptor inhibitor therapy: Bleeding, reversal, thrombocytopenia, and retreatment. Am Heart J 2000;139:S38-S45.
Yusuf S, Zhao F, Mehta SR, Chrolavicius S, Tognoni G, Fox KK; The Clopidogrel in Unstable Angina to Prevent Recurrent Events Trial Investigators. Effects of clopidogrel in addition to aspirin in patients with acute coronary syndromes without ST-segment elevation. N Engl J Med 2001 Aug 16;345(7):494-502.
Packer M, Poole-Wilson PA, Armstrong PW, Cleland JG, Horowitz JD, Massie BM, Ryden L, Thygesen K, Uretsky BF. Comparative effects of low and high doses of the angiotensinconverting enzyme inhibitor, lisinopril, on morbidity and mortality in chronic heart failure. ATLAS Study Group. Circulation 1999 Dec 7;100(23):2312-8.

[105] 2011 ACCF/AHA Focused Update of the Guidelines for the Management of Patients With Unstable Angina/Non-ST-Elevation Myocardial Infarction.

[106] Widmer et al. "The Evolving Face of Myocardial Reperfusion in Acute Coronary Syndromes: A Primer for the Internist." Mayo Clinic Proceedings , Volume 93 , Issue 2 , 199 – 216.

[107] MIAMI trial research group

[108] Mandrola John. "Beta-Blockade After MI: No Practice Should Be Set in Stone ." Medscape. September, 13, 2018.

[109] GISSI-3. Lancet. 1994, 343: 1115-1122

[110] Hunt SA, Abraham WT, Chin MH, et al. 2009 Focused update incorporated into the ACC/AHA 2005 guidelines for the diagnosis and management of heart fail- ure in adults: a report of the American College of Cardiology Foundation/Ameri- can Heart Association Task Force on Prac- tice Guidelines developed in collabora- tion with the International Society for Heart and Lung Transplantation. J Am Coll Cardiol 2009;53(15):e1-e90. [Erra- tum, J Am Coll Cardiol 2009;54:2464.]

[111] MKSAP 15

[112] Consensus Panel statement on Cardiac Rehabilitation of the AHA, the U.S. Department of Health and Human Services, and the Agency for Health Care Policy and Research.

[113] Bradley, John. "Orthostatic Hypotension" American Family Physician. Volume 68:12. December 2003

[114] Wu, Audrey. "Management of Patients with Non-ischaemic Cardiomyopathy." Heart. 2007; 93. 403-408.

[115] UCLA Inpatient Handbook 2010-2011

[116] Zaghlol RY et al. "A 71-year-old woman with shock and a high INR." Cleveland Clinic Journal of Medicine. 2018 April;85(4):303-312.

[117] Charles et al. "Secondary Hypertension: Discovering the Underlying Cause." Am Fam Physician. 2017 Oct 1;96(7):453-461.

[118] Reference card from the Seventh Report of the Joint National Committee on Prevention, Detection, Evaluation, and Treatment of High Blood Pressure (JNC 7)

[119] DynaMed

[120] Diamond GA. A clinically relevant classification of chest discomfort. *J Am Coll Cardiol* 1983;1:574–575.

[121] Gibbons RJ, Balady GJ, Bricker JT, et al. ACC/AHA 2002 guideline update for exercise testing: A report of the American College of Cardiology/American Heart Association Task Force on practice guidelines (Committee on Exercise Testing). 2002. Available at: www.acc.org/qualityandscience/clinical/guidelines/exercise/exercise_clean.pdf. Accessed on March 6, 2007.

[122] Askew et al. Selecting the optimal cardiac stress test. UpToDate. Last update: 15FEB2013

[123] Garner et al. "Exercise Stress Testing: Indications and Common Questions." Am Fam Physician. 2017 Sep 1;96(5):293-299A.

[124] Six (2008) Neth Heart J 16(6):191-6 [PubMed]

[125] Bouida W et al. LOw dose MAGnesium sulfate versus HIgh dose in the early management of rapid atrial fibrillation: Randomised controlled double blind study. Acad Emerg Med 2018 Jul 19

[126] Alboni et al. "Outpatient Treatment of Recent-Onset Atrial Fibrillation with the "Pill-in-the-Pocket" Approach." N Engl J Med 2004;351:2384-91.

[127] Gonsalves et al. "The New Oral Anticoagulants in Clinical Practice." Mayo Clinic Proceedings. May 2013; 88(5): 495-511.

[128] Mandell et al. "Selecting antithrombotic therapy for patients with atrial fibrillation." CCJM. 2015: 82(1)

[129] Pisters R, Lane DA, Nieuwlaat R, de Vos CB, Crijns HJ, Lip GY. A novel user-friendly score (HAS-BLED) to assess 1-year risk of major bleeding in patients with atrial fibrillation: the Euro Heart Survey. Chest. 2010 Nov;138(5):1093-100. Epub 2010 Mar 18. PubMed PMID: 20299623. Lip GY, Frison L, Halperin JL, Lane DA. Comparative validation of a novel risk score for predicting bleeding risk in anticoagulated patients with atrial fibrillation: the HAS-BLED (Hypertension, Abnormal Renal/Liver Function, Stroke, Bleeding History or Predisposition, Labile INR, Elderly, Drugs/Alcohol Concomitantly) score. J Am Coll Cardiol. 2011 Jan 11;57(2):173-80. Epub 2010 Nov 24. PubMed PMID: 21111555.

[130] UCLA CCU Resident Housebook Version 3

[131] Zeiger et al. "American Association of Clinical Endocrinologists and American Association of Endocrine Surgeons Medical Guidelines for the Management of Adrenal Incidentalomas." Endocrine practice vol 15 (suppl 1) july/august 2009

[132] A. El Maghraoui and C. Roux. "DXA scanning in clinical practice" QJM (2008) 101(8): 605-617 first published online March 10, 2008 doi:10.1093/qjmed/hcn022

[133] South-Paul, Jeanette. "Osteoporosis: Part II. Nonpharmacologic and Pharmacologic Treatment." American Family Physician. March 15, 2001 / volume 63, number 6

[134] Lyles KW.Have we learned how to use bisphosphonates yet? *J Am Geriatr Soc* 2017 Sep; 65:1902. (http://dx.doi.org/10.1111/jgs.14948)

[135] AACE Male Sexual Dysfunction Task Force. AMERICAN ASSOCIATION OF CLINICAL ENDOCRINOLOGISTS MEDICAL GUIDELINES FOR CLINICAL PRACTICE FOR THE EVALUATION AND TREATMENT OF MALE SEXUAL DYSFUNCTION: A COUPLE'S PROBLEM–2003 UPDATE.

[136] Schnipper JL. Chapter 149. Inpatient Management of Diabetes and Hyperglycemia. In: Lawry GV, Matloff J, Dressler DD, Brotman DJ, Ginsberg JS, eds. Principles and Practice of Hospital Medicine. New York: McGraw-Hill; 2012.

[137] AACE. "American Association of Clinical Endocrinologists' Comprehensive Diabetes Management Algorithm 2013." Endocr Pract. 2013;19:327-336.

[138] American Diabetes Association. Older adults. Sec. 10. In Standards of Medical Care in Diabetesd2016. Diabetes Care 2016;39(Suppl. 1):S81–S85.

[139] Summary of revisions for the 2013 clinical practice recommendations. Diabetes Care. January 2013 vol. 36 no. Supplement 1 S3.

[140] Qaseem A, Barry MJ, Humphrey LL, Forciea MA; Clinical Guidelines Committee of the American College of Physicians. Oral Pharmacologic Treatment of Type 2 Diabetes Mellitus: A Clinical Practice Guideline Update From the American College of Physicians. Ann Intern Med. 2017 Jan 3.

[141] Ingham M, Lefebvre P, Pilon D, et al. Glycaemic control, weight loss, and use of other antihyperglycaemics in patients with type 2 diabetes initiated on canagliflozin or sitagliptin: a real-world analysis. Paper presented at: European Association for the Study of Diabetes (EASD) 53rd Annual Meeting 2017; September 11-15, 2017. Lisbon, Portugal. http://www.abstractsonline.com/pp8/ - !/4294/presentation/5259. Accessed on September 18, 2017.

[142] Ou SM, Shih CJ, Chao PW, et al. Effects on clinical outcomes of adding dipeptidyl peptidase-4 inhibitors versus sulfonylureas to metformin therapy in patients with type 2 diabetes mellitus. *Ann Inter Med.* 2015;163:663-672. doi:10.7326/M15-0308.

[143] Ian Blumer, Eran Hadar, David R. Hadden, Lois Jovanovič, Jorge H. Mestman, M. Hassan Murad, Yariv Yogev; Diabetes and Pregnancy: An Endocrine Society Clinical Practice Guideline, *The Journal of Clinical Endocrinology & Metabolism*, Volume 98, Issue 11, 1 November 2013, Pages 4227–4249, https://doi.org/10.1210/jc.2013-2465

[144] Hermida RC, Ayala DE, Mojón A, Fernández JR. Bedtime ingestion of hypertension medications reduces the risk of new-onset type 2 diabetes: a randomized controlled trial. Diabetologia. 2016 Feb;59(2):255-65. Erratum in: Diabetologia. 2016 Feb;59(2):395. PMID: 26399404.

[145] le Roux CW, Astrup A, Fujioka K, et al. 3 years of liraglutide versus placebo for type 2 diabetes risk reduction and weight management in individuals with prediabetes: A randomised, double-blind trial. *Lancet.* 2017;389:1399-1409. doi:10.1016/S0140-6736(17)30069-7.

[146] Dobri et al. "How should we manage insulin therapy before surgery?" Cleveland Clinic Journal of Medicine. 80(11). November 2013.

[147] Kapoor A, Page S, LaValley M, Gale DR, Felson DT. Magnetic Resonance Imaging for Diagnosing Foot Osteomyelitis: A Meta-analysis. *Arch Intern Med.* 2007;167(2):125-132. doi:10.1001/archinte.167.2.125.
[148] USMLEWorld
[149] Kitabachi et al. "Hyperglycemic Crises in Adult Patients With Diabetes. DIABETES CARE, VOLUME 32, NUMBER 7, JULY 2009.
[150] Schmeltz, Lowell. "Management of Inpatient Hyperglycemia." Lab Med. 2011;42(7):427-434.
[151] McNaughton et al. "Diabetes in the Emergency Department: Acute Care of Diabetes Patients." Clinical Diabetes April 2011 vol. 29 no. 2 51-59
[152] Adams PC, Barton JC. Lancet 2007;370:1855-60
[153] Hordinsky, Maria. "Primary Care Dermatology Roundtable: Common Dermatologic Conditions..." Medscape.
[154] Mounsey et al. "Diagnosing and Treating Hair Loss." Am Fam Physician. 2009;80(4):356-362, 373-374.
[155] Alkhalifah A et al. "Alopecia areata update: part II. Treatment." J Am Acad Dermatol. 2010 Feb;62(2):191-202, quiz 203-4. doi: 10.1016/j.jaad.2009.10.031.
[156] McPhee, SJ. Current Medical Diagnosis and Treatment 2010. 49th Edition.
[157] Carroll et al. "Evaluation of Hypercalcemia." AFP. May 1, 2003: 67(9)
[158] 61-Year-Old Man With Hypercalcemia and Generalized Lymphadenopathy Egan, Ashley M. et al. Mayo Clinic Proceedings , Volume 0 , Issue 0.
[159] Maier et al. "Hypercalcemia in the Intensive Care Unit: A Review of Pathophysiology, Diagnosis, and Modern Therapy." J Intensive Care Med published online 15 October 2013.
[160] Kovesdy, Csaba. "Management of Hyperkalemia: An Update for the Internist." The American Journal of Medicine (2015) 128, 1281-1287
[161] Spasovski et al. "Clinical practice guideline on diagnosis and treatment of hyponatraemia." Eur J Endocrinol March 1, 2014 170 G1-G47
[162] Gardner DG. Chapter 24. Endocrine Emergencies. In: Gardner DG, Shoback D.eds. *Greenspan's Basic & Clinical Endocrinology, 9e.* New York, NY: McGraw-Hill; 2011
[163] Braun et al. "Diagnosis and Management of Sodium Disorders: Hyponatremia and Hypernatremia." Am Fam Physician. 2015;91(5):299-307.
[164] Sterns et al. "The Treatment of Hyponatremia." Seminars in Nephrology. 29(3) May 2009
[165] Tandon, Nikhil. "Management of Hypothyroidism in Adults." SUPPLEMENT TO JAPI. JANUARY 2011. VOL. 59.
[166] Oxford Handbook of Clinical Medicine 10th edition and Pocket Medicine 6th Edition
[167] Freda et al. "Pituitary Incidentaloma: An Endocrine Society Clinical Practice Guideline." JCEM. July 02, 2013.
[168] http://www.mayoclinic.com/health/prednisone-withdrawal/AN01624
[169] The Endocine Society. "Testosterone Therapy in Adult Men with Androgen Deficiency Syndromes: An Endocrine Society Clinical Practice Guideline." 2010.
[170] Tsametis CP, Isidori AM. Testosterone Replacement Therapy: for whom, when and how?" Metabolism. 2018 Mar 9. pii: S0026-0495(18)30073-8.
[171] Welker, Mary Jo. "Thyroid Nodules" AAFP Practical Therapeutics. FEBRUARY 1, 2003 / VOLUME 67, NUMBER 3
[172] Hegedus, Laszlo. "The Thyroid Nodule." NEJM 2004; 351:1764-71
[173] Katz S., Down, TD, Cash, HR, et al. (1970) progress in the development of the index of ADL. *Gerontologist* 10:20-30
[174] "Mini-mental state." a practical method for grading the cognitive state of patients for the clinician. Journal of Psychiatric Research, 12(3): 189-198, 1975.
[175] Sink et al. Pharmacological Treatment of Neuropsychiatric Symptoms of Dementia: A Review of the Evidence. JAMA, February 2, 2005—Vol 293, No. 5 (Reprinted)
[176] Kao, Amy. Fast Five Quiz: Test Your Knowledge on Key Aspects of Alzheimer Disease - Medscape - Sep 14, 2017.
[177] ACP Smart Medicine. "Dementia."
[178] Geschwind, Michael D. "Rapidly Progressive Dementia." Continuum 2016; 22(2): 510-537.
[179] Ronald C. Petersen, Oscar Lopez, Melissa J. Armstrong, Thomas S.D.Getchius, Mary Ganguli, David Gloss, Gary S. Gronseth, DanielMarson, Tamara Pringsheim, Gregory S. Day, Mark Sager, JamesStevens, Alexander Rae-Grant. "Practice guideline update summary: Mild cognitive impairment." Neurology Jan 2018, 90 (3) 126-135; DOI: 10.1212/WNL.0000000000004826
[180] http://medschool.slu.edu/agingsuccessfully/pdfsurveys/slumsexam_05.pdf
[181] Buss, Mary K. Mayo Clinic Proceedings. 92(2). 280-286.
[182] Chapter 5. Laboratory Diagnosis: Clinical Hematology. In: Gomella LG, Haist SA. eds. *Clinician's Pocket Reference: The Scut Monkey, 11e* New York, NY: McGraw-Hill; 2007. http://accessmedicine.mhmedical.com/content.aspx?bookid=365§ionid=43074914. Accessed November 10, 2018.
[183] Blood. In: Mescher AL. eds. Junqueira's Basic Histology: Text and Atlas.
[184] Fischer, Conrad. "USMLE:Master the Boards Step 3." Kaplan Medical.
[185] Wan et al. "83-Year-Old Man With Chest Pain, Exertional Dyspnea, and Anemia." Mayo Clinic Proceedings Residents Clinic. November 2013;88(11):e129-e133
[186] Tirona, Maria Taria. Breast Cancer Screening Update. *Am Fam Physician.* 2013;87(4):274-278
[187] Ezekial, Mark. "Current Clinical Strategies: Handbook of Anesthesia" 2007-2008
[188] Carson JL, Reynolds RC. In search of the transfusion threshold. Hematology. 2005;10(Suppl 1):86-88.
[189] Carson JL, Duff A, Poses RM, et al. Effect of anemia and cardiovascular disease on surgical mortality and morbidity. Lancet. 1996;348(9034):1055-1060.
[190] Herbert. et al. "A Multicenter, Randomized, Controlled Clinical Trial of Transfusion Requirements In Critical Care." NEJM. 11FEB1999. 340(6).
[191] Federici et al. "Transfusion issues in cancer patients." Thrombosis Research. 2012. S60-5.
[192] Klein et al. "Red blood cell transfusion in clinical practice." The Lancet. Vol 370 (4AUG2007)
[193] Frontera et al. "Guideline for Reversal of Antithrombotics in Intracranial Hemorrhage." Neurocrit Care (2016) 24:6–46.
[194] Sangle et al. "Antiphospholipid Antibody Syndrome." Archives of Pathology and Laboratory Medicine. 135 (9/2011)
[195] Larson RA, Hall MJ. Chapter 71. Acute Leukemia. In: Hall JB, Schmidt GA, Wood LD, eds. Principles of Critical Care. 3rd ed. New York: McGraw-Hill; 2005.
[196] Habermann, Thomas M. Mayo Clinic Internal Medicine Concise Textbook. Edition 1. 2008
[197] PL Detail-Document, How to Manage High INRs in Warfarin Patients. Pharmacist's Letter/Prescriber's Letter. May 2012.

[198] Holbrook A, Schulman S, Witt DM, et al. Evidence-Based Management of Anticoagulant Therapy. Chest 2012. February 1, 2012;141(2 suppl):e152S-e84S.

[199] Freifeld et al. "Clinical Practice Guideline for the Use of Antimicrobial Agents in Neutropenic Patients with Cancer: 2010 Update by the Infectious Diseases Society of America"CID. 2011:52

[200] Bergstrom C, Nagalla S, Gupta A. Management of Patients With Febrile NeutropeniaA Teachable Moment. JAMA Intern Med. Published online February 12, 2018. doi:10.1001/jamainternmed.2017.8386

[201] Cedars-Sinai Medical Center Intern Survival Guide

[202] Wilbur et al. "Deep Venous Thrombosis and Pulmonary Embolism: Current Therapy." *Am Fam Physician.* 2017 Mar 1;95(5):295-302.

[203] Kearon et al. "Antithrombotic Therapy for VTE Disease: CHEST Guideline and Expert Panel Report." CHEST 2016; 149(2):315-352.

[204] Agnelli et al. "Oral Apixaban for the Treatment of Acute Venous Thromboembolism." N Engl J Med 2013;369:799-808

[205] Pflipsen et al. Am Fam Physician. 2016 Jun 15.

[206] Azari et al. "Conjunctivitis A Systematic Review of Diagnosis and Treatment." JAMA. 2013;310(16):1721-1729.

[207] Abbatemarco et al. "Acute monocular vision loss: Don't lose sight of the differential." Cleveland Clinic Journal of Medicine. 2017 October;84(10):779-787.

[208] Special Operations Forces Medical Handbook. 1 June 2001.

[209] Editorial Board. In: Gomella LG, Haist SA. eds. *Clinician's Pocket Reference: The Scut Monkey, 11e* New York, NY: McGraw-Hill; 2007.

[210] Quizlet Oncology Flashcards <http://quizlet.com/37408090/oncology-flash-cards/>

[211] De Fer et al. "Washington Manual Internship Survival Guide, The." 2013:4.

[212] https://web.stanford.edu/group/ccm_echocardio/cgibin/mediawiki/index.php/Parasternal_long_axis_view

[213] Textbook of Diagnostic Ultrasonography; Sandra L. Hagen-Ansert; 2001

[214] Perron, Andrew. How to Read a Head CT Scan. Chapter 69.

[215] Worsley, DF. Comprehensive analysis of the results of the PIOPED Study. Prospective Investigation of Pulmonary Embolism Diagnosis Study. J Nucl Med. 1995 Dec;36(12):2380-7.

[216] Hooten et al. "Evaluation and Treatment of Low Back Pain: A Clinically Focused Review for Primary Care Specialists." Mayo Clin Proc. 2015;90(12):1699-1718.

217 Van Tulder MW, Touray T, Furlan AD, Solway S, Bouter LM. Muscle relaxants for non-specific low back pain. *Cochrane Database Syst Rev*. 2003;(2):CD004252.

218 Schraeder et al. Clinical Evaluation of the Knee. N Engl J Med 2010;363(4):e5.

219 Helfenstein et al. "Anserine syndrome" Bras J Rheumatology. 2010; 50(3). 313-27

220 Jones et al. "Nonsurgical Management of Knee Pain in Adults." Am Fam Physician. 2015 Nov 15;92(10):875-883.

221 McGahan JP, Shoji H. Knee effusions. J Fam Practice 1977;4:141–4

222 Johnson MW. Acute knee effusions: a systematic approach to diagnosis. Am Fam Physician. 2000 Apr 15;61(8):2391-400.

[223] Woodward TW, Best TM. The painful shoulder: part I. Clinical evaluation. Am Fam Physician. 2000 May 15;61(10):3079-88.

[224] Greenberg, Deborah. "Evaluation and Treatment of Shoulder Pain." Med Clin N Am 98 (2014) 487–504.

[225] Cooper et al. Synopsis of the National Institute for Health and Clinical Excellence Guideline for Management of Transient Loss of Consciousness. Ann Intern Med. 2011;155:543-549

[226] Brignole et al. European Heart Journal, Volume 39, Issue 21, 1 June 2018.

[227] Michele Brignole, Angel Moya, Frederik J de Lange, Jean-Claude Deharo, Perry M Elliott, Alessandra Fanciulli, Artur Fedorowski, Raffaello Furlan, Rose Anne Kenny, Alfonso Martín, Vincent Probst, Matthew J Reed, Ciara P Rice, Richard Sutton, Andrea Ungar, J Gert van Dijk, ESC Scientific Document Group; 2018 ESC Guidelines for the diagnosis and management of syncope, European Heart Journal, , ehy037

[228] Matuszak JM, McVige J, McPherson J, Willer B, Leddy J. A Practical Concussion Physical Examination Toolbox: Evidence-Based Physical Examination for Concussion. Sports Health. 2016;8:260-269.

[229] Matuszak JM, McVige J, McPherson J, Willer B, Leddy J. A Practical Concussion Physical Examination Toolbox: Evidence-Based Physical Examination for Concussion. Sports Health. 2016;8:260-269.

[230] Stillman et al. "Concussion: Evaluation and management." *Cleveland Clinic Journal of Medicine*. 2017 August;84(8):623-630.

[231] Watto, M. (2018, November 5). #123 Sleep Apnea Pearls and Pitfalls [Audio blog post]. Retrieved November 5, 2018, from https://thecurbsiders.com/podcast/123-sleep-apnea-pearls-and-pitfalls

[232] Robbins et al. "Migraine Treatment From A to Z." Practical Pain Management. April 2012.

[233] Charles, Andrew. "Migraine." NEJM. 2017: 377; 553-561.

[234] Watto, M. (n.d.). #122 Headaches Advanced Class: Migraines, medication overuse, and more! [Audio blog post]. Retrieved from https://thecurbsiders.com/podcast/122-headaches-advanced-class

[235] Faubion et al. "Migraine Throughout the Female Reproductive Life Cycle." Mayo Clin Proc. 2018;93(5):639-645.

[236] Taggart et al. "Ketorolac in the treatment of acute migraine: a systematic review." Headache. 2013 Feb;53(2):277-87.

[237] Chou, Kelvin et al. "Diagnosis of Parkinson disease. " UpToDate 20JUL2012

[238] Wills AJ, Stevens DL. Epilepsy in the accident and emergency department. Br J Hosp Med 1994;52:42–5.
Morrison AD, McAlpine CH. The management of first seizures in adults in a district general hospital. Scot Med J 1997;42:73–5.
Pellegrino TR. An emergency department approach to first-time seizures. Emerg Med Clin North Am 1994;12:925–39.

[239] Greenberg DA, Aminoff MJ, Simon RP. Chapter 12. Seizures & Syncope. In: Greenberg DA, Aminoff MJ, Simon RP, eds. Clinical Neurology. 8th ed. New York: McGraw-Hill; 2012.

[240] Adapted from Status Epilepticus/Stroke 2/22/01 by Dr. Steve Lee and Stroke 2006 by Nereses Sanossian, MD

[241] Rob's Pearls

[242] Go S, Worman DJ. Chapter 161. Stroke, Transient Ischemic Attack, and Cervical Artery Dissection. In: Tintinalli JE, Stapczynski JS, Cline DM, Ma OJ, Cydulka RK, Meckler GD, eds. *Tintinalli's Emergency Medicine: A Comprehensive Study Guide*. 7th ed. New York: McGraw-Hill; 2011

[243] Badruddin A, Gorelick PB. Antiplatelet therapy for prevention of recurrent stroke. Curr Treat Options Neurol. 2009 Nov;11(6):452-9. PMID: 20848331 [PubMed]

[244] Adams et al. "Guidelines for the Early Management of Adults With Ischemic Stroke : A Guideline From the American Heart Association/ American Stroke Association Stroke Council, Clinical Cardiology Council, Cardiovascular Radiology and Intervention Council, and the Atherosclerotic Peripheral Vascular Disease and Quality of Care Outcomes in Research Interdisciplinary Working Groups: The American Academy of Neurology affirms the value of this guideline as an educational tool for neurologists." Stroke. 2007;38:1655-1711

[245] Goldstein, Larry B. Blood Pressure Management in Patients With Acute Ischemic Stroke. Hypertension. 2004;43:137-141

[246] Powers et al. "2018 Guidelines for the Early Management of Patients With Acute Ischemic Stroke: A Guideline for Healthcare Professionals From the American Heart Association/American Stroke Association." Stroke; a Journal of Cerebral Circulation 2018 January 24.

[247] Oxford Handbook of Clinical Medicine (10th Edition)

[248] *Circulation* 2005;112:IV-111–IV-120

[249] Saposnik et al. "AHA/ASA Scientific Statement. Diagnosis and Management of Cerebral Venous Thrombosis" Stroke. 2011; 42: 1158-1192

[250] Cumbler E, Glasheen J. "Management of Blood Pressure after Acute Ischemic Stroke: An Evidenced-Base Guide for the Hospitalist." Journal of Hospital Medicine 2007;2: 261–267.

[251] Prasad K, Siemieniuk R, Hao Q, et al. Dual antiplatelet therapy with aspirin and clopidogrel for acute high risk transient ischaemic attack and minor ischaemic stroke: a clinical practice guideline [published online Decembre 18, 2018]. BMJ.

[252] Morgenstern LB, Hemphill JC 3rd, Anderson C, et al; American Heart Association Stroke Council and Council on Cardiovascular Nursing. Guidelines for the management of spontaneous intracerebral hemorrhage: a guideline for healthcare professionals from the American Heart Association/American Stroke Association. Stroke. 2010 Sep;41(9): 2108-29.

[253] Neligan, Patrick. Subarachnoid Hemorrhage. CCMTutorials.com

[254] McGirt et al. "Risk of cerebral vasopasm after subarachnoid hemorrhage reduced by statin therapy: a multivariate analysis of an institutional experience." Journal of Neurosurgery. November 2006. Vol. 105 (5) 671-674.

[255] Kumar et al. "Medical complications after stroke." Lancet Neurology. 2010: 9. 105-108.

[256] Lansberg et al. "Antithrombotic and thrombolytic therapy for ischemic stroke, Ninth Edition" *Chest*. 2012: 141(2).

[257] Johnston et al. "National Stroke Association Guidelines for the Management of TIAs." Ann Neurol 2006. Vol 60 (301-313).

[258] Giles M, Rothwell P. Transient ischaemic attack: clinical relevance, risk prediction and urgency of secondary prevention. Current Opinion in Neurology. 2009, 22:46–53

[259] Gomella L.G., Haist S.A. (2007). Chapter 21. Common Medical Emergencies. In L.G. Gomella, S.A. Haist (Eds), *Clinician's Pocket Reference: The Scut Monkey*, 11e. Retrieved May 5, 2012

[260] Arnold JJ, Williams PM. "Anaphylaxis: recognition and management." Am Fam Physician. 2011 Nov 15;84(10):1111-8.

[261] Andreas Achilleos, Evidence-based Evaluation and Management of Chronic Cough, Medical Clinics of North America, Volume 100, Issue 5, September 2016, Pages 1033-1045, ISSN 0025-7125, http://dx.doi.org/10.1016/j.mcna.2016.04.008.

[262] Alhajjaj MS, Bhimji SS. Cough, Chronic. [Updated 2017 Feb 10]. In: StatPearls [Internet]. Treasure Island (FL): StatPearls Publishing; 2018 Jan-. Available from: https://www.ncbi.nlm.nih.gov/books/NBK430791/

[263] Davids, Susan. "The Respiratory System." Conn's Current Therapy 2013.

[264] Kinkade S, Long NA. "Acute Bronchitis." Am Fam Physician. 2016 Oct 1;94(7):560-565.

[265] Fan et al. "Acute Respiratory Distress Syndrome Advances in Diagnosis and Treatment." JAMA. 2018;319(7):698-710.

[266] Ventilation with lower tidal volumes as compared with traditional tidal volumes for acute lung injury and the acute respiratory distress syndrome. The Acute Respiratory Distress Syndrome Network. N Engl J Med. 2000 May 4;342(18):1301-8. PubMed PMID: 10793162

[267] Martin et al. "A randomized, controlled trial of furosemide with or without albumin in hypoproteinemic patients with acute lung injury." Critical Care Medicine. 2005. 33(8).

[268] Evensen AE. "Management of COPD exacerbations." Am Fam Physician. 2010 Mar 1;81(5):607-13.

[269] Vogelmeier et al. "Global Strategy for the Diagnosis, Management, and Prevention of Chronic Obstructive Lung Disease 2017 Report: GOLD Executive Summary." European Respiratory Journal Mar 2017, 49 (3) 1700214

[270] Craddock et al. "ACUTE EXACERBATIONS OF COPD: AVOIDING DANGER AND DEATH." Consultant. 2016;56(8):740-745.

[271] Khilnani et al. "Noninvasive ventilation in patients with chronic obstructive airway disease." International Journal of COPD. 2008: 3(3).

[272] Edvardsen et al. "Air travel and chronic obstructive pulmonary disease: a new algorithm for pre-flight evaluation." Thorax 2012;67:964–969.

[273] Weiler et al. "Exercise-induced bronchoconstriction update—2016." J Allergy Clin Immunol 2016.

[274] Barreirotin et al. An Approach to Interpreting Spirometry. Am Fam Physician 2004;69:1107-14

[275] John A Gjevre, MD FRCPC, Thomas S Hurst, MVetSc FCCP, Regina M Taylor-Gjevre, MD MSc FRCPC, and Donald W Cockcroft, MD FRCPC. The American Thoracic Society's spirometric criteria alone is inadequate in asthma diagnosis. Can Respir J. 2006 Nov-Dec; 13(8): 433–437.

[276] Dempsey TM et al. "Pulmonary Function Tests for the Generalist: A Brief Review." Mayo Clinic Proceedings , Volume 93 , Issue 6 , 763 - 771.

[277] Case Approach Resident Guide to IM (UH Case Medical Center) 2015-2016.

[278] Case Approach Resident Guide to IM (UH Case Medical Center) 2015-2016.

[279] Case Approach Resident Guide to IM (UH Case Medical Center) 2015-2016.

[280] Dettbarn, Kyle MD. "Bi-Level Ventilation/APRV." http://www.wsrconline.org/read/Bi-Level%20Ventilation.pdf

[281] Peter JV, Moran JL, Phillips-Hughes J, et al. Effect of non-invasive positive pressure ventilation (NIPPV) on mortality in patients with acute cardiogenic pulmonary oedema: a meta-analysis. *Lancet*. 2006;367:1155-63.

[282] Kirkland, Lisa. "Noninvasive positive-pressure ventilation." ACP Hospitalist. September. 2010.

[283] Tobin MJ. Advances in mechanical ventilation. N Engl J Med 2001; 344:1986-96.

[284] Chesnutt MS, Chesnutt MC, Prendergast TJ, Tavan ET, Tavan ET. Chapter 9. Pulmonary Disorders. In: McPhee SJ, Papadakis MA, Rabow MW, eds. *CURRENT Medical Diagnosis & Treatment 2012*. New York: McGraw-Hill; 2012.

[285] Strange, Charlie et al. "Parapneumonic effusion and empyema in adults." In: UpToDate, Basow, DS (Ed), UpToDate, Waltham, MA, 2012.

[286] Jaff et al. Management of Massive and Submassive Pulmonary Embolism, Iliofemoral DVT, and Chronic Thromboembolic Pulmonary Hypertension. Circulation. 2011: 123; 1788-1830

[287] Jeikai Liang et al. "A 51-year-old woman with dyspnea" CCJM. August 2013: 80(8)

[288] Latifi et al. "Is spirometry necessary to diagnose and control asthma?" Cleveland Clinic Journal of Medicine. 2017 August;84(8):597-599.

[289] Dellinger et al. "Surviving Sepsis Campaign: International Guidelines for Management of Severe Sepsis and Septic Shock: 2012." Critical Care Medcine. February 2013 • Volume 41 • Number 2

[290] 2012 Society of Critical Care Meeting

[291] Dellinger et al. "Surviving Sepsis Campaign: International Guidelines for Management of Severe Sepsis and Septic Shock: 2012" CCJM. February 2013 • Volume 41 • Number 2

[292] Watto, M. (2018, November 5). #123 Sleep Apnea Pearls and Pitfalls [Audio blog post]. Retrieved November 5, 2018, from https://thecurbsiders.com/podcast/123-sleep-apnea-pearls-and-pitfalls

[293] Balachandran JS, Patel SR. Obstructive Sleep Apnea. Ann Intern Med. ;161:ITC1. doi: 10.7326/0003-4819-161-9-201411040-01005

[294] Batlle et al. "The use of the urinary anion gap in the diagnosis of hyperchloremic metabolic acidosis." N Engl J Med. 1988 Mar 10;318(10):594-9.

[295] Simon, James. Interpreting the estimated glomerular filtration rate in primary care: Benefits and pitfalls." CCJM. 78(3). March, 2011.

[296] Fenske W, Allolio B. Clinical review: Current state and future perspectives in the diagnosis of diabetes insipidus: a clinical review. J Clin Endocrinol Metab. 2012 Oct;97(10):3426-37

[297] http://medicine.ucsf.edu/education/resed/Chiefs_cover_sheets/nephrotic.pdf

[298] Gottlieb M, Long B, Koyfman A. "The evaluation and management of urolithiasis in the emergency department: A review of the literature." Am J Emerg Med. 2018 Jan 5. pii: S0735-6757(18)30003-2.

[299] Sur et al. "Treatment of Allergic Rhinitis." Am Fam Physician. 2015;92(11):985-992.

[300] Battisti AS, Pangia J. Sinusitis. [Updated 2018 Jan 29]. In: StatPearls [Internet]. Treasure Island (FL): StatPearls Publishing; 2018 Jan-. Available from: https://www.ncbi.nlm.nih.gov/books/NBK470383/

[301] Cots JM, Alós JI, Bárcena M, Boleda X, Ca˜nada JL, Gómez N, et al. Recomendaciones para el manejo de la faringoamigdalitis aguda del adulto. Acta Otorrinolaringol Esp. 2015;66:159---170.

[302] McGinnis HD. Nose and Sinuses. In: Tintinalli JE, Stapczynski J, Ma O, Yealy DM, Meckler GD, Cline DM. eds. *Tintinalli's Emergency Medicine: A Comprehensive Study Guide, 8e* New York, NY: McGraw-Hill; 2016. http://accessmedicine.mhmedical.com/content.aspx?bookid=1658§ionid=109387197. Accessed November 26, 2017

[303] Audiodigest.com

[304] El-Zawawy et al. "Managing gout: How is it different in patients with chronic kidney disease?" CCJM. 77(12). 12/2010.

[305] Burns et al. " Latest evidence on gout management: what the clinician needs to know." Ther Adv Chronic Dis. 2012 Nov; 3(6): 271–286.

[306] Siva et al. "Diagnosing acute monoarthritis in adults: a practical approach for the family physician." Am Fam Physician. 2003 Jul 1;68(1):83-90.

[307] Pujalte, George et al. Am Fam Physician. 2015.

[308] Journal of General Internal Medicine 1999;14:27.

[309] Josephson SA, Miller BL. Chapter 25. Confusion and Delirium. In: Longo DL, Fauci AS, Kasper DL, Hauser SL, Jameson JL, Loscalzo J, eds. *Harrison's Principles of Internal Medicine*. 18th ed. New York: McGraw-Hill; 2012.

[310] Reuben DB, Herr KA, Pacala JT, Pollock BG, Potter JF, Semla TP. Dementia. In: Geriatrics At Your Fingertips: 2009.11th ed. New York: The American Geriatrics Society; 2009:54-59.

[311] Imm et al. "Postoperative delirium in a 64-year-old woman." Cleveland Clinic Journal of Medicine. 2017 September;84(9):690-698.

[312] Abad, V. C., & Guilleminault, C. (2018). Insomnia in Elderly Patients: Recommendations for Pharmacological Management. Drugs & Aging. doi:10.1007/s40266-018-0569-8

[313] Riemann, D.; Spiegelhalder, K.; Espie, C.; Pollmächer, T.; Léger, D.; Bassetti, C.; van Someren, E. Chronic insomnia: Clinical and research challenges—An agenda. Pharmacopsychiatry 2011, 44, 1–14. Buysse, D.J. Insomnia. JAMA 2013, 309, 706–716. Krystal, A.D.; Durrence, H.H.; Scharf, M.; Jochelson, P.; Rogowski, R.; Ludington, E.; Roth, T. Efficacy and safety of doxepin 1 mg and 3 mg in a 12-week sleep laboratory and outpatient trial of elderly subjects with chronic primary insomnia. Sleep 2010, 33, 1553–1561. Michelson, D.; Snyder, E.; Paradis, E.; Chengan-Liu, M.; Snavely, D.B.; Hutzelmann, J.; Walsh, J.K.; Krystal, J.D.; Benca, R.M.; Cohn, M.; et al. Safety and efficacy of suvorexant during 1-year treatment of insomna with subsequent abrupt treatment discontinuation: A phase 3 randomised, double-blind, placebo-controlled trial. Lancet Neurol. 2014, 13, 461–471. Mayer, G.; Wang-Weigand, S.; Roth-Schechter, B.; Lehmann, F.; Staner, C.; Partinen, M. Efficacy and safety of 6-month nightly ramelteon administration in adults with chronic primary insomnia. Sleep 2009, 32, 351–360. Roehrs, T.A.; Randall, S.; Harris, E.; Maan, R.; Roth, T. Twelve months of nightly zolpidem does not lead to dose escalation: A prospective placebo-controlled study. Sleep 2011, 34, 207–212. Krystal, A.D.; Erman, M.; Zammit, G.K.; Soubrane, C.; Roth, T. Long-term efficacy and safety of zolpidem extended-release 12.5 mg, administered 3 to 7 nights per week for 24 weeks, in patients with chronic primary insomnia: A 6-month, randomized, double-blind, placebo-controlled, parallel-group, multicenter study. Sleep 2008, 31, 79–90. Roth, T.; Walsh, J.K.; Krystal, A.; Wessel, T.; Roehrs, T.A. An evaluation of the efficacy and safety of eszopiclone over 12 months in patients with chronic primary insomnia. Sleep Med. 2005, 6, 487–495.

[314] McCarron et al. ACP Smart Medicine: Depression. May 2014.

[315] Armstrong, Carrie. "APA Releases Guideline on Treatment of Patients with Major Depressive Disorder." *Am Fam Physician*. 2011 May 15;83(10):1219-1227.

[316] Lang, Michael. "Managing Depression in Primary Care." AudioDigest Volume 62 (16).

[317] Bostwick, Michael. A Generalist's Guide to Treating Patients With Depression With an Emphasis on Using Side Effects to Tailor Antidepressant Therapy." Mayo Clin Proc. 2010;85(6):538-550.

[318] Keks et al. "Switching and stopping antidepressants." Aust Prescr 2016;39:76–83.

[319] Serafini et al. Curr Neuropharmacol. 2014 Sep; 12(5): 444–461.

[320] Ogle et al. "Guidance for the Discontinuation or Switching of Antidepressant Therapies in Adults." Journal of Pharmacy Practice 26(4) 389-396.

[321] Berman BD. "Neuroleptic malignant syndrome: a review for neurohospitalists." Neurohospitalist. 2011 Jan;1(1):41-7.

[322] Martin, Thomas G. "Serotonin Syndrome." Ann Emerg Med. 1996 Nov;28(5):520-6.

[323] Savel et al. "Alcohol Withdrawal in the ICU - Practice and Pitfalls." SCCM. 2010.

[324] Marinella MA. "Refeeding syndrome and hypophosphatemia." J Intensive Care Med. 2005 May-Jun;20(3):155-9.

[325] Shuk-Ling Wong et al. "Treatment of Delirium Tremends." USPharmacist.com

[326] Rayner et al. "Dexmedetomidine as adjunct treatment for severe alcohol withdrawal in the ICU." Annals of Intensive Care 2012, 2:12

[327] Vieweg, W. Victor R. et al. "Posttraumatic Stress Disorder: Clinical Features, Pathophysiology, and Treatment." The American Journal of Medicine , Volume 119 , Issue 5 , 383 – 390.

[328] Schneier, Franklin. "Social Anxiety Disorder." N Engl J Med 2006; 355:1029-1036.

[329] Dunlop BW, Davis PG. Combination Treatment With Benzodiazepines and SSRIs for Comorbid Anxiety and Depression: A Review. *Primary Care Companion to The Journal of Clinical Psychiatry*. 2008;10(3):222-228.

[330] Schneier, Franklin. "Social Anxiety Disorder." N Engl J Med 2006; 355:1029-1036.

[331] Donaldson et al. "Oral Sedation: A Primer on Anxiolysis for the Adult Patient." Anesth Prog. 2007 Fall; 54(3): 118–129.

[332] Lader, Malcolm, Andre Tylee, and John Donoghue. "Withdrawing benzodiazepines in primary care." CNS drugs 23.1 (2009): 19-34.

[333] Smith et al. Am J Psychiatry 1998; 155:1339–1345.
[334] Hirschfeld, Robert. "The Comorbidity of Major Depression and Anxiety Disorders: Recognition and Management in Primary Care." Primary Care Companion J Clin Psychiatry 2001;3:244–254.
[335] Wigle et al. Updated Guidelines on Outpatient Anticoagulation. Am Fam Physician. 2013;87(8):556-566.
[336] Moll. Stephan. "New insights into treatment of venous thromboembolism." Hematology 2014.
[337] Dubois et al. "Perioperative management of patients on direct oral anticoagulants." Thrombosis Journal. 2017. 15:14.
[338] American Society of Anesthesiologists
[339] Cohn SL. Preoperative Evaluation for Noncardiac Surgery. Ann Intern Med. ;165.
[340] UCSF Hospitalist Handbook 2002
[341] Alexandra Dretler MD, Dominique Williams MD, Mark Gdowski MD, Pavat Bhat MD, Rajeev Ramgopal MD, eds. 2016. Washington Manual® of Medical Therapeutics, The - 35th Ed.
[342] Smetana GW. Preoperative pulmonary evaluation. N Engl J Med 1999; 340:937-44.
[343] TAMC Preoperative Medicine Handbook 2010
[344] Frank J. Domino, MD, ed. 2014. 5-Minute Clinical Consult - 22nd Ed. Philadelphia, PA. Lippincott Williams & Wilkins Health. ISBN-10: 1-4511-8850-1, ISBN-13: 978-1-4511-8850-9. STAT!Ref Online Electronic Medical Library. https://online.statref.com/Document.aspx?fxId=31&docId=200. 8/12/2013 2:38:53 AM CDT (UTC -05:00).
[345] Long D, et al, The emergency medicine management of severe alcohol withdrawal, American Journal of Emergency Medicine (2017).
[346] Frank J. Domino, MD, Jeremy Golding, MD, FAAFP, Mark B. Stephens, MD, Robert A. Baldor MD, FAAFP, eds. 2019. 5-Minute Clinical Consult - 27th Ed. Philadelphia, PA. Lippincott Williams & Wilkins Health.
[347] Moeller, Karen E. et al. "Clinical Interpretation of Urine Drug Tests." Mayo Clinic Proceedings. Volume 92 , Issue 5 , 774 – 796.
[348] Hadland et al. "OBJECTIVE TESTING – URINE AND OTHER DRUG TESTS." Child Adolesc Psychiatr Clin N Am. 2016 Jul; 25(3): 549–565.
[349] Armstrong C. ACOG guidelines on noncontraceptive uses of hormonal contraceptives. Am Fam Physician. 2010;82(3):288-295. doi:10.1097/AOG.0b013e3181cb50b5.
[350] Polycystic Ovary Syndrome (Persistent Anovulation). In: Papadakis MA, McPhee SJ, Bernstein J. eds. Quick Medical Diagnosis & Treatment 2018 New York, NY: McGraw-Hill; . http://accessmedicine.mhmedical.com/content.aspx?bookid=2273§ionid=178303475. Accessed March 25, 2018.
[351] ACOG Practice Bulletin No. 141: Management of menopausal symptoms. (2014, January). Retrieved from https://www.ncbi.nlm.nih.gov/pubmed/24463691
[352] Contraceptive Use, Centers for Disease Control and Prevention, http://www.cdc.gov/reproductivehealth/unintendedpregnancy/usmec.htm. 11Sept2015.
[353] Kiefer et al. "Pocket Primary Care."
[354] Raymond EG, Cleland K. Emergency contraception. *N Engl J Med* 2015;372:1342-1348. doi:10.1056/NEJMcp1406328.
[355] Practice Bulletin No. 152: Emergency Contraception. Obstet Gynecol. 2015;126(3):e1-11.
[356] Raymond EG, Cleland K. Emergency contraception. *N Engl J Med* 2015;372:1342-1348. doi:10.1056/NEJMcp1406328.
[357] Davies, Joanna et al. "Heavy menstrual bleeding: An update on management." Thrombosis Research. Volume 151 , S70 - S77.
[358] Diagnosis, Evaluation and Follow-Up of Asymptomatic Microhematuria (AMH) in Adults: AUA Guideline Algorithm (2012)
[359] Sarma et al. "Benign Prostatic Hyperplasia and Lower Urinary Tract Symptoms." NEJM. 2012. 367: 248-257.
[360] Matsukawa Y et al. Effects of withdrawing α1-blocker from combination therapy with α1-blocker and 5α-reductase inhibitor in patients with lower urinary tract symptoms suggestive of benign prostatic hyperplasia: A prospective and comparative trial using urodynamics. J Urol 2017 Oct; 198:905.
[361] Sarma, RVSN. "Algorithmic Approach for the Diagnosis of Polyuria." Accessed December 21, 2017. <http://www.apiindia.org/medicine_update_2013/chap69.pdf>
[362] "Diagnosis and Treatment of Non-Neurogenic Overactive Bladder (OAB) in Adults: AUA/SUFU Guideline." AUA/SUFU Guideline: Published 2012; Amended 2014.
[363] Adopted from the ICU Book (Tripler)
[364] Lande et al. "Nicotine Addiction Treatment & Management." Medscape.
[365] Bornemann et al. "Smoking cessation: What should you recommend?" J Fam Pract. 2016 January;65(1):22-29B.

Made in the USA
Monee, IL
26 February 2021